ONCOLOGY AND BASIC SCIENCE

ORTHOPAEDIC SURGERY ESSENTIALS

ONCOLOGY AND BASIC SCIENCE

ORTHOPAEDIC SURGERY ESSENTIALS

Adult Reconstruction
Daniel J. Berry, MD
Scott P. Steinmann, MD

Foot and Ankle
David B. Thordarson, MD

Hand and Wrist
James R. Doyle, MD

Oncology and Basic Science
Timothy A. Damron, MD

Pediatrics
Susan A. Scherl, MD
Kathryn E. Cramer, MD

Spine
Christopher M. Bono, MD
Steven R. Garfin, MD

Sports Medicine
Anthony A. Schepsis, MD
Brian D. Busconi, MD

Trauma
Charles Court-Brown, MD
Margaret M. McQueen, MD
Paul Tornetta III, MD

ORTHOPAEDIC SURGERY ESSENTIALS

ONCOLOGY AND BASIC SCIENCE

Series Editors

PAUL TORNETTA III, MD

Professor
Department of Orthopaedic Surgery
Boston University School of Medicine
Director of Orthopaedic Trauma
Boston University Medical Center
Boston, Massachusetts

THOMAS A. EINHORN, MD

Professor and Chairman
Department of Orthopaedic Surgery
Boston University School of Medicine
Boston, Massachusetts

Book Editor

TIMOTHY A. DAMRON, MD

David G. Murray Endowed Professor of Orthopedic Surgery
Vice Chairman, Department of Orthopedic Surgery
State University of New York Upstate Medical University
Adjunct Professor, Department of Biomedical and
  Chemical Engineering
Syracuse University
Syracuse, New York

Wolters Kluwer | Lippincott Williams & Wilkins
Health
Philadelphia • Baltimore • New York • London
Buenos Aires • Hong Kong • Sydney • Tokyo

Acquisitions Editor: Robert Hurley
Managing Editor: David Murphy
Developmental Editor: Grace R. Caputo, Dovetail Content Solutions
Marketing Director: Sharon Zinner
Project Manager: Nicole Walz
Manufacturing Manager: Kathy Brown
Creative Director: Doug Smock
Compositor: Maryland Composition
Printer: Gopsons

Library of Congress Cataloging-in-Publication Data
Oncology and basic science / [edited by] Timothy A. Damron.
p. ; cm. — (Orthopaedic surgery essentials)
Includes bibliographical references and index.
ISBN-13: 978-0-7817-8045-2
ISBN-10: 0-7817-8045-4
1. Musculoskeletal system—Tumors. 2. Orthopedics. 3. Orthopedic surgery. I. Damron, Timothy A. II. Series.
[DNLM: 1. Bone Neoplasms. 2. Orthopedic Procedures—methods. 3. Soft Tissue Neoplasms. WE 258 O58 2008]
RC280.M83O53 2008
616.99'4—dc22

2006100177

Dedicated to the many students, residents, attendings, and researchers—past, present, and future—whom I have worked with, learned from, and taught. Thank you.

CONTENTS

SECTION I: EVALUATION AND MANAGEMENT OF MUSCULOSKELETAL ONCOLOGY PROBLEMS

SECTION II: SPECIFIC BONE NEOPLASMS AND SIMULATORS

SECTION III: SPECIFIC SOFT TISSUE NEOPLASMS AND SIMULATORS

SECTION IV: BASIC SCIENCE

CONTRIBUTING AUTHORS

Answorth A. Allen, MD
Associate Professor of Orthopaedic Surgery
Weill Medical College of Cornell University
Associate Attending Orthopaedic Surgeon
Hospital for Special Surgery
New York, New York

Matthew J. Allen, VetMB, PhD
Associate Professor
Department of Orthopaedic Surgery
SUNY Upstate Medical University
Syracuse, New York

Edward A. Athanasian, MD
Associate Professor of Orthopaedic Surgery
Weill Medical College of Cornell University
Associate Attending Orthopaedic Surgeon
Hospital for Special Surgery
Surgeon
Memorial Sloan-Kettering Cancer Center
New York, New York

Joseph W. Bergman
Division of Orthopaedic Surgery
Department of Surgery
Edmonton, Alberta, Canada

Patrick Boland, MD
Memorial Sloan-Kettering Cancer Center
New York, New York

Mathias Bostrom, MD
Associate Professor
Weill Medical College of Cornell University
Hospital for Special Surgery
New York, New York

Susan V. Bukata, MD
Assistant Professor
Department of Orthopaedics and Rehabilitation
Director, Osteoporosis Center
University of Rochester Medical Center
Rochester, New York

Michael T. Clarke, MD
Department of Orthopaedic Surgery
SUNY Upstate Medical University
Syracuse, New York

Christian Custodio, MD
Memorial Sloan-Kettering Cancer Center
New York, New York

Timothy A. Damron, MD
David G. Murray Professor of Orthopaedics
SUNY Upstate Medical University
University Hospital
Syracuse, New York

Gustavo de la Roza
Associate Professor
Department of Pathology
SUNY Upstate Medical University
Syracuse, New York

Paul E. Di Cesare, MD, FACS
Director, Musculoskeletal Research Center
Hospital for Joint Diseases
Professor of Orthopaedic Surgery and Cell Biology
New York University School of Medicine
New York, New York

Mark C. Drakos, MD
Department of Sports Medicine
Hospital for Special Surgery
New York, New York

Donald Flemming, MD
Penn State Milton S. Hershey Medical Center
Hershey, Pennslyvania

C. Parker Gibbs, MD
University of Florida
Department of Orthopaedic Surgery
Gainesville, Florida

Brian J. Harley, MD, FRCSC
Associate Professor
Department of Orthopaedic Surgery
SUNY Upstate Medical University
Syracuse, New York

Julie M. Hasenwinkel, PhD
Assistant Professor
Department of Biomedical and Chemical Engineering
Syracuse University
Syracuse, New York

John Heiner, MD
Department of Orthopaedic Surgery and Rehabilitation
University of Wisconsin—Madison
Madison, Wisconsin

Alexia Hernandez-Soria, MD
Hospital for Special Surgery
New York, New York

Kenneth J. Hunt, MD
Sarcoma Services
Huntsman Cancer Institute and Primary Children's
Medical Center
Department of Orthopaedic Surgery
University of Utah
Salt Lake City, Utah

Kirill Ilalov, BS
Research Associate
Musculoskeletal Research Center
NYU Hospital for Joint Diseases
Department of Orthopaedic Surgery
New York, New York

Samuel A. Joseph, Jr, MD
Memorial Sloan-Kettering Cancer Center
New York, New York

Danielle A. Katz, MD, FACS
Assistant Professor
Department of Orthopaedic Surgery
SUNY Upstate Medical University
Syracuse, New York

Bryan T. Kelly, MD
Assistant Attending Physician
Hospital for Special Surgery
New York, New York

Cynthia M. Kelly, MD
Colorado Limb Consultants
Presbyterian/St. Luke's Medical Center
Denver, Colorado

Francis Young-In Lee, MD
Assistant Professor
Department of Orthopaedic Surgery
Children's Hospital of New York
Tumor and Bone Disease Service
College of Physicians and Surgeons of Columbia University
New York, New York

Valerae O. Lewis, MD
Assistant Professor of Orthopaedic Oncology
MD Anderson Cancer Center
Houston, Texas

Sean V. McGarry, MD
University of Florida
Department of Orthopaedic Surgery
Gainesville Florida

Young Lae Moon, MD
Associated Professor
Chief of Shoulder and Elbow Services
Orthopaedic Department
Chosun University Hospital
Gwangju, Korea

Hannah D. Morgan, MD
University of Washington
Department of Orthopaedics
Seattle, Washington

Carol D. Morris, MD
Assistant Professor
Department of Orthopaedic Surgery
Weill Medical College
Cornell University
Attending Surgeon
Memorial Sloan-Kettering Cancer Center
New York, New York

Kathryn Palomino, MD
Assistant Professor
Pediatric Orthopaedic Surgery
SUNY Upstate Medical University
Syracuse, New York

Francis R. Patterson, MD
Assistant Professor
Department of Orthopaedics
Division of Musculoskeletal Oncology
New Jersey Medical School
Newark, New Jersey

Robert Quinn, MD
Associate Professor of Orthopaedic Surgery
Director, Orthopaedic Oncology
Residency Program Director
University of New Mexico School of Medicine
Albuquerque, New Mexico

R. Lor Randall, MD, FACS
Director, Sarcoma Service
Chief, SARC Lab
Huntsman Cancer Institute and Primary Children's Medical
Center
University of Utah
Salt Lake City, Utah

William J. Robertson, MD
Orthopaedic Resident
Hospital for Special Surgery
New York, New York

Peter J. Roughley, PhD
Shriners Hospital for Children
Montreal, Quebec, Canada

Bruce Rougraff, MD
Ortho Indy
Indianapolis, Indiana

Sathappan S. Sathappan, MD
Adult Reconstruction Fellow
NYU Hospital for Joint Disease
Department of Orthopaedic Surgery
New York, New York

Sung Wook Seo, MD
Fellow, Department of Orthopaedic Surgery
Columbia University Medical School
New York, New York

Shikha Sethi, MD
Electrodiagnostic Services
Department of Physiatry
Hospital for Special Surgery
New York, New York

Kris Shekitka, MD
St. Agnes Hospital
Baltimore, Maryland

Thomas V. Smallman, MD
Assistant Professor
Department of Orthopaedic Surgery
SUNY Upstate Medical University
Syracuse, New York

Joseph A. Spadaro, MD
Professor (Research)
Department of Orthopaedic Surgery
SUNY Upstate Medical University
Syracuse, New York

Michael Stubblefield, MD
Department of Physical Medicine and Rehabilitation
New York-Presbyterian Medical Center
New York, New York

Donald E. Sweet, MD
Armed Forces Institute of Pathology
Washington, DC

Frederick W. Werner, MME
Professor (Research)
Department of Orthopaedic Surgery
SUNY Upstate Medical University
Syracuse, New York

Jeremy White, MD
Department of Orthopaedics and Rehabilitation
University of Wisconsin, Madison
Madison, Wisconsin

Felasfa M. Wodajo, MD
Clinical Assistant Professor, Orthopaedics
Georgetown University and Howard University
Director, Orthopaedic Oncology
Inova Fairfax Hospital and Hospital for Children
Consultant, National Cancer Institute, NIH
Bethesda, Maryland

SERIES PREFACE

Most of the available resources in orthopaedic surgery are very good, but they either present information exhaustively—so that the reader has to wade through too many details to find what he or she seeks—or they assume too much knowledge, making the information difficult to understand. Moreover, as residency training has advanced, it has become more focused on the individual subspecialties. Our goal was to create a series at the basic level that residents could read completely during a subspecialty rotation to obtain the essential information necessary for a general understanding of the field. Once they have survived those trials, we hope that *Orthopaedic Surgery Essentials* books will serve as a touchstone for future learning and review.

Each volume is to be a manageable size that can be read during a resident's tour. As a series, they will have a consistent style and template, with the authors' voices heard throughout. Content will be presented more visually than in most books on orthopaedic surgery, with a liberal use of tables, boxes, bulleted lists, and algorithms to aid in quick review. Each topic will be covered by one or more authorities, and each volume will be edited by experts in the broader field.

But most importantly, each volume—*Pediatrics, Spine, Sports Medicine,* and so on—will focus on the requisite knowledge in orthopaedics. Having the essential information presented in one user-friendly source will provide the reader with easy access to the basic knowledge needed in the field, and mastering this content will give him or her an excellent foundation for additional information from comprehensive references, atlases, journals, and on-line resources.

We would like to thank the editors and contributors who have generously shared their knowledge. We hope that the reader will take the opportunity of telling us what works and does not work.

—Paul Tornetta III, MD
—Thomas A. Einhorn, MD

PREFACE

The latest addition to the *Orthopaedic Surgery Essentials* series, *Oncology and Basic Science*, provides the orthopaedic resident, medical student, or bioengineering graduate student with the essential information needed to understand the areas of musculoskeletal oncology and the fundamental science of orthopaedics. In keeping with the goal of the series, it is intended to be a single volume that a resident or student would be able to read during an orthopaedic tumor rotation and then use as a reference for later study.

Although other musculoskeletal oncology texts exist, they are usually devoted exclusively to bone tumors, soft tissue tumors, surgical procedures, or basic science as single topics. Thus, the exhaustive information contained therein is useful for reference but difficult to use as a study tool. This text is unique in providing a comprehensive but concise presentation of the essential information for both bone *and* soft tissue tumors as well as clinical aspects, surgical options, and the underlying science. Beyond just providing the basic science of tumors, however, the text presents a complete spectrum of orthopaedic basic science topics.

In addition to the classic teaching, *OSE: Oncology and Basic Science* includes pertinent cutting-edge clinical and basic research findings. Clinical practice and research in musculoskeletal oncology and orthopaedic basic science are being driven by recent advances in the understanding of the humane genome and evolving techniques in molecular biology, including microarray and proteomics. The basic science section includes chapters on topics most acutely affected by this ever-expanding knowledge base, including molecular and cellular biology, growth and development, the genetic basis of musculoskeletal disorders, biomaterials and biologic response to orthopaedic implants, and neoplastic disorders.

While being comprehensive in its scope, *OSE: Oncology and Basic Science* is presented in an easy-to-use outline format and contains dozens of tables and boxes for quick reference and review as well as literally hundreds of figures to enhance understanding. The inclusion of color figures with histopathology for key orthopaedic oncology conditions is a unique addition to the series that will enhance learning and exam preparation.

When selecting authors, we intentionally included representatives of the finest musculoskeletal oncology and orthopaedic research facilities across the country to reflect the breadth of training and experience in those varied settings. Their excellent work is a testament not only to their passion but also to the importance of these topics in the advancement of musculoskeletal oncology as a subspecialty and of orthopaedics overall.

The book will be of benefit as a concise reading source during an orthopaedic oncology clinical rotation, as a study tool for the in-training examination and boards review, as a concise guide to basic science topics for clinicians and graduate students involved in orthopaedic research, and as a reference resource for orthopaedic surgeons in clinical practice. Others who will find it useful include orthopaedic laboratory personnel and affiliated orthopaedic health care providers (physician assistants, nurse practitioners). From an institutional standpoint, the text has a place in orthopaedic residency programs, medical schools, and graduate bioengineering programs.

We hope that *Orthopaedic Surgery Essentials: Oncology and Basic Science* can serve as a springboard to more in-depth study and research for those who develop or already have an interest in these critical areas.

—Timothy A. Damron, MD

ACKNOWLEDGMENTS

As in all such endeavors, many people contributed to the completion of this book. My thanks go out to each of the chapter authors for their excellent work through the preparation and review process. Both Carol Morris and Tom Smallman deserve special mention for their willingness to complete multiple chapters. Special thanks to Matthew Allen, John Heiner, Cynthia Kelly, and Robert Quinn for their willingness to commit to and complete chapters on short notice. Thanks to Aaron Anderson, Andrew Evans, and Jennifer Lisle for their requested reviews and input from an orthopaedic residents' perspective. Matthew Allen, Brian Harley, Danielle Katz, David Lehmann, Matthew Scuderi, and Michael Sun from our Department of Orthopedic Surgery and from the Pharmacology Department here at SUNY Upstate were gracious to lend their expertise in providing editing input on specific chapters. Much of the artwork was done by Kit Hefner in our Medical Illustration Department. Additional artwork for Lippincott was created by Jennifer Smith. Special thanks to my secretary Julie Davila and my clinic nurse Sandy Telonis for tolerating me during the time of book preparation.

This book would not have been possible without the sometimes gentle, sometimes firm, always experienced hand of Grace Caputo, who has carried through to the end where others before her could not. Thanks to my family and friends for their understanding and support.

EVALUATION AND MANAGEMENT OF MUSCULOSKELETAL ONCOLOGY PROBLEMS

EVALUATION OF BONE TUMORS

TIMOTHY A. DAMRON

Bone lesions can be difficult to identify specifically, and arriving at a specific diagnosis can elude even the most experienced orthopaedic oncologist. However, by using a systematic approach to the evaluation of these tumors, including consideration of the pathogenesis, often a narrow enough differential diagnosis may be arrived at by clinical and radiological means to allow specific treatment (often observation) or to guide the subsequent evaluation and care. This chapter discusses pathogenesis and an approach to evaluation of bone tumors.

PATHOGENESIS

Etiology

- The vast majority of bone tumors arise de novo with no identifiable predisposing precursor lesion or associated agent. However, well-defined clinical precursor lesions have been established (Box 1-1).
- Established etiologic agents for osteosarcoma are given in Box 1-2.
- Implicated but unproven causes:
  - Chromium, nickel, cobalt, aluminum, titanium, methyl-methacrylate, polyethylene
  - Trauma

Epidemiology

- Incidence of bone sarcomas
  - 0.2% of all cancers

- 0.8 new cases per 100,000 population per year in North America and Europe
- Most common bone sarcomas
  - #1: Osteosarcoma
  - #2: Chondrosarcoma
  - #3: Ewing sarcoma
- Age distribution is bimodal
  - First peak: Second decade of life
    - Osteosarcoma predominates at this age
    - Ewing sarcoma #2
  - Second peak: >60 years old
    - Chondrosarcoma predominates
    - Secondary osteosarcomas #2
      - Paget's osteosarcoma
      - Postradiation osteosarcoma

Pathophysiology

- Unknown for most bone tumors
- Best described for congenital and inherited syndromes (Table 1-1)

CLASSIFICATION

Current classification systems are derived from the type of cell or tissue involved. Hence, bone tumors are divided into osseous, cartilaginous, cystic, myogenic, lipogenic, epithelial, neural, notochordal, fibrous, fibrohistiocytic, giant cell, round cell, and vascular categories as well as those of undefined neoplastic nature. The organization of the subsequent chapters follows this classification scheme.

BOX 1-1 PRECURSOR LESIONS FOR DEVELOPMENT OF BONE SARCOMA

Low Risk
Fibrous dysplasia
Bone infarct
Chronic osteomyelitis
Metallic and polyethylene implants
Osteogenesis imperfecta
Giant cell tumor
Osteoblastoma
Chondroblastoma
Intermediate Risk
Multiple osteochondromas
Polyostotic Paget disease
Radiation osteitis
High Risk
Ollier's disease (enchondromatosis)
Maffucci syndrome
Familial retinoblastoma syndrome
Rothmund-Thompson syndrome

Adapted from Fletcher DM, Unni KK, Merlens F, eds. *Tumours of Soft Tissue and Bone. World Health Organization Classification of Tumours.* Lyon: IARC Press, 2002:228.

DIAGNOSIS

For bone lesions, one of the primary goals of the history, physical examination, and radiological evaluation is to at least classify the lesion into one of three categories of biological behavior: latent, active, or aggressive (Table 1-2). The last category includes both aggressive benign lesions and malignancies. In some cases, a specific diagnosis may be attainable, but if not, this classification provides some guide to the need for diagnostic evaluation and treatment.

History and Physical Examination

The patient with a bone lesion in general presents in one of four clinical scenarios: (1) incidentally noted bone lesions, (2) painless bony masses, (3) painful bone lesions, and (4) pathologic fractures. The differential diagnosis and

BOX 1-2 ETIOLOGIC AGENTS IN THE DEVELOPMENT OF OSTEOSARCOMA

Chemical Agents
Methylcholanthrene
Beryllium oxide
Zinc beryllium silicate
Radiation
Radium dye workers
Thorotrast radioactive contrast medium
Therapeutic radiotherapy
Viruses
Rous sarcoma virus (v-Src gene)
FBJ virus (c-Fos gene)

approach are guided by which of these scenarios applies. Hence, the clinical features are divided into those four categories.

Incidentally Noted Bone Lesions

This very frequent scenario in musculoskeletal tumors occurs commonly in a number of ways, such as when a minor injury leads to an x-ray that reveals a bone lesion, shoulder pain from impingement leads to discovery of a proximal humeral bone lesion, or a bone scan done for an entirely different purpose lights up unexpectedly at the site of a previously unrecognized bone lesion not associated with the original problem.

Differential Diagnosis
- Common bone lesions discovered incidentally
  - Adults: enchondroma
  - Pediatrics: nonossifying fibroma

History
- Injury leading to discovery
  - Did pain precede the injury? Pain preceding the injury may indicate an active or aggressive lesion rather than the typical latent lesion discovered incidentally.
  - Is pain resolving since injury? Complete resolution of the injury-related pain supports the incidental nature of the bone lesion.
- Pain leading to discovery. The key is to determine whether the pain is more likely to be from a common cause of pain at the affected anatomic site or from the bone lesion itself.
  - Shoulder: Elicit exacerbating features such as overhead activity as an indicator of impingement. Consider subacromial injection.
  - Knee: Elicit exacerbating features such as going up and down stairs and sitting for long periods with knees flexed as indications of patellar-femoral discomfort. Consider intra-articular injection.
- Bone scan leading to discovery
  - Has there ever been pain or local tenderness at the site of the bone lesion? Some patients may have had a mild aching pain at the site of a low-grade malignancy that they never sought medical attention for in the past.

Physical Examination
- Bone tenderness (tumor) versus joint line tenderness (intra-articular pathology) is an important distinguishing feature.
- Signs of the possible joint problem causing pain (if any) should be elicited.

Diagnostic Workup
- Blood work: No role unless infection suspected (obtain complete blood count [CBC] with differential, erythrocyte sedimentation rate [ESR], C-reactive protein [CRP])
- If suspected cartilage neoplasm, consider computed tomography (CT) or magnetic resonance imaging (MRI)
  - CT scan: Delineates endosteal scalloping, periosteal reaction best

TABLE 1-1 CONGENITAL AND INHERITED SYNDROMES PREDISPOSING TO BONE SARCOMAS

Syndrome	Inheritance Pattern	Typical Tumors/ Findings	Malignancy	Implicated Genes	Pathophysiology
Ollier's disease and Maffucci syndrome	Mostly sporadic Some families suggest AD	Multiple enchondromas (hemangiomas in Maffucci syndrome)	Chondro-sarcoma in Ollier's disease; multiple malignancies in Maffucci syndrome	Unknown	Unknown
McCune-Albright syndrome (MAS), polyostotic fibrous dysplasia, monostotic fibrous dysplasia	Sporadic	Multiple lesions of fibrous dysplasia (endocrine abnormalities and coast of Maine pigmented skin lesions with MAS)		GNAS1 (guanine nucleotide-binding protein, α-stimulating activity polypeptide 1)	Extent of disease dependent upon how large of a cell mass is affected by somatic mutation during embryogenesis
Multiple osteochondromas	50% sporadic 50% AD	Osteochondromas	Chondrosarcoma	EXT1, EXT2 (exostosin)	Mutant exostosin glycoproteins alter heparin sulfate proteoglycans, affecting FGF and Ihh signaling
Retinoblastoma syndrome	60% sporadic 40% AD	Retinoblastoma	Osteosarcoma Other cancers	RB1	Mutant RB1 tumor suppressor gene allows tumor development
Rothmund-Thomson syndrome	AR	Poikiloderma Short stature Sparseness of eyebrows/lashes Juvenile cataracts Sunlight sensitivity Hypogonadism Defective dentition Nail problems	Osteosarcoma Cutaneous epitheliomas Gastric adenocarcinomas Fibrosarcomas	RECQL4	Mutant helicase gene
Bloom syndrome		Telangiectatic erythema resembling SLE Dwarfism Thin, triangular face	Osteosarcoma Other cancers	BME	Mutant RECQ helicase gene
Li-Fraumeni syndrome		<45 with sarcoma and first-degree relative <45 with any cancer and another first- or second-degree relative in same lineage with any cancer at any age	Osteosarcoma Soft tissue sarcoma Breast cancer Brain tumors Acute leukemia Adrenal cortical cancers Gonadal giant cell tumors	TP53 gene (71%)	Mutant p53 tumor suppressor gene

TABLE 1-2 CLASSIFICATION OF BONE TUMORS ACCORDING TO BIOLOGICAL BEHAVIOR

Classification	Symptoms	Type of Bone Lesion	Radiographic Features	Common Examples
Latent	Asymptomatic No pain preceding fracture	Benign	Narrow zone of transition	Nonossifying fibroma* (fibrous cortical defect) Unicameral bone cyst* Adult osteochondroma*
Active	Painful Pain preceding fracture	Benign	Intermediate zone of transition Expansion	Fibrous dysplasia Osteoid osteoma Osteochondroma
Aggressive or malignant	Painful Pain preceding fracture	Benign or malignant	Broad zone of transition Cortical destruction Soft tissue extension	**Benign** Aneurysmal bone cyst# Chondroblastoma# Giant cell tumor# Osteoblastoma# **Malignant** Sarcoma Metastatic carcinoma Lymphoma

*Classic latent lesions such as these may be active during childhood.
#Some tumors, such as aneurysmal bone cyst, chondroblastoma, and giant cell tumor, may have a spectrum of clinical behavior patterns.

- MRI scan: Helps differentiate features of hyaline cartilage
    - Lobular organization pattern, bright with T2 weighting, dark with T1 weighting
- If fibrous dysplasia or enchondroma considered, consider total body bone scan to establish solitary or polyostotic process
    - Enchondroma versus Ollier's disease/enchondromatosis
    - Monostotic versus polyostotic fibrous dysplasia or McCune-Albright syndrome
- If presumptive diagnosis of latent lesion is established on plain radiographs, key is serial clinical and radiographic follow-up.
    - Common serial follow-up plan: 3 months, 6 months, 1 year, and 2 years after discovery
    - If lesion behaves more aggressively than expected, biopsy and appropriate surgical treatment may be necessary.
    - In most cases, the lesion will remain unchanged (e.g., enchondroma) or go on to heal (e.g., nonossifying fibroma), and after 2 years of follow-up, most asymptomatic lesions may be considered stable.
- Biopsy is usually unnecessary.

Painless Bony Masses
Differential Diagnosis
- Osteochondroma (most common by far)
- Low-grade malignancies with associated soft tissue mass
    - Parosteal osteosarcoma
    - Periosteal chondrosarcoma
    - Secondary chondrosarcoma arising in osteochondroma

History
- Age
    - Pediatric patient: Osteochondroma grows during skeletal immaturity
    - Adult patients: Osteochondromas should not grow once growth has ceased. Consider other diagnoses.
- Pain
    - Osteochondroma typically painless unless pressure on other structures
    - Pain may be associated with low-grade malignancies.
- Family history of osteochondromatosis
    - Half of cases are spontaneous mutations, so many patients will have negative family history despite autosomal-dominant (AD) mode of transmission.

Physical Examination
- Bone versus soft tissue origin
    - Soft tissue masses close to bone may mimic surface bone lesions (myositis ossificans).
- Signs of multiple osteochondromatosis
    - Other bony masses
    - Short stature
- Findings that might warrant surgical excision of osteochondroma
    - Local tenderness, limited motion, nerve compression

Diagnostic Workup
- Blood work: No role unless infection suspected (obtain CBC with differential, ESR, CRP)
- Total body bone scan: establish monostotic versus polyostotic process

- Solitary osteochondroma versus osteochondromatosis
- If distinction between benign and malignant lesions necessary, consider CT scan.
  - Myositis ossificans shows peripherally mature mineralization.
  - Osteochondroma shows continuity of cortical and medullary bone from stalk to adjacent bone.
  - Parosteal osteosarcoma gives a "stuck-on" appearance, often with a very thin radiolucency between the lesion and the underlying bone.
- If osteochondroma or parosteal osteosarcoma suspected, MRI scan should be obtained.
  - For osteochondroma: assess thickness of cartilage cap, especially in adults, to differentiate from peripheral chondrosarcoma.
    - Cap thickness >2 cm is consistent with a chondrosarcoma.
    - Cap thickness 1 to 2 cm in adults is concerning for chondrosarcoma.
  - For parosteal osteosarcoma, MRI determines both soft tissue extent and involvement of underlying medullary cavity.
- If parosteal osteosarcoma is a diagnostic consideration or if the diagnosis cannot be established with imaging studies, a biopsy is needed.

Painful Bone Lesions
Differential Diagnosis
- Pediatric patients (<20)
  - Painful active lesions
    - Osteoid osteoma
  - Painful aggressive benign lesions
    - Osteoblastoma
    - Aneurysmal bone cyst
    - Langerhans cell histiocytosis
  - Painful malignant lesions
    - Osteosarcoma
    - Ewing sarcoma
- Young adult patients (20 to 40)
  - Giant cell tumor of bone
  - Lymphoma
  - Ewing sarcoma (5 to 30 years)
- Adult patients (>40)
  - Metastatic carcinoma
  - Myeloma
  - Lymphoma
  - Chondrosarcoma and other sarcomas

History
- If osteoid osteoma suggested, seek typical pain pattern (worse at night, relieved by nonsteroidal anti-inflammatory agents [NSAIDs]).
- Pain at rest in addition to mechanical pain suggests tumor-related pain.
  - Tumor-related causes of rest pain
    - Bone destruction
    - Intraosseous pressure
    - Proteinases
    - Inflammatory cytokine response
  - Tumor-related causes of activity-related pain

- Advanced bone destruction
- Extra-osseous soft tissue pressure
- If malignancy suspected, check for systemic symptoms, more common with disseminated malignancies.
  - Fevers, chills, unintentional weight loss, anorexia, fatigue
- In adults, elicit risk factors for and signs of systemic malignancies:
  - Family history of breast cancer
  - Prostate symptoms for prostate cancer
  - Smoking history for lung cancer
  - Hematuria for renal cancer
  - Thyroid masses/symptoms for thyroid cancer
  - Complete review of systems

Physical Examination
- Adults (also see section on metastatic disease)
  - Potential sources of primary carcinoma (especially breast, prostate, lung, kidney, thyroid)
  - Other evidence of metastatic disease (lymph nodes, soft tissues)
- All: Site of primary symptoms

Diagnostic Workup
- Blood work
  - Pediatrics: Infection is always a consideration, so CBC with differential, ESR, and CRP are needed.
  - Adults (also see Chapter 8, Metastatic Disease)
    - CBC, ESR, serum calcium and phosphorus, alkaline phosphatase, lactate dehydrogenase, serum protein electrophoresis, prostate-specific antigen, urinalysis
- Bone scan
  - Assesses for multifocal disease in potentially polyostotic pediatric processes and in metastatic or multifocal adult tumors
  - Identifies potential sites of referred pain
  - Identifies intense uptake within osteoid osteomas, which is needed to support this presumptive clinicoradiographic diagnosis
  - Stages for potential bone metastases in suspected primary sarcomas
- CT scan of primary site
  - Identifies scalloping and cortical destruction better than MRI
  - Useful for cartilage tumors and giant cell tumors
  - May be used to complement MRI
- MRI of primary site
  - Best identifies intramedullary and extramedullary extent and relationship to surrounding structures
  - Should be done prior to biopsy
- CT of chest
  - Primary staging study for sarcomas
    - Lung metastases most common site of metastases from sarcomas
  - Part of metastatic work-up for adults with aggressive bone lesions and suspected metastatic disease (also see Chapter 8)
- CT of abdomen and pelvis
  - Part of metastatic work-up for adults with aggressive

bone lesions and suspected metastatic disease (also see Chapter 8)
  - Allows identification of renal cell carcinoma prior to biopsy
- Mammography
  - Part of metastatic work-up in adult women with aggressive bone lesions and suspected metastatic disease (also see Chapter 8)
- Biopsy: After completion of all imaging studies, biopsy is necessary in most painful bone lesions.

Pathologic Fracture (also see Chapter 4.5, Pathologic Fractures)

Differential Diagnosis

- Most common bone lesions associated with pathologic fractures in pediatric patients
  - Benign tumors (Figs. 1-1 and 1-2)
    - Unicameral bone cyst
    - Nonossifying fibroma
    - Fibrous dysplasia
  - Malignant tumors (Figs. 1-3 and 1-4)
    - Osteosarcoma
    - Ewing sarcoma
- Most common bone lesions associated with pathologic fractures in adults
  - Young adults
    - Giant cell tumor (Fig. 1-5)
    - Lymphoma
  - Adults >40
    - Metastatic carcinoma
    - Myeloma
    - Lymphoma (Figs. 1-6 and 1-7)

History

- Key question: Did the patient have pain at the site leading up to the time of the fracture?

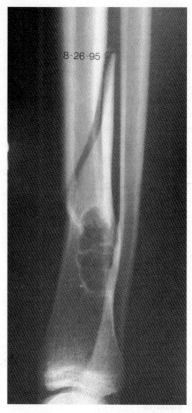

Figure 1-2   Pathologic fracture through nonossifying fibroma typically occurs without preceding pain.

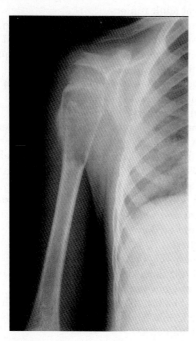

Figure 1-1   Pathologic fracture through unicameral bone cyst typically occurs without preceding pain.

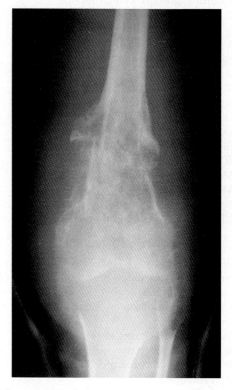

Figure 1-3   Pathologic fracture through an osteosarcoma is usually preceded by progressively worsening pain.

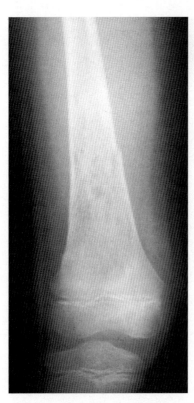

Figure 1-4 Pathologic fracture through aggressive lesions such as this Ewing sarcoma is usually preceded by pain.

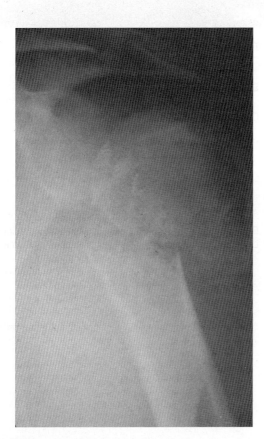

Figure 1-5 Pathologic fractures through giant cell tumors are usually preceded by pain, as was the case here.

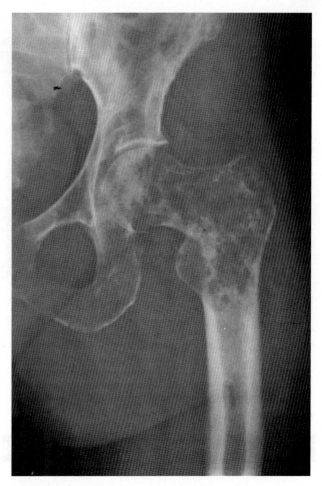

Figure 1-6 Pathologic fractures through lesions created by metastatic carcinoma are often preceded by pain.

- "No" implies a latent lesion without progressive destruction. Most of these lesions can be diagnosed by radiograph alone without biopsy. This situation is most common in the pediatric population. Many of these fractures may be allowed to heal before addressing the lesion itself, unless there is the potential for deformity.
- "Yes" implies a potentially aggressive or malignant lesion. These lesions usually require a biopsy to establish the diagnosis. This situation includes most malignant primary bone tumors and metastatic lesions.

Physical Examination
- Site of pathologic fracture: Open? Neurovascular status intact distally?
- General examination to elicit source of metastatic disease and other evidence of disseminated malignancy (see section above on painful bone lesions)

Radiologic Examination

X-Ray Evaluation and Classic Features
- Radiographic differential diagnosis by age (Table 1-3)
- Location

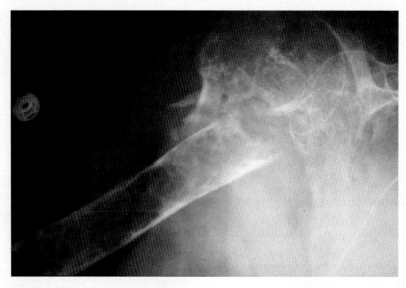

Figure 1-7   Pathologic fractures through multiple myeloma lesions are often preceded by pain.

TABLE 1-3 RADIOGRAPHIC DIFFERENTIAL DIAGNOSIS BY AGE

Differential Diagnosis	Age Range (yr)			
	0 to 5	>5 to Skeletal Maturity	Skeletal Maturity to 40	>40
Benign	Langerhans cell histiocytosis Osteomyelitis	Nonossifying fibroma Unicameral bone cyst Aneurysmal bone cyst Osteoid osteoma Osteochondroma Fibrous dysplasia Langerhans cell histiocytosis Numerous others	Giant cell tumor of bone Fibrous dysplasia Enchondroma	Enchondroma
Malignant	Metastatic neuroblastoma	Osteosarcoma Ewing sarcoma Lymphoma	Ewing sarcoma (up to age 30) Lymphoma	Metastatic carcinoma Multiple myeloma Lymphoma Chondrosarcoma Osteosarcoma MFH Fibrosarcoma

BOX 1-3 DIFFERENTIAL DIAGNOSIS ACCORDING TO LOCATION WITHIN LONG BONE

Epiphyseal: PGCAT
PVNS
Giant cell tumor
Chondroblastoma
Clear cell chondrosarcoma
Aneurysmal bone cyst
Tuberculosis and other infections
Metaphyseal
Nonossifying fibroma
Unicameral bone cyst
Osteosarcoma
Chondrosarcoma
Numerous others
Diaphyseal
Ewing sarcoma
Langerhans cell histiocytosis
Osteoid osteoma
Metastases

- Epiphyseal, metaphyseal, and diaphyseal locations in long bones (Box 1-3)
  - Epiphyseal sites are an uncommon site of bone lesions and are affected by a relatively short list of potential lesions.
  - Similarly, the diaphysis is a less common site for bone lesions.
  - By contrast, the metaphysis is the most common site of long bone involvement, and most lesions can affect the metaphysis.
- Surface bone lesions
  - Specific osseous and cartilaginous lesions arise from the surface of the bone or are intracortical.
  - A CT scan is often helpful to better define the relationship of these lesions to the bone cortex (Table 1-4 and Fig. 1-8).

TABLE 1-4 DIFFERENTIAL DIAGNOSIS OF SURFACE AND INTRACORTICAL ECCENTRIC BONE LESIONS

	Osseous Lesions	Cartilaginous Lesions
Surface bone lesions	Parosteal osteosarcoma Periosteal osteosarcoma High-grade peripheral osteosarcoma	Osteochondroma Periosteal chondroma Periosteal chondrosarcoma
Intracortical lesions	Osteoid osteoma	Periosteal chondroma Chondromyxoid fibroma Nonossifying fibroma

- Axioms of tumor location
  - Most common bone lesion in the phalanges: enchondromas
  - Two tumors with a very strong predilection for the tibia: osteofibrous dysplasia and adantinoma
  - Most common locations for aggressive benign and primary malignant bone tumors in children and young adults involve areas of rapid longitudinal growth: distal femur, proximal tibia, proximal femur, proximal humerus.
  - Chondrosarcomas have a predilection for the proximal peripheral skeleton: pelvis, scapula, proximal humerus, femur.
  - Chordoma usually occurs in sacrum or base of skull.
  - Three most common bone tumors in patients >40: metastases, metastases, metastases!
  - Most metastases occur proximal to knees and elbows: those distal to knees and elbows are usually due to lung or renal metastases or melanoma.
  - Common anterior spine lesions: metastases, hemangiomas of bone, Langerhans cell histiocytosis, osteomyelitis, giant cell tumor
  - Common posterior spine lesions: aneurysmal bone cyst, osteoid osteoma, osteoblastoma
  - Bone lesions that skip across joints to involve adjacent bones are frequently vascular: angiosarcoma and Gorham's disease (disappearing bone disease).
- Three key questions
1. What is the lesion doing to bone? This question can also be asked as, "What is the border of the lesion?" Three types of borders are defined by the width of the zone of transition with normal bone. Each type of border leads to a differential diagnosis of latent, active, or aggressive bone lesions (Table 1-5 and Figs. 1-9 and 1-10).
2. How is the bone responding to the lesion (Table 1-6 and Figs. 1-11 and 1-12)?
3. What matrix, if any, makes up the lesion?
   - Matrix refers to the pattern of mineralization within a lesion that is not purely radiolucent.
   - The specific pattern of mineralization helps point to a specific category of bone lesions (Table 1-7 and Fig. 1-13).

Bone Scans and Skeletal Surveys
- Bone scans are invaluable in determining whether a bone lesion is solitary or one of a larger number of bone lesions throughout the skeleton (Table 1-8).
- Skeletal surveys may be necessary in conditions where the bone scan may be "cold," such as myeloma and Langerhans cell histiocytosis.

Computed Tomography and Magnetic Resonance Imaging
- Common differential diagnoses
  - Holes in bone: FEGNOMASHIC or FOGMACHINE (Box 1-4)
  - Epiphyseal lesions. Lesions of the epiphysis may either be isolated to one side of the joint or involve both sides. The differential diagnosis differs for these two general groups, although for those lesions

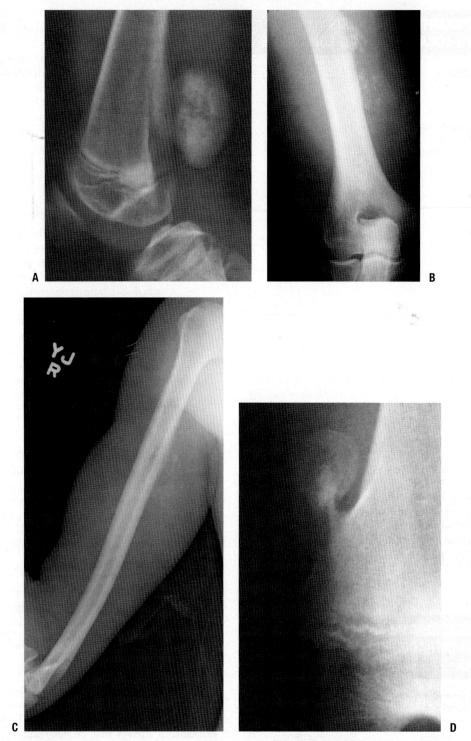

Figure 1-8   Common surface and intracortical eccentric bone lesions are displayed radiographically. (**A**) Parosteal osteosarcoma, (**B**) periosteal osteosarcoma, (**C**) high-grade surface osteosarcoma, (**D**) osteochondroma,

(continues)

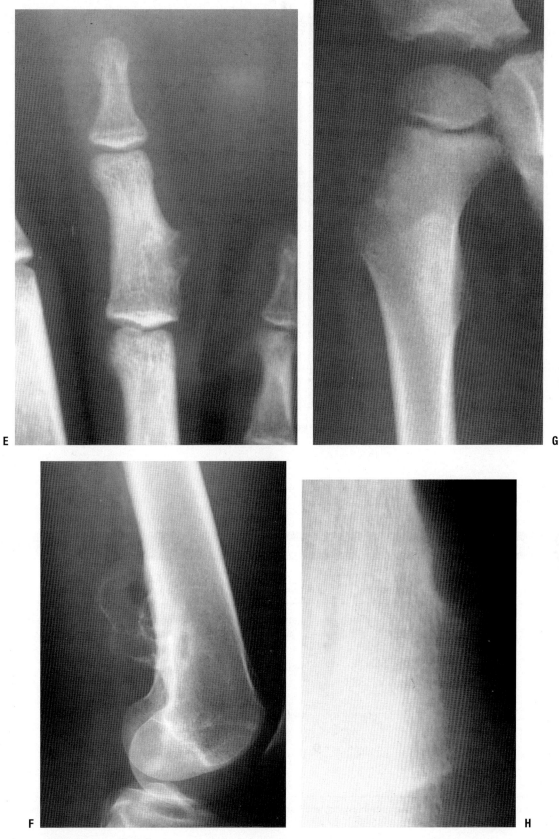

Figure 1-8 *(continued)*   (E) periosteal chondroma, (F) periosteal chondrosarcoma, (G) osteoid osteoma, (H) chondromyxoid fibroma,

(continued)

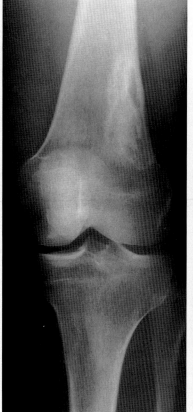
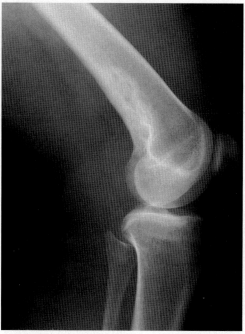

Figure 1-8 *(continued)*   **(I)** nonossifying fibroma.

TABLE 1-5 TYPES OF BORDERS THAT DEFINE BONE LESIONS

Border	Type of Transition	Width of Transition	Type of Bone Lesion	Common Examples
Geographic	Narrow	Pencil-thin line	Latent benign vs. active	Nonossifying fibroma (fibrous cortical defect) Chondromyxoid fibroma Unicameral bone cyst
Moth-eaten	Intermediate	Millimeters	Active benign	Aneurysmal bone cyst[*] Chondroblastoma[*] Giant cell tumor[*]
Permeative	Broad	Centimeters	Aggressive benign vs. malignant	Aneurysmal bone cyst[*] Chondroblastoma[*] Giant cell tumor[*] Sarcoma Metastatic carcinoma Lymphoma

[*]Some tumors, such as aneurysmal bone cyst, chondroblastoma, and giant cell tumor, may have a spectrum of clinical behavior patterns.

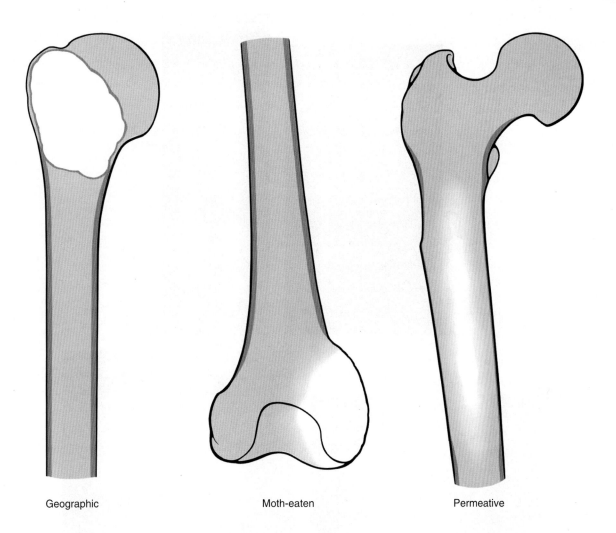

Geographic   Moth-eaten   Permeative

Figure 1-9 Border types. The interface at the edge of any given bone lesion on plain radiographs may be classified as geographic, moth-eaten, or permeative. A geographic border, as illustrated by the proximal humeral tumor on the left, has a very narrow zone of transition (able to be traced with a pencil-thin line) between normal and abnormal bone and usually represents an indolent benign process, such as a unicameral bone cyst. A moth-eaten border, as illustrated by the distal femoral tumor in the center, has a slightly blurred zone of transition (typically a few millimeters) and may reflect a more active process, such as a giant cell tumor of bone. A permeative border, as illustrated by the proximal femoral diaphyseal tumor on the right, is typified by a broad zone of transition (usually 1 cm or greater) and usually represents a more aggressive process, such as a sarcoma or metastatic carcinoma. These border types are only one piece of the radiographic interpretation, and they cannot be relied upon wholly to determine biologic activity.

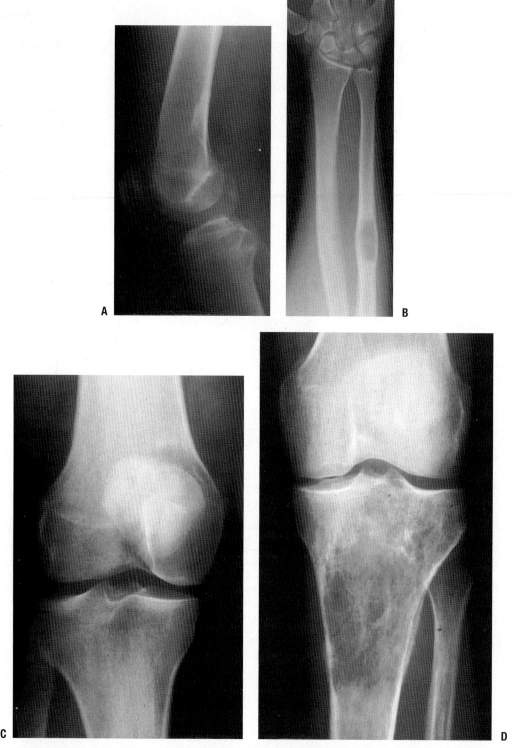

Figure 1-10   Bone lesions with a spectrum of borders. (**A**) Nonossifying fibroma with a geographic border. (**B**) Fibrous dysplasia with a geographic to slightly moth-eaten border. (**C**) Giant cell tumor of bone with a moth-eaten border. (**D**) Lytic osteosarcoma with a permeative border.

TABLE 1-6 RADIOGRAPHIC TYPES OF RESPONSES TO BONE LESIONS

Types of Response	Definition	Classic Examples
Marginal sclerosis	Dense peripheral medullary lamellar bone margin to inactive, active, or very slowly expansile aggressive lesions	Nonossifying fibroma Fibrous dysplasia
Cortical thickening	Sometimes massive cortical response to very slow-growing lesions	Osteoid osteoma Osteomyelitis
Orderly periosteal new bone	Regular laminar periosteal response without accompanying aggressive features	Stress fracture
Endosteal expansion	Combination of orderly periosteal bone formation with endosteal erosion (scalloping)	Low- to intermediate-grade chondrosarcoma
Periosteal neocortical response	Rapid expansion of bone and destruction of overlying cortex remains contained by periosteum and thin neocortex	Aneurysmal bone cyst Giant cell tumor of bone
Poorly organized new bone	Inability of periosteal response to contain rapid destruction Soft tissue mass extends beyond the intact cortex	Osteosarcoma: Codman's triangle Ewing sarcoma: sunburst appearance, onion-skinning

Adapted from Levesque J, Marx R, Bell RS, et al. *A Clinical Guide to Primary Bone Tumors.* Philadelphia: Williams & Wilkins, 1998.

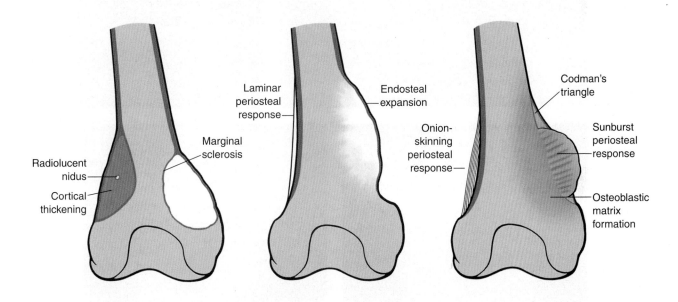

Figure 1-11 Varying types of bony response are seen in association with different tumors of bone. On the left, a distal femur shows typical benign types of bone response. The lateral bone lesion, with a central nidus surrounded by a dense cortical thickening or hyperostosis, is typical for an osteoid osteoma. On the same femur, there is also a medial lesion with a reactive sclerotic rim and slight endosteal expansion. This appearance in the distal femoral metaphysis of a child is typical for a non-ossifying fibroma. In the center femur, there is an aneurysmal dilatation or ballooning of the cortex with an eggshell-thin rim of peripheral bone that is typical of an aneurysmal bone cyst. On the right femur, aggressive types of periosteal reaction are shown, including onion-skinning periosteal reaction on the lateral distal femoral metaphysis and a medial sunburst osteoblastic response with bordering Codman's triangles proximally and distally. These aggressive types of periosteal response may be seen independently or together. Although onion-skinning is often associated with Ewing sarcoma, sunburst response with osteosarcoma, and Codman's triangle with osteosarcoma, each type of response may be seen in other conditions as well, including osteomyelitis, Langerhans cell histiocytosis, lymphoma, and metastatic carcinoma, among others.

Figure 1-12 Bone lesions with a spectrum of responses in the surrounding bone. (**A**) A proximal femoral fibrous dysplasia lesion shows marginal sclerosis. (**B**) A humeral diaphyseal region of cortical thickening is seen here in association with an area of chronic osteomyelitis. (**C**) Poorly organized new bone formation demonstrating both Codman's triangle and a sunburst appearance is shown here in an osteosarcoma.

(continues)

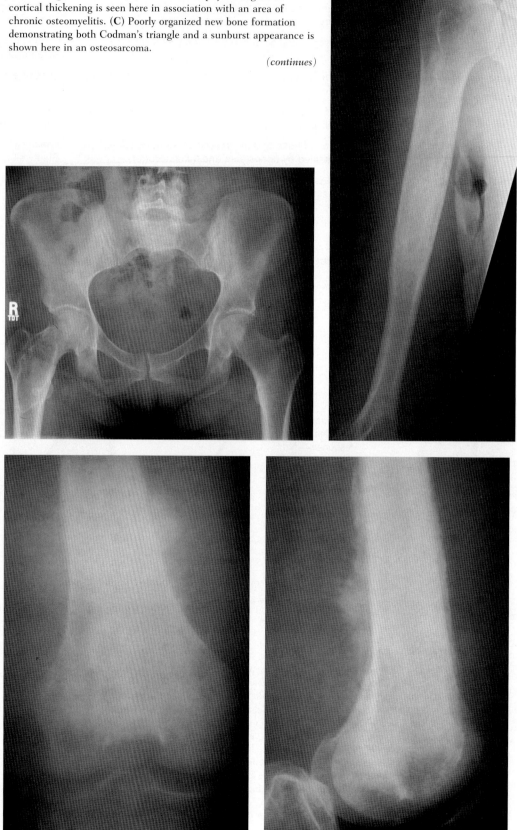

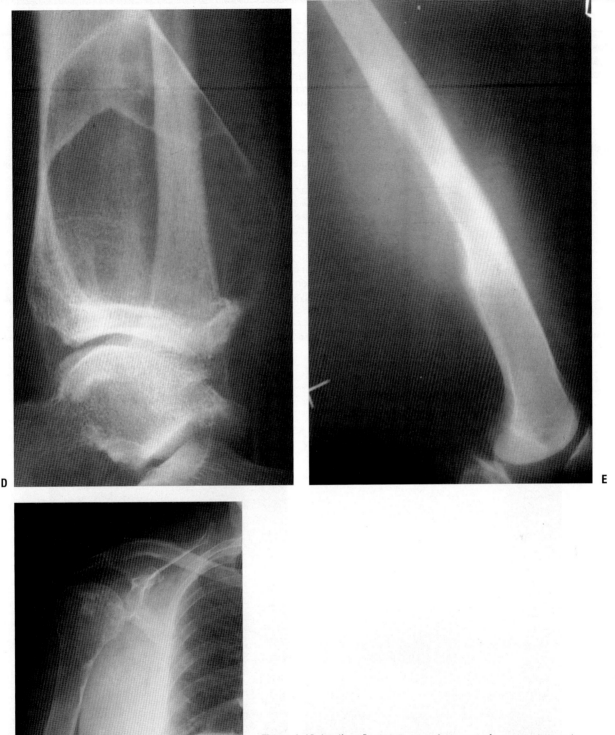

D

E

F

Figure 1-12 *(continued)*   (**D**) Periosteal neocortical response is seen in the posterior cortex of the distal tibia due to this aneurysmal bone cyst. (**E**) Onion-skinning periosteal reaction with Codman's triangle and an associated soft tissue mass is shown in this Ewing sarcoma. (**F**) Endosteal expansion and erosions are seen with this low-grade chondrosarcoma.

TABLE 1-7 PATTERNS OF MINERALIZATION WITHIN BONE LESIONS

	Description	Typical Lesions	Other Distinguishing Features
Radiolucent (lytic)	Absence of matrix	Numerous (nonspecific)	Numerous
Mineralized			
Calcified	Punctate rings and arcs	Hyaline cartilage lesions*	
		Enchondroma	Geographic
		Chondrosarcoma	Permeative zone of transition
			Endosteal erosions
			Periosteal reaction
Ossified	More organized pattern of bone formation	Osseous lesions	
		Osteoid osteoma	Reactive peripheral bone, central nidus
		Osteoblastoma	Scant to densely sclerotic lesions
		Osteosarcoma	Scant to densely sclerotic lesions
		Lesions with marked sclerotic response	
		Breast carcinoma metastases	Permeative destructive lesions
		Prostate carcinoma metastases	Variable sclerotic response in surrounding bone
		Lymphoma	
	Blurring of trabeculae	Fibrous dysplasia	Geographic long lesion in long bone
			Ground glass

* Immature cartilage lesions, such as chondroblastoma and periosteal chondroma, do not show the degree of mineralization characteristic of mature hyaline lesions.

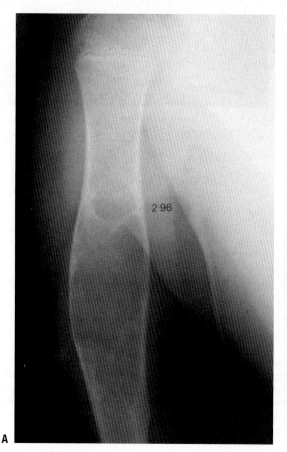
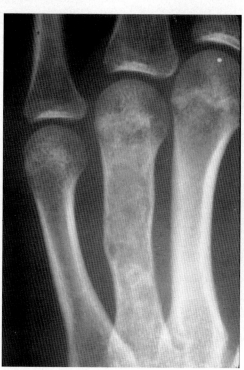

Figure 1-13   Bone lesions with a spectrum of types of matrix mineralization. (**A**) Absence of matrix mineralization is seen in a lucent lesion from a unicameral bone cyst. (**B**) The typical rings and arcs of hyaline cartilage matrix mineralization are seen in this metacarpal enchondroma.

(continues)

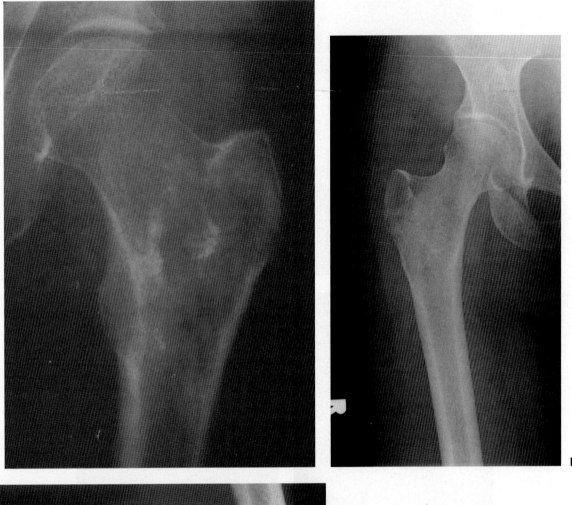

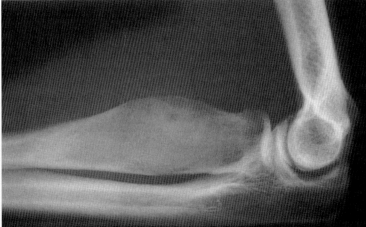

Figure 1-13 *(continued)*   **(C)** The same type of hyaline cartilage matrix mineralization is apparent in this chondrosarcoma. **(D)** Ground glass appearance is typical of fibrous dysplasia, as in this lesion of the proximal radius. **(E)** A mixed sclerotic and partially lytic lesion of the proximal femur, which is frequently seen in the setting of metastatic breast cancer.

(continued)

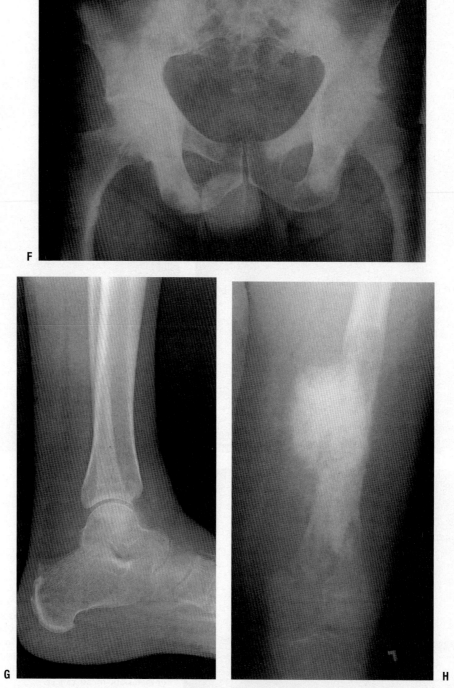

Figure 1-13 *(continued)*   (**F**) Densely sclerotic metastases are the most common appearance in bony metastatic prostate carcinoma. (**G**) Lytic metastases are the most common appearance for metastatic lung cancer, which is also the most common primary source for metastases distal to the elbows and knees, as shown in this tarsal navicular metastatic deposit from lung carcinoma. (**H**) A cumulus cloud pattern of matrix mineralization is most characteristic of osteosarcoma.

TABLE 1-8 MULTIFOCAL BONE LESIONS

	Pediatrics	Adults
Metabolic bone diseases		Multifocal Paget's disease of bone
Infections	Chronic recurrent multifocal osteomyelitis	
Malignant neoplasms	Metastases (neuroblastoma, rhabdomyosarcoma, osteosarcoma) Multifocal osteosarcoma	Metastases Myeloma
Endocrinopathies		Hyperparathyroidism (brown tumors)
Vascular conditions	Disappearing bone disease (Gorham's disease) Skeletal/extraskeletal lymphangiomatosis Angiosarcoma Multifocal bone infarcts	
Congenital diseases	Osteochondromatosis (multiple hereditary exostoses)	
Developmental skeletal dysplasias	Ollier's disease (multiple enchondromatosis) Maffucci syndrome (multiple enchondromatosis with hemangiomas) Polyostotic fibrous dysplasia McCune-Albright syndrome (polyostotic fibrous dysplasia with endocrinopathy)	
Other diseases	Langerhans cell histiocytosis	Erdheim-Chester disease

that may involve both sides of the joint, an isolated lesion early on in the disease process may involve only one side. PGCAT is a convenient mnemonic to recall the most common lesions in both of these categories, but it does not distinguish between lesions that are always solitary and those that may involve one or both sides of the joint (Figs. 1-14 and 1-15 and Box 1-5).

■ As a subset of epiphyseal lesions, juxta-articular lesions may involve one or both sides of the joint and typically represent non-neoplastic arthropathies.

BOX 1-4 DIFFERENTIAL DIAGNOSIS FOR HOLES IN BONE: FOGMACHINE

Fibrous dysplasia
Osteoid osteoma, osteoblastoma, osteosarcoma, osteofibrous dysplasia
Giant cell tumor
Myeloma
Aneurysmal bone cyst, adamantinoma
Chondromyxoid fibroma, chondroblastoma, chondrosarcoma
Histiocytosis
Infection
Nonossifying fibroma
Enchondroma, Ewing sarcoma

- ■ Inflammatory arthropathies
- ■ Infectious arthropathy
- ■ Crystal-induced arthropathy (gout, pseudogout)
- ■ Pigmented villonodular synovitis
- ■ Synovial chondromatosis
- ■ Intraosseous ganglions
- ■ Degenerative cysts (geodes)

■ Isolated epiphyseal lesions (as a subset of the larger group of epiphyseal lesions) are neoplastic conditions that involve only one side of the joint.
- ■ Aneurysmal bone cysts
- ■ Chondroblastoma (confined to epiphysis; pediatrics or adults)
- ■ Giant cell tumor (meta-epiphyseal; mostly adults)
- ■ Clear cell chondrosarcoma (adults)

■ Spine lesions
- ■ Other than metastatic disease, which often begins its destruction in the pedicle, and hence may enlarge to affect either the anterior or posterior elements or both, there is a sharp delineation between the processes that affect the vertebral body from those that affect the posterior elements. Infections and pediatric malignancies, for instance, nearly always affect the anterior spine, and the benign tumors that characteristically involve the two anatomic regions do not overlap (Table 1-9).

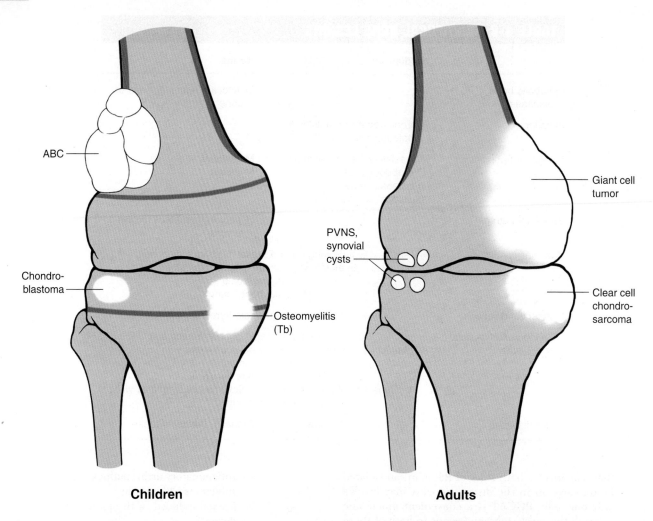

ABC

Chondro-
blastoma

Osteomyelitis
(Tb)

PVNS,
synovial
cysts

Giant cell
tumor

Clear cell
chondro-
sarcoma

Children   **Adults**

Figure 1-14 PGCAT lesions. Epiphyseal lesions have a relatively narrow differential diagnosis that can be recalled using the mnemonic PGCAT, which includes such common epiphyseal lesions as PVNS (pigmented villonodular synovitis), GCT (giant cell tumor of bone), chondroblastoma, ABC (aneurysmal bone cyst), and Tb (tuberculosis). In the figure, the femur on the left, with open growth plates shown, illustrates common pediatric epiphyseal lesions. Chondroblastoma is represented by the purely epiphyseal radiolucency without sclerotic borders. Aneurysmal bone cyst is represented by the septated, expansile lesion centered in the meta-epiphysis. Osteomyelitis, of which tuberculosis is only a representative example, may manifest itself as a metaphyseal radiolucency eroding across into the epiphysis, as shown on the pediatric figure. The femur on the right, without open growth plates, illustrates the common adult epiphyseal lesions. Synovial processes, of which PVNS is only a representative example, are relatively common. Degenerative geodes and intraosseous ganglions are more common examples of such processes. Giant cell tumor of bone has its epicenter in the metaphysis but classically erodes down to subchondral bone within the epiphysis.

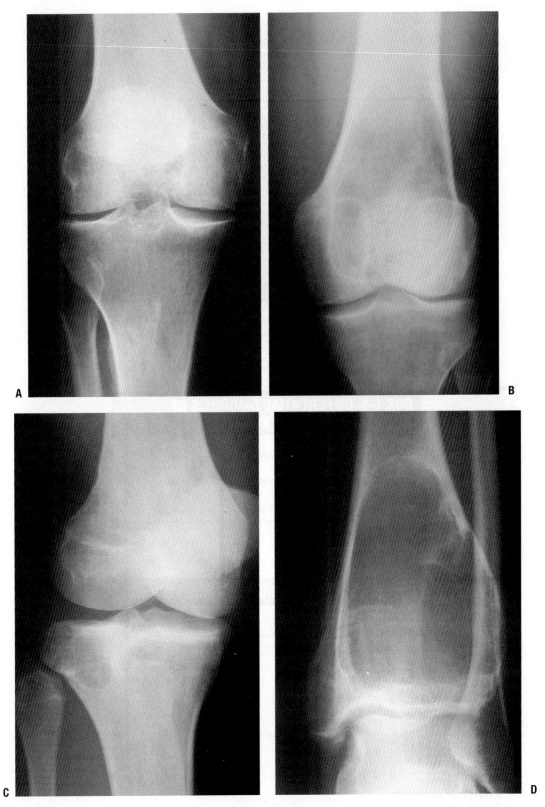

Figure 1-15   Bone lesions that frequently occur in the epiphyseal region. **(A)** Pigmented villonodular synovitis may show juxta-articular erosions. **(B)** Giant cell tumor of bone frequently extends from the metaphyseal region into the epiphysis and down to subchondral bone. **(C)** Chondroblastoma has its epicenter within the epiphysis and extends into the metaphysis occasionally. **(D)** Most commonly, when aneurysmal bone cyst is seen in the epiphysis, it occurs as a secondary lesion within a chondroblastoma or giant cell tumor, although the lesion shown was a primary aneurysmal bone cyst extending into the epiphysis.

(continued)

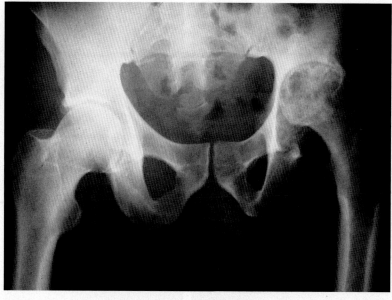

E

Figure 1-15 *(continued)* (E) Infections, such as tuberculosis, can cause juxta-articular cysts in an epiphyseal location. This immunosuppressed patient had tuberculous left hip arthritis.

BOX 1-5 DIFFERENTIAL DIAGNOSIS OF EPIPHYSEAL LESIONS: PGCAT

Pigmented villonodular synovitis
Giant cell tumor
Chondroblastoma and clear cell chondrosarcoma
Aneurysmal bone cyst
Tuberculosis and other infections

TABLE 1-9 DIFFERENTIAL DIAGNOSIS FOR SPINE LESIONS

	Pediatrics	Adults
Anterior elements (vertebral body)		
Infections		Bacterial infection (discitis)
		Tuberculosis (Pott's disease)
Benign tumors	Histiocytosis	Hemangioma
		Giant cell tumor
Malignancies	Ewing sarcoma	Metastases
		Myeloma
	Lymphoma	
Posterior elements		
Benign tumors		Aneurysmal bone cyst
		Osteoid osteoma
		Osteoblastoma
		Osteochondroma
Malignancies		Metastases

TABLE 1-10 MUSCULOSKELETAL TUMOR SOCIETY STAGING SYSTEM

Stage	Anatomic Extent	Histologic Grade*	Presence of Metastases	Treatment
0	—	Benign	None	Curettage or marginal excision
IA	Intraosseous	Low	None	Wide resection of involved bone
IB	Extraosseous extension	Low	None	Wide resection of involved bone and soft tissue
IIA	Intraosseous	High	None	Wide resection of involved bone Chemotherapy
IIB	Extraosseous	High	None	Wide resection of involved bone and soft tissue Chemotherapy
III	Either	Either low or high	Present	Wide resection of involved bone and soft tissue and metastases Chemotherapy

*Low-grade tumors by definition have <15% chance of metastasis; high-grade tumors have >15% chance of metastasis. Ewing sarcoma is high grade by definition, and its treatment differs in that radiotherapy is an alternative to wide resection for nonexpendable, nonreconstructible bone sites.

- Sacral lesions
  - Dural cysts
  - Giant cell tumors
  - Aneurysmal bone cysts
  - Chordoma
  - Chondrosarcoma
  - Metastases
- Mineralized bone lesions
  - Central lesions
    - Enchondroma (popcorn; rings and arcs)
    - Bone infarct (smoke up the chimney)
    - Fibrous dysplasia (ground glass)
    - Intraosseous lipoma (cockade sign)
    - Osteoblastoma
    - Chondrosarcoma
    - Osteosarcoma, high-grade conventional
    - Osteosarcoma, low-grade central
    - Metastatic carcinoma (especially prostate, breast, less commonly lung)
    - Lymphoma (variably)
  - Eccentric lesions
    - Osteochondroma (stalk, cortical continuity)
    - Periosteal chondroma (heaped-up borders)
    - Myositis ossificans (peripheral ossification)
    - Periosteal chondrosarcoma
    - Parosteal osteosarcoma (stuck on cortex)

- Recommended tests
  - Suspected bone sarcoma
    - CT chest (#1 site of sarcoma metastases is lung)
    - Bone scan (#2 site of sarcoma metastases is bone)
  - Suspected metastatic carcinoma (see Chapter 8)

STAGING

The purpose of staging for bone tumors is to guide treatment. Staging describes both the extent of the tumor and the potential for development of metastatic disease. Staging in general involves determining the specific diagnosis, histologic grade, local extent and/or size of tumor, and the presence (and type) or absence of metastatic disease. Various staging systems exist, but that of the Musculoskeletal Tumor Society is commonly employed (Table 1-10).

SUGGESTED READING

Aboulafia AJ, Kennon RE, Jelinek JS. Benign bone tumors of childhood. *J Am Acad Orthop Surg* 1999;7(6):377–388.

Bibbo C, Patel DV, Benevenia J. Perioperative considerations in patients with metastatic bone disease. *Orthop Clin North Am.* 31(4):577–95.

Bolling WS, Beauchamp CP. Presentation and evaluation of bone tumors. *AAOS Instr Course Lect* 1999;48:607–612.

Levine SM, Lambiase RE, Petchprapa CN. Cortical lesions of the tibia: characteristic appearances at conventional radiography. *Radiographics* 2003;23(1):157–177.

Rougraff BT. Evaluation of the patient with carcinoma of unknown origin metastatic to bone. *Clin Orthop Relat Res* 2003;(415 Suppl):S105–109.

Rougraff BT, Kniesl JS, Simon MA. Skeletal metastases of unknown origin: prospective study of a diagnostic strategy. *J Bone Joint Surg [Am]* 1993;75:1276.

Rybak LD, Rosenthal DI. Radiological imaging for the diagnosis of bone metastases. *Q J Nucl Med* 2001;45(1):53–64.

Sanders TG, Parsons TW 3rd. Radiographic imaging of musculoskeletal neoplasia. *Cancer Control* 2001;8(3):221–231.

Simon MA, Finn HA. Diagnostic strategy for bone and soft-tissue tumors. *J Bone Joint Surg [Am]* 1993;75(4):622–631.

Sundaram M. Magnetic resonance imaging for solitary lesions of bone: when, why, how useful? *J Orthop Sci* 1999;4(5):384–396.

Temple HT, Bashore CJ. Staging of bone neoplasms: an orthopedic oncologist's perspective. *Semin Musculoskelet Radiol* 2000;4(1):17–23.

Wenaden AE, Szyszko TA, Saifuddin A. Imaging of periosteal reactions associated with focal lesions of bone. *Clin Radiol* 2005;60(4):439–456.

Woertler K. Benign bone tumors and tumor-like lesions: value of cross-sectional imaging. *Eur Radiol* 2003;13(8):1820–1835. Epub 2003 Apr 17.

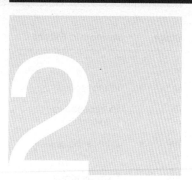

EVALUATION OF SOFT TISSUE TUMORS

CAROL D. MORRIS

Soft tissue tumors are heterogeneous in their behavior and management. The vast majority of soft tissue tumors are benign, with benign tumors outnumbering malignant tumors by a factor of at least 100. This chapter deals with the general diagnostic and management guidelines for both benign and malignant soft tissue tumors. More specific information is available in each tumor-specific chapter.

PATHOGENESIS

Etiology

The etiology of most soft tissue tumors is largely unknown. Environmental exposures, radiation, viral infection, and genetic associations have all been implicated, though the developmental associations are casual in most instances (Box 2-1).

Epidemiology

- Benign
  - True incidence is poorly reported
    - ~300/100,000
  - Outnumber malignant soft tissue sarcomas by 100:1

- Malignant
  - ~8,700 cases/year in the U.S.
  - Annual incidence ~1.5/100,000
    - 8/100,000 in individuals >80 years old
  - Accounts for <1% of all cancers

Pathophysiology

While the pathophysiology of most soft tissue tumors remains ambiguous, the past two decades have provided considerable insight into the biology of these tumors in the form of cytogenetic and molecular information. Chromosomal translocations or other chromosomal aberrations have been reported for virtually every type of soft tissue tumor. The more consistent genetic findings are outlined in Tables 2-1 and 2-2. In addition, a number of inherited conditions are associated with the development of soft tissue tumors (Table 2-3).

Classification

Soft tissue tumors are most commonly characterized histologically according to the type of tissue they most closely resemble. The most widely recognized classification is that

BOX 2-1 ETIOLOGIC FACTORS REPORTED IN THE DEVELOPMENT OF SOFT TISSUE TUMORS

Environmental
  Trauma
  Chemical carcinogens
    (dioxin)
  Asbestos
  Surgical implants
Radiation
  Therapeutic
Viral Infection
  Human immunodeficiency
    virus (HIV)
  Cytomegalovirus (CMV)
  Human herpes virus
    (HHV)-8
  Epstein-Barr virus (EBV)

Genetic
  Neurofibromatosis
  Retinoblastoma
  Gardner's syndrome
  Li-Fraumeni
    syndrome
Immunologic
  Therapeutic
    immunosuppression
  Stewart-Treves
    syndrome

TABLE 2-1 CYTOGENETIC AND MOLECULAR GENETIC ALTERATIONS SEEN IN BENIGN SOFT TISSUE TUMORS

Tumor	Genetic Alterations
Lipoma	12q13–15, 6p21–23, 13q11–22, 13q del
Desmoid	Trisomy 8, trisomy 20, APC gene mutations
Schwannoma	Monosomy 22
Neurofibroma	t(12;14)

of the World Health Organization (WHO), which was first published in 1969 and most recently updated in 2002.

The major histologic categories are:

- Adipocytic
- Fibroblastic
- Fibrohistiocytic
- Smooth muscle
- Perivascular
- Skeletal muscle
- Vascular
- Chondro-osseous
- Uncertain differentiation

The major histologic categories are then divided into benign, intermediate, and malignant groups. WHO recognizes over 60 subtypes of benign soft tissue tumors and over 50 subtypes of malignant soft tissue tumors (sarcomas). It is not thought that the malignant subtypes arise from the benign forms. For example, liposarcoma does not arise from benign fat in lipoma but rather histologically exhibits lipoblastic differentiation.

DIAGNOSIS

Benign soft tissue tumors are fairly common and rarely problematic. In contrast, soft tissue sarcomas are exceedingly rare but diagnostically and therapeutically challenging. Unfortunately both benign soft tissue tumors and soft tissue sarcomas have a deceptively similar presentation, and as such a delay in the diagnosis of soft tissue sarcoma is not uncommon (Table 2-4). While clinical and imaging features will help guide an appropriate work-up, any suspicious soft tissue mass must be biopsied.

TABLE 2-2 CYTOGENETIC AND MOLECULAR GENETIC ALTERATIONS SEEN IN MALIGNANT SOFT TISSUE TUMORS

Tumor	Translation	Involved Genes
Primitive neuroectodermal tumor (PNET)	t(11;22)	FLI1, EWS
Clear cell sarcoma	t(12;22)	ATF1, EWS
Extraskeletal myxoid chondrosarcoma	t(9;22)	CHN, EWS
Synovial sarcoma	t(X;18)	SSX1 or SSX2, SYT
Myxoid liposarcoma	t(12;16)	CHOP, TLS
Alveolar rhabdomyosarcoma	t(2;13)	PAX3, FKHR
Alveolar soft part sarcoma	t(X;17)	TFE3, ASPL
Dermatofibrosarcoma protuberans*	t(17;22)	COL1A1, PDGFB1

* In the WHO classification, dermatofibrosarcoma protuberans is classified as a skin tumor, but it may be encountered in the orthopaedic oncology setting.

TABLE 2-3 INHERITED SYNDROMES ASSOCIATED WITH SOFT TISSUE TUMORS

Syndrome	Associated Tumors
Bannayan-Riley-Ruvalcaba syndrome	Lipoma, hemangioma (hamartoma syndrome)
Beckwith-Wiedemann syndrome	Rhabdomyosarcoma, myxoma, fibroma (overgrowth syndrome)
Costello syndrome	Rhabdomyosarcoma (congenital anomaly/mental retardation syndrome)
Cowden disease	Lipoma, hemangioma (hamartoma syndrome)
Familial fibromatosis	Desmoid tumors
Li-Fraumeni syndrome	Various soft tissue sarcomas (or bone sarcomas)
Maffucci syndrome	Hemangioma, angiosarcoma (with enchondromas)
Mazabraud syndrome	Intramuscular myxoma (with fibrous dysplasia)
Neurofibromatosis-1	Neurofibromas, malignant peripheral nerve sheath tumors (MPNST)
Neurofibromatosis-2	Schwannoma
Proteus syndrome	Lipoma (overgrowth syndrome)
Retinoblastoma syndrome	Various soft tissue sarcomas
Rubinstein-Taybi syndrome	Myogenic sarcoma
Werner syndrome	Various soft tissue sarcomas

Physical Examination and History

Clinical Features
History.

- How long has the mass been present?
  - Masses present for long periods of time are most likely benign.

- New masses arising over a short period of time raise malignancy suspicion.
- Synovial sarcoma and clear cell sarcoma are classic exceptions (may be present for many years).
- Any mass that persists for >4 weeks in the absence of clear-cut trauma warrants consideration of biopsy.

TABLE 2-4 GUIDELINES FOR THE CLINICAL PRESENTATION OF EXTREMITY SOFT TISSUE MASSES

Parameter	Benign	Malignant	Comments
Pain	Rare*	Rare	Uncommon in the absence of nerve or bone invasion
Size	<5 cm	>5 cm	
Location	Superficial (subcutaneous)	Deep to fascia	1/3 of soft tissue sarcomas are superficial.
Mobility	Mobile**	Fixed	
Consistency	Soft	Firm	
Growth	Stable	Enlarging	Synovial sarcoma and clear cell sarcoma can be very slow-growing.

* One benign soft tissue mass that typically presents with pain is an intramuscular hemangioma.
** Benign peripheral nerve sheath tumors are tethered to the nerve and therefore are mobile only medially and laterally but not proximally/distally.

- Is the mass enlarging?
    - Enlarging masses indicate an active process.
    - Patients often have difficulty assessing growth patterns, especially axial lesions (buttock, pelvis, shoulder girdle); they may not be noticed until of substantial size.
- Is there any history of cancer?
    - Certain malignancies may metastasize to the soft tissues with greater frequency:
        - Lung carcinoma
        - Melanoma
        - Lymphoma

Physical Examination.

- Always measure the size of the mass.
    - Any mass >5 cm warrants biopsy!
    - Any mass that increases in size over time warrants a biopsy!
- Always assess depth.
    - Any deep mass (involving fascia or deeper) warrants consideration of biopsy!
- Determine mobility relative to surrounding structures.
    - Any fixed mass warrants a biopsy!
- Transilluminate superficial masses (rule out ganglion).
- Palpate for tenderness.
- Palpate to determine consistency (soft versus firm).
- Check for pulsations, bruit.
- Palpate adjacent blood vessels and bones.
- Perform complete neurological examination.
- Examine the abdomen for hepatomegaly or splenomegaly.
- Examine entire extremity; check for satellite lesions.
- Examine regional lymph nodes.

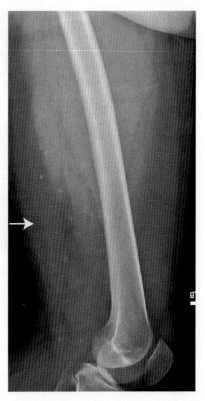

Figure 2-1   Soft tissue phleboliths. *Diagnosis*: Hemangioma.

Radiographic Features
Plain Radiographs.

- Plain radiographs of the affected area are important for the evaluation of soft tissue mineralization and bony involvement. In addition, any patient with a mass suspicious for soft tissue sarcoma should have a chest x-ray.
- *Any* soft tissue sarcoma can present with soft tissue calcifications.
- The most common masses with soft tissue mineralization:
    - Myositis ossificans (more mature mineralization around periphery)
    - Hemangioma (small, round, well-defined phleboliths; Fig. 2-1)
    - Synovial sarcoma (variable pattern of mineralization)
    - Well-differentiated liposarcoma
    - Extraskeletal chondrosarcoma
    - Extraskeletal osteogenic sarcoma (centrally mature mineralization; Fig. 2-2)

Computed Tomography (CT).

- There are four main reasons to obtain a CT scan in patients with soft tissue masses:
    - CT scan of the chest for staging in soft tissue sarcoma

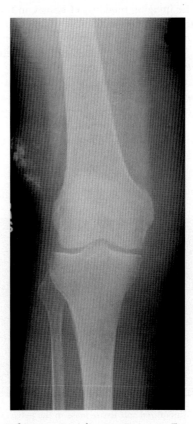

Figure 2-2   Soft tissue mineralization. *Diagnosis*: Extraskeletal osteogenic sarcoma.

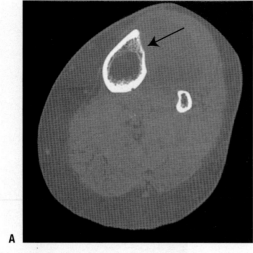
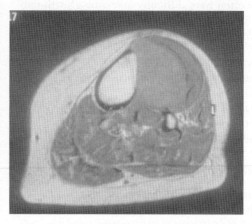

Figure 2-3   MRI versus CT scan in the evaluation of adjacent bone involvement in a patient with soft tissue sarcoma in the leg. The CT scan (**A**) clearly shows loss of cortex, whereas the MRI (**B**) is more ambiguous.

- Evaluation of underlying bony involvement (Fig. 2-3)
- Evaluation of the primary tumor in patients with contraindication to magnetic resonance imaging (MRI)
- Evaluation of pattern of mineralization (Fig. 2-4)

Magnetic Resonance Imaging.

- MRI is the imaging modality of choice in the diagnosis and therapeutic planning of soft tissue tumors. It is superior to other imaging modalities in determining size, location, and anatomic relationships to neurovascular structures in multiple planes.
- For soft tissue sarcomas, MRI is useful for evaluating preoperative radiation or chemotherapy responses and for detecting local recurrences.
- In general, most tumors demonstrate dark signal on T1-weighted images and bright signal on T2-weighted images (Fig. 2-5).

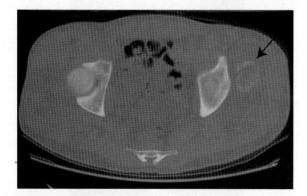

Figure 2-4   Mineralized soft tissue mass in the pelvis. CT scan nicely demonstrates a zonal pattern of ossification with more mature mineralization peripherally, consistent with myositis ossificans.

- Tumors that do not follow this usual signaling pattern have a narrow differential (Table 2-5).
- MRI alone cannot differentiate benign tumors from malignant ones. Lipomas and synovial cysts/ganglions are exceptions.
  - Lipomas have a characteristic appearance on MRI, with uniform homogenous fatty signal on all sequences and loss of signal on the fat-suppression sequences (Fig. 2-6).
  - Cysts have homogenous fluid signal with only peripheral enhancement.
- Helpful hints when evaluating soft tissue masses on MRI:
  - *Any* deep heterogeneous mass or *any* heterogeneous mass >5 cm regardless of location is a soft tissue sarcoma until proven otherwise.
  - Cysts do not demonstrate central enhancement with gadolinium (Fig. 2-7).
  - Not all small masses near a joint (especially the knee and wrist) are ganglions. Unfortunately, small soft tissue sarcomas can occur in and around joints. When in doubt, obtain an MRI with contrast to differentiate cystic masses from solid masses (Fig. 2-8).
  - Just because some of the tissue has the same signal as fat does not make it a lipoma. True lipomas are homogenous on all sequences, are isointense with the subcutaneous fat on all sequences, and uniformly suppress with fat suppression (see Fig. 2-6). Well-differentiated to moderately differentiated liposarcomas have areas of signal consistent with normal fat but admixed with nonfatty signal (Fig. 2-9).

STAGING

Staging systems are a way to predict a tumor's biological potential and hence its clinical behavior, which in turn aids

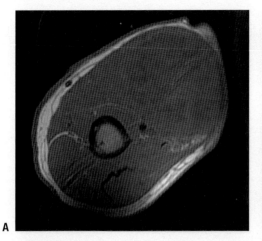 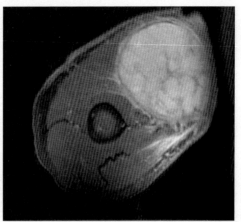

Figure 2-5   A typical MRI appearance of a soft tissue sarcoma in the arm. (**A**) The mass displays dark signal on the T1-weighted image, which is isointense with the adjacent muscle. (**B**) On the T2-weighted image, the mass displays bright signal relative to the surrounding normal tissues. On both sequences, there is considerable heterogeneity, which is more obvious on the T2 image.

clinicians in outlining treatment strategies for a given patient. Staging systems guide the diagnostic work-up, the type of local control, the need for adjuvant treatments, and a long-term follow-up strategy.

- All patients with suspicious soft tissue masses require MRI and biopsy. (The importance of biopsy choice and technique is discussed in Chapter 3.)
- All patients with suspected sarcoma require MRI, chest x-ray, CT scan of the chest, and biopsy.

Benign

- Staging systems for benign soft tissue tumors are not well developed or widely used.
- Most benign tumors have limited local recurrence potential and distant metastases are exceedingly rare. As

such, evaluations of the extent of disease are unnecessary, and when surgery is necessary, local excision alone is usually curative.

Intermediate

- In 2002, WHO subdivided intermediate tumors into two categories: intermediate–locally aggressive and intermediate–rarely metastasizing.
- Intermediate–locally aggressive tumors tend to cause local problems and recur locally.
  - Examples include desmoid tumors and atypical lipomatous tumors.
  - Histologically, they demonstrate an infiltrative pattern.
  - Often, wide surgical excision is necessary, particularly with desmoid tumors, although on occasion even this is inadequate to achieve local control.
- Intermediate–rarely metastasizing tumors can also display locally aggressive characteristics but demonstrate the ability to give rise to distant disease, though to a lesser degree than fully malignant tumors (on the order of ~2%).
  - Examples of such tumors are hemangiopericytoma and giant cell tumor of soft tissues.

Malignant

- Staging systems for soft tissue sarcomas rely on histologic grade, size of the tumor, anatomic location of the tumor, and the degree of regional and distant disease.
- The primary staging system used for soft tissue sarcomas was developed by the American Joint Committee on Cancer (AJCC) (Table 2-6).
- The histologic grading is a complex endeavor that has evolved through the years.

TABLE 2-5 TUMORS OTHER THAN THOSE WITH LOW T1/HIGH T2* THAT HAVE SPECIFIC MRI SIGNALING CHARACTERISTICS

High T1	Low T1, Low T2
Lipoma	Fibromatosis
Well-differentiated liposarcoma	Diffuse giant cell tumor (pigmented villonodular synovitis)
Hemangioma (with serpiginous vascular channels)	Clear cell sarcoma
Acute hemorrhage	Rind around chronic hematoma

* The only tumor with low T1/high T2 that can be specifically diagnosed by MRI is a cyst, the diagnosis of which is confirmed by the absence of any central enhancement after gadolinium administration.

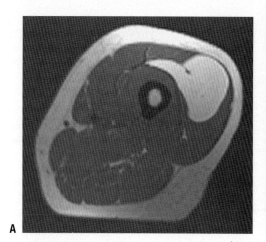 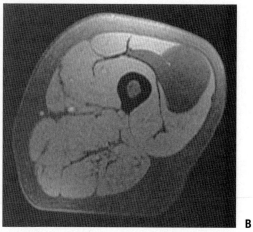

Figure 2-6 Intramuscular lipoma. (**A**) On the T1-weighted image, the intramuscular mass is the same signal as the subcutaneous fat. (**B**) On the fat-suppression T2 image, the mass remains homogenous with a uniform loss of signal. Post-contrast enhanced images would not show any enhancement.

■ Grading incorporates the mitotic index (number of mitoses per high-power field), extent of spontaneous necrosis, and the degree of tumor differentiation, cellularity, and pleomorphism.

■ The anatomic location of the tumor refers to the location of the tumor relative to the deep fascia and is termed superficial or deep.

■ The size of the tumor has significant prognostic importance.
  ■ For the purposes of the AJCC staging system, tumors >5 cm are deemed large and those <5 cm are deemed small.
  ■ Tumors >10 cm have been shown to carry an even worse prognosis, but this information has not for-

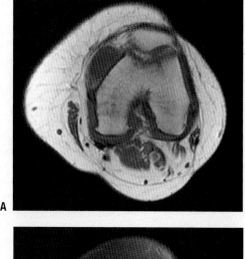 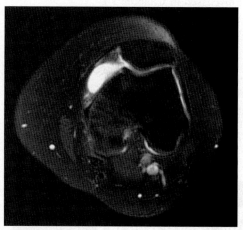

Figure 2-7 This parameniscal cyst demonstrates homogenous dark signal and bright signal on the T1-weighted (**A**) and T2-weighted (**B** and **C**) images, respectively. (**C**) With the administration of gadolinium contrast, note the lack of central enhancement, with enhancement peripherally only. The enhancement pattern is characteristic for cystic structures.

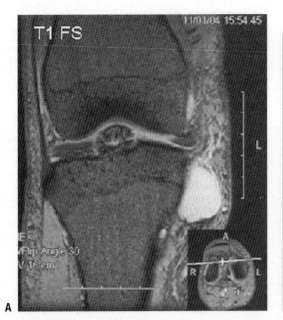
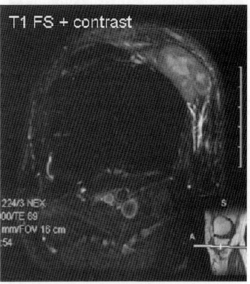

Figure 2-8   (A) This small, well-encapsulated mass near the knee joint demonstrating homogenous high signal on the T1-weight fat-suppressed image could easily be mistaken for a cyst. (B) Contrast administration reveals heterogeneous, central enhancement, proving this is a solid mass. Biopsy revealed an extraskeletal myxoid chondrosarcoma.

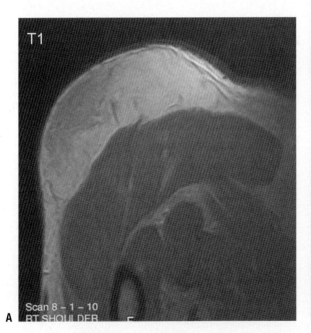
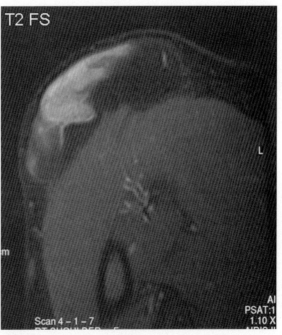

Figure 2-9   (A) On this T1-weighted image, the subcutaneous soft tissue mass overlying the deltoid displays areas of high signal with intensity similar to the adjacent subcutaneous fat. (B) On the fat-suppression image, while some of the mass displays similar loss of signal, there are persistent areas of high signal, which indicates the mass is not simply a lipoma. *Diagnosis*: Well-differentiated liposarcoma.

TABLE 2-6 AJCC STAGING SYSTEM FOR SOFT TISSUE SARCOMA

Stage	Size	Depth*	Grade	Metastases
I	Any	Any	Low	No
II	<5 cm, any depth OR >5 cm, superficial		High	No
III	>5 cm	Deep	High	No
IV	Any	Any	Any	Yes

* Depth is termed superficial (above the deep fascia) or deep (deep to the deep fascia). Retroperitoneal tumors are considered deep.
From *AJCC Cancer Staging Handbook,* 6th ed. New York: Springer, 2002.

mally been incorporated into a formal staging system, though it is used for stratification in clinical trials.

■ The presence or absence of distant metastases carries tremendous prognostic significance.

   ■ Most distant spread from soft tissue sarcomas occurs in the lungs, while lymph node, bone, and other organ involvement is far less common.

SUGGESTED READING

Aflatoon K, Aboulafia AJ, McCarthy EF Jr, et al. Pediatric soft-tissue tumors. *J Am Acad Orthop Surg* 2003;11(5):332–343.

AJCC Cancer Staging Handbook, 6th ed. New York: Springer, 2002.

Damron TA, Rougraff BT, Ward Sr WG. Soft-tissue lumps and bumps. *AAOS Instr Course Lect* 2004;53:625–637.

Damron TA, Sim FH. Soft-tissue tumors about the knee. *J Am Acad Orthop Surg* 1997;5(3):141–152.

Fletcher JA. Molecular biology and cytogenetics of soft tissue sarcomas: relevance for targeted therapies. *Cancer Treat Res* 2004; 120:99–116.

Frassica FJ, Khanna JA, McCarthy EF. The role of MR imaging in soft tissue tumor evaluation: perspective of the orthopedic oncologist and musculoskeletal pathologist. *Magn Reson Imaging Clin North Am* 2000;8(4):915–927.

Heslin MJ, Lewis JJ, Woodruff JM, et al. Core needle biopsy for diagnosis of extremity soft tissue sarcoma. *Ann Surg Oncol* 1997;4(5): 425–431.

Mankin HJ, Mankin CJ, Simon MA. The hazards of the biopsy, revisited. Members of the Musculoskeletal Tumor Society. *J Bone Joint Surg [Am]* 1996;78(5):656–663.

Siegel MJ. Magnetic resonance imaging of musculoskeletal soft tissue masses. *Radiol Clin North Am* 2001;39(4):701–720.

Skrzynski MC, Biermann JS, Montag A, et al. Diagnostic accuracy and charge-savings of outpatient core needle biopsy compared with open biopsy of musculoskeletal tumors. *J Bone Joint Surg [Am]* 1996;78(5):644–649.

Weiss SW. *Enzinger and Weiss's Soft Tissue Tumors*, 4th ed. St. Louis: Mosby, 2001.

World Health Organization Classification of Tumors: Pathology and Genetics of Tumors of Soft Tissue and Bone. Lyon, France: IARC Press, 2002.

BIOPSY OF MUSCULOSKELETAL TUMORS

EDWARD A. ATHANASIAN

Biopsy of musculoskeletal bone and soft tissue tumors may appear to be a deceptively easy technical surgical procedure. Patients may also perceive biopsy as a relatively straightforward, low-risk procedure. While many aspects of the biopsy procedure require only basic technical skills, the proper execution of biopsy of extremity lesions requires careful preparation and planning, plus exacting technique. Errors made at the time of biopsy may not become apparent until the time of surgical resection or recurrence.

RISKS OF IMPROPER BIOPSY

Most extremity bone and soft tissue tumors are benign. Fortunately, the risks of suboptimal biopsy when performed on benign lesions are minimal. The risks of biopsy of malignant lesions are much greater. Insufficient planning and poor execution have the potential to complicate subsequent definitive treatment if the lesion under consideration must be definitively treated surgically. Inadequate biopsy has the potential to increase the risk to the patient's life, as demonstrated in studies performed by the American Musculoskeletal Tumor Society. If the risks of biopsy are carefully considered, it becomes very clear that fundamental understanding of planning and executing a biopsy is imperative to maximize the ability to perform limb salvage surgery and maximize patient survival.

- Improper incision placement or orientation
  - May compromise and complicate attempts at subsequent limb salvage
  - May result in need for performing amputation specifically as a result of the biopsy
    - In studies reported by the American Musculoskeletal Tumor Society, amputation was required specifically because of improper biopsy placement in as many as 18% of patients.
  - May result in need for more extensive amputation than otherwise might have been necessary
- Improper excisional biopsy
  - Associated with greater risks than incision biopsy or needle biopsy
  - Specific anatomic regions such as the axilla, antecubital fossa, carpal tunnel, groin, and popliteal fossa are specifically at risk for contamination when excisional biopsy is performed.
  - Soft tissue contamination produced following marginal excision of malignant lesions must be excised at the definitive surgical excision.
    - Extensive contamination increases the amount of soft tissue that needs to be resected.
    - Results in a greater need for soft tissue coverage to close wounds
    - While more extensive surgical excisions and liberal use of soft tissue coverage may compensate in the effort to achieve negative margins, it is

not clear that this compensates in reducing local recurrence risk.

INDICATIONS FOR BIOPSY

Lesions That Do Not Require Biopsy

■ Many benign bone and soft tissue tumors can be readily recognized clinically or radiographically and do not require biopsy to establish a diagnosis (Table 3-1).

Lesions That Require Biopsy

■ Lesions that are not readily recognized based on clinical examination or radiographic assessment should be considered for biopsy. Even innocuous-appearing soft tissue lesions that are painless and may have been present for a long period of time without growth must be considered for biopsy if a differential diagnosis limited to benign lesions only cannot be made. The rule of thumb is that *if the clinical and radiographic diagnosis cannot be limited to benign lesions only, biopsy or referral to a specialist is indicated.*
■ Soft tissue sarcomas frequently present as painless masses that have been present for a long period of time with recent change in size. Synovial sarcomas are notorious for this sort of behavior.

TYPES OF BIOPSIES

Box 3-1 lists the types of biopsies used for musculoskeletal tumors, some of which are discussed in detail below.

BOX 3-1 BIOPSY TYPES EMPLOYED FOR MUSCULOSKELETAL TUMORS

Fine-needle aspiration/biopsy	Open incisional biopsy
Core-needle biopsy	Open excisional biopsy
	Primary wide excision

Fine Needle Aspiration (FNA)/Biopsy (Skinny Needle)

Setting
■ In the office under local anesthetic
■ In the radiology suite
  ■ Under ultrasound guidance for soft tissue biopsy
  ■ Under computed tomography (CT) guidance for bone lesion biopsy

Technique
■ Soft tissue
  ■ Small-gauge needle on syringe used to aspirate cells during multiple passes in several directions via single entry site
  ■ Cells collect in syringe or hub of needle and are examined on glass slides, often immediately after biopsy performed
■ Bone
  ■ Fine-needle aspiration biopsy of bone tumors may require additional anesthetic, depending upon site and need to enter bone.
  ■ If no soft tissue extension of process from bone, may require larger-gauge needle or drill to enter bone
  ■ Usually done under CT guidance

TABLE 3-1 SOFT TISSUE AND BONE LESIONS THAT CAN USUALLY BE RECOGNIZED CLINICALLY OR RADIOGRAPHICALLY

Tumor/Lesion	Typical Location	Suggestive Findings	Additional Tests if Diagnosis Not Clear
Ganglion cyst	Mid-dorsal hand Volar radial wrist	Transillumination on physical examination	Magnetic resonance imaging (MRI) or ultrasound shows cystic features
Subcutaneous lipoma	Subcutaneous tissue	Soft, doughy feel <5 cm	MRI shows fatty tissue blending with surrounding fat
Nonossifying fibroma (fibrous cortical defect)	Metaphysis of long bone	Asymptomatic, discovered incidentally on plain films as geographic eccentric partially intracortical lesion	MRI shows fibrous low-signal center and absence of surrounding marrow edema
Fibrous dysplasia	Long lesion in metaphysis or diaphysis of long bone	Ground glass matrix within geographic centrally located lesion	MRI
Enchondroma	Metaphysis of long bones	Asymptomatic Rings and arcs of stippled mineralization within geographic lytic lesion without endosteal scalloping	Computed tomography (CT) or MRI to delineate absence of associated endosteal scalloping

General Principles

■ Provides cells (cytology) but no true pattern of organization

■ Site and pathway for the needle need to be planned such that they can be incorporated into a standard limb salvage incision in the event wide excision of the tumor is subsequently required.

■ Needle placement must not compromise amputation flaps in the event amputation is chosen as the most appropriate treatment for the lesion in question.

Advantages

■ Principal advantage is the rapidity with which lesional tissue can be obtained and the histologic diagnostic process started.

■ Less costly than a hospital-based procedure

■ Limited discomfort for the patient

■ Limited soft tissue contamination

■ Limited risk as long as the biopsy site, needle entry point, and needle course are carefully planned

Disadvantages

■ Limited material to examine means lower likelihood of achieving specific diagnosis.

■ Usually performed by radiologist without detailed knowledge of need for appropriate placement of needle tract

■ Negative biopsy does not reliably exclude neoplasm.

■ Negative result often requires repeat aspiration or biopsy by another technique.

Indications

■ Relatively inaccessible lesions of bone and soft tissue

■ Confirmation of strong clinical suspicion of metastatic disease or sarcoma recurrence

Results

■ Diagnostic accuracy rate 64% to 88% for musculoskeletal tumors

■ Diagnostic accuracy is lower for benign tumors.

Needle Biopsy (Core-Needle Biopsy)

Setting

■ Same as for fine-needle biopsy

Technique

■ Soft tissue

  ■ A special hollow needle with a cutting mechanism retrieves a cylindrical core of tissue approximately 2 mm in diameter and several millimeters in length, depending upon the specific type of needle used.

  ■ Typically two or three passes of the needle are made.

■ Bone

  ■ Core-needle biopsy of bone tumors usually requires a heavier anesthetic.

■ Performed with a hollow trephine-type needle with much larger diameter (4 to 7 mm)

■ Usually done under fluoroscopic guidance, often with frozen section analysis done to confirm the presence of lesional tissue

General Principles

■ Provides for evaluation of pattern of tissue organization and cellular features

■ Placement of needle should follow same principles as for skinny needle.

Advantages

■ Provides more tissue for evaluation than fine-needle aspiration, with additional component of the pattern of organization

■ Otherwise same advantages as for fine-needle aspiration/biopsy (rapidity of diagnosis; limited cost, discomfort, contamination, risk)

Disadvantages

■ Principal disadvantage pertains to the limited size of the tissue sample obtained, which has the potential to reduce accuracy and result in sampling error.

■ Molecular diagnostic testing, which can be particularly useful in difficult cases, may not be able to be done if inadequate tissue has been obtained to allow initial processing to prepare for this potential need.

Indications

■ Core-needle biopsy is most often indicated for superficial or accessible deep extremity lesions that are of sufficient size to allow needle placement (>3 cm) and that do not involve major neurovascular structures.

Results

■ Diagnostic accuracy rate 83% to 93% for musculoskeletal tumors

■ Diagnostic accuracy is lower if the lesion is thought to be benign.

Open Biopsy (Incisional or Excisional)

Setting

■ Typically in the operating room under general anesthetic with pathologist standing by for frozen section analysis to confirm adequacy of tissue

Advantages

■ Principal advantage relates to the larger size of the tissue sample obtained, reducing the risk of sampling error and allowing for more extensive histologic assessment as well as molecular diagnostic assessment when needed.

■ Gold standard in achieving high diagnostic accuracy

Disadvantages

■ Principal disadvantage of open biopsy is potential for improper execution by surgeon.

■ Potential adverse consequences of tissue contamination/ exposure during open biopsy

- ▪ Any tissue exposed or manipulated at the time of biopsy is potentially contaminated with tumor cells.
- ▪ Any hematoma or seroma that develops has the potential to further contaminate local soft tissues.
- ▪ Any tissue contaminated as the result of biopsy of a malignant lesion should be carefully considered for resection in continuity with the major tumor mass at that time of definitive treatment if the lesion's definitive treatment requires surgery with widely negative margins.
- ▪ Need for greater soft tissue excision than would be required with needle biopsy
- ▪ Potential adverse consequences of poorly placed open biopsy incision
  - ▪ If not placed in line with or immediately parallel to a standard limb salvage incision, may result in need to resect more soft tissue than might otherwise have been necessary had the biopsy incision been ideally placed
  - ▪ May result in need to sacrifice functional tissues, including tendon, nerve, and vessels, in an effort to achieve negative margins
  - ▪ Commonly results in the need for soft tissue coverage in the form of skin graft, rotation flap, or free flap
- ▪ Poorly performed open biopsy increases the risk of positive margins at the time of definitive treatment and increases risk of local recurrence.

Indications

- ▪ Many bone and less accessible deep soft tissue tumors are best approached with open biopsy (see details below for incisional versus excisional biopsy).

Results

- ▪ Accuracy rates of 96% for extremity bone and soft tissue lesions following final analysis have been reported at major cancer centers.

BIOPSY TECHNIQUE

Biopsy Incision Placement

- ▪ Biopsy incisions must be carefully planned and placed.
- ▪ As a general rule, biopsy incisions for extremity lesions should be *longitudinal* (Box 3-2 and Figs. 3-1 and 3-2)
  - ▪ Incisions that incorporate limited oblique segments can be used at major flexion creases such as the

BOX 3-2 THREE MOST IMPORTANT PRINCIPLES OF BIOPSY INCISION ORIENTATION

Longitudinal, *not transverse*, incisions

Longitudinal, *not transverse*, incisions

Longitudinal, *not transverse*, incisions

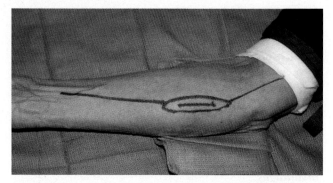

Figure 3-1 Longitudinal biopsy incision is drawn over the medial proximal forearm. The potential limb salvage incision is drawn at the time of the biopsy to ensure that it can be incorporated into a future planned wide excision if this is subsequently needed.

  popliteal fossa, antecubital fossa, volar wrist flexion crease, and palmar surface of the hand.
  - ▪ Transverse incisions and palmar oblique Z-Brunner incisions should specifically be *avoided* due to the extent of soft tissue contamination these will produce.
  - ▪ Oblique incisions may be used over the clavicle and ilium in line with planned line of resection of those bones.
- ▪ Planning for biopsy incision placement requires a basic knowledge of limb salvage incisions and procedures.
  - ▪ Biopsy incisions should be placed in line with or immediately parallel to the limb salvage incision that would be required at definitive treatment.
  - ▪ If the treating physician is not familiar with the appropriate limb salvage incision or amputation flaps, consideration should be given to referral to a musculoskeletal tumor specialist.
- ▪ Common incisions for *bone* tumor biopsy are demonstrated in Figure 3-3.
- ▪ Incision placement for *soft tissue* tumors is more dependent on the primary location of the tumor, the most direct route to the tumor, which will limit contamination to a single plane or compartment, and proximity of major neurovascular structures.
- ▪ Areas at high risk for contamination are depicted in Figure 3-4.

Incisional Biopsy

Incisional biopsy refers to the procedure where the biopsy is performed by cutting directly into the tumor tissue and removing a wedge of the tumor for analysis while leaving the majority of the tumor intact and untouched. This is a relatively safe and accurate form of biopsy; it carries relatively low risk when carefully planned and properly executed. Any tissue that is touched or manipulated at the time of biopsy will be contaminated with tumor tissue and may have to be excised at the time of definitive tumor treatment if the lesion is malignant. The lesion is approached by the most direct means while limiting contamination to a planned region and avoiding exposure and contamination of major neurovascular structures.

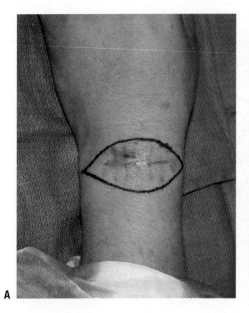
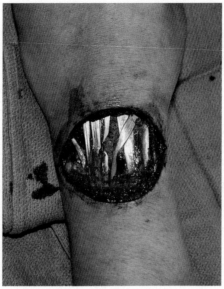

Figure 3-2 (**A**) A malignant fibrous histiocytoma was approached with marginal excision biopsy prior to referral. Note the suture marks, which were placed far from the incision. (**B**) Wide excision of the tumor bed and all contaminated tissue from the biopsy results in a large soft tissue defect, which may commit the patient to a soft tissue coverage procedure that might not have been otherwise needed.

Indications

- Most commonly done for lesions >3 to 4 cm in maximum dimension
- In certain situations, incisional biopsy may be the best approach for even smaller lesions, perhaps 1 to 2 cm.
  - Distal aspect of the arm or leg
  - Lesion in close proximity to a major neurovascular bundle
  - Lesion arises in a high-risk region such as the axilla, antecubital fossa, carpal tunnel, groin, popliteal fossa, medial malleolus, or plantar aspect of the foot.
    - Alternative biopsy type in these high-risk regions is primary wide excision (see below), which may also carry significant morbidity due to the associated requirement for sacrifice of additional soft tissue to act as margin at the time of biopsy. The determination of which type of biopsy is best in a high-risk region may be best done by a musculoskeletal oncologist.
- Importance of frozen section during incisional biopsy
  - Main purpose is to confirm presence of diagnostic tissue, not necessarily to establish definitive diagnosis on which to base treatment.
  - Potential for inaccuracy of frozen section analysis may lead to inappropriate initial surgical procedure.
    - No potential during frozen section for immunohistochemical or molecular analysis
    - Crucial for potentially malignant lesions
    - Less important for benign conditions
  - A second-stage procedure may be required for definitive treatment after initial impression under frozen section is confirmed on further review of permanently fixed tissue.
    - Particularly true for suspected primary malignancy

Excisional Biopsy

Excisional biopsy refers to the procedure where the entire lesion is excised in one piece while dissecting at the margin through the reactive zone surrounding the lesion, accomplishing a "marginal" excision. This type of biopsy is usually best done for small soft tissue lesions that appear to be benign, such as lipomas.

Advantage

- Lesion is removed in one stage and the full lesion is available for pathologic analysis, thereby maximizing accuracy and eliminating the potential for sampling error.

Disadvantages

- Associated with significant risks, particularly when done for malignant lesions
  - Produces extensive contamination of all tissues exposed, retracted, or manipulated at the time of the procedure
  - If done for a soft tissue sarcoma, residual microscopic disease will be left in the patient that will require subsequent wide excision to minimize local recurrence risk.
  - When done for large lesions, large amounts of otherwise uninvolved tissues will need to be sacrificed to achieve negative margins. Additional need to sacrifice uninvolved soft tissues is greater than would be required in the setting of needle or incision biopsy.
  - If major nerves or vessels are exposed at biopsy, definitive treatment may require excision of those vital structures, thereby increasing the morbidity of definitive treatment.
  - Suboptimal placement of biopsy incision will increase the need for soft tissue coverage at definitive treatment and might even preclude limb salvage procedures.
  - The larger the size of the lesion and the more distal in the extremity the tumor arises, the greater the risks associated with excisional biopsy.

Indications

- Best reserved for small lesions (<3 to 4 cm) arising within muscle of the proximal portions of the extremities.

ANTERIOR VIEW

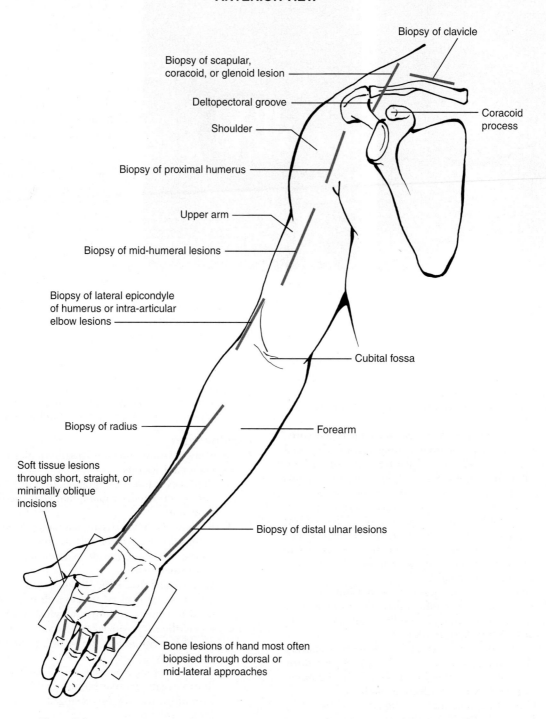

Figure 3-3 Common incisions for bone tumor biopsy in the upper right (**A** and **B**) and lower left (**C**) extremities. (*continues*)

POSTERIOR VIEW

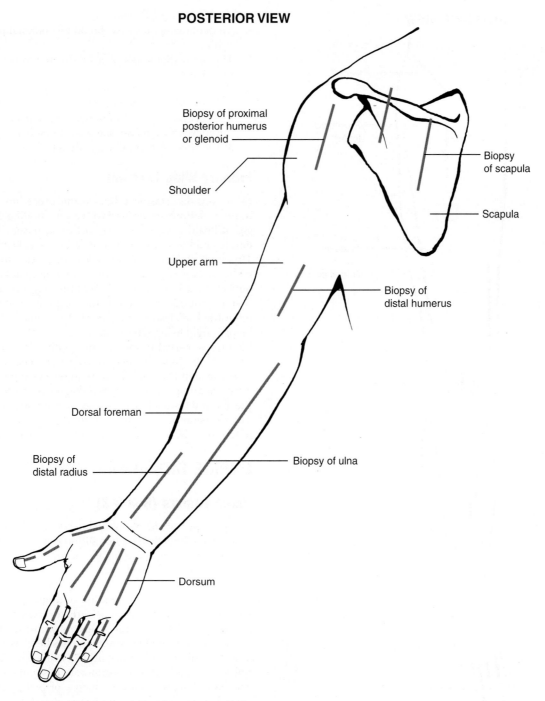

Biopsy of proximal
posterior humerus
or glenoid

Shoulder

Biopsy
of scapula

Scapula

Upper arm

Biopsy of
distal humerus

Dorsal foreman

Biopsy of
distal radius

Biopsy of ulna

Dorsum

Figure 3-3 (*continued*)

ANTERIOR VIEW

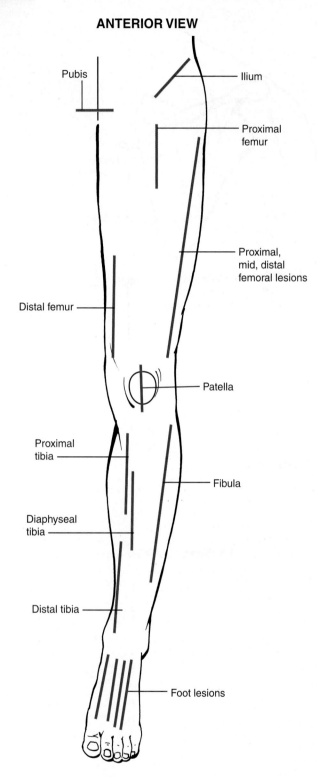

Pubis

Ilium

Proximal femur

Proximal, mid, distal femoral lesions

Distal femur

Patella

Proximal tibia

Fibula

Diaphyseal tibia

Distal tibia

Foot lesions

Figure 3-3 (continued)

Drain Usage and Placement
- Meticulous hemostasis should be obtained prior to closure.
- The drain should not be a substitute for meticulous hemostasis.
- If a drain is used, it should exit the patient immediately in line with the more distal end of the incision.
- Lateral drain placement or placement at a distance from the incision increases the need for soft tissue sacrifice at the time of definitive treatment.

Primary Wide Excision

Primary wide excision refers to the procedure where the tumor is definitively excised with a surrounding cuff or margin of healthy, uninvolved, nonreactive tissue. This procedure should be considered as a definitive cancer operation. This type of biopsy is performed when the suspicion for malignancy is high and the risks of contamination of biopsy outweigh the morbidity of the additional soft tissue sacrifice that is required to achieve the desired negative margins upon final analysis of the resected specimen. This type of biopsy might be used for lesions arising in the axilla, antecubital fossa, carpal tunnel, groin, popliteal fossa, or plantar aspect of the foot. The decision of when to perform primary wide excision is complex and requires considerable knowledge regarding the differential diagnosis of the lesion and the morbidity of biopsy for the specific anatomic region. The decision of when to perform this biopsy is often best determined by an experienced musculoskeletal oncologist.

UNIQUE CONSIDERATIONS FOR BIOPSY

Nerve Tumors (Box 3-3)

The presence of the peripheral nerve sheath tumor may be suspected clinically based on differential mobility, as nerve lesions tend to be more mobile in the medial lateral plane than the proximal distal plane (being tethered by their neural attachment). Confirmation of the presence of the lesion arising in a major nerve requires a unique preparation and technical approach. There are greater risks for permanent nerve injury following the biopsy of nerve-related lesions. Marginal excision of schwannoma has been associated with a permanent risk of injury of 4%, while the risk of injury following excision of neurofibroma is significantly higher. The risk of injury following biopsy of malignant nerve lesions has not been well characterized and is superseded by the need to widely excise the lesion and nerve in an effort to achieve local control of the tumor. It may be impossible to determine whether a specific nerve lesion is benign or malignant based on preoperative testing, including magnetic resonance imaging. Lesions are often best approached through a direct approach to the nerve with minimal dissection of the surrounding tissues. Dissection is done under magnification when necessary while mobilizing healthy fascicles to accomplish a marginal excision. If the lesion is not readily dissected from the normal nerve fascicles, an incisional biopsy should be performed, with subsequent treatment determined by frozen section or permanent analysis.

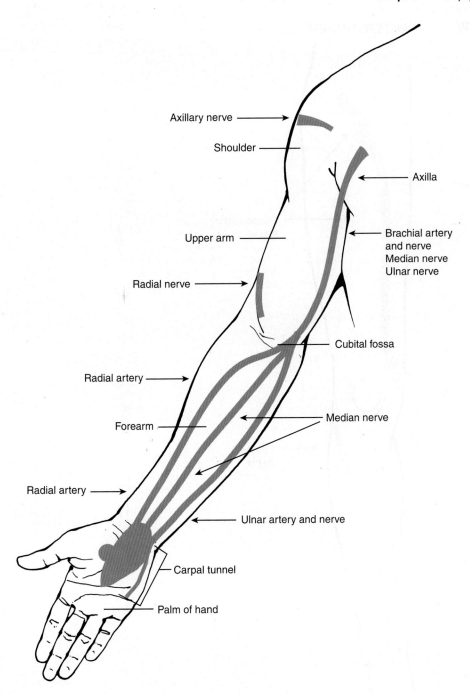

Axillary nerve

Shoulder

Axilla

Upper arm

Brachial artery
and nerve
Median nerve
Ulnar nerve

Radial nerve

Cubital fossa

Radial artery

Median nerve

Forearm

Radial artery

Ulnar artery and nerve

Carpal tunnel

Palm of hand

Figure 3-4 The areas shown in blue are at high risk for contamination during biopsy in the upper right (**A**) and lower left (**B**) extremities. (*continues*)

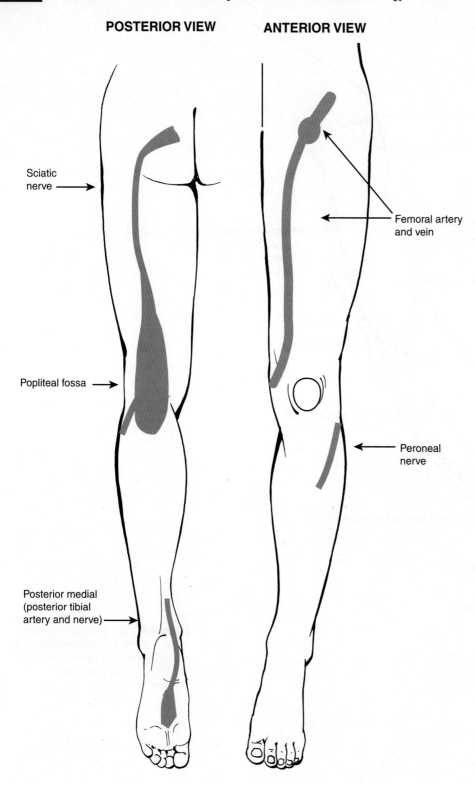

POSTERIOR VIEW   **ANTERIOR VIEW**

Sciatic nerve

Femoral artery and vein

Popliteal fossa

Peroneal nerve

Posterior medial (posterior tibial artery and nerve)

Figure 3-4 (*continued*)

BOX 3-3 TUMORS ARISING IN MAJOR PERIPHERAL NERVES

Benign	**Malignant**
Schwannoma (neurilemoma)	Malignant peripheral nerve
Neurofibroma	sheath tumor

Scapular Lesions with Anterior Extension

Scapular lesions with anterior extension present unique risks for biopsy due to the proximity of the brachial plexus. The approach for biopsy is dependent upon the extent of soft tissue involvement and the primary location within the scapula.

■ Scapular body lesions: Best approached through a posterior incision, particularly if scapular resection might ultimately be required

■ Lesions in the region of the glenoid neck or base of the coracoid: Can be approached anteriorly by dissecting along the superior aspect of the coracoid while meticulously maintaining hemostasis to reduce the risks of soft tissue contamination. The biopsy site can subsequently be incorporated into an extended deltopectoral approach, which can readily be extended posteriorly if needed.

Proximal Humerus Lesions

Most proximal humerus lesions can be biopsied through an incision placed 1 to 2 cm lateral to the deltopectoral groove. If the incision is extended distally beyond 5 cm from the acromion, the terminal portion of the axillary nerve will be transected or injured. This will result in denervation of only the most medial portion of the deltoid without significant functional impairment. Placement of the incision at this location reduces the risk of spread of hematoma medially along the course of the cephalic vein and pectoralis major and reduces the risk of contamination of the major neurovascular structures.

Intra-articular Lesions of the Elbow

Biopsy of lesions arising in or near the elbow is particularly difficult. There are limited windows for biopsy that allow access to the joint without contaminating major nerves. Posterior biopsy carries little risk but might impair attempts at limb salvage if anterior exposure is required to resect the lesion. There is a large window of potential exposure near the lateral epicondyle, but this approach might also impair limb salvage if mobilization of the median and ulnar nerves is required at definitive treatment. At times, separate biopsy and limb salvage incisions might be required where the biopsy incision and contaminated tissues from biopsy are dissected separately from the limb salvage incision and left attached to the major tumor mass while the limb salvage approach is performed through a separate incision on the opposite side of the elbow. Lesions in this region require detailed planning and often unique approaches.

Distal Radius Lesions

The approach to the distal radius is complicated by the compact arrangement of functional tissues surrounding this

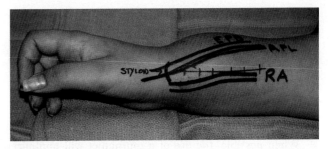

Figure 3-5 Biopsy incision for distal radius lesions with volar soft tissue extension.

structure at the level of the distal forearm. The optimal site for biopsy placement is often determined by the planned definitive treatment or limb salvage incision. For example, lesions requiring wide excision of the distal radius and carpus are best approached through a dorsal biopsy incision. The window for biopsy at the level of Lister's tubercle is 4 mm between the third and fourth dorsal compartments. There is a substantial risk of contamination of the extensor tendons at biopsy. Contamination of these structures will require their subsequent excision in the event of a malignant diagnosis. When intralesional treatment of a distal radius tumor such as giant cell tumor of bone is anticipated, the volar radial approach between the radial artery and the first dorsal compartment allows excision of any volar soft tissue extension and excellent exposure of the distal radius. This approach, however, is not easily extended distally should additional exposure be required (Fig. 3-5).

Carpal Tunnel, Axilla, and Popliteal Fossa Lesions

Soft tissue contamination following excision biopsy or marginal excision of malignant lesions in the carpal tunnel can produce contamination that eliminates the possibility of limb salvage and commits the patient to amputation of the hand. Even small lesions are often best approached with either incisional biopsy or primary wide excision. The risks of contamination of major nerves and blood vessels are similar in the axilla and popliteal fossa, as well as other extracompartmental sites.

BIOPSY PLANNING AND PROCEDURE

Biopsy should be performed as the final step in the analysis of a specific patient and lesion after complete history, physical examination, laboratory and radiographic assessment have been performed.

Communication with the Pathologist

■ A differential diagnosis should be formulated in advance of the procedure and communicated to the pathologist.
■ Review of imaging studies will often assist the pathologist in generating a differential diagnosis.
■ When malignancy is suspected or considered in the dif-

ferential diagnosis, the pathologist should be notified in advance to ensure appropriate tissue handling and assessment (e.g., lymphoma protocols and molecular studies require unique tissue processing protocols).
- Need for frozen section should be established in advance of the case.

Tourniquet Usage

- When possible, the use of a tourniquet will minimize blood loss and assist in visualization at the time of biopsy.
- Excellent hemostasis should be achieved following release of the tourniquet prior to definitive closure to limit the potential for hematoma and its attendant risks.
- Exsanguination of the limb with an elastic bandage should be avoided owing to the risk of dislodging tumor cells and causing venous embolization; gravity exsanguination is preferred.

Planning the Incision

- A final exercise that confirms appropriate preparation for biopsy is to *draw the limb salvage incision or anticipated amputation flaps at the time of the biopsy* prior to drawing the biopsy incision.
- The biopsy incision should be placed in line with a portion of the limb salvage incision or away from the amputation flaps.
- This approach minimizes the risks of improper biopsy incision placement and assists in the attempt to maximize limb salvage options in the event of a malignant final diagnosis.

Dissection Technique

- Following incision, dissection to the biopsy should be made using the most direct approach.
- Dissection should be through tissues as opposed to usual surgical dissection, which is between tissue planes.
- The dissection technique used should minimize the extent of contamination caused by the biopsy and limit the spread of hematoma.
  - All tissues contaminated at the time of biopsy will need to be excised at the time of definitive excision if the lesion is malignant on final analysis.
- Biopsy is usually best performed at the periphery of the lesion.
  - Lesion is directly entered and a wedge of tissue excised.

Histologic Tissue and Culture Processing

- If there is sufficient tissue available, frozen section analysis is performed to determine a preliminary diagnosis and to confirm the presence of lesional tissue.
- Additional tissue is sent for permanent analysis (1 cc minimum).
- Tissue cultures are also taken and sent to the laboratory for analysis ("culture all tumors, biopsy all infections").

Hemostasis

- In most instances the tourniquet should be released prior to closure.
- Means to achieve hemostasis: electrocautery, gelatin sponge, methyl-methacrylate cement for bone windows, or direct closure of the pseudocapsule or periosteum

Drain Usage and Placement

- If a drain is required, it is placed with an exit point directly in line with the incision, usually at the distal aspect.

Wound Closure

- Wound is closed in layers, with attention to suture placement.
- Sutures should be placed close to the wound margin to limit contamination and the extent of skin excision that will be required at definitive treatment.

Instrument Handling

- It is useful to use an instrument basin for contaminated instruments during the procedure.
- Used operative instruments are placed in the basin with contaminated ends pointing in one direction.
- Operative personnel limit the handling of instruments to the noncontaminated end.
- If concurrent surgery is to be performed, operative clothing and instruments should be changed for use in a separately draped field to reduce the risk of cross-contamination.

Postoperative Care

If bone biopsy has been performed, measures should be taken to protect the limb from intraoperative and postoperative fracture.

PATHOLOGIC ASSESSMENT AND LIMITATIONS

Most patients consider pathologic assessment to be a definitive "black-or-white" process. Patients should be specifically counseled prior to the biopsy procedure regarding accuracy rates for frozen section analysis and permanent analysis of biopsy tissue.

- Accuracy of frozen section analysis for bone and soft tissue tumors is approximately 80%. If definitive treatment is being considered based on frozen section analysis, the surgeon must incorporate the possibility of an incorrect diagnosis into the treatment plan. The potential for inaccuracy should be discussed with the patient in advance.
- When is it reasonable to proceed with definitive treatment based upon frozen section?
  - If the primary considerations in the differential diag-

nosis are benign based on preoperative assessment and the frozen section analysis supports this.

■ When is it not reasonable to proceed based upon frozen section?

   ■ When malignancy is a major consideration in the differential diagnosis, it is often best to defer treatment until the final analysis is completed. The accuracy of a final pathologic analysis at a tumor center is approximately 96%. Preoperative discussion with the pathologist ensures the availability of appropriate diagnostic testing, which can aid in maximizing the effort to establish an accurate diagnosis and maximize patient care.

SUGGESTED READING

Domanski HA, Akerman M, Carlen B, et al. Core-needle biopsy performed by the cytopathologist: a technique to complement fine-needle aspiration of soft tissue and bone lesions. *Cancer* 2005; 105(4):229–239.

Donner TR, Voorhies RM, Kline DG. Neural sheath tumors of major nerves. *J Neurosurg* 1994;81:362–373.

Heslin MJ, Lewis JJ, Woodruff JM, et al. Core needle biopsy for diagnosis of extremity soft tissue sarcoma. *Ann Surg Oncol* 1997;4: 425–431.

Mankin HJ, Lange TA, Spanier SS. The hazards of biopsy in patients with malignant primary bone and soft tissue tumors. *J Bone Joint Surg [Am]* 1982;64:1121–1127.

Ogilvie CM, Torbert JT, Finstein JL, et al. Clinical utility of percutaneous biopsies of musculoskeletal tumors. *Clin Orthop Relat Res* 2006;450:95–100.

Scarborough MT. The biopsy. *AAOS Instr Course Lect* 2004;53: 639–644.

Simon MA. Biopsy of musculoskeletal tumors. *J Bone Joint Surg* 1982; 64:1253–1257.

Skrzynski MC, Biermann JS, Montag A, et al. Diagnostic accuracy and charge savings of outpatient core needle biopsy compared with open biopsy of musculoskeletal tumors. *J Bone Joint Surg [Am]* 1996; 78:644–649.

Trigg SD. Biopsy of hand, wrist, and forearm tumors. *Hand Clin* 2004; 20(2):v, 131–135.

Yang YJ, Damron TA. Comparison of needle core biopsy and fine-needle aspiration for diagnostic accuracy in musculoskeletal lesions. *Arch Pathol Lab Med* 2004;128(7):759–764.

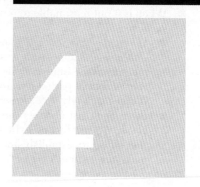

TREATMENT PRINCIPLES

4.1 SURGICAL MARGINS

ROBERT QUINN

Appropriate surgical planning for the treatment of musculo-skeletal tumors requires proper histologic diagnosis and staging. The type of surgical margin most appropriate for a given tumor is, to a large extent, dictated by the appropriate stage.

TERMINOLOGY

■ The pathologic definitions in Table 4.1-1 are essential to the understanding of surgical margins.

SURGICAL MARGINS

■ The surgical procedures and margins are defined in Table 4.1-2.

SURGICAL PROCEDURES

Principles of Selecting the Appropriate Surgical Procedure

■ Selection of the most appropriate surgical margin is dependent upon the overall treatment goals of the patient.
■ Table 4.1-3 shows some example tumor types according to surgical stage for each type of surgical procedure.
■ If the goal of treatment is to establish the best chance of cure, then the most appropriate margin is that which will provide the lowest risk of local recurrence.
　■ Life-threatening malignancy: successful limb salvage is a secondary goal, and margins should not be

TABLE 4.1-1 TERMS PERTAINING TO SURGICAL MARGINS

Term	Definition
Reactive zone	Area, or potential area, between the tumor and normal tissue; it may be composed of variable amounts of pseudocapsule, satellite tumor lesions, and reactive tissue, including edema
Satellite lesion	Nodules of isolated tumor within the reactive zone
Skip lesion	Nodule of isolated tumor within the same compartment as the primary tumor but separated by an interval of normal tissue beyond the reactive zone

compromised in an effort to save a limb or improve its function.

- Most aggressive benign tumors: rarely life- or limb-threatening, and these are often best treated with a less aggressive procedure, accepting a low rate of local recurrence in exchange for improved functional outcome

Types of Surgical Procedures

- Figures 4.1-1 and 4.1-2 illustrate the respective planes of dissection that would be performed with these types of resections and amputations.

Intralesional Procedure

- Debulking or curettage of a tumor from within the tumor itself

Indications

- This type of procedure may be performed for diagnosis (i.e., with an open biopsy), for cure, or for palliation.
  - Biopsy
    - When surgery is to be performed for sarcomas with curative intent, the carefully planned biopsy is an acceptable initial intralesional procedure.
    - An intralesional margin obtained following resection is generally unplanned and unlikely to be curative.
  - Palliation
    - An intralesional procedure might be performed in the presence of metastatic disease where the primary goal of surgery is palliation and the secondary goal is tumor removal.
    - Example: Impending pathologic fracture of the femur
      - Primary goal of the procedure is stabilization

TABLE 4.1-2 DEFINITIONS OF SURGICAL PROCEDURES RELATED TO MARGINS

Procedure	Definition
Intralesional	Procedure performed within the capsule or pseudocapsule of the tumor. This is generally a curettage type of procedure for bone tumors and piecemeal excision for soft tissue tumors. By definition, macroscopic disease is left behind. An intralesional margin is obtained when the plane of dissection passes within the lesion.
Extended intralesional	Procedure performed intralesionally but extended beyond the confines of the tumor reactive zone into normal tissue by use of mechanical or other adjunctive means. This usually applies to low-grade aggressive bone lesions, where the outer border of a standard curettage is extended mechanically with aggressive use of curettes, a high-speed bur, or both, into normal surrounding bone. The bone margin may also be extended by the use of chemical (phenol), electrical, or laser cauterization, thermal effect of curing bone cement, and freezing effect of liquid nitrogen.
Marginal	Procedure performed within the reactive zone of the lesion. This is typically an *en bloc* type of resection for soft tissue tumors such as excision of a lipoma. For intraosseous bone tumors, a marginal excision would be an "extended curettage." For surface bone tumors, a marginal excision would be accomplished by simple excision of the lesion without any surrounding tissue. A marginal margin is obtained when the plane of dissection passes through the reactive zone. Microscopic disease may be left behind where portions of the tumor itself extend into the reactive zone or where satellite lesions are present. A marginal resection or amputation risks leaving satellite lesions behind.
Wide	Procedure performed entirely through normal tissue beyond the reactive zone. It reflects not the amount of normal tissue that makes up the margin but simply the presence of some amount of normal tissue between the reactive zone and the plane of dissection. A wide procedure only risks leaving skip lesions behind.
Radical	Procedure in which the entire compartment of origin is removed
Contaminated margin	If, during the process of performing a wide or radical resection, the tumor is inadvertently entered and local normal tissue exposed, the area is at increased risk for local recurrence of the tumor. If the at-risk tissues are then removed with a wide margin, the ultimate margin is said to be a contaminated wide margin. If the at-risk tissues are not removed, the ultimate margin is intracapsular.

TABLE 4.1-3 SURGICAL MARGINS AS A FUNCTION OF TUMOR STAGE

Musculoskeletal Tumor Society Stage	Example		Typical Desired Surgical Margin
	Bone Tumor	Soft Tissue Tumor	
Benign 1 (latent)	Enchondroma, nonossifying fibroma, solitary eosinophilic granuloma, unicameral bone cyst	Lipoma, ganglion, giant cell tumor of tendon sheath	Intralesional
Benign 2 (active)	Aneurysmal bone cyst, chondroblastoma, osteoblastoma	Hemangioma, myxoma	Marginal
Benign 3 (aggressive)	Giant cell tumor	Fibromatosis (desmoid type)	Extended intralesional curettage (bone) or wide (soft tissue or expendable bone)
Malignant IA/B	Low-grade osteosarcoma, conventional chondrosarcoma	Low-grade soft tissue sarcoma*	Wide
Malignant IIA/B	High-grade osteosarcoma, Ewing sarcoma	High-grade soft tissue sarcoma	Wide
Malignant III	High-grade osteosarcoma, Ewing sarcoma	High-grade soft tissue sarcoma	Wide with metastatectomy for cure if resectable

* Some soft tissue tumors that may be considered low-grade sarcomas by some, such as atypical lipomatous tumor (low-grade well-differentiated lipoma-like liposarcoma), are most often excised with a marginal margin.

with an intramedullary rod, but intralesional curettage of the tumor is performed for two reasons:

- To allow further strengthening of the construct by replacing tumor with polymethylmethacrylate
- To afford potentially greater efficacy of adjuvant radiation or chemotherapy

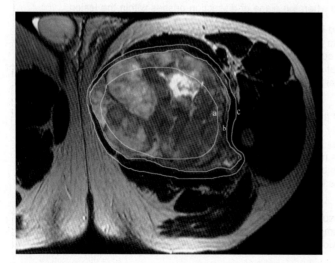

Figure 4.1-1 Magnetic resonance imaging of a soft tissue sarcoma in the adductor compartment of the thigh demonstrating potential surgical margins. Dissection along line *a* would constitute an intralesional margin, along line *b* would be a marginal resection, and along line *c* would be a wide margin. A radical margin would entail removal of the entire adductor compartment.

Residual Disease and Risk of Recurrence

- By definition this type of procedure leaves behind macroscopic, or at least microscopic, disease. This is acceptable for benign nonaggressive lesions (stage 1 or 2), but it is not desirable for aggressive benign or malignant lesions except when palliation is the goal.
- For many benign bone and soft tissue tumors (enchondroma, nonossifying fibroma, eosinophilic granuloma), this procedure will result in a very small risk of local recurrence.
- For most malignancies, this procedure will result in a high rate of local recurrence.

Marginal Procedure

- A more aggressive excision performed through the reactive zone to minimize the amount of residual microscopic tumor, but leaving the potential for both satellite and skip lesions
- For soft tissue tumors an *en bloc* excision ("shell-out" procedure) is performed.
- For more aggressive benign tumors of bone (aneurysmal bone cyst, chondroblastoma, osteoblastoma) and even some low-grade chondrosarcomas, acceptance of a marginal margin by way of an extended intralesional curettage will result in a measurable risk of local recurrence but not high enough to warrant the additional morbidity of obtaining a wide margin except occasionally in expendable bones such as the fibula, rib, or ilium.
  - Extended intralesional curettage procedure: A marginal curettage is performed, and the margin is then extended into the reactive zone or even into normal tissue mechanically with a bur and/or using cytostatic or cytocidal agents such as liquid nitrogen, phenol, laser, or alcohol.

bone metastases (such as renal carcinoma), and for some particularly aggressive benign tumors such as desmoid-type fibromatosis
- Palliation: Occasionally wide resection will also be performed for the treatment of metastatic disease when the tumor is felt to be poorly responsive to other adjuvant measures.

Amputation With Wide Margins
- Performed with curative intent when limb salvage is not indicated
- When limb-sparing surgery would leave an extremity with compromised vascularity or limited function inferior to that which would be obtained with a prosthesis
- If a patient would prefer amputation in deference to the more complex nature of a reconstructive procedure and the potential associated complications

Radical Resection
- Removal of the entire compartment(s) involved by the tumor, including the entire bone for bone tumors and the entire muscle compartment from origin to insertion for soft tissue tumors or soft tissue extension from bone tumors
- Radical resections are largely of historical importance but were thought to be necessary in some cases to eliminate both satellite and skip lesions. In practice, skip lesions are rare, probably represent metastatic disease, and can generally be recognized on imaging studies provided the entire compartment is visualized. Hence, prophylactic removal of the entire compartment without evidence of skip lesions is rarely indicated.
  - If the skip lesion is in close proximity to the primary, both will generally be resected with a single wide margin.
  - If the skip lesion is more remote from the primary, two separate wide resections will generally suffice and often allow better functional outcome than a radical resection.

SUGGESTED READING

Enneking WF, Maale GE. The effect of inadvertent tumor contamination of wounds during the surgical resection of musculoskeletal neoplasms. *Cancer* 1988;62(7):1251–1256.
Enneking WF, Spanier SS, Goodman MA. A system for the surgical staging of musculoskeletal sarcoma. *Clin Orthop Relat Res* 1980;(153):106–120.
Enneking WF, Spanier SS, Malawer MM. The effect of the anatomic setting on the results of surgical procedures for soft parts sarcoma of the thigh. *Cancer* 1981;47(5):1005–1022.
Rydholm A. Surgical margins for soft tissue sarcoma. *Acta Orthop Scand Suppl* 1997;273:81–85.
Rydholm A, Rooser B. Surgical margins for soft-tissue sarcoma. *J Bone Joint Surg [Am]* 1987;69(7):1074–1078.
Virkus WW, Marshall D, Enneking WF, et al. The effect of contaminated surgical margins revisited. *Clin Orthop Relat Res* 2002;(397):89–94.
Wolf RE, Enneking WF. The staging and surgery of musculoskeletal neoplasms. *Orthop Clin North Am* 1996;27(3):473–481.

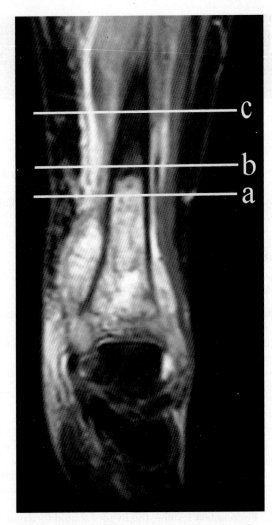

Figure 4.1-2 Magnetic resonance imaging of a high-grade osteosarcoma of the distal tibia illustrating margins possible obtained at different levels of amputation: intralesional (*a*), marginal (*b*), and wide (*c*). A radical margin would be obtained with a knee disarticulation.

- Amputations that achieve marginal margins
  - May be performed as a palliative procedure
  - May result from unsuccessful attempt at a wide margin amputation
  - May be performed with plans to use adjunctive treatment to minimize recurrence

Wide Margins
- When the plane of dissection passes through normal tissue some distance beyond the reactive zone, theoretically eliminating satellite lesions but potentially leaving skip lesions behind

Indications
- Cure: Appropriate margin to achieve cure for majority of bone and soft tissue sarcomas, for occasional isolated

4.2 BENIGN TUMORS OF BONE

CYNTHIA M. KELLY

Musculoskeletal tumors are, in general, uncommon problems, and malignant tumors of bone are considered rare. Comparatively speaking, benign tumors of bone are more commonly seen by orthopaedic surgeons and primary care practitioners. Benign tumors of bone may exhibit various biologic and clinical behaviors that require a broad spectrum of treatment options. Management of these lesions is best handled by an orthopaedic surgeon and, in certain instances, by a fellowship-trained orthopaedic oncologist. Many benign tumors of bone are incidental findings, noted during radiographic evaluation of an extremity for an unrelated complaint such as a sports injury or other trauma. It is important to recognize lesions that are most likely benign processes that can be observed versus those that need to be treated surgically. In rare instances benign lesions have the potential to undergo malignant transformation. It is therefore important for the physician to understand these variations in biological behavior in order to care for patients appropriately.

PATHOGENESIS

Etiology

- Most bone tumors, either benign or malignant, have no identifiable etiology.
- Few benign bone lesions are associated with preexisting conditions or have a hereditary or familial pattern.

Pathophysiology

- Unknown for most benign tumors of bone and is best described for congenital and inherited syndromes (Table 4.2-1)

Classification

- Classification terms for benign bone tumors are based on their biological behavior, tissue of origin, or syndrome names generally associated with polyostotic diseases.
- Based on biologic behavior
  - Stage of the lesion
  - Latent, active, and aggressive (see Box 4.2-1; see also Chapter 1, Evaluation of Bone Tumors)
- Based on tissue of origin
  - World Health Organization classifies tumors into general categories based on the type of neoplastic tissue within the lesion (Table 4.2-2).

- Other lesions of bone that mimic tumors (Box 4.2-2)
- Syndromes associated with polyostotic disease (Table 4.2-3)

DIAGNOSIS

History and Physical Examination

- History: including presenting complaint and past medical history
- Patients with benign bone lesions generally present with one of four scenarios:
  - Painless bone mass
  - Incidental radiographic finding
  - Painful bone lesion
  - Pathologic fracture
- An important early factor in evaluation of a patient with a benign tumor of bone is: "Is the lesion associated with pain?"
  - For those with pain, consideration should be given to the patient's pain complaints and exacerbating activities.
  - For painless lesions, the history should focus on the means of discovery.

Clinical Features
- Painless bone mass
  - Painless bone masses are usually noted as a bump on the affected bone and may be solitary or multiple.
  - Most common example: osteochondroma
- Incidental radiographic finding
  - A common scenario is that a patient injures an area, an x-ray is obtained, and an asymptomatic bony lesion is noted. These incidentally identified lesions generally are benign, and important radiographic features to be considered in these situations will be discussed below.
  - Most common example: nonossifying fibroma (fibrous cortical defect)
- Painful bone lesion
  - When a patient presents with pain as the primary complaint and an underlying tumor of bone is identified, a more thorough evaluation is warranted to rule out an aggressive benign tumor that is associated with structural compromise of the bone or even a malignancy.
  - Differential diagnosis in this situation may be extensive.
- Pathologic fracture

BOX 4.2-1 STAGING OF BENIGN BONE LESIONS*

Stage 1 (latent)	Chondromyxoid fibroma
Nonossifying fibroma	Fibrous dysplasia
Enchondroma	Eosinophilic granuloma
Unicameral bone cyst	(Langerhans cell
Osteochondroma	histiocytosis)
Osteoid osteoma	Aneurysmal bone cyst
Fibrous dysplasia	Unicameral bone cyst
Eosinophilic granuloma	Osteofibrous dysplasia
(Langerhans cell	Juxtacortical chondroma
histiocytosis)	Chondroblastoma
Stage 2 (active)	**Stage 3 (aggressive)**
Enchondroma	Giant cell tumor
Osteochondroma	Osteoblastoma
Osteoid osteoma	Chondroblastoma
Osteoblastoma	Aneurysmal bone cyst
Giant cell tumor	

*Many types of benign bone lesions may be classified in more than one stage based on their biologic behavior.

- Most children with a pathologic fracture through an underlying benign tumor of bone can be managed conservatively initially to allow for fracture healing, and then a biopsy may be performed in a delayed fashion if appropriate.
- Key question in determining whether there is cause for concern: Was pain present preceding the time of the fracture?
  - Preceding pain: Possible aggressive benign or malignant lesion: may warrant biopsy/surgical intervention
  - No preceding pain: Very likely a benign, inactive lesion
    - Common examples: nonossifying fibroma, simple bone cyst

Physical Examination
- General physical examination
  - Look for signs of multifocal disease (café-au-lait spots, axillary freckling, multiple bony masses, soft tissue myxomas, soft tissue hemangiomas, short stature, limb deformities), generalized lymphadenopathy.
  - Examine for possible sites of referred pain.
- Focused examination concentrating on the area of concern
  - Specific findings to assess are the presence of a visible mass, limb length discrepancy, overlying skin changes, increased tactile temperature, presence of a soft tissue mass, tenderness on palpation of the area, compromised joint range of motion, surrounding muscle atrophy, neurovascular status of the limb and any lymphadenopathy.

Radiographic Evaluation
- X-ray films are a necessary part of the work-up of any patient with a musculoskeletal complaint.
  - At a minimum, two orthogonal view x-rays of the affected area should be obtained, an AP and a lateral view.
  - Oblique views may also be of assistance.
    - Example: avulsive cortical irregularity (periosteal desmoid), which always occurs at the posteromedial distal femoral metaphysis
- Compare to old radiographs, when available, in order to establish natural history.

TABLE 4.2-1 BENIGN BONE LESIONS WITH CONSISTENT GENETIC DEFECTS AND/OR HEREDITARY OR FAMILIAL INHERITANCE PATTERNS

Lesion	Description
Aneurysmal bone cyst	Sporadic rearrangement of the chromosome 17 short arm
Fibrous dysplasia	Activating GNAS1 gene mutations in G alpha protein
Solitary (monostotic)	
Polyostotic	
McCune-Albright syndrome	
Mazabraud syndrome	Gene mutation only in myxoma cells
Multiple hereditary osteochondromatosis	Autosomal dominant; EXT1 or EXT2 gene mutations
Multiple enchondromatosis (Ollier's disease)	Mostly sporadic; genetic defect unknown but now known *not* to be PTHR1
Maffucci syndrome	Mostly sporadic; genetic defect unknown but known *not* to be PTHR1

TABLE 4.2-2 WORLD HEALTH ORGANIZATION BENIGN BONE TUMOR CATEGORIES

Category	Examples
Cartilage tumors	Chondroma (enchondroma, periosteal chondroma, multiple chondromatosis, osteochondroma, chondroblastoma, chondromyxoid fibroma)
Osteogenic tumors	Osteoma, osteoid osteoma, osteoblastoma
Fibrogenic tumors	Desmoplastic fibroma
Fibrohistiocytic tumors	Benign fibrous histiocytoma
Giant cell tumors	Giant cell tumor, osteoclastoma
Vascular tumors	Hemangioma
Smooth muscle tumors	Leiomyoma
Lipogenic tumors	Lipoma
Neural tumors	Neurilemoma
Miscellaneous lesions	Aneurysmal bone cyst, simple cyst, fibrous dysplasia, osteofibrous dysplasia, Langerhans cell histiocytosis, Erdheim-Chester disease, chest wall hamartoma
Joint lesions	Synovial chondromatosis

No benign counterparts are recognized currently by the World Health Organization for the following bone tumor disease categories: Ewing sarcoma/primitive neuroectodermal tumors, hematopoietic tumors, notochordal tumors, or miscellaneous tumors (adamantinoma).

■ In the case of an inactive lesion that is an incidental radiographic finding, observation and serial x-rays are often all that is warranted. This regimen affords the opportunity to observe the natural history of the process.
■ Consider proximal x-ray evaluation of an area that can be associated with a referred pain pattern (e.g., hip pathology presenting as knee pain, spine pathology presenting as hip pain).
■ Size of the lesion on initial evaluation is generally of limited help in establishing a diagnosis.

BOX 4.2-2 LESIONS THAT SIMULATE BONE TUMORS

Solitary bone cyst
Aneurysmal bone cyst
Nonossifying fibroma
Fibrous cortical defect
Avulsive cortical
 irregularity (periosteal
 desmoid)
Eosinophilic granuloma
 (Langerhans cell
 histiocytosis)

Erdheim-Chester disease
Fibrous dysplasia
Osteofibrous dysplasia
Giant cell reparative
 granuloma
Myositis ossificans
Osteomyelitis

Adapted from Schajowicz F, Ackerman LV, Sissons HA. Histologic typing of bone tumors. In *International Histologic Classification of Tumors*, vol. 6. Geneva: World Health Organization, 1972.

■ Systematic review of the x-ray is essential.
   ■ The soft tissues should be evaluated for mineralization or other significant findings.
   ■ The bone then should be evaluated with attention to the following (also see Chapter 1):
      ■ Location of the lesion
      ■ What the lesion is doing to the bone
      ■ What the bone is doing in response to the lesion
      ■ Any other characteristic findings that may suggest a given diagnosis, especially matrix mineralization

Specific Radiographic Findings (also see Table 1-6)
■ **Dense sclerotic margin** around the tumor is a characteristic sign of a benign tumor of bone. (Fig. 4.2-1).
■ **Mature periosteal reaction.** If the periosteum has had an opportunity to react to the expansion of the bone by forming mature bone, a benign process is favored.
■ **Lack of sclerotic rim** suggests more rapid growth of the underlying lesion (Fig. 4.2-2).
■ **Soft tissue extension:** Any extension of the lesion into the surrounding soft tissues is an ominous sign and suggests a rapidly growing process—a malignancy, an infection, or an aggressive benign process.
■ **Onion-skinning, sequential periosteal elevation,** is also indicative of a rapidly growing process; it can be seen in both benign and malignant tumors.
■ **Codman's triangles** are a result of rapid periosteal elevation indicative of a rapidly growing process such as an infection or malignancy.

TABLE 4.2-3 POLYOSTOTIC DISEASES

Disease	Associated Conditions
Polyostotic fibrous dysplasia	Endocrine abnormalities in McCune-Albright syndrome or soft tissue myxomas in Mazabraud syndrome
Eosinophilic granuloma (Langerhans cell histiocytosis)	Hand-Schuller-Christian disease and Letterer-Siwe disease
Enchondromatosis (Ollier's disease)	Vascular abnormalities (hemangiomas) in Maffucci syndrome
Chronic recurrent multifocal osteomyelitis (CRMO)	
Multiple nonossifying fibromas	Type I peripheral neurofibromatosis or Jaffe-Campanacci syndrome

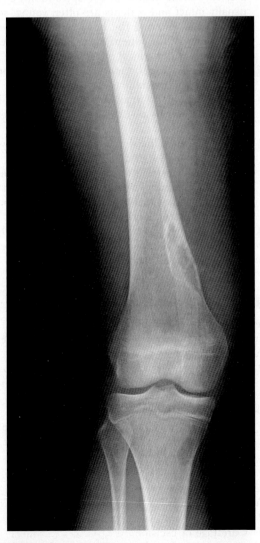

Figure 4.2-1   Benign nonossifiying fibroma of femur. Note sclerotic margins.

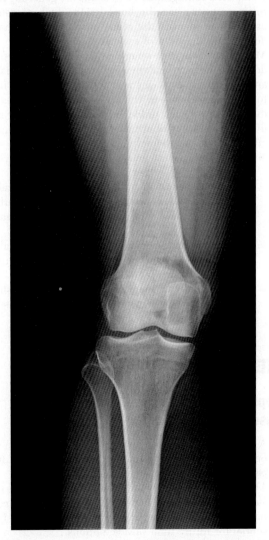

Figure 4.2-2   Lytic epiphyseal and metaphyseal lesion of distal femur without sclerotic margins, consistent with giant cell tumor of bone.

- **Location of the lesion** within the bone is important in the formulation of the differential diagnosis.
  - Majority of lesions occur within the **metaphysis.**
  - Neoplasms that arise in the **epiphysis** are giant cell tumor, chondroblastoma, and clear cell chondrosarcoma. In addition, juxta-articular cysts such as those from pigmented villonodular synovitis and degenerative geodes are often located in the epiphysis of adult bones. Aneurysmal bone cysts rarely occur in the epiphysis. Brodie's abscesses often are located in the epiphysis of children, and tuberculosis may cause epiphyseal "kissing cysts" in adults (Fig. 1-14 and Box 1-5).
  - Benign-appearing **diaphyseal** lesions tend to be eosinophilic granuloma, fibrous dysplasia, "inactive" positioned simple bone cysts, and osteomyelitis.

Other Imaging Studies

- **Technetium-99m bone scan** may be helpful in identifying other sites of skeletal involvement.
- **Computed tomography (CT) scans** are generally helpful in assessing specific bone lesions such as osteoid osteoma (to identify the nidus) and enchondroma (to determine the extent of endosteal scalloping).
- **Magnetic resonance imaging (MRI)** is more useful to delineate the extent of any associated soft tissue masses and the intraosseous extent of the process. It also helps to distinguish between tissues of similar densities but different histologies, unlike CT scanning, which primarily evaluates tissue densities. In certain situations, specific findings may be helpful:
  - Fluid–fluid levels are associated with aneurysmal bone cyst.
  - Perilesional edema is often seen with osteomyelitis, osteoid osteoma, eosinophilic granuloma (Langerhans cell histiocytosis), and chondroblastoma and may be extensive.
  - Peripheral enhancement alone (without central enhancement) is seen with simple cysts, degenerative geodes, or intraosseous synovial cysts.
  - Fat, especially surrounding a central area of ossification (the cockade sign), is diagnostic of intraosseous lipoma.

TREATMENT

Biopsy (also see Chapter 3, Biopsy of Musculoskeletal Tumors)

- A biopsy should be the last step in the evaluation of a benign bone tumor and is to be performed only after careful planning.
- There is always the remote possibility that what is considered to be a benign tumor may ultimately be a malignancy, and therefore a properly performed biopsy is essential for future limb salvage options.
- It is recommended that the surgeon who would perform the ultimate limb-sparing surgical procedure also be the one to perform the biopsy so that the biopsy track may

be placed in the appropriate location for a definitive orthopaedic surgery.
  - If a radiologist is to perform the biopsy, guidance for needle placement is recommended from the orthopedist.
- Biopsies are performed to confirm the diagnosis as suspected by the orthopaedic surgeon.
  - Adequate tissue from representative areas of the tumor is necessary for the pathologist to render the appropriate diagnosis.
  - A multidisciplinary approach to the biopsy is also helpful for the pathologist, who then has an understanding of the physical examination and x-ray findings with which to correlate the histologic appearance of the lesion.

Technique

- There are several ways in which to biopsy a bone tumor: skinny needle, core needle, and open incisional or excisional biopsy
  - Benign bone lesions usually do not afford easy access for needle biopsy, as the surrounding bone is usually intact and patients are often young, so the difficulty of entering the bone is compounded by the inability of the patient to tolerate any procedure performed under a local anesthetic.
  - Skinny needles may be appropriate tools for inaccessible lesions (especially the spine and pelvis).
  - Core-needle biopsy may be appropriate for a bone lesion with soft tissue extension in an adolescent or adult patient.
  - Otherwise, open incisional bone biopsy is the workhorse tool for benign bone lesions.
  - Excisional biopsies are performed when the entire lesion is to be removed and are practical when limb function will not be impaired over an incisional biopsy (e.g., osteochondroma).
- "Culture all tumors and biopsy all infections." Osteomyelitis is the great imposter, often mimicking the presentation and appearance of bone tumors.

Surgical Management

General Principles

- Treatment options for benign tumors of bone are matched to the aggressiveness of the lesion.
  - Specific treatment considerations may apply to individual tumor types and the stage of the lesion (see Box 4.2-1).
- Other variables affecting treatment choices
  - Clinical picture, radiographic evaluation, physician's judgment and experience, patient and/or family goals/desires

Stage 1 Lesions

- Treatment options for Stage 1 lesions
  - Observation with serial radiographs
  - Curettage or excision
  - Curettage and grafting with autograft, allograft, or bone graft substitute products

- Stage 1 lesions identified as an incidental finding: Observation is appropriate in most cases.
  - Serial radiographic and clinical evaluation
  - The potential for these lesions to remain stable or resolve on their own is greater than for a lesion associated with symptoms or a more active radiographic appearance.
- Stage 1 lesions in high-stress areas (proximal femur) and those that are symptomatic or cause structural compromise to the bone should be considered for surgical intervention.
  - Generally, curettage and grafting with or without stabilization is elected in these cases.
  - Need for stabilization is determined by the presence or absence of fracture, anatomic site, risk of subsequent fracture, activity level, and ability to comply with postoperative restrictions.

Stage 2 Lesions

- Concerns: Stage 2 lesions often pose a greater risk of pathologic fracture based on the location and size of the lesion as well as activity and age of the patient.
- Standard of care: Generally treated with an intralesional procedure (with the exception of juxtacortical chondroma), with the defect filled with bone graft, bone graft substitute materials, or cementation
- Specific exceptions
  - Juxtacortical chondroma: Recurrence rate is less following *en bloc* excision.
  - Osteoid osteoma: Radiofrequency ablation has generally supplanted curettage: medical management with nonsteroidal anti-inflammatory agents is also an option.

Stage 3 Lesions

- Concerns: Stage 3 lesions continue their growth unless treated. Their biological behavior is more aggressive and they therefore have a greater risk of pathologic fracture, local recurrence, and in some cases (giant cell tumors and chondroblastomas) a risk of metastatic disease.
- Standard of care: Generally treated with an extended curettage with or without adjuvant agents (phenol, laser, liquid nitrogen) and with or without stabilization
  - Defect may be filled with bone graft or bone graft substitute products, bone cement, or structural grafts.
  - Indications for stabilization same as for stage 1 and 2 lesions (above)
- Exceptions
  - Expendable bone or multiply recurrent tumors with extensive bone destruction: wide *en bloc* excision
  - In the case of wide excision, reconstruction commences in a similar fashion to that following removal of a sarcoma, including a megaprosthesis or allograft prosthetic composite reconstruction (see Chapter 4.3, Malignant Bone Lesions).

Reconstruction

- Removal of large, active, or aggressive lesions may result in a large structural defect that warrants additional consideration for reconstructive options.

- None of the commercially available bone graft substitute materials are approved by the Food and Drug Administration for reconstruction of structural defects in bone.
- A combination of an osteoinductive agent, an osteoconductive product, and a source of osteoprogenitor cells (bone marrow aspirate) recreates the elements contained in an autograft.
- Autograft bone may be in limited supply for treatment of large defects, and either allograft or bone graft substitute products are often used as supplement or alone in these situations.
- Methylmethacrylate bone cement has been useful in reconstruction of major structural defects in the bone and also in the subchondral and periarticular areas, particularly in the treatment of giant cell tumors of the bone.
  - Advantages
    - Immediate structural stability
    - Exothermic reaction may kill cells at periphery.
    - Provides clear radiographic interface with surrounding normal bone, facilitating recognition of local recurrence

Results and Outcomes

- Results of treatment for benign tumors of bone are generally favorable, barring any complications of a surgical procedure or pathologic fracture through a lesion.
- Local recurrence rates vary according to the underlying diagnosis.
- Many assessment tools are available for functional outcome, including the Musculoskeletal Tumor Society Rating Scale, The Hospital for Special Surgery Knee and Harris Hip scores, as well as the Health Satisfaction Questionnaire (SF-36).

Postoperative Management and Follow-Up

- Variables important in determining postoperative management (including activity, weight bearing)
  - Surgical procedure performed, upper versus lower extremity, specific location, size of defect, type of reconstruction, presence or absence of stabilization device, underlying disease process, medical comorbidities, and compliance
- Stage 3 (aggressive) lesions merit a closer follow-up, much like a sarcoma, particularly for the first 2 years postoperatively, to evaluate for local recurrence and metastatic foci of disease.
- Benign bone lesions with a high risk of local recurrence
  - Giant cell tumor of bone: near 50% recurrence if treated with simple curettage and bone grafting and as low as 3% to 17% when adjuvant agents, extended curettage, and cementation are used
  - Aneurysmal bone cysts: Risk of recurrence for secondary aneurysmal bone cyst depends on the accompanying lesion. Primary aneurysmal bone cysts have a local recurrence rate as high as 32%.
  - Chondroblastomas: 5% local recurrence risk

■ Benign bone tumors with risk of pulmonary metastases: giant cell tumor, chondroblastoma

SUGGESTED READING

Aboulafia AJ, Temple HT, Scully SP. Surgical treatment of benign bone tumors. *AAOS Instr Course Lect* 2002;51:441–450.

American Academy of Orthopaedic Surgeons Instructional Lecture Series, Chapters 45–48. Volume 51, 2002.

Enneking WF, Dunham W, Gebhardt MC, et al. A system for the functional evaluation of reconstructive procedures after surgical treatment of tumors of the musculoskeletal system. *Clin Orthop* 1993;(286):241–246.

Gitelis S, Wilkins RM, Conrad E. Benign bone tumors. *J Bone Joint Surg [Am]* 1995;77:1756–1782.

Harris WH. Traumatic arthritis of the hip after dislocation and acetabular fractures: treatment by mold arthroplasty. An end-result study using a new method of result evaluation. *J Bone Joint Surg [Am]* 1969;51:737–755.

Insall JN, Dorr LD, Scott RD, et al. Rationale of the Knee Society Clinical Rating System. *Clin Orthop* 1989;(248):13–14.

Lewis M. *Musculoskeletal Oncology: A Multidisciplinary Approach.* Philadelphia: WB Saunders, 1992:1–73.

Menendez LR. Musculoskeletal tumors. *Orthopaedic Knowledge Update.* Rosemont, IL: AAOS, 2002:113–117.

Mirra JM. *Bone Tumors: Clinical, Radiographic and Pathologic Correlations.* Philadelphia: Lea & Febiger, 1989.

Schajowicz F, Ackerman LV, Sissons HA. Histologic typing of bone tumors. In *International Histologic Classification of Tumors,* vol. 6. Geneva: World Health Organization, 1972.

Ware JE Jr, Sherbourne CD. The MOS 36-item Short-Form Health Survey (SF-36). I. Conceptual framework and item selection. *Med Care* 1992;30(6):473–483.

Wetzel LH, Levine E, Murphey MD. A comparison of MR imaging and CT in the evaluation of musculoskeletal masses. *Radiographics* 1987;7:851–874.

4.3 MALIGNANT BONE LESIONS

FRANCIS R. PATTERSON ■ TIMOTHY A. DAMRON ■ CAROL D. MORRIS

Malignancies involving bone include metastatic disease, myeloma, lymphoma, and bone sarcoma. Treatment options include surgery, radiotherapy, and chemotherapy. This chapter will focus on the treatment principles involved in choosing the appropriate surgical treatment along with appropriate adjuvant radiotherapy and/or chemotherapy according to the diagnosis.

SURGICAL TREATMENT

Surgical Indications/Contraindications

Indications for surgical intervention of bone malignancies vary according to the underlying disease process (Table 4.3-1).

■ Biopsy for diagnosis
  ■ Indications: plays a role in diagnosing nearly all bone malignancies, although multiple myeloma may often be diagnosed by serum or urine protein electrophoresis (SPEP or UPEP).
■ Prophylactic stabilization
  ■ Indications: Impending pathologic fractures merit prophylactic fixation in many cases of metastatic disease, myeloma, and lymphoma.
  ■ Contraindications: Except in unusual circumstances, bone sarcomas should be treated by wide excision, as instrumentation will potentially disseminate tumor locally and possibly systemically.
■ Open reduction and internal fixation (ORIF) pathologic fractures

  ■ Same as for prophylactic stabilization
■ Extended intralesional curettage with adjuncts
  ■ Indication: low-grade chondrosarcomas without soft tissue extension (as an alternative to wide resection)
  ■ Contraindication: more aggressive-appearing chondrosarcomas (soft tissue extension and/or intermediate or high grade), all other bone sarcomas
■ Resection for extensive destruction
  ■ Indications: Extensive symptomatic bony destruction that is not amenable to stabilization may warrant resection and reconstruction in the setting of metastatic disease, myeloma, and lymphoma.
    ■ Especially proximal femur and proximal humerus
    ■ Endoprosthetic reconstructions favored
    ■ Appropriate surgical margins range from intralesional to marginal or wide in this situation, as resection is not for cure.
  ■ Contraindications: When internal fixation will suffice in metastatic disease, myeloma, and lymphoma, ORIF is preferred.
■ Resection for cure
  ■ Indications
    ■ Solitary bone metastases (Box 4.3-1)
    ■ Most bone sarcomas (except intraosseous low-grade chondrosarcomas)

Resection of major segments of bone should not be undertaken without considering (1) whether limb-sparing surgery or amputation should be done, (2) whether reconstruction will be needed for the defect left after limb-sparing surgery, and (3) what reconstructive options should be considered.

TABLE 4.3-1 ROLES FOR SURGICAL TREATMENT ACCORDING TO DISEASE PROCESS

Disease	Roles for Surgical Treatment	Appropriate Surgical Margin
Metastatic disease	Biopsy for diagnosis	Intralesional
	Prophylactic stabilization	Intralesional
	ORIF pathologic fractures	Intralesional
	Resection for extensive destruction	Marginal or wide
	Resection for cure (e.g., isolated renal carcinoma metastasis)	Wide
Multiple myeloma	Biopsy for diagnosis	Intralesional
	Prophylactic stabilization	Intralesional
	ORIF pathologic fractures	Intralesional
	Resection for extensive destruction	Marginal
Lymphoma	Biopsy for diagnosis	Intralesional
	Prophylactic stabilization	Intralesional
	ORIF pathologic fractures	Intralesional
Bone sarcoma	Biopsy for diagnosis	Intralesional
	Extended intralesional curettage of low-grade chondrosarcoma	Intralesional
	Resection for cure of most sarcomas	Wide

Limb Salvage Versus Amputation

The most important goal of the surgical treatment of bone sarcoma is complete resection of the tumor with a wide margin. Maximizing function and salvaging the limb are secondary but important considerations in surgical planning. The decision to perform limb salvage versus amputation is dependent on several factors.

Indications for Limb-Sparing Surgery
- Wide resection (complete resection of the tumor) must be attainable.
- Function of the salvaged limb must be at least as good as the function of the limb after amputation at the appropriate level required for complete tumor resection (Fig. 4.3-1).
- Reconstructed limb must be stable and durable.
- There must be adequate skin and soft tissue after resection of the tumor to allow for coverage of the limb/reconstruction.
  - Local rotation of tissues and the use of free tissue transfer have broadened the indications for limb salvage.

BOX 4.3-1 DIAGNOSES FOR WHICH RESECTION OF A SOLITARY BONE METASTASIS MAY BE CONSIDERED FOR ONCOLOGIC PURPOSES

Renal carcinoma	Bone sarcoma
Thyroid carcinoma	Soft tissue sarcoma

- Usually major neurovascular bundles must not be involved or surrounded by tumor.

Evaluation and Management of Possible Neurovascular Involvement
- Magnetic resonance imaging (MRI) is the gold standard for imaging to determine the relationship of the tumor to the surrounding structures.
- Major vessel resection *en bloc* with the sarcoma and reconstruction with vein graft or artificial vessel graft is possible.
- Resection of major nerves is allowable as long as the predicted function of the limb is at least as good as an amputation with prosthesis.
  - Upper extremity: As a general rule, any function saved is better than an amputation
  - Lower extremity
    - Patients without a sciatic nerve can walk; may require ankle–foot orthosis (AFO) and/or assistive device.
    - Femoral nerve resection/loss of extensor mechanism is not an indication for amputation, as patients can walk without active knee extension.

Relative Contraindications to Limb Salvage
- Displaced pathologic fracture, due to tumor contamination throughout extent of fracture hematoma
  - Not absolute, as there is literature to support limb salvage after pathologic fracture if there is a good response to chemotherapy and the fracture heals
- Misplaced biopsy site or prior "nononcologic" procedure performed with contamination of surrounding tissues
- Reconstruction of limb not possible to allow function equivalent to an amputation

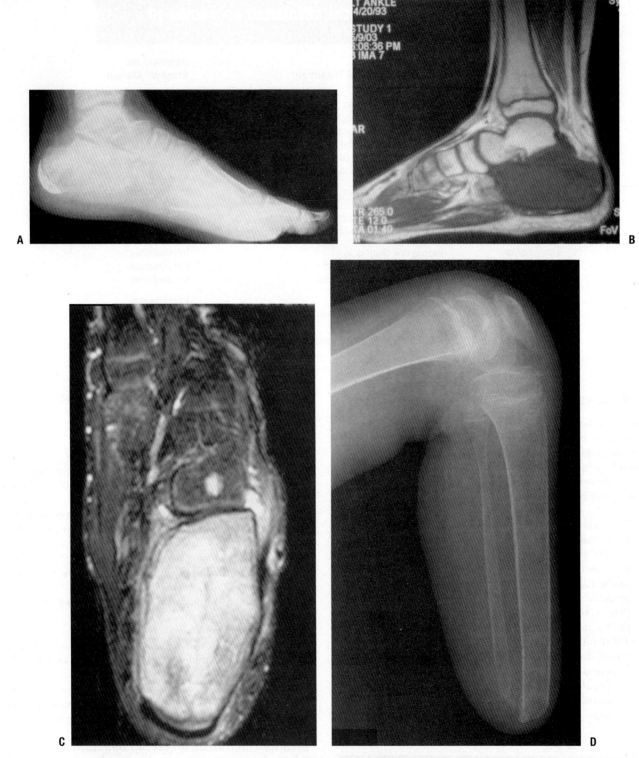

Figure 4.3-1 When the expected function following limb preservation is worse than that following amputation, the latter is preferred, as in this patient with a Ewing sarcoma of the calcaneus. Preoperative lateral foot radiograph (**A**) and sagittal T1-weighted (**B**) and coronal T2-weighted magnetic resonance images (**C**) are shown. This patient underwent below-knee amputation (**D**).

- Poor response to chemotherapy
- Vital neurovascular structures encased by tumor and not reconstructible or amenable to bypass

Amputation

- Primary goal of amputation, like limb salvage surgery, is to resect the entire tumor with adequate "wide" margins.
- Secondary goals of amputation are functional:
  - Must result in a stump that will allow for fitting of a prosthesis
  - Prosthetic fitting and rehabilitation is an important part of recovery and can be difficult while patient is still undergoing postoperative chemotherapy.
- Risk of surgical complications is lower than for limb-sparing surgery.
  - Sometimes required after failed limb salvage attempts (e.g., infection, prosthesis failure, fracture)

Expendable Bone

After determining that limb-sparing surgery is indicated, the decision of whether to reconstruct or not must be weighed next. The specific sites of bone that are generally considered expendable, and therefore not in need of reconstruction, are those listed.

- Fibula: usually no bony reconstruction required (lateral collateral ligament [LCL] stabilization proximally or augmentation distally is sometimes required)
- Iliac wing: when acetabulum not involved (some surgeons advocate reconstruction to restore pelvic continuity)
- Pubis: if hip joint maintained, no bone reconstruction of inferior pelvis usually necessary
- Rib: no bone reconstruction necessary
- Distal ulna: no bone reconstruction is necessary, but soft tissue repair of the triangular fibrocartilage is recommended (Fig. 4.3-2)

Limb Reconstruction

Generalities of Available Options

There are several options for reconstructing skeletal defects after resection of malignant or aggressive benign bone tumors. Each has inherent advantages and disadvantages, and these should be considered when planning limb salvage surgery. The seven "A's" of limb reconstruction are:

- Amputation
- Autograft
- Arthrodesis
- Allograft
- Arthroplasty
- Allograft-prosthetic composites (APC)
- Alternative reconstructions

Amputation (see Fig. 4.3-1)

- Advantages
  - Lowest complication rate
  - Least chance of requiring reoperation for failure of reconstruction

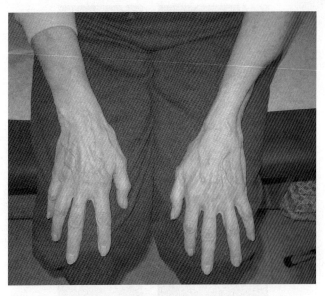

Figure 4.3-2 This patient underwent resection of the left distal ulna for a malignant fibrous histiocytoma adjacent to the bone. The distal ulna is an example of an expendable bone, since it does not require reconstruction.

- Disadvantages
  - Body image issues
  - Function of upper extremity or proximal lower extremity may be fair to poor.

Autograft (Fig. 4.3-3)

- Vascularized (e.g., free fibula) or nonvascularized (iliac crest, rib, fibula)
- Advantages
  - "Normal" bone
  - Durable reconstruction
  - No risk of disease transmission
- Disadvantages
  - Limited by size of defect and amount of bone available
  - Additional morbidity from donor site
  - Risk of cross-contamination (small)

Arthrodesis: Fusion of Bone With Elimination of Joint (Fig. 4.3-4)

- Advantages
  - Stable reconstruction after union
  - No need for revision/repeat surgery after union
- Disadvantages: does not allow immediate function/weight bearing, may require additional bone graft (auto- or allograft), delayed union/nonunion rates can be high depending on site

Allograft

- Supplied by "bone bank": sterilization with or without radiation (weakens), processing required for storage and transplantation
- "Rejection" of transplanted bone does not occur, but role of "histocompatibility" is currently being evaluated.

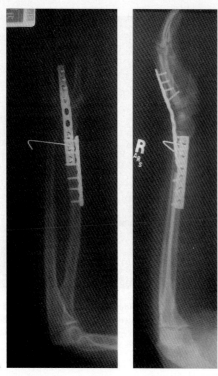

Figure 4.3-3 These early postoperative radiographs show an autograft nonvascularized proximal fibula that has been used to reconstruct the defect following resection of a distal radius for a giant cell tumor of bone. In this case, the fibula was used to achieve an intercalary arthrodesis. A proximal fibula may also be used with ligament reconstruction to replace the distal radius and allow some wrist motion.

- Intercalary: segment of bone between joints maintained; host joint surfaces maintained; cylinder versus hemicylinder (Fig. 4.3-5)
- Osteoarticular: articular surface of allograft used to reconstruct at least part of the joint surface (Fig. 4.3-6)
- Advantages
  - Stable reconstruction after union
  - Not limited by size of reconstruction required
  - No donor morbidity
- Disadvantages
  - Infection up to 20%
  - Nonunion/delayed union of host–graft junctions up to 20%
  - Fracture of allograft up to 15% to 20%
  - Disease transmission possible
  - Size of allograft needs to be matched to host.

Arthroplasty
- Usually by "megaprostheses"; modular endoprosthesis that can replace segments of bone and adjacent joint(s) (Fig. 4.3-7)
- Advantages
  - Stable reconstruction that usually allows early weight bearing
  - Implant failure short term is low (less than fracture, nonunion of allograft)
  - No disease transmission
  - Size of reconstruction less of a problem (e.g., "total femur" and variable sizing of implant possible)
- Disadvantages
  - Will likely require (several) revisions over lifetime

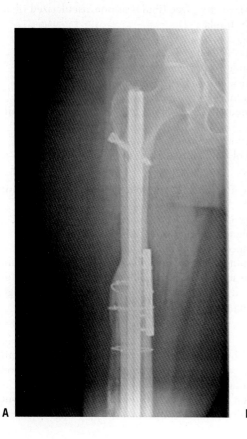

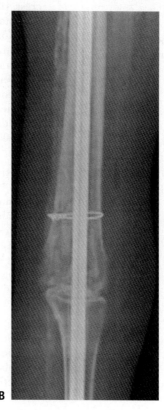

Figure 4.3-4 Radiographs of the proximal femur (**A**) and knee (**B**). An extra-articular resection of the distal femur was performed secondary to extensive tumor extension into the knee joint. An intercalary allograft fusion of the knee with a long intramedullary fusion nail was performed.

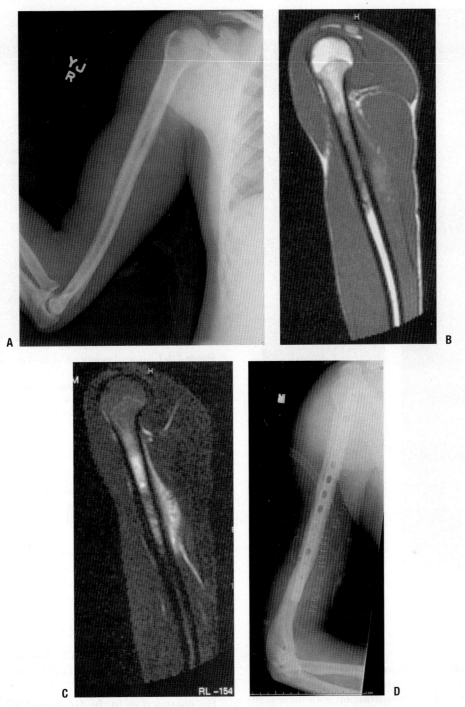

Figure 4.3-5 Intercalary allograft reconstruction of a right proximal humeral diaphyseal osteosarcoma. Preoperative studies include radiograph (**A**) and T1-weighted sagittal (**B**) and T2-weighted sagittal (**C**) magnetic resonance images. (**D**) Postoperative radiograph shows dual 90:90 plate fixation spanning the intercalary allograft, which is filled with antibiotic-loaded cement.

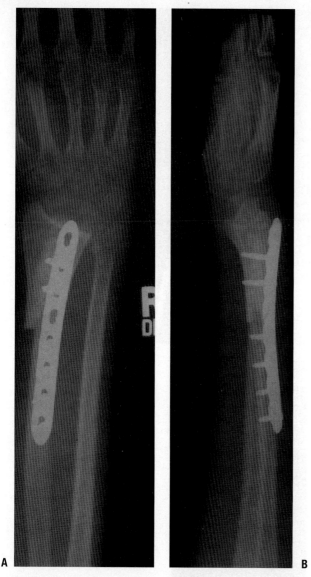

A **B**

Figure 4.3-6 Following resection of a giant cell tumor of the distal radius, this patient underwent reconstruction using a distal radius osteoarticular allograft.

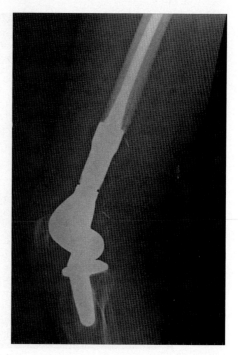

Figure 4.3-7 Lateral radiograph of the knee shows a rotating-hinge distal femoral replacement endoprosthesis. Both the femoral stem and tibial stem are cemented. The surgical clips are seen that were used to ligate the multiple branches off the popliteal artery at the time of resection of this distal femur osteosarcoma.

Allograft-Prosthetic Composite (APC)
- Combines segmental reconstruction of bone with allograft and joint surface reconstruction with more standard arthroplasty (cemented) components (Fig. 4.3-8)
- Advantages
    - *May* allow for better soft tissue (tendon) attachment about the joint and therefore more stability (e.g., host rotator cuff to proximal humeral APC or host patellar tendon to proximal tibial APC or host gluteus medius tendon to proximal femoral APC)
    - Some surgeons believe this allows better function of that joint (controversial).
- Disadvantages
    - Technically more difficult
    - All the risks of allograft and arthroplasty combined,

though stems of prosthesis should cross host allograft junction to make nonunion and fracture less of a clinical problem
- Disease transmission

Alternative Reconstructions
- Site-specific options may have advantages over other types of reconstructions.
    - Rotationplasty: for resections about the knee (Fig. 4.3-9)
    - Single-bone forearm after radial/ulnar tumor resection (Fig. 4.3-10)
    - Bone transport/limb lengthening
    - Physeal distraction in children

Reconstruction in the Growing Child
Since bone sarcomas can occur at ages where there is more bone growth left, resection of bone can result in significant leg length discrepancies. This needs to be considered in the treatment of these young patients. One indication for amputation is significant limb length inequality after treatment. However, options do exist for limb salvage surgery in growing children:

- Expandable prostheses can be "lengthened" as the child grows (Fig. 4.3-11).
- Rotationplasty requires preoperative planning to achieve both knees being at same level at skeletal maturity (see Fig. 4.3-9).

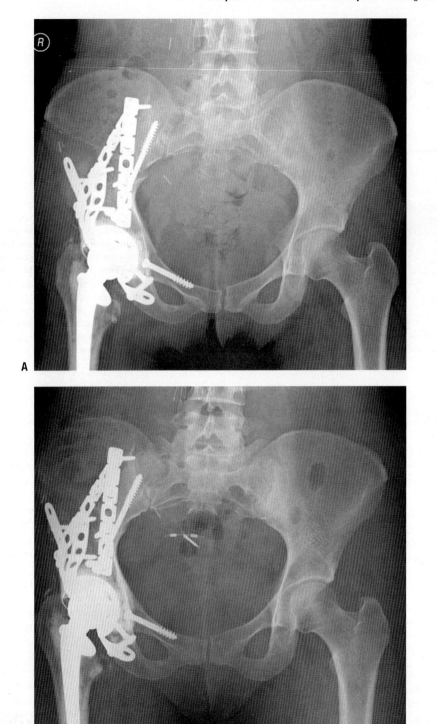

Figure 4.3-8   After resection of an acetabular sarcoma, an allograft–prosthetic composite of the acetabulum was used for reconstruction. (**A**) An anteroposterior (AP) radiograph soon after surgery shows the acetabular cage and constrained cup cemented into the acetabular allograft and the cemented femoral stem. The allograft is secured with interfragmentary lag screws and pelvic reconstruction plates. (**B**) The allograft–host junctions are healed at 9 months postoperatively.

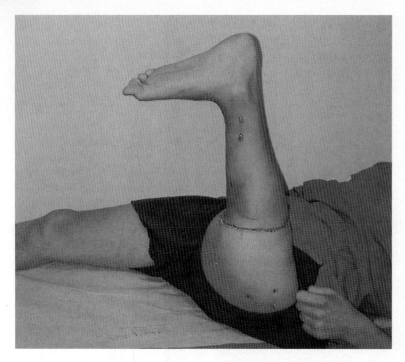

Figure 4.3-9 A postoperative picture of a skeletally immature patient after rotationplasty was performed following extra-articular resection of a distal femur osteosarcoma. The tibia has been turned 180 degrees and osteosynthesis between the proximal femur and proximal tibia was performed. The sciatic nerve and femoral arteries and veins were preserved, as was active motion at the ankle. This allowed what would have been an above-knee amputation to potentially function as a below-knee amputation.

- Limb lengthening after treatment (e.g., bone transport or Ilizarov technique)
- Claviculo-pro-humero (autograft clavicle used to replace proximal humerus)
- Proximal fibular autograft

Location-Specific Reconstructive Options
There are unique anatomic considerations to each site of bone tumor resection. Those, along with the reconstructive options, are discussed below.

Scapula (Fig. 4.3-12)
Many patients with scapular bone sarcomas undergo resection without reconstruction, but scapular endoprostheses are available; proponents cite improved functional outcome through lateralization of the shoulder joint.

- Unique anatomic considerations
  - Soft tissue extent determines feasibility of scapular endoprosthetic reconstruction.
- Reconstructive options
  - Flail shoulder reconstruction
  - Scapular endoprostheses (see Fig. 4.3-12)
    - Need rhomboids, trapezius, latissimus dorsi, serratus anterior, some of rotator cuff

Proximal Humerus (Figs. 4.3-13 and 4.3-14)
- Unique anatomic considerations
  - Intra-articular involvement
    - Some surgeons feel the shoulder joint should be routinely resected *en bloc* with the proximal humerus due to a purported high incidence of intra-articular tumor extension.

  - Many surgeons feel the resection should be based upon individual radiographic assessment.
  - Rotator cuff tendon insertion at tuberosities
    - Any resection of the proximal humerus entails sacrifice of the native rotator cuff attachments, and only osteoarticular allograft and allograft prosthetic composite reconstructions allow the potential for suturing of the host tendons to the reconstruction.
  - Axillary nerve and deltoid muscle insertion at deltoid tuberosity
    - Axillary nerve and/or deltoid muscle resection is sometimes needed for tumor resection based upon soft tissue extension.
    - Without the axillary nerve and/or deltoid function, the best reconstructive options are arthrodesis or proximal humeral spacer.
    - If axillary nerve and deltoid function can be preserved, mobile reconstructive options (osteoarticular allograft, allograft prosthetic composite, and megaprosthesis) are viable alternatives.
  - Glenohumeral joint stability
- Reconstructive options (Table 4.3-2)
  - Osteoarticular allograft
  - Allograft prosthetic composite (see Fig. 4.3-13)
  - Proximal humeral megaprosthesis (see Fig. 4.3-14)
  - Proximal humeral spacer prosthesis (Fig. 4.3-15)

Humeral Shaft (Figs. 4.3-5 and 4.3-16)
- Unique anatomic considerations
  - Deltoid muscle insertion at deltoid tuberosity
    - Remaining deltoid may be sewn to allograft soft tissue or to a sleeve of synthetic material around prosthesis.

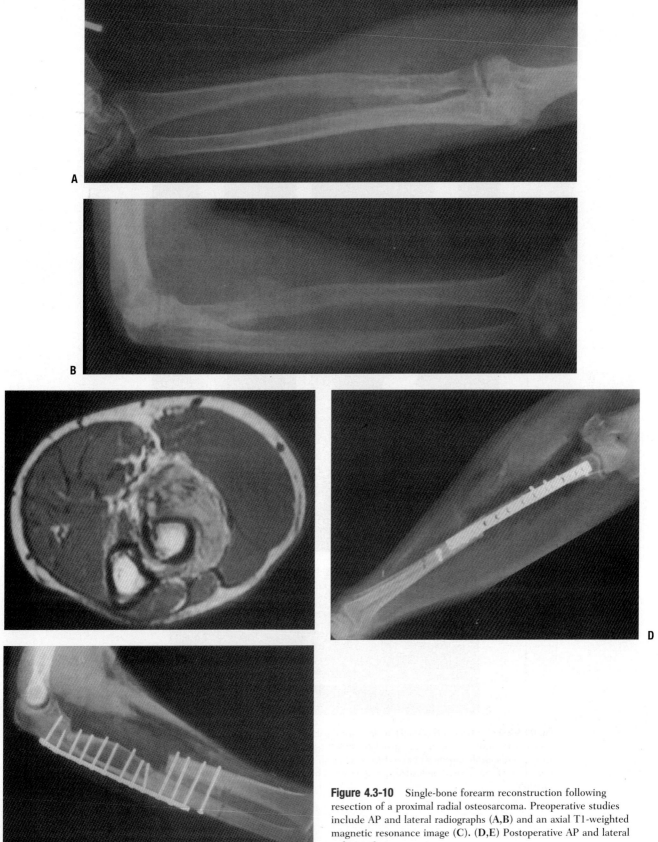

Figure 4.3-10   Single-bone forearm reconstruction following resection of a proximal radial osteosarcoma. Preoperative studies include AP and lateral radiographs (**A,B**) and an axial T1-weighted magnetic resonance image (**C**). (**D,E**) Postoperative AP and lateral radiographs.

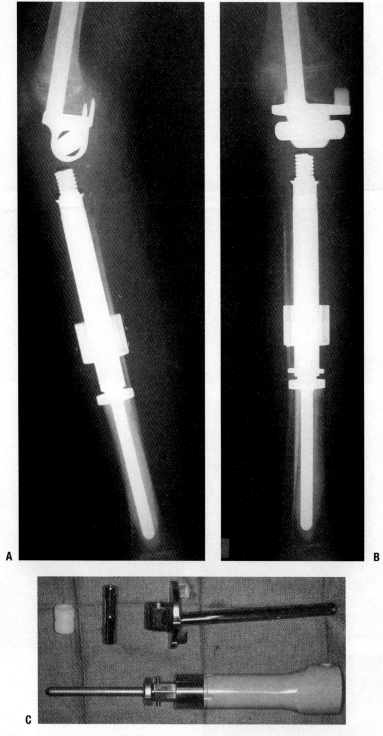

Figure 4.3-11 (**A,B**) In this skeletally immature patient with a proximal tibial Ewing sarcoma, the tibia was reconstructed using an expandable prosthesis, maintaining the distal femoral physis. (**C**) This specific expandable prosthesis has a deformable resin, which, when placed in a magnetic coil, allows expansion of the encased preloaded spring device. The expansion procedure does not require a skin incision.

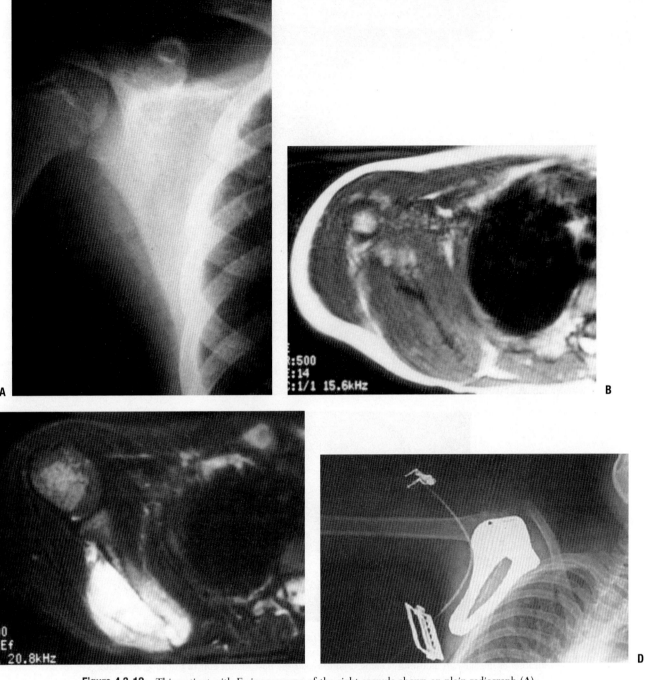

Figure 4.3-12   This patient with Ewing sarcoma of the right scapula shown on plain radiograph (**A**) and T1-weighted (**B**) and T2-weighted (**C**) axial magnetic resonance images underwent scapulectomy and prosthetic scapular reconstruction (**D**), maintaining the integrity of the proximal humeral metaphysis following neoadjuvant chemotherapy.

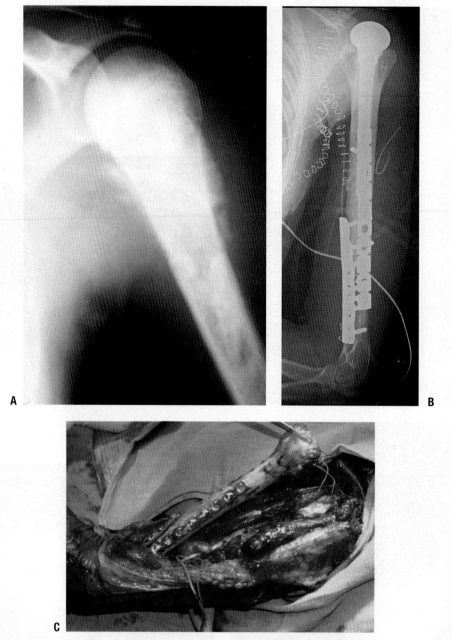

Figure 4.3-13   A proximal humeral osteosarcoma (**A**) has been reconstructed using an allograft–prosthetic composite reconstruction (**B,C**). The intraoperative photo shows dual 90:90 plate fixation of the allograft and sutures being used to repair the host rotator cuff to the allograft rotator cuff (**C**).

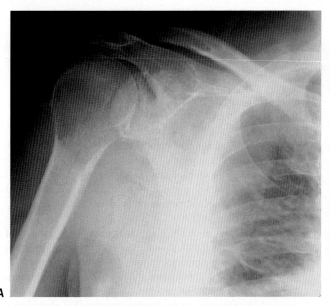
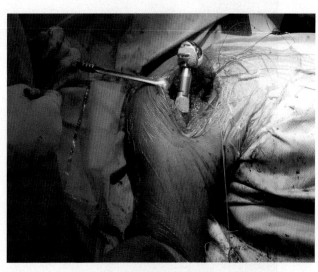

Figure 4.3-14 This patient with metastatic renal carcinoma to the right proximal humerus (**A**) underwent resection and reconstruction using a proximal humeral replacement endoprosthesis, shown here intraoperatively prior to reduction and closure (**B**).

- Reconstructive options (Table 4.3-3)
  - Intercalary allograft (see Fig. 4.3-5)
  - Intercalary metallic spacer (see Fig. 4.3-16)

Distal Humerus
- Unique anatomic considerations
  - Elbow joint
    - Use of osteoarticular allografts in this site is usually limited to partial distal humeral resections and requires soft tissue repair.
- Reconstructive options (Table 4.3-4)
  - Distal humeral osteoarticular allograft

- Custom distal humeral megaprosthesis total elbow replacement
- Rehabilitative considerations
  - Early range of motion is crucial to maximize function.

Distal Radius (see Figs. 4.3-3 and 4.3-6)
- Unique anatomic considerations
  - Wrist joint instability
- Reconstructive options
  - Mobile wrist reconstruction (see Fig. 4.3-6)
  - Wrist fusion (see Fig. 4.3-3)

TABLE 4.3-2 RECONSTRUCTIVE OPTIONS FOR THE PROXIMAL HUMERUS

Reconstructive Option	Advantages	Disadvantages	Unique Issues
Osteoarticular allograft	Allows rotator cuff repair	Potential for late subchondral collapse	
Allograft prosthetic composite	Allows rotator cuff repair		Eliminates potential for subchondral collapse
Proximal humeral megaprosthesis	Less technically difficult	No rotator cuff repair Potential instability	Potential for shoulder function controversial
Proximal humeral spacer prosthesis		No rotator cuff repair Potential instability	Only provides stable post for distal function
Intercalary allograft arthrodesis	Stable, durable function achieved	Technically very difficult May require vascularized fibula graft	Scapulothoracic motion preserved

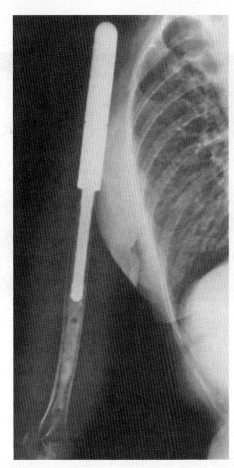

Figure 4.3-15 A proximal humeral spacer prosthesis has been cemented into the remaining humerus and used to suspend the limb to the chest wall following an extensive resection of the shoulder girdle, including the deltoid musculature. In this case, the prosthesis helps to provide a stable post for distal upper extremity function, but essentially no shoulder function is achieved.

For each of the reconstructions, either an allograft or the proximal fibula may be used. Mobile wrist reconstructions require meticulous soft tissue repair to avoid instability. Proximal fibular grafts rarely need to be vascularized, as the total length of the graft needed is rarely long enough to encompass the region where the vascular supply enters the proximal fibula. The lateral collateral ligament must be repaired at the donor site.

Periacetabular Region
- Unique anatomic considerations
  - Hip joint instability
- Reconstructive options (Fig. 4.3-8 and Table 4.3-5)
  - Resection arthroplasty (flail hip reconstruction)
  - Hip arthrodesis (ischiofemoral or iliofemoral, depending upon resection and remaining bone; with or without intercalary allograft)
  - Allograft prosthetic composite total hip replacement (see Fig. 4.3-8)
  - Saddle prosthesis
- Rehabilitative considerations
  - Period of bracing (hip abduction orthosis) to allow

for soft tissue healing used by some surgeons routinely
- Weight bearing may be delayed to allow for healing of the allograft–host junction in a composite reconstruction.

Proximal Femur (Fig. 4.3-17)
- Unique anatomic considerations
  - Gluteus medius tendon insertion
    - Level of tendon resection dictated by soft tissue extent of tumor
    - Even for completely intraosseous sarcoma, approximately 2-cm cuff of tendon generally left with resected femur to achieve wide margin
  - Hip joint instability
    - Degree of instability dependent on extent of bone and soft tissue resection, including capsule, hip abductor, iliopsoas, and adductors
    - Standard soft tissue closure should attempt to restore stability.
      - Bipolar components generally considered more stable than total hip arthroplasty
      - Cerclage closure of remaining capsule when remains
      - Synthetic substitution when no remaining capsule (synthetic aortic grafts commonly used)
      - Gluteus medius tendon reefed into allograft tendon, abductor attachment device on prosthesis, and/or vastus lateralis muscle when feasible
- Reconstructive options (Table 4.3-6)
  - Allograft–prosthetic composite
  - Proximal femoral megaprosthesis (see Fig. 4.3-17)
- Rehabilitative considerations same as for periacetabular region

Femoral Shaft
- Reconstructive options (Table 4.3-7)
  - Intercalary femoral allograft
  - Custom intercalary femoral metallic spacer
- Rehabilitative considerations
  - Intercalary femoral allograft reconstruction requires prolonged period of limited weight bearing until radiographic signs of healing evident.
  - Cemented custom intercalary femoral spacer allows immediate full weight bearing.

Distal Femur (Fig. 4.3-18)
- Unique anatomic considerations
  - Ligamentous stability of knee joint
    - Most easily substituted for by use of rotating hinge knee components (fully constrained), but this increases stresses at bone–cement or bone–prosthesis (for cementless) stemmed components
    - Use of allograft–prosthetic composite reconstruction with repair of allograft–host collateral ligament(s) or capsule may allow use of a less constrained device than a hinge (usually a constrained condylar type).

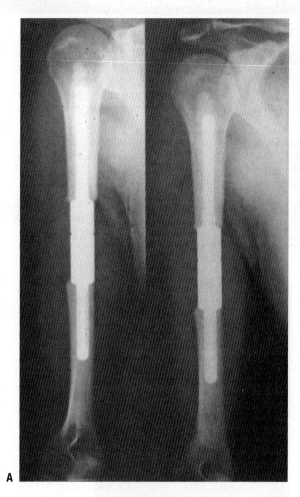

A

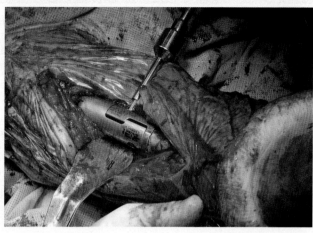

B

Figure 4.3-16 Intercalary humeral metallic spacers have been used predominately for reconstruction of segmental diaphyseal defects in patients with metastatic carcinoma and myeloma. (**A**) The radiograph shows the early male–female taper device with both components cemented and reduced. (**B**) This intraoperative photograph shows the current lap joint with Morse taper and compression set screw.

TABLE 4.3-3 RECONSTRUCTIVE OPTIONS FOR THE HUMERAL SHAFT

Reconstructive Option	Advantages	Disadvantages	Unique Issues
Intercalary allograft	Biologic reconstruction Allows deltoid repair	Allograft fracture Allograft–host nonunion Higher infection risk	Higher fracture risk with plate/screws Higher nonunion risk with intramedullary fixation
Intercalary metallic spacer	Immediate stability Avoids allograft risks	Less durable	Usually reserved for patients with limited life expectancy

TABLE 4.3-4 RECONSTRUCTIVE OPTIONS FOR THE DISTAL HUMERUS

Reconstructive Option	Advantages	Disadvantages	Unique Issues
Distal humeral osteoarticular allograft	Biological reconstruction	Allograft fracture Allograft–host nonunion Infection risk	Extremely difficult to achieve size matching
Custom distal humeral megaprosthesis	Avoids allograft risks	Potential for aseptic loosening	Usually custom component required

TABLE 4.3-5 COMMON RECONSTRUCTIVE OPTIONS FOR THE PERIACETABULAR REGION

Reconstructive Option	Advantages	Disadvantages	Unique Issues
Resection arthroplasty	Minimizes complications	Least potential functional outcome	
Hip arthrodesis	Stable hip	Technically demanding Difficult to achieve union	Intercalary allograft more common for iliofemoral fusion
Allograft–prosthetic composite	Best potential functional outcome	Extremely high risk: instability, allograft fracture, allograft–host nonunion, infection	Cement cup into allograft acetabulum
Saddle prosthesis	Stable hip but preservation of some motion	May dislocate from iliac notch	Mersilene tape through drill holes in ilium often used to increase initial stability

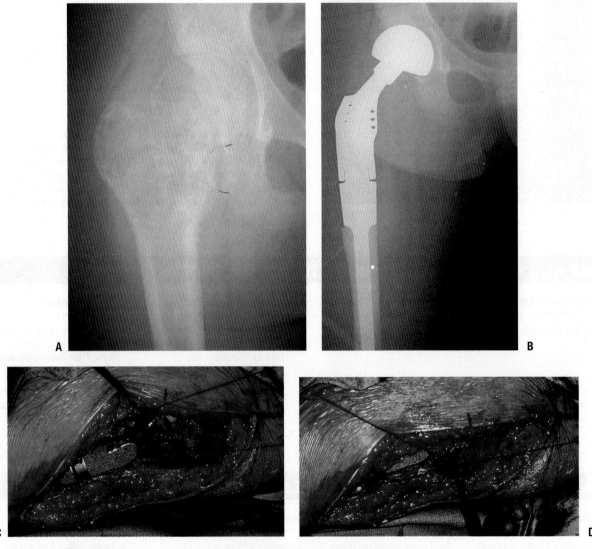

A

B

C

D

Figure 4.3-17 A proximal femoral Ewing sarcoma (A) was treated with neoadjuvant chemotherapy followed by resection and reconstruction with a proximal femoral prosthesis (B). (C) Intraoperative photos show the prosthesis in place with the bipolar component reduced in the acetabulum. (D) Sutures attached to the remaining hip abductors proximally and to the vastus lateralis distally have been pulled in the direction of closure. When possible, these structures are reefed together and may be attached to the prosthesis with tape or nonabsorbable suture.

TABLE 4.3-6 COMMON RECONSTRUCTIVE OPTIONS FOR THE PROXIMAL FEMUR

Reconstructive Option	Advantages	Disadvantages	Unique Issues
Allograft–prosthetic composite	Allows reattachment of hip abductors Potential improvement in hip abductor function Potential improvement in hip stability	Allograft fracture Allograft–host nonunion Infection risk PLUS all of prosthetic risks	Bipolar components favored for stability Capsular reconstruction beneficial
Proximal femoral megaprosthesis	Avoids allograft risks	Hip instability Aseptic loosening	

- Reconstructive options (Table 4.3-8)
  - Allograft–prosthetic composite
  - Distal femoral megaprosthesis (see Fig. 4.3-18)
- Rehabilitative considerations
  - Many surgeons rehabilitate these patients similar to a standard total knee replacement, with early weight bearing for cemented components and early aggressive range of motion.
  - Weight bearing may be delayed to allow for healing of the allograft–host junction in a composite reconstruction.

Proximal Tibia (Figs. 4.3-19 and 4.3-20)
- Unique anatomic considerations
  - Patellar tendon insertion/extensor mechanism
    - Level of reconstruction is dictated by level of resection and may be through the patellar tendon (most common), transpatellar, or through the quadriceps tendon.
    - Level of resection is dictated by tumor extent.
  - Limited native soft tissue coverage
    - Medial gastrocnemius muscle flap is used by many surgeons for routine coverage of reconstruction.
- Reconstructive options (Table 4.3-9)
  - Allograft–prosthetic composite (see Fig. 4.3-19)
  - Proximal tibial megaprosthesis (see Fig. 4.3-20)

- Rehabilitative considerations are same as for distal femoral reconstruction.

Tibial Shaft (Fig. 4.3-21)
- Unique anatomic considerations
  - Limited native soft tissue coverage
- Reconstructive options (Table 4.3-10)
  - Intercalary allograft (see Fig. 4.3-21)
  - Fibular interposition graft (single or double barrel)
  - Custom tibial metallic prosthesis

Distal Tibia (see Fig. 4.3-1)
Most patients with high-grade distal tibial bone sarcomas warrant below-knee amputation for the prime reason that function is better with the use of a prosthesis than after reconstruction.

- Unique anatomic considerations
  - Ankle joint
  - Soft tissue coverage of distal third of leg
    - Free-flap coverage should be considered.
    - Too distal for soleus flap
- Reconstructive options
  - Distal tibial allograft–arthrodesis
    - May be accomplished with retrograde intramedullary nail fixation through calcaneus, talus, and across intercalary segmental allograft into proximal host bone

TABLE 4.3-7 COMMON RECONSTRUCTIVE OPTIONS FOR THE FEMORAL SHAFT

Reconstructive Option	Advantages	Disadvantages	Unique Issues
Intercalary femoral allograft	Biological reconstruction	Allograft fracture Allograft–host nonunion Infection risk	Higher fracture risk with plate fixation Higher nonunion risk with intramedullary fixation
Custom intercalary femoral metallic spacer	Avoids allograft risks	Less durable Usually reserved for patients with limited life expectancy	Usually available only on custom basis

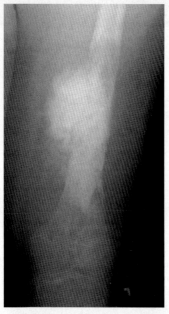

Figure 4.3-18 A distal femoral osteosarcoma is shown on an AP plain radiograph (**A**) and sagittal fat-suppressed inversion recovery magnetic resonance image (**B**). (**C,D**) After preoperative chemotherapy and resection, the distal femur was reconstructed using a distal femoral megaprosthesis rotating hinge knee replacement. Postoperative radiographs also show screw fixation of a slipped capital femoral epiphysis, which occurred during postoperative chemotherapy.

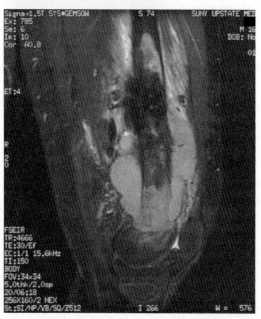

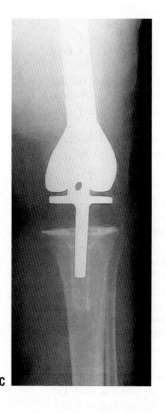

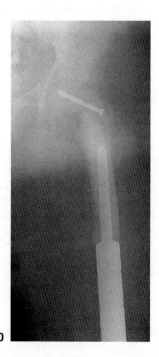

TABLE 4.3-8 COMMON RECONSTRUCTIVE OPTIONS FOR THE DISTAL FEMUR

Reconstructive Option	Advantages	Disadvantages	Unique Issues
Allograft–prosthetic composite	Partial biological reconstruction May allow less constrained total knee to be used	Allograft fracture Allograft–host nonunion Infection risk Technically more difficult	Long-stem femoral component should bypass allograft–host junction
Distal femoral megaprosthesis	Avoids allograft risks Technically easier	Aseptic loosening	

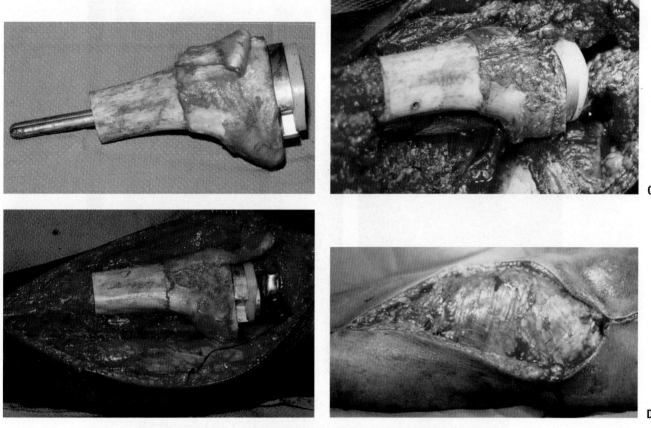

Figure 4.3-19 Intraoperative photographs during a proximal tibial allograft–prosthetic composite reconstruction. (**A**) The allograft has been prepared on the back table, and the trial tibial component has been placed through the bone. (**B**) The rotating hinge tibial and femoral components have been cemented into place. (**C**) The host and allograft patellar tendons have been sutured together. (**D**) Finally, the medial gastrocnemius muscle flap has been closed over the construct in preparation for split-thickness skin grafting.

- Prolonged limited weight bearing needed until signs of allograft–host healing
- Normal allograft risks apply: fracture, delayed union, nonunion, and infection

CHEMOTHERAPY

Prior to 1970, the 5-year survival of patients with nonmetastatic osteogenic sarcoma treated with surgical ablation of the tumor was less than 20%. The primary mechanism of failure for these patients was the development of fatal pulmonary metastases. In the 1970s, the benefit of adjuvant chemotherapy started to emerge, with individual institutional protocols reporting increased survival in patients treated with both surgery and chemotherapeutic agents. Unfortunately, early trials provided conflicting results and confusion. As a result, two prospective randomized trials were designed to define the role of adjuvant chemotherapy in the treatment of osteosarcoma. Both the Multi-Institutional Osteosarcoma Study Group and the UCLA group unequivocally demonstrated that the addition of chemother-

apy to surgical excision of the tumor significantly improved survival. In the modern era, standard treatment for nonmetastatic osteogenic sarcoma consists of a combination of chemotherapy and surgery resulting in 5-year survival rates of 60% to 65%. Ewing sarcoma enjoys similar survival statistics when chemotherapy is used along with local control.

Indications/Contraindications

Indications
Chemotherapy has been shown to be effective in improving survival for the majority of malignant bone tumors:

- Osteogenic sarcoma (high-grade conventional)
- Ewing sarcoma
- Malignant fibrous histiocytoma of bone
- Fibrosarcoma of bone
- Leiomyosarcoma of bone
- Lymphoma of bone

Relative Contraindications
- High-grade chondrosarcoma
  - Some have advocated chemotherapy for the spindle

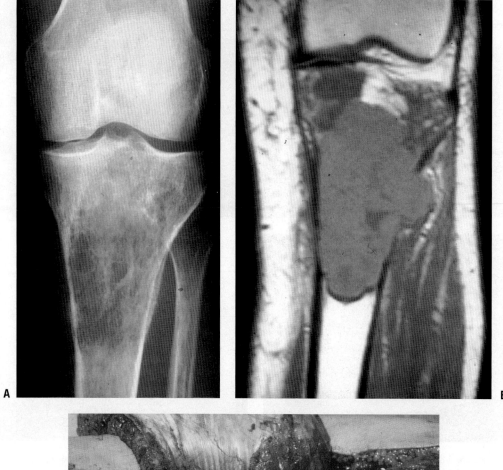

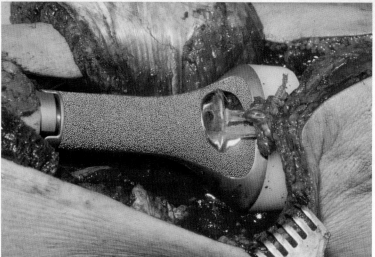

Figure 4.3-20   A proximal tibial endoprosthetic reconstruction following resection of an osteosarcoma. Preoperative anteroposterior radiograph (**A**) and coronal T1-weighted magnetic resonance image (**B**). (**C**) Intraoperative photograph shows the cemented proximal tibial megaprosthetic rotating hinge total knee replacement in place. The remaining host patellar tendon has been sutured with Mersilene tape to the polished loop prior to coverage with the medial gastrocnemius flap, which has been mobilized and is laid back medially (top) in this figure.

TABLE 4.3-9 COMMON RECONSTRUCTIVE OPTIONS FOR THE PROXIMAL TIBIA

Reconstructive Option	Advantages	Disadvantages	Unique Issues
Allograft–prosthetic composite	Partial biological reconstruction Allows repair of host–allograft patellar tendon or through patellar osteotomy	Allograft fracture Allograft–host nonunion Infection risk Technically more difficult	Long-stem tibial component should bypass allograft–host junction
Proximal tibial megaprosthesis	Avoids allograft risks Technically easier	Doesn't allow biologic repair of extensor mechanism	

cell component of dedifferentiated chondrosarcoma and for mesenchymal chondrosarcoma, though no improvement in survival has ever been demonstrated.

Absolute Contraindications

- Nonmetastatic low-grade sarcomas (no role for chemotherapy)
  - Low-grade parosteal osteogenic sarcoma
  - Low-grade central osteosarcoma
  - Low-grade chondrosarcomas

Chemotherapeutic Drugs

In general, chemotherapy works by damaging DNA or halting the cell cycle. It preferentially targets rapidly dividing cells, those of both high-grade tumors and normal cells with high division rates. Affected normal cells manifest some of the commonly seen side effects from chemotherapy: alopecia from hair follicles, mucositis from gastrointestinal mucosa, and myelosuppression from the hematopoietic system. Fortunately, great strides have been made in supportive measures to decrease the intensity of adverse side effects, thereby allowing for clinically effective chemotherapeutic dosing (Table 4.3-11).

The best outcomes in bone sarcoma treatment are associated with multiagent or combination chemotherapy as opposed to single-agent regimens. Most patients with malignant bone tumors are treated in the setting of a clinical trial or on established protocols. Table 4.3-12 outlines the most commonly used chemotherapy agents for specific malignant bone tumors. While there is some institutional variability

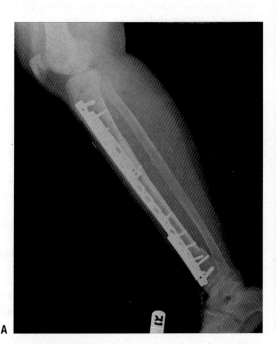
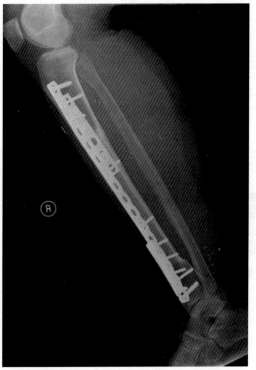

Figure 4.3-21   (A) A lateral postoperative radiograph of the tibia shows an intercalary allograft fixed with multiple plates and screws. Graft–host junctions are still visible. (B) A radiograph obtained 9 months after surgery reveals complete healing of the proximal and distal graft junctions. The patient obtained near-normal postoperative function of the ipsilateral ankle and knee joints.

TABLE 4.3-10 COMMON RECONSTRUCTIVE OPTIONS FOR THE TIBIAL SHAFT

Reconstructive Option	Advantages	Disadvantages	Unique Issues
Intercalary tibial allograft	Biological reconstruction	Allograft fracture Allograft–host nonunion Infection risk	Higher fracture risk with plate fixation Higher nonunion risk with intramedullary fixation Sometimes combined with vascularized fibular grafts to facilitate healing
Fibular interpositional graft	Autogenous biological reconstruction	Donor site morbidity	Fibular grafts hypertrophy over time
Custom intercalary tibial metallic spacer	Avoids allograft risks	Less durable Usually reserved for patients with limited life expectancy	Usually available only on custom basis

for a given tumor, the tumor cytotoxicity of the drugs listed below has been well established. The exact drugs, duration, and dosing used remain controversial.

Important Chemotherapy Concepts

Induction Chemotherapy
- Definition: chemotherapy administered before gross total resection of the tumor
  - Synonyms: neoadjuvant or preoperative chemotherapy
- Historical perspective: Originally administered during the advent of limb salvage surgery in order to treat patients while custom prostheses were being manufactured
- Advantages
  - Immediate treatment of micrometastases and potential metastatic sites
  - Reduces surrounding tumor edema and in some instances shrinks the tumor, facilitating surgical resection
  - Causes tumor necrosis, providing important prognostic information (see *Assessment of Chemotherapy Response* below)
- While induction chemotherapy has become the standard of care for osteogenic sarcoma and Ewing sarcoma, the administration of chemotherapy prior to surgical removal of the tumor has never been shown to improve patient survival.

Pathologic Assessment of Chemotherapy Response
- Aside from the presence of metastatic disease at presentation, histologic necrosis following induction chemotherapy is the most powerful predictor of disease-free survival available.
  - Synonyms: Huvos grading system
- Prognostic value has been established for both osteogenic sarcoma and Ewing sarcoma.
- Calculated by quantifying tumor viability on grid constructed from cut sections of the tumor (Fig. 4.3-22)
- Theoretically, the amount of necrosis reflects the effectiveness of the therapy.
- Consists of a four-tiered grading system
  - Grade I (0% to 50% necrosis)
  - Grade II (51% to 90% necrosis)
  - Grade III (91% to 99% necrosis)
  - Grade IV (100% necrosis)
- Clinical significance
  - "Good response" (grade III and IV) is associated with superior survival outcomes (as high as 89% at 5 years).
  - Grade I and II responders are at increased risk of relapse.
    - A grade I response is superior to no chemotherapy (5-year survival of 50% versus 17%, respectively).
  - Increasing necrosis by prolonging chemotherapy induction time or dose intensification does not correlate with increased survival (i.e., the grading system loses its prognostic power).

TABLE 4.3-11 BIOLOGIC RESPONSE MODIFIERS USED TO TREAT CHEMOTHERAPY TOXICITIES

Protective Agent	Use
Dexrazoxane	Cardiac
Erythropoietin	Anemia
Granulocyte colony-stimulating factor (G-CSF)	Neutropenia
Leucovorin	Rescue normal cells from methotrexate effects
Mesna	Hemorrhagic cystitis

Clinical and Radiographic Assessment of Chemotherapy Response
- Decreased pain and swelling
- Decreased alkaline phosphatase

TABLE 4.3-12 CHEMOTHERAPY AGENTS USED TO TREAT MALIGNANT BONE TUMORS

Sarcoma Type	Commonly Used Chemotherapy Agents	Mechanism of Action	Associated Major Toxicity
Osteogenic sarcoma	Doxorubicin	1. Binds DNA via intercalation on the DNA helix, blocking DNA and RNA synthesis 2. Inhibits topoisomerase II 3. Produces free radicals, cleaving DNA and the cell membrane	Cardiomyopathy, myelosuppression
	Cisplatin	Covalently binds DNA, disrupting DNA function	Renal failure, neuropathy, ototoxicity, myelosuppression
	High-dose methotrexate	Inhibits dehydrofolate reductase, thereby blocking thymidine synthesis and hence DNA synthesis	Mucositis, renal toxicity
	Ifosfamide	Alkylates DNA, leading to cross-linking	Cystitis, renal failure, encephalopathy
Ewing sarcoma	Vincristine	Prevents the polymerization of tubulin to form microtubules, thereby blocking mitosis	Peripheral neuropathy
	Doxorubicin	1. Binds DNA via intercalation on the DNA helix, blocking DNA and RNA synthesis 2. Inhibits topoisomerase II 3. Produces free radicals, cleaving DNA and the cell membrane	Cardiomyopathy, myelosuppression
	Cyclophosphamide	Alkylates DNA, leading to cross-linking	Cystitis, renal failure, encephalopathy
	Ifosfamide	Structural analogue of cyclophosphamide with same mechanism of action	Same as cyclophosphamide
	Etoposide	Inhibits DNA topoisomerase II, thereby inhibiting DNA synthesis	Neutropenia
Malignant fibrous histiocytoma, fibrosarcoma, and leiomyosarcoma of bone	Same as for osteogenic sarcoma		
Lymphoma (also see Chapter)	CHOP (cyclophosphamide, hydroxydoxorubicin, Oncovin [vincristine], prednisone)	See above	

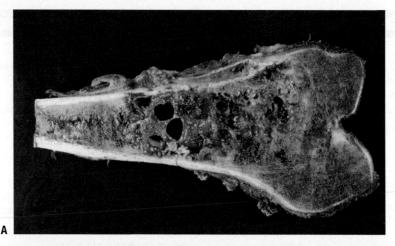

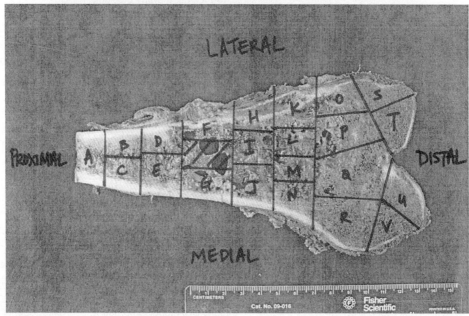

Figure 4.3-22   Pathologic assessment of chemotherapy response. (**A**) Gross photograph of a distal femoral osteogenic sarcoma. (**B**) Mapping of the gross specimen for histologic analysis.

- "Normalization" of the tumor on x-ray (Fig. 4.3-23)
- Decreased uptake on Tc-99 bone scan and thallium scan
- Decreased edema on magnetic resonance imaging (Fig. 4.3-24)
- Decreased size of the tumor
  - Most commonly seen in Ewing sarcoma
  - Seldom seen in osteogenic sarcoma secondary to osteoid matrix

Chemotherapy Tailoring
- Definition: Refers to modifying the postoperative chemotherapy regimen for an inferior histologic response to chemotherapy
- Most studies have failed to increase survival by changing or intensifying chemotherapeutics.

RADIATION THERAPY

Radiation therapy is a local treatment modality. The most commonly used form of radiotherapy is a high-energy photon beam delivered by a linear accelerator. When the beam collides with its target, it "ionizes" its target by removing an orbiting electron from an atom or group of atoms. In tumors, the target is water in the tumor cells, which creates highly reactive free radicals capable of causing DNA stand breaks and eventually cell death. For bone tumors, radiation is usually delivered as fractionated (small doses) external beam radiation administered on consecutive days for a specified period of time. Fractionation allows for a large total dose to be delivered without exceeding the threshold of the normal surrounding tissues.

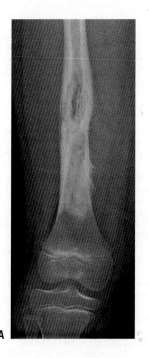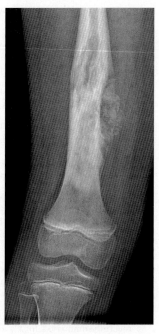

Figure 4.3-23   Normalization of the tumor following induction chemotherapy. **(A)** Preoperative x-ray of a diaphyseal femoral osteogenic sarcoma demonstrating periosteal elevation with soft tissue extension. **(B)** Following induction chemotherapy, there is increased sclerosis in the femur and thickening of the periosteum.

Dosage

Radiation dose is typically reported as the absorbed dose, which is measured in grays (Gy).

- 1 Gy = 1 J/kg
- 1 centigray (cGy) = 1/100 of a Gy
- 1 rad = 1 cGy

For bone tumors, a total dose of 4,500 to 6,000 cGy is delivered in fractionated doses of 180 to 200 cGy per day, 5 days per week.

While the role of radiation is well established in the management of soft tissue sarcomas, it has a less defined role in the management of bone malignancies.

Use in Specific Tumors

Osteogenic Sarcoma
- Very limited role for radiation
- Primary indications
  - Anatomic locations where complete surgical resection is not feasible
  - Palliate symptomatic metastases

Ewing Sarcoma
- Very radiosensitive
- Radiation is a standard local control option, achieving local control rates of greater than 70%.
- Overall survival is similar for patients treated with radiation compared to surgery.

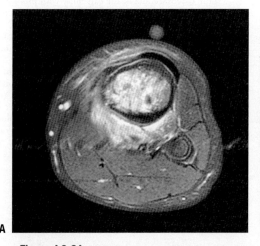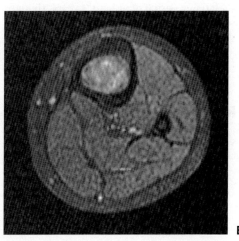

Figure 4.3-24   MRI assessment of chemotherapy response. T1-weighted fat-suppressed MR images of an osteogenic sarcoma of the proximal tibia. **(A)** Considerable edema surrounds the tumor at presentation. **(B)** The same tumor following 9 weeks of induction chemotherapy.

- Local recurrence rate is likely greater in irradiated patients compared to surgically treated patients.
- Primary indications
  - When surgical treatment would cause unacceptable disfigurement, functional deficit, morbidity, or mortality
  - When surgical margins are positive or close
  - Metastases

Chondrosarcoma
- Radioresistant
- May have a role to palliate unresectable tumors

Chordoma
- Definitive local control has been reported with highly conformal therapy such as high-dose proton/photon-beam radiation and intensity-modulated radiation therapy (IMRT).
- Requires very high doses (>7,000 cGy) to maximize local control
- For large tumors, preoperative radiation may facilitate surgical resection.
- Postoperative radiation has been associated with improved local control.

Lymphoma of Bone
- Used as the primary local control measure

Side Effects

- Dermatologic
  - Acutely: erythema, desquamation, wound dehiscence
  - Long-term: hyperpigmentation
- Myelosuppression (acutely)
- Muscle fibrosis
- Extremity edema
- Joint contractures
- Growth arrest
- Fracture
- Avascular necrosis
- Secondary malignancy
  - Requires a latency period of at least 3 years, though typically occurs 10 to 20 years after radiation
  - Risk is ~1% following treatment for all childhood cancers.
  - Risk is ~5% following treatment for Ewing sarcoma.

SUGGESTED READING

Bacci G, Ferrari S, Bertoni F, et al. Neoadjuvant chemotherapy for osseous malignant fibrous histiocytoma of the extremity: results in 18 cases and comparison with 112 contemporary osteosarcoma patients treated with the same chemotherapy regimen. *J Chemother* 1997;9(4):293–299.

Bramwell VH, Steward WP, Nooij M, et al. Neoadjuvant chemotherapy with doxorubicin and cisplatin in malignant fibrous histiocytoma of bone: A European Osteosarcoma Intergroup study. *J Clin Oncol* 1999;17(10):3260–3269.

DeLaney TF, Park L, Goldberg SI, et al. Radiotherapy for local control of osteosarcoma. *Int J Radiat Oncol Biol Phys* 2005;61(2):492–498.

Donaldson SS, Torrey M, Link MP, et al. A multidisciplinary study investigating radiotherapy in Ewing's sarcoma: end results of POG #8346. Pediatric Oncology Group. *Int J Radiat Oncol Biol Phys* 1998;42(1):125–135.

Eilber F, Giuliano A, Eckardt J, et al. Adjuvant chemotherapy for osteosarcoma: a randomized prospective trial. *J Clin Oncol* 1987;5(1):21–26.

Ferrari S, Smeland S, Mercuri M, et al. Neoadjuvant chemotherapy with high-dose ifosfamide, high-dose methotrexate, cisplatin, and doxorubicin for patients with localized osteosarcoma of the extremity: a joint study by the Italian and Scandinavian Sarcoma Groups. *J Clin Oncol* 2005;23(34):8845–8852.

Goorin AM, Schwartzentruber DJ, Devidas M, et al. Presurgical chemotherapy compared with immediate surgery and adjuvant chemotherapy for nonmetastatic osteosarcoma: Pediatric Oncology Group Study POG-8651. *J Clin Oncol* 2003;21(8):1574–1580.

Gorlick R, Anderson P, Andrulis I, et al. Biology of childhood osteogenic sarcoma and potential targets for therapeutic development: meeting summary. *Clin Cancer Res* 2003;9(15):5442–5453.

Kolb EA, Kushner BH, Gorlick R, et al. Long-term event-free survival after intensive chemotherapy for Ewing's family of tumors in children and young adults. *J Clin Oncol* 2003;21(18):3423–3430.

Krasin MJ, Rodriguez-Galindo C, Davidoff AM, et al. Efficacy of combined surgery and irradiation for localized Ewing's sarcoma family of tumors. *Pediatr Blood Cancer* 2004;43(3):229–236.

Link MP, Goorin AM, Miser AW, et al. The effect of adjuvant chemotherapy on relapse-free survival in patients with osteosarcoma of the extremity. *N Engl J Med* 1986;314(25):1600–1606.

Meyers PA, Gorlick R, Heller G, et al. Intensification of preoperative chemotherapy for osteogenic sarcoma: results of the Memorial Sloan-Kettering (T12) protocol. *J Clin Oncol* 1998;16(7):2452–2458.

Meyers PA, Heller G, Healey J. Retrospective review of neoadjuvant chemotherapy for osteogenic sarcoma. *J Natl Cancer Inst* 1992;84(3):202–204.

Meyers PA, Schwartz CL, Krailo M, et al. Osteosarcoma: a randomized, prospective trial of the addition of ifosfamide and/or muramyl tripeptide to cisplatin, doxorubicin, and high-dose methotrexate. *J Clin Oncol* 2005;23(9):2004–2011.

Paulino AC. Late effects of radiotherapy for pediatric extremity sarcomas. *Int J Radiat Oncol Biol Phys* 2004;60(1):265–274.

Provisor AJ, Ettinger LJ, Nachman JB, et al. Treatment of nonmetastatic osteosarcoma of the extremity with preoperative and postoperative chemotherapy: a report from the Children's Cancer Group. *J Clin Oncol* 1997;15(1):76–84.

Samson IR, Springfield DS, Suit HD, et al. Operative treatment of sacrococcygeal chordoma. A review of twenty-one cases. *J Bone Joint Surg [Am]* 1993;75(10):1476–1484.

Wexler LH, DeLaney TF, Tsokos M, et al. Ifosfamide and etoposide plus vincristine, doxorubicin, and cyclophosphamide for newly diagnosed Ewing's sarcoma family of tumors. *Cancer* 1996;78(4):901–911.

Wunder JS, Paulian G, Huvos AG, et al. The histological response to chemotherapy as a predictor of the oncological outcome of operative treatment of Ewing sarcoma. *J Bone Joint Surg [Am]* 1998;80(7):1020–1033.

4.4 SOFT TISSUE TUMORS

JOHN HEINER ▪ JEREMY WHITE

The treatment of soft tissue tumors is dictated strictly by the diagnosis. Based on the pathology of the tumor, appropriate treatment can involve observation, surgery, radiation and/or chemotherapy. This chapter will discuss the general treatment principles.

SURGICAL MANAGEMENT

Benign Soft Tissue Tumors

Benign tumors represent the vast majority of soft tissue lesions. Often, the diagnosis of a benign tumor can be made based on physical examination findings and imaging studies. If there is confidence that a tumor is benign, treatment can be either observation or excision.
- **Indications for excision of a benign lesion**
  - Unacceptable symptoms from mass effect
  - Known aggressiveness of the tumor type (Box 4.4-1)
  - Uncertainty in the diagnosis (e.g., rapidly enlarging mass)

Malignant Soft Tissue Tumors

Almost all soft tissue sarcomas are treated with surgical excision. Widespread metastatic disease where local control provides no benefit is a relative contraindication to surgery. Historically, soft tissue sarcomas were treated with amputation. Improvements in radiation, chemotherapy, and imaging and a better understanding of surgical margins have made limb salvage possible in the majority of cases. For limb salvage to be pursued, the excision should give equal local control and function as good as or better than that of an amputation.

General Principles of Soft Tissue Sarcoma Surgery

- Vascular involvement
  - If a major vessel is contained within the wide surgical margin, excision and reconstruction of the vessels are indicated.
- Neural involvement
  - If major nerves are contained within the wide surgical margin, necessitating resection of the nerve(s),

the functional result must be weighed against amputation.
  - If the function of the residual limb is likely to be very poor, amputation may be a better option.
- Osseous involvement
  - If cortical destruction is present, the bone must also be excised and reconstructed as indicated.
- Dead-space management and soft tissue coverage
  - The defect should be closed to minimize the space for fluid collections, which may impair wound healing. Surgical drains are frequently used.
  - Large defects may require rotational or free flaps for closure (Fig. 4.4-1).
  - Split-thickness skin grafts can be used when there is a skin defect over healthy muscle.

Surgical Margins (For more extensive discussion, please see Chapter 4.1, Surgical Margins)

A benign soft tissue tumor (i.e., lipoma) is often surrounded by a capsule, whereas a sarcoma is surrounded by a pseudocapsule and a reactive zone. The types of surgical excisions are defined as intralesional, marginal, wide, or radical according to the relation of the excised tumor to the surrounding tissue (Fig. 4.4-2).

Intralesional Excision of Soft Tissue Tumors
- Definition: Dissection plane is carried directly into the tumor; removal is piecemeal
- Recurrence rate: As gross tumor is left behind, results in 100% recurrence rate in malignancies
- Indications
  - Often used for biopsy purposes
  - Rarely indicated in treatment of sarcomas
  - Can rarely be used for debulking to relieve mass effect of tumor in palliative surgery

Marginal Excision of Soft Tissue Tumors
- Definition: Tumor is excised along with the pseudocapsule, with the dissection carried through the reactive zone
- Recurrence rate: Recurrence rate for soft tissue sarcoma approximately 25% to 50%
- Indications
  - Used predominantly for treatment of benign lesions (Fig. 4.4-3)
  - Rarely used alone for sarcoma treatment, as tumor will extend to the margin of the resection
  - If necessary because of anatomic limitations, marginal excision with radiation may potentially provide equivalent local control as wide excision.

BOX 4.4-1 LOW-GRADE SOFT TISSUE TUMORS THAT MAY EXHIBIT AGGRESSIVE BEHAVIOR

Extra-abdominal fibromatosis	Atypical lipomatous tumors
Active hemangiomas	

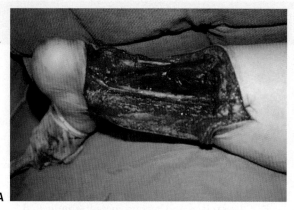
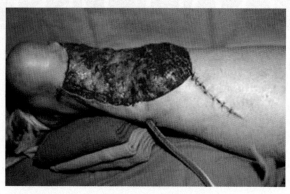

Figure 4.4-1 A synovial cell sarcoma was treated with wide resection (**A**) and required a free tissue flap for coverage (**B**).

Wide Excision of Soft Tissue Tumors

- Definition
  - Tumor is excised along with pseudocapsule, reactive zone, and cuff of normal tissue.
  - Width of normal tissue that needs to be excised is variable and often dictated by anatomic location and aggressiveness of tumor.
- Recurrence rate: Approximately 10% or less in general
- Indications
  - The basis of surgical treatment for most soft tissue sarcomas (Fig. 4.4-4)
  - Used for aggressive benign lesions (extra-abdominal fibromatosis, active hemangiomas)

Radical Excision of Soft Tissue Tumors

- Definition
  - Excision of the tumor and the anatomical compartment in which it is contained
  - Can be excision of a muscle compartment (i.e., anterior compartment of thigh) or amputation
  - Results in a larger functional deficit than lesser excisions
- Recurrence rate: Leaves no potential for local recurrence, but does not appear to provide any benefit over wide excision in terms of overall survival
- Indications
  - Used if wide excision cannot be achieved otherwise

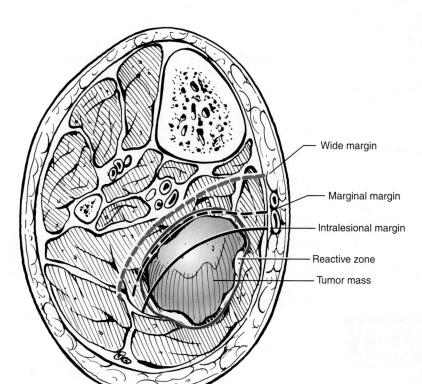

Wide margin

Marginal margin

Intralesional margin

Reactive zone

Tumor mass

Figure 4.4-2 Different types of surgical margins. (Adapted from Sim FH, Frassica FJ, Frassica DA. Soft-tissue tumors: diagnosis, evaluation, and management. *J Am Acad Orthop Surg* 1994;2: 202–211.)

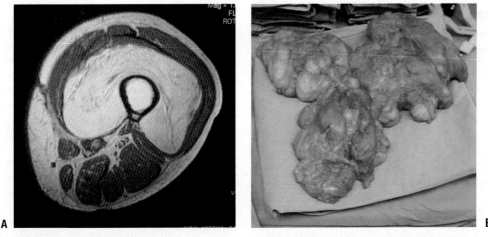

Figure 4.4-3 (A) Magnetic resonance image of a large, deep lipoma in the thigh. (B) Specimen after treatment with marginal excision.

- Not as commonly performed as wide excision and radiation
- Amputation, a form of radical excision, is often used to treat very aggressive disease.

However, radical surgery doesn't always achieve radical margins (Box 4.4-2).

RADIATION THERAPY

Radiation plays a major role in soft tissue sarcoma treatment. Wide resection of sarcomas is often difficult to achieve because of anatomic proximity of tumor to bone and major neurovascular structures. Radiotherapy is an in-

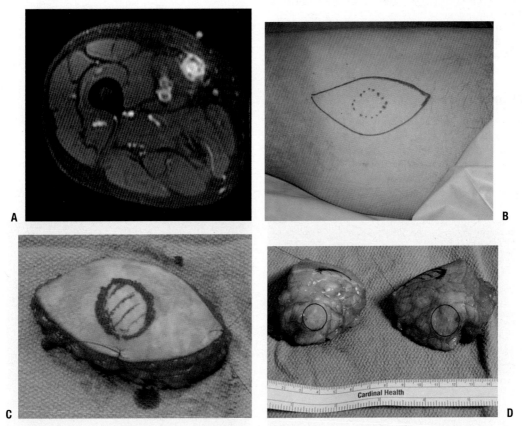

Figure 4.4-4 (A) Magnetic resonance imaging shows a soft tissue lesion in the medial thigh. (B) Skin markings showing the limits of the lesion (*dashed line*) and planned wide resection (*solid line*). (C) Tissue after wide resection showing sutures marking the orientation. (D) Specimen has been hemisected, showing the normal tissue margins around the tumor (*circle*).

BOX 4.4-2 AMPUTATION DOES NOT IMPLY A RADICAL MARGIN!

- Amputation *through the tumor* is **intralesional.**
- Amputation *through the reactive zone* is **marginal.**

- Amputation *through normal tissue* but leaving a portion of the involved compartment is **wide.**
- Amputation *involving the entire compartment(s) involved* is **radical.**

valuable adjunctive treatment in these instances to augment surgical margins, to allow a more conservative resection, and therefore to improve the residual function of the salvaged limb. There is strong evidence that radiotherapy improves local control rates in combination with conservative surgery with negative, marginal, or minimal microscopic positive margins.

- Indications
  - In current practice, radiation therapy is commonly used as adjuvant therapy for most soft tissue sarcomas.
  - Soft tissue sarcomas that don't always require radiotherapy
    - Low-grade soft tissue sarcomas
    - Small lesions with very wide surgical margins
- Techniques
  - Radiation therapy can be delivered with external beam, brachytherapy, or intraoperative methods. External beam may be delivered before or after surgery (Fig. 4.4-5).

External Beam Radiation

- Preoperative external beam radiation
  - Administration
    - Usually given as a daily fraction over 5 to 7 weeks
    - Surgical resection carried out 3 to 6 weeks following radiation treatment
    - Typical dose is 50 Gy in 2-Gy fractions.

- Based on pathological findings, a postoperative boost of 10 to 15 Gy can be given.
- Rationale: In comparison to postoperative radiation, has the potential benefit of improving the resectability of lesions and decreasing treatment volumes and local recurrence rates for large lesions
- Randomized prospective comparison to postoperative external beam:
  - Higher incidence of wound complications (short-term)
  - Lower incidence of edema and fibrosis (long-term)
- Postoperative external beam radiation
  - Administration
    - Includes the entire surgical bed with a margin including biopsy site, drain site, and surgical scar
    - Often involves radiation to wider area of nontumor tissue than with preoperative radiotherapy
    - With negative margins, total radiation dose of 50 to 60 Gy
    - With residual tumor or intralesional margin, total dose of 65 to 70 Gy
    - Can combine therapy with a radiation sensitizer to decrease necessary dose
  - Rationale: Minimizes wound healing complications, but late adverse effects, including edema and fibrosis, are greater

Brachytherapy

- Administration
  - Local delivery of radiation through catheters placed at the time of surgery
  - If used alone, a typical dose is 40 to 45 Gy over 4 to 6 days in the perioperative period.
  - If used to augment external beam radiation, a typical dose is 15 to 20 Gy.
- Rationale
  - Allows use of a lower dose because radiation is delivered in close proximity to tissues
  - Delivers radiation dose in shorter time period

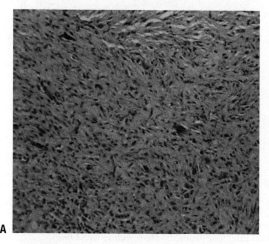
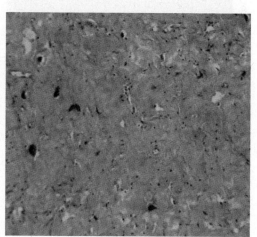

Figure 4.4-5 Histological slide of a sarcoma at the time of initial biopsy (**A**) and after a preoperative course of radiation (**B**), which resulted in cytoreduction of the tumor.

- Indications
  - Can be used as alternative or in addition to external beam radiation
  - No randomized trials comparing efficacy to external beam radiation, but appears to have equivalent efficacy

Intraoperative Radiation Therapy

- Administration
  - Treatment given at the time of surgery to the tumor bed
  - Typical dose: 10 to 20 Gy, which is equivalent to 20 to 40 Gy of external beam radiation
  - Can be given in two forms
    - High-dose brachytherapy
      - Catheters used intraoperatively to selectively deliver high-dose radiation to tissue of interest
      - Similar to standard brachytherapy, but higher doses given over a few minutes
    - Low-penetration beam (electron beam)
      - The penetration is limited to the first few centimeters of tissue based on energy of beam.
      - Allows use of lower doses than external beam radiation
  - Rationale: Can move vital structures out of the field of radiation

Complications of Radiotherapy

- Common complications
  - Skin necrosis: the most common major complication
  - Wound dehiscence (Fig. 4.4-6)
  - Soft tissue fibrosis
  - Decreased range of motion
  - Decreased muscle strength
  - Edema
  - Bone fracture
  - Postirradiation sarcoma (very poor prognosis)
- Techniques used to minimize soft tissue damage
  - Conformal radiation
  - Intensity-modulated radiation therapy

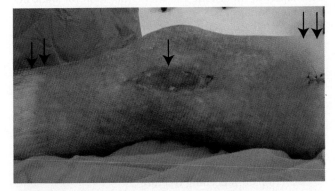

Figure 4.4-6 Wound breakdown after external beam radiation and surgical resection (*single arrow*). The margins of the irradiated field and subsequent skin changes can also be seen (*double arrows*).

- Factors affecting complication rate
  - Total dose of radiation
  - Dose per fraction
  - Relative volume of organ that is irradiated
  - Sensitivity of the specific tissue to radiation

CHEMOTHERAPY

The role of chemotherapy in the treatment of soft tissue sarcomas is not as well established as that of surgery or radiation. Promising local control and recurrence rates have been reported for preoperative chemotherapy combined with radiation and surgery in certain series. However, limitations in study design, including small sample size, variation in treatment protocols, tumor type, tumor stage, and lack of control groups, have made it difficult to draw definitive conclusions on the efficacy of chemotherapy protocols. Based on building evidence in the literature, systemic chemotherapy in combination with local control is used in situations where distant metastases are likely or already present.

Indications/Contraindications for Systemic Chemotherapy

- Relative indications
  - High-grade extremity sarcomas >5 cm
  - Intermediate-grade extremity sarcomas >10 cm
  - Locally recurrent disease
  - Known metastatic disease
  - Small cell sarcomas of any size (primitive neuroectodermal tumor/Ewing sarcoma, rhabdomyosarcoma)
- Relative contraindications
  - Chemoresistant tumors
  - Poor general health that would not tolerate side effects
  - Low-grade nonmetastatic sarcomas
  - Small nonmetastatic sarcomas

Specific Chemotherapy Agents

A multitude of chemotherapy agents have been studied as potential treatments for soft tissue sarcomas. The two agents that show the greatest activity are doxorubicin and ifosfamide. There is building evidence that these agents improve local control and overall survival in patients with extremity soft tissue sarcomas.

Doxorubicin

- Cytotoxic anthracycline antibiotic that exerts its effect on malignant cells through two mechanisms of action:
  - Intercalates between nucleotide bases, blocking DNA synthesis and transcription
  - Interacts with topoisomerase type II, leading to formation of DNA cleavable complexes
- Tumor response rate is dose-dependent.
- Cardiac toxicity is a serious side effect and can lead to arrhythmias and congestive heart failure.

Ifosfamide

◼ An alkylating agent that exerts its effects through active metabolites that alkylate, or bind, many intracellular molecules, including DNA and RNA

◼ Cytotoxic effect is thought to be secondary to cross-linking of DNA and RNA as well as inhibition of protein synthesis.

◼ Tumor response is dose-dependent.

◼ Used alone or in combination with doxorubicin

◼ Side effects include myelosuppression, nephrotoxicity, and neurotoxicity.

SUGGESTED READING

Buesa JM, Lopez-Pousa A, Martin J, et al. Phase II trial of first-line high-dose ifosfamide in advanced soft tissue sarcomas of the adult: a study of the Spanish Group of Research on Sarcomas (GEIS). *Ann Oncol* 1999;10(1):123–124.

Davis AM. Functional outcome in extremity soft tissue. *Semin Radiat Oncol* 1999;9:360–368.

Einck JP, Schwartz D. Radiation therapy for malignant soft-tissue tumors. *OKU: Musculoskeletal Tumors* 2002;289–299.

Kraybill WG, Harris J, Spiro IJ, et al. Study of neoadjuvant chemotherapy and radiation therapy in the management of high-risk, high-grade, soft tissue sarcomas of the extremities and body wall: Radiation Therapy Oncology Group Trial 9514. *J Clin Oncol* 2006;24(4):619–625.

Nathan PC, Tsokos M, Long L, et al. Adjuvant chemotherapy for the treatment of advanced pediatric nonrhabdomyosarcoma soft tissue sarcoma: the National Cancer Institute experience. *Pediatr Blood Cancer* 2005;45(2):226–227.

O'Sullivan B, Davis AM, Turcotte R, et al. Preoperative versus postoperative radiotherapy in soft-tissue sarcoma of the limbs: a randomised trial. *Lancet* 2002;359(9325):2235–2241.

Patel SR, Vadhan-Raj S, Papadopolous N, et al. High-dose isofosfamide in bone and soft tissue sarcomas: results of phase II and pilot studies—dose response and schedule dependence. *J Clin Oncol* 1997;15(6):2378–2384.

Pisters PW. Preoperative chemotherapy and split-course radiation therapy for patients with localized soft tissue sarcomas: home run, base hit, or strike out? *J Clin Oncol* 2006;24(4):549–551.

Pisters PW, Ballo MT, Patel SR. Preoperative chemoradiation treatment strategies for localized sarcoma. *Ann Surg Oncol* 2002;9(6):535–542.

Sarcoma Meta-analysis Collaboration. Adjuvant chemotherapy for localised resectable soft-tissue sarcoma of adults: meta-analysis of individual data. *Lancet* 1997;350:1647–1654.

Sim FH, Frassica FJ, Frassica DA. Soft-tissue tumors: diagnosis, evaluation, and management. *J Am Acad Orthop Surg* 1994;2:202–211.

Strander H, Turesson I, Cavallin-Stahl E. A systemic overview of radiation therapy effects in soft tissue sarcomas. *Acta Oncol* 2003;42(5/6):526–531.

Suit HD, Spiro I. Role of radiation in the management of adult patients with sarcoma of soft tissue. *Semin Surg Oncol* 1994;10(5):347–356.

Suit HD, Spiro I. Soft tissue sarcomas: radiation as a therapeutic option. *Ann Acad Med Singapore* 1996;25(6):855–861.

Weiss SW, Goldblum JR. *Enzinger and Weiss's Soft Tissue Tumors*, 4th ed. Mosby: 2001, pp. 21–42.

4.5 PATHOLOGIC FRACTURES

TIMOTHY A. DAMRON

A pathologic fracture is defined as one occurring in abnormal bone. The abnormality in the bone may be due to metabolic diseases (such as osteoporosis, osteomalacia, or Paget's disease), benign lesions, sarcomas, lymphoma, metastatic disease, and myeloma. This section focuses on management of pathologic fractures in bone sarcomas and in disseminated malignancy (metastatic disease and myeloma).

DIAGNOSTIC WORK-UP

Because treatment differs according to diagnosis, the underlying diagnosis should be established prior to embarking on a treatment plan (Algorithm 4.5-1). The most serious mistake one can make is to assume that a pathologic fracture is due to a disseminated malignancy only to find out after the surgical procedure that the actual diagnosis is that of a bone sarcoma.

The work-up of an aggressive-appearing bone lesion suspected of being due to disseminated malignancy is detailed in Chapter 8, Metastatic Disease. Other than for some benign bone lesions and very carefully selected cases of widely disseminated metastatic disease, biopsy is often necessary to establish the diagnosis.

General Principles of Work-up

◼ Presence of a fracture should not preclude an adequate preoperative work-up.

◼ Many benign bone lesions can be managed without biopsy initially, allowing healing of fracture if specific criteria are met:
  ◼ No pain preceding fracture
    ◼ Pain preceding fracture should elicit concern for active or aggressive lesion, and biopsy should be considered.

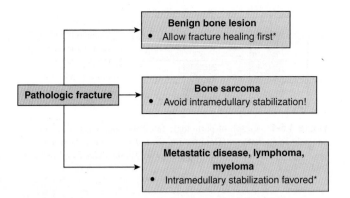

Algorithm 4.5-1. General treatment of pathologic fractures.
*General treatment principles only.

- Recognizable radiographic features of an indolent lesion
  - Nonossifying fibroma
  - Unicameral bone cyst
  - Enchondroma
- Proximal femoral benign lesions with displaced pathologic fractures heal with malunion if not treated operatively.
- Intramedullary reamings are not a good source of biopsy material.
- Await final frozen section diagnosis before proceeding with operative intervention.

PATHOLOGIC FRACTURES IN BONE SARCOMAS

Pathologic fractures through bone sarcomas present the clinician with two difficult decisions. First, initial fracture management must be carefully executed to minimize complications and, in the case of high-grade sarcomas, to allow completion of neoadjuvant chemotherapy. Second, since pathologic fracture has been associated with a poorer overall prognosis, a decision must be made between amputation and limb-sparing surgery, taking into account the associated fracture and its initial treatment.

Initial Bone Sarcoma Pathologic Fracture Management (Table 4.5-1)

Goals
- Minimize tumor contamination of uninvolved areas
  - Avoid spreading tumor proximally and distally within intramedullary canal.
  - Avoid exposure of vital neurovascular structures to tumor.
  - Avoid spreading tumor to uninvolved muscle compartments.
  - Avoid loading pulmonary vasculature with tumor-laden reamings.
- Allow completion of neoadjuvant chemotherapy.

Approaches
- Preferred: casting or traction
- Less viable alternatives
  - Spanning external fixation
  - Limited internal fixation with plate/screws
- Contraindicated: intramedullary stabilization
  - Contaminates uninvolved proximal and distal bone, soft tissues
  - Reamings may disseminate tumor into pulmonary vasculature.

Limb-Sparing Versus Amputation for Bone Sarcoma Pathologic Fracture

Theoretical Concerns
- Fracture hematoma increases local tumor dissemination.

TABLE 4.5-1 ALTERNATIVES FOR INITIAL MANAGEMENT OF PATHOLOGIC FRACTURE THROUGH BONE SARCOMA

Management Option	Advantages	Disadvantages	Indication
Traction or casting	Minimizes contamination	Possibly more challenging pain control; Prolonged immobilization	Nondisplaced or minimally displaced stable fracture *Preferred*
Spanning external fixation	Minimizes contamination	Pin sites create potential area for tumor implantation; Prolonged immobilization	Displaced or unstable fracture *Use with caution*
Limited internal fixation	Better pain control; Early joint motion	Increased potential for contamination of local tissues	Displaced or unstable fracture *Use with caution*
Intramedullary stabilization	None	Unacceptable contamination/dissemination	*Contraindicated*

- Difficulty predicting extent of tumor
- Consequent increased risk for local recurrence
- More difficult to manage resection intraoperatively, particularly with unstable fracture or deformity
  - Consequent increased risk of tumor spillage or positive margin

Outcome
- With adjuvant chemotherapy, osteosarcoma and Ewing sarcoma oncologic survival outcome equivalent between amputation and limb-sparing surgery

PATHOLOGIC FRACTURES IN DISSEMINATED MALIGNANCY

The goals of treatment for patients with disseminated malignancies, including metastatic disease, myeloma, and lymphoma, are to relieve pain, preserve function, and maintain independence. These goals may be accomplished by means of surgery, bracing, radiotherapy, chemotherapy, bisphosphonates, or a combination. Consideration for nonorthopaedic care should be given in consultation with medical and/or radiation oncologists. Medical oncologists should be consulted to estimate expected survival.

Surgical Principles

Surgical principles are summarized in Table 4.5-2. Figure 4.5-1 summarizes the healing rates associated with pathologic fractures based on underlying disease.

Preoperative Planning
- X-rays of entire long bones and adjacent joints should be obtained to evaluate for other lesions.
- Consider complete staging to assess for extent of disease.
  - Extent influences the prognosis, which should be considered prior to operative intervention.

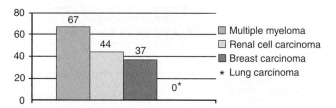

Figure 4.5-1   Graph of pathologic fracture healing rates according to underlying disease. (Data from Gainor BJ, Buchert P. Fracture healing in metastatic bone disease. *Clin Orthop Relat Res* 1983;178: 297–302.)

- Impending pathologic fractures may become apparent in other bones.
- Consider preoperative embolization for renal cell metastases due to their high propensity for intraoperative hemorrhage (Fig. 4.5-2).

Complications Unique to Metastatic Disease Pathologic Fracture Fixation

- Disease recurrence
  - Radiosensitive tumors are less likely to recur locally following postoperative irradiation (especially breast cancer, myeloma; Fig. 4.5-3).
  - Relatively radioresistant tumors must be watched closely (especially renal cell carcinoma; see Fig. 4.5-2).
- Failure of fixation
  - Tumors with higher potential to heal fractures are less likely to incur fixation failure (e.g., myeloma; see Fig. 4.5-1).
  - Tumors with lower potential to heal fractures are more likely to incur fixation failure (e.g., lung carcinoma), but patients may not live long enough to have a problem.

TABLE 4.5-2 SURGICAL PRINCIPLES FOR PATHOLOGIC FRACTURES DUE TO DISSEMINATED MALIGNANCY

Problem Unique to Metastatic Disease	Corresponding Surgical Fixation Principle(s)	Technique to Achieve Principle
Shortened life expectancy	Achieve immediately stable fixation durable enough to last patient's remaining lifetime	Rigid fixation supplemented sometimes with bone cement
	Patients should have enough expected survival time left to benefit from operation	Minimum 6 weeks expected survival, 3 to 6 months for more extensive procedures
Subsequent metastases may develop elsewhere along bone	Protect entire long bone when possible	Intramedullary rods and long-stem prostheses preferred
Decreased potential for fracture healing due to tumor and radiotherapy	Do not rely on fracture healing for a stable construct	Have a low threshold to substitute metal prostheses for compromised bone

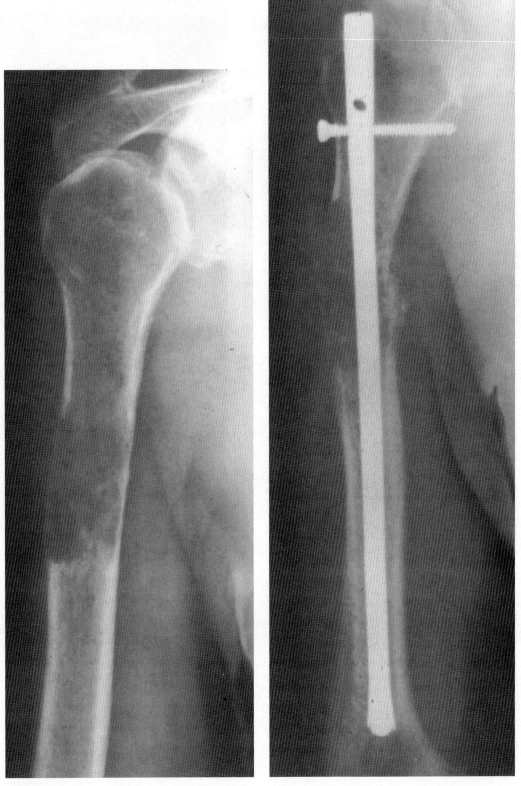

A   B

Figure 4.5-2   A lytic lesion secondary to metastatic renal cell carcinoma (A) has been treated with intramedullary stabilization and radiotherapy (B). Due to progression of the tumor, embolization and resection was elected. (*continues*)

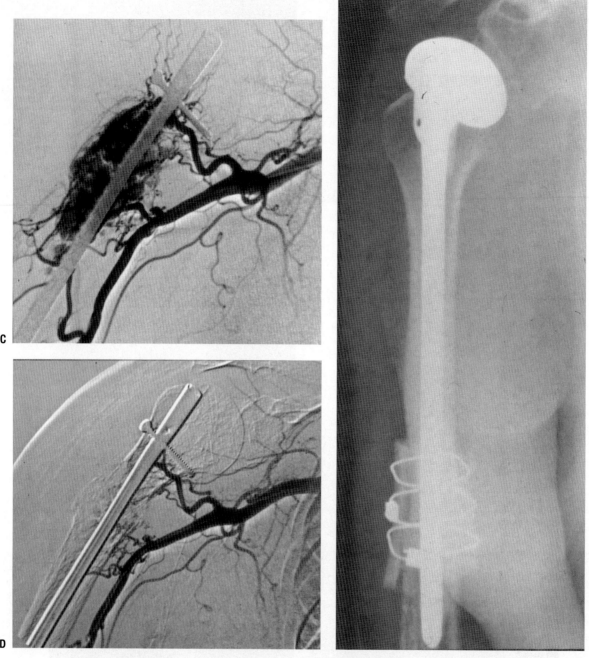

Figure 4.5-2 (*continued*)   Pre-embolization (**C**) and post-embolization (**D**) angiography of the lesion shows the diminished tumor blush. (**E**) The proximal humerus has been resected and reconstructed with an allograft prosthetic composite reconstruction.

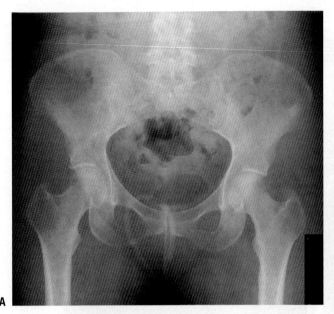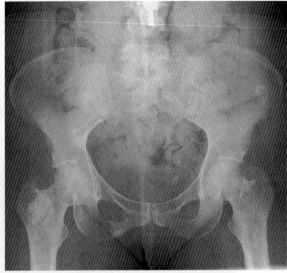

A   B

Figure 4.5-3   Anteroposterior view of pelvis in woman with a lytic metastatic breast cancer lesion in the right intertrochanteric region (**A**) responded well to radiotherapy, with a sclerotic healing response (**B**).

Postoperative Management

- Goal should be to allow full weight bearing immediately postoperatively.
- Importance of postoperative radiotherapy
  - Lower chance of disease recurrence
  - Lower chance of hardware failure and need for second operative intervention
  - Better functional outcome

Surgical and Nonoperative Options

Femur
- Proximal femur
  - Femoral neck
    - Long-stem cemented hemiarthroplasty is the gold standard for both impending fractures and after the fact.
      - Long stem is absolutely indicated when there are distal shaft lesions, as these lesions serve as stress risers and may progress. The long stem protects the remainder of the femur.
      - Cementing provides immediate stability.
      - Hemiarthroplasty is inherently more stable than total hip arthroplasty.
      - Total hip arthroplasty is not needed unless there is a significant acetabular lesion that requires operative fixation (see acetabular section).
  - Potential complications
    - Embolization has been reported, sometimes with catastrophic consequences, so adequate

precementing hydration, oxygenation, canal lavage, and consideration of venting should be done.
  - Occult penetration of the femoral cortex by guide rods, reamers, broaches, and/or femoral stems may occur through unrecognized distal lesions.
- Intertrochanteric region (Figs. 4.5-4 to 4.5-6)
  - Surgical options: Depend on extent of destruction, adequacy of proximal femoral bone to accept internal fixation (Table 4.5-3)
- Subtrochanteric region
  - Gold standard is the proximally and distally locked intramedullary reconstruction nail.
  - Bone cement is absolutely indicated only if screw fixation is inadequate or when segmental destruction creates loss of femoral continuity, but bone cement can be used at the surgeon's discretion.
  - When subtrochanteric lesions extend proximally to the point that inadequate fixation will be achieved with an intramedullary nail, a proximal femoral replacement long-stem cemented endoprosthetic hemiarthroplasty should be considered.
- Femoral diaphysis
  - Gold standard is the proximally and distally locked intramedullary reconstruction nail. (Fig. 4.5-7).
  - Rationale: Proximal prophylactic fixation of the neck region protects a common site of femoral metastases, where a standard intramedullary nail would leave the femoral neck unprotected.

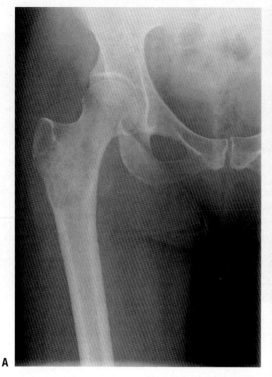

Figure 4.5-4   A woman with an impending pathologic right intertrochanteric femur fracture due to metastatic breast carcinoma (**A**) underwent prophylactic stabilization with a cephalomedullary locked nail (**B**).

■ Distal femur
   ■ Surgical options: Depend on exact location of lesion, extent of destruction (Table 4.5-4)
      ■ Distal femoral plate and screw options are dictated by availability of distal bone.
         ■ Dynamic condylar screw requires approximately 5 cm of intact distal bone.
         ■ Distal femoral blade plate requires approximately 3 cm of intact distal bone.
         ■ Condylar buttress plates, particularly newer locking condylar plates, are necessary for severely compromised distal bone with less intact bone or partially compromised distal bone; these plates are generally preferred for pathologic distal femur fractures.
         ■ Bone cement is generally indicated as an adjunct to these fixation options.

Pelvis
■ Nonacetabular (ilium, pubic ramus)
   ■ Nonoperative care: observation, irradiation

   ■ Operative care: usually not indicated
■ Acetabulum (Table 4.5-5 and Fig. 4.5-8)

Humerus
■ Proximal humerus
   ■ Nonoperative treatment: Sarmiento-type fracture brace with proximal Galveston extension, irradiation
   ■ Prophylactic stabilization and fracture fixation depend upon location and extent of bone destruction (Table 4.5-6 and Fig. 4.5-9).
■ Humeral diaphysis
   ■ Nonoperative care: Sarmiento clamshell fracture brace, irradiation
   ■ Operative care: depends on location and presence or absence of segmental destruction (Table 4.5-7 and Fig. 4.5-10)

Scapula
■ First-line care should be nonoperative with local irradiation and/or systemic agents.

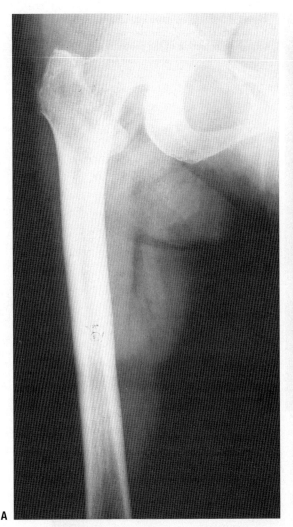
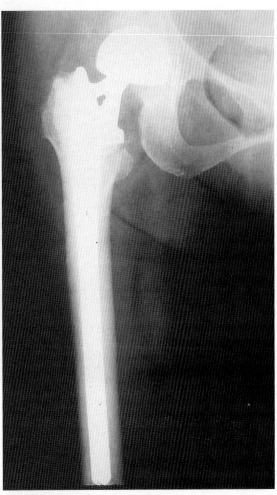

Figure 4.5-5 Another patient with intertrochanteric disease felt too extensive to be amenable to stabilization (**A**) was treated with a calcar replacement cemented long-stem hemiarthroplasty (**B**).

- Surgical options, which consist of subtotal or total scapulectomy, are reserved for failure of nonoperative care or when a solitary metastasis from renal cell carcinoma can be resected for potential cure.

Clavicle
- First-line care should be nonoperative with local irradiation and/or systemic agents and a sling or figure-of-eight immobilizer as needed.
- Resection should be reserved for failure of nonoperative care.

Spine
- General considerations
  - Anterior spinal involvement far outweighs posterior element involvement.
  - Cervical spine metastases result in a lower incidence of neurologic deficit than thoracic or lumbar spinal metastases.

- Plain films and bone scan may miss lesions, so magnetic resonance imaging (MRI) is the test of choice when spine metastases are suspected.
- Because of the overlap in radiographic features between metastatic disease and benign degenerative conditions and hemangiomas, a tissue diagnosis should almost always be obtained prior to *any* treatment.
- Indications for surgical treatment
  - Failure of nonoperative treatment (bracing, radiation, chemotherapy, hormonal manipulation) to relieve pain
  - Need for diagnostic tissue
  - Spinal instability (pathologic fracture, progressive deformity, or neurologic deficit)
  - Clinically significant neural compression
- Spiegel showed a significantly shorter survival duration for vertebral metastases patients with more than one site of visceral metastases, so surgical intervention was not recommended in those patients.

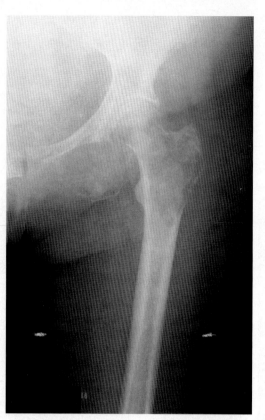

Figure 4.5-6 Even more extensive proximal femoral metastatic destruction here (**A**) was treated by resection of the proximal femur with a megaprosthesis reconstruction (**B,C**).

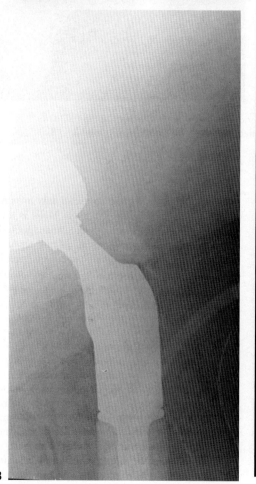

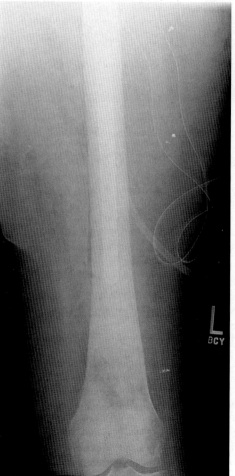

TABLE 4.5-3 SURGICAL OPTIONS FOR PATHOLOGIC FRACTURE OF THE INTERTROCHANTERIC FEMUR

Surgical Option	Immediate Stability?	Protects Entire Bone?	Unique Potential Complications	Indication
Dynamic hip screw, side plate, and cement	Technique-dependent; requires bone cement	No	Device failure if fracture nonunion	Adequate proximal bone to achieve fixation
Femoral reconstruction nailing	Depends on bone quality, cement supplementation	Yes	Device failure if fracture nonunion	Adequate proximal bone to achieve fixation
Calcar replacement long-stem cemented hemiarthroplasty	Yes	If long stems are used	Embolization, instability	Inadequate proximal bone for fixation
Proximal femoral replacement megaprosthesis hemiarthroplasty	Yes	If long stems used	Embolization, instability	Extensive destruction to below lesser trochanter

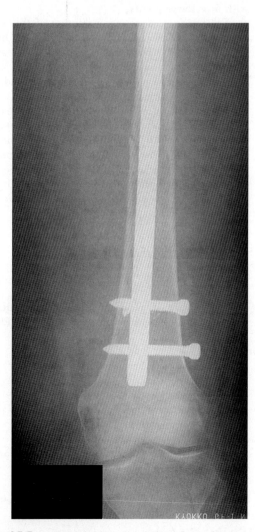

Figure 4.5-7   A distal diaphyseal pathologic femur fracture secondary to metastatic disease was stabilized with a proximally and distally locked cephalomedullary nail.

- Cervical spine
  - Nonoperative treatment
    - Bracing, irradiation, chemotherapy, hormonal manipulation, bisphosphonates
  - "Patient at risk" for developing progressive neurologic deficit will have three characteristics and should be treated surgically:
    - >50% vertebral body involvement
    - Exceeding White and Panjabi criteria for instability
      - >3.5 mm of subluxation
      - >11 degrees of adjacent angulation
    - Crescendo pain
  - Surgical options
    - Anterior corpectomy and stabilization is the procedure of choice for solitary or two-level C3–C7 anterior lesions.
    - Indications for posterior approach with laminectomy and stabilization
      - Occiput to C3 lesions
      - Cervicothoracic junction
      - Multilevel involvement with posterior epidural lesions (common in prostate carcinoma)
- Thoracic spine
  - Nonoperative treatment
    - Bracing (Jewett brace for T7–L2), irradiation, or medical measures, as for cervical spine
  - Thoracic spinal instability criteria
    - Translational deformity
    - Collapse of >50%
    - Denis three-column involvement
    - Involvement of same column in adjacent levels
  - Surgical options
    - Anterior approaches for anterior lesions: corpectomy and polymethylmethacrylate (PMMA), cage, or allograft reconstruction, depending upon patient prognosis.
    - Posterior approaches for posterior lesions: laminectomy and stabilization with or without fusion

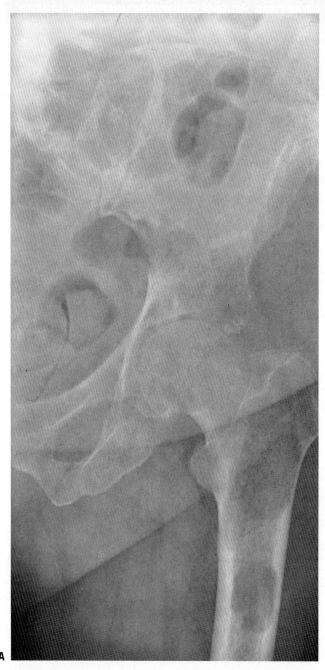

A

Figure 4.5-8   A patient with metastatic breast cancer involving the superior and medial acetabulum as well as the proximal femur (**A**) underwent reconstruction using a protrusio cage, reinforced cement, and a long-stem cemented femoral prosthesis (**B**). (*continues*)

- Combined approaches for anterior corpectomy and posterior stabilization are generally preferred if multiple-level disease and instability exist.
- Lumbar spine
  - Nonoperative treatment
    - Bracing (Jewett brace for T7–L2, lumbosacral corset for L3–S1), irradiation, or medical measures, as for other levels)

- Surgical options
  - Upper lumbar lesions: anterior approach, corpectomy and PMMA, cage, or allograft reconstruction with or without plate stabilization
  - Lower lumbar lesions: posterior decompression and stabilization or combined anterior corpectomy and reconstruction with posterior stabilization
- Classification systems designed to provide guidance for intervention in spinal metastases are as follows:
  - Harrington classification (Table 4.5-8)
  - Kostuik two-column, six-segment concept of stability, defined instability, and hence the need for surgical intervention, as destruction of three or more segments
  - Tokuhashi's six variables (general medical condition, number of extraspinal bone metastases, number of vertebral metastases, visceral metastases, primary tumor type, presence of neurologic deficit), with 0 to 2 points assigned per variable, suggested that an excisional operation be done for cases with 9 or more points and a palliative operation be done for those with 5 or fewer points.
    - Enkaoua's prospective evaluation of the Tokuhashi system revealed median survival of 24 months if the Tokuhashi score is above 7 and 5 months for a score of 7 or less, but the series was limited to patients with renal, thyroid, and unknown primary carcinomas.
  - Tomita's 2001 scoring system consists of three prognostic factors (grade of malignancy 1/2/4 points, visceral metastases 0/2/4 points, number of bone metastases 1 or 2 points), totaling 2 to 10 points. Patients with 2 or 3 points are recommended for wide or marginal excision, 4 or 5 points marginal or intralesional excision, 6 or 7 points palliative surgery, 8 to 10 points nonoperative approach.

Sites Distal to the Elbow
- Distal humerus
  - Nonoperative care: Sarmiento-type hinged elbow brace, irradiation
  - Operative care: depends on extent of destruction, presence of proximal lesions (Table 4.5-9 and Fig. 4.5-11)
- Forearm
  - Nonoperative care: bracing, irradiation and/or medical management
  - Operative care: rarely indicated
  - Surgical options: intramedullary nailing, plate/screw, or combination
- Wrist and hand
  - Nonoperative care: observation, irradiation and/or medical management
  - Operative care: rarely indicated
  - Surgical options: palliative amputation, resection

Sites Distal to the Knee
- Tibia and fibula
  - General considerations

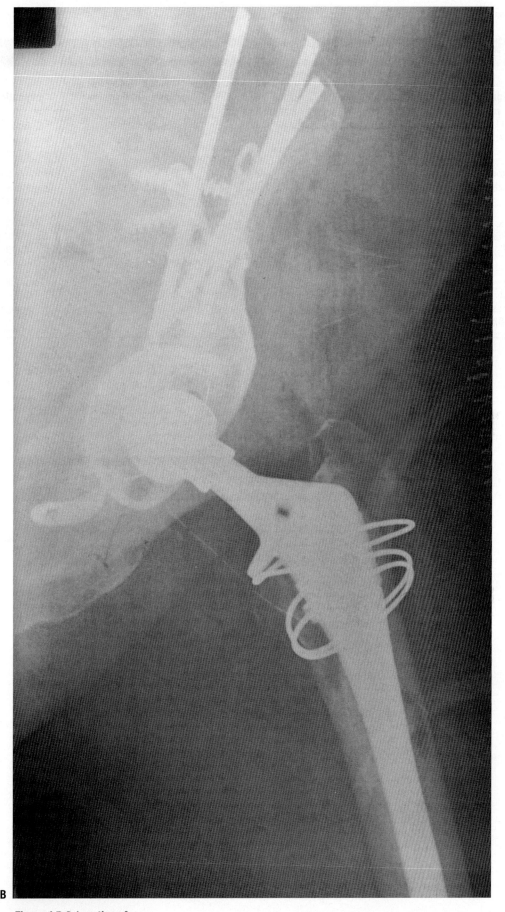

B

Figure 4.5-8 (*continued*)

TABLE 4.5-4 SURGICAL OPTIONS FOR PATHOLOGIC FRACTURE OF THE DISTAL FEMUR

Surgical Option	Immediate Stability?	Protects Entire Bone?	Unique Potential Complications	Indication
Curettage and cementing	Only for impending pathologic fractures	No	Fracture if lesion progresses	Small metaphyseal or epiphyseal eccentric defects
Curettage, cementing, and plate/screw fixation	Depends on bone quality, cement supplementation	No	Device failure if fracture nonunion	Adequate distal bone to achieve fixation; no proximal lesions
Retrograde intramedullary femoral nail	Depends on bone quality	No	Fracture proximal to end of nail	Distal diaphyseal lesion not amenable to antegrade nailing; no proximal lesions
Distal femoral replacement megaprosthesis total knee arthroplasty	Yes	If long stems used	Embolization	Extensive destruction distal femur precluding other options

TABLE 4.5-5 MODIFIED HARRINGTON CLASSIFICATION OF PELVIC INSUFFICIENCY AND SUGGESTED MANAGEMENT

Class	Description	Management
0	Supra-acetabular defect that does not penetrate acetabular subchondral plate	Nonoperative care vs. curettage, cementation, and reinforcement pins/mesh
I	Contained defect involving acetabulum with intact rim and superior dome	Curettage and cementing of defect with cemented cup total hip arthroplasty with or without protrusio ring
II	Medial wall acetabular defect	Cemented protrusio cage total hip arthroplasty
III	Deficiency of rim or dome	Option 1: Cemented protrusio cage total hip arthroplasty with curettage of supra-acetabular bone and reinforcement pins (Fig. 4.5-8)
		Option 2: Saddle prosthesis
IV	Resection of lesion required for cure	Option 1: Saddle prosthesis
		Option 2: Allograft acetabular prosthetic total hip arthroplasty composite reconstruction

TABLE 4.5-6 SURGICAL OPTIONS FOR PATHOLOGIC FRACTURE OF THE PROXIMAL HUMERUS

Surgical Option	Immediate Stability?	Protects Entire Bone?	Unique Potential Complications	Indication
Long-stem cemented hemiarthroplasty	Yes	Yes	Shoulder instability	Epiphyseal and limited metaphyseal involvement
Plate, screws, and bone cement	Dependent on bone quality, cement supplementation	No	Loss of fixation, fracture below device	Metaphyseal lesions with enough intact proximal bone
Endoprosthetic proximal humeral replacement (EPHR)	Yes	If long stems used	Poor shoulder function	Extensive epiphyseal/ metaphyseal and proximal diaphyseal destruction
Allograft prosthetic composite (Fig. 4.5-2)	Yes, but must protect cuff reconstruction	If long stems used	Allograft infection and fracture risk	Same as EPHR but patient with longer potential survival

- Tibial metastatic lesions far outweigh pathologic fractures, likely because tibial lesions become symptomatic earlier than femoral lesions.
- Protection of the entire tibia is of less concern than in femur or humerus due to the less frequent occurrence of distal lesions.
- Proximal tibia
  - Nonoperative care: bracing (patellar tendon–bearing orthosis or knee–ankle–foot orthosis, often with drop-lock knee hinges), irradiation/chemotherapy/hormone manipulation/bisphosphonates
  - Surgical options: depend on location, extent of bone destruction (Table 4.5-10)

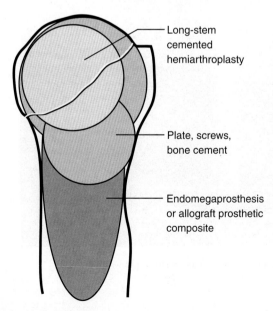

Figure 4.5-9 Proximal humeral surgical options according to location.

Labels in figure:
- Long-stem cemented hemiarthroplasty
- Plate, screws, bone cement
- Endomegaprosthesis or allograft prosthetic composite

- Tibial diaphysis
  - Nonoperative care: patellar tendon–bearing orthosis, irradiation, chemotherapy, hormone manipulation, bisphosphonates
  - Gold standard is antegrade proximally and distally locked tibial nail.
  - Need for cement depends on need to re-establish continuity of the bone; cement is indicated for segmental destruction of the bone.
- Distal tibia
  - Nonoperative care: patellar tendon–bearing orthosis or ankle–foot orthosis, irradiation, chemotherapy, hormone manipulation, bisphosphonates
  - Surgical options depend upon exact location and extent of destruction. The techniques parallel those of the proximal tibia in concept. Small lesions can be curetted and cemented, and larger lesions require plate fixation to complement the cemented defect.
- Ankle and foot
  - General considerations
    - Rare site of metastatic disease
  - Gold standard is nonoperative care with short-leg boots or pressure-relief shoes combined with irradiation, chemotherapy, hormone manipulation, and bisphosphonates.
  - Surgical options include amputation for palliation.

EVALUATION AND TREATMENT OF IMPENDING FRACTURES

Prediction of risk for fracture in the setting of destructive bone involvement by metastatic disease and myeloma is important in order to educate the patient and to give him or her the opportunity to potentially avoid an emergent hospitalization and the added pain of a fracture. Furthermore,

TABLE 4.5-7 SURGICAL OPTIONS FOR PATHOLOGIC FRACTURE OF THE HUMERAL DIAPHYSIS

Surgical Option	Immediate Stability?	Protects Entire Bone?	Unique Potential Complications	Biomechanical Properties	Indication
Intramedullary nailing (Fig. 4.5-2)	Yes, unless segmental bone loss	Yes	Insertion site rotator cuff pain	Intermediate	Mid-diaphyseal lesions
Plate, screws, and bone cement	Dependent on bone quality, cement supplementation	No	Loss of fixation, fracture at ends of device	Worst	Too proximal or distal for intramedullary nailing
Intercalary spacer endoprostheses (Fig. 4.5-10)	Yes	If long stems used	Dissociation, rotational malalignment	Best	Segmental bone loss

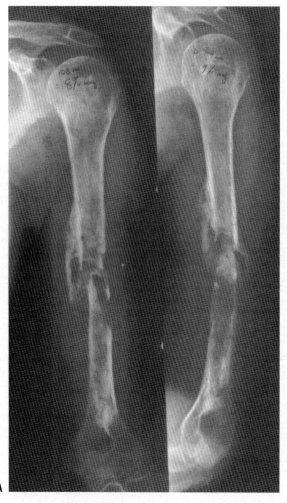 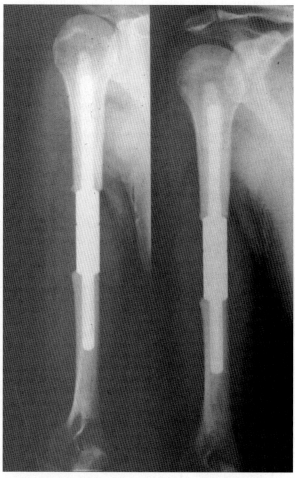

Figure 4.5-10 Failure of earlier plate fixation of this pathologic humeral shaft fracture (**A**) was salvaged with a cemented intercalary humeral spacer (**B**).

TABLE 4.5-8 HARRINGTON CLASSIFICATION OF METASTATIC SPINE TUMORS AND SUGGESTED MANAGEMENT

Class	Description	Management
I	Asymptomatic spine lesion	Nonoperative treatment (chemotherapy, hormonal manipulation, or local irradiation)
II	Painful lesion with/without minor neurologic defect; no collapse or instability	As for class I
III	Major neurologic impairment (motor or sensory) without significant collapse (often due to epidural tumor extension)	Gray area
IV	Vertebral collapse, pain due to mechanical causes or instability, no significant neurologic impairment	Surgical intervention indicated if patient factors allow
V	Vertebral collapse, instability, and major neurologic impairment	As for class IV

TABLE 4.5-9 SURGICAL OPTIONS FOR PATHOLOGIC FRACTURES OF THE DISTAL HUMERUS

Surgical Option	Immediate Stability?	Protects Entire Bone?	Unique Potential Complications	Biomechanical Properties	Indication
Retrograde dual Rush rods, bone cement (Fig. 4.5-11)	Technique-dependent; requires bone cement	Yes	Rod migration	Intermediate	Distal-third fracture with lesions proximal
90:90 dual plates, screws, and bone cement	Dependent on bone quality, cement supplementation	No	Loss of fixation, fracture at ends of device	Best	Distal-third fracture
Single plate, screw, and bone cement	Dependent on bone quality, cement supplementation	No	Loss of fixation, fracture at ends of device	Worst	Unable to use other technique
Distal humeral replacement total elbow arthroplasty	Yes	If long stems used	Instability, loosening	N/A	Extensive distal destruction precludes fixation

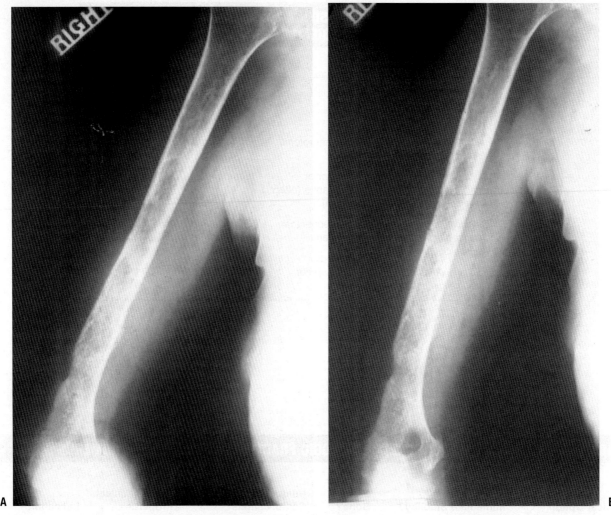

Figure 4.5-11 A patient with metastatic breast carcinoma involving much of the humerus with an impending distal third fracture (**A,B**) (*continues*)

because of the lower likelihood of fracture healing in the setting of malignancy, potential long-term complications of fracture fixation in these patients may be avoided by prophylactic stabilization. Guidelines for prediction of pathologic fracture risk continue to evolve.

Classic indications of impending pathologic fracture are as follows:

- More than half of width of bone destroyed
- >2.5 cm of bone destruction
- Avulsion of lesser trochanter
- Pain unresponsive to radiotherapy

Mirel's classification of impending pathologic fractures is covered in Tables 4.5-11 and 4.5-12. This classification scheme is sensitive and poorly specific for prediction of pathologic fracture risk, but nonetheless it remains a useful objective tool.

MEDICAL MANAGEMENT OF METASTATIC DISEASE AND RELATED CONDITIONS

Therapy to Decrease Bone Resorption

- Osteoclasts are the cellular mediator of bone resorption in metastatic disease and myeloma.
- Osteoclast inhibitor drug class: bisphosphonates
  - Etidronate (Didronel)
  - Pamidronate (Aredia)
  - Alendronate (Fosamax)
  - Risedronate (Actonel)
  - Zoledronate (Zometa)
  - Ibandronate (Boniva)
- Types of efficacy demonstrated for bisphosphonates
  - Fewer skeletal complications

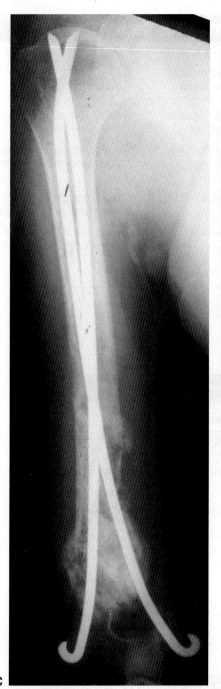

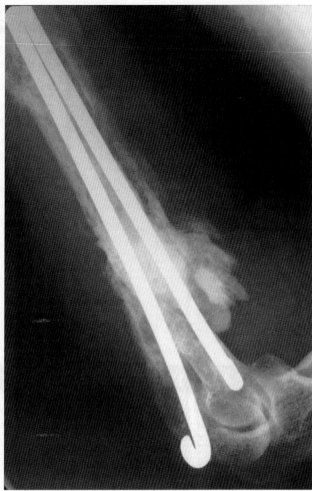

Figure 4.5-11 (*continued*)   was treated with dual cemented Rush rod fixation, with good results (**C,D**).

- Increased time to progression of disease
- Decreased time to first skeletal event
- Less bone pain
- Tumors with documented efficacy of bisphosphonates
  - Breast carcinoma
  - Multiple myeloma
  - Prostate carcinoma
  - Lung carcinoma
  - Renal carcinoma
- Indications for bisphosphonates in metastatic disease
  - Hypercalcemia

- Bone metastases in breast, prostate, lung, or renal carcinoma
- Multiple myeloma

Medical Management of Metastases According to Specific Primary Tumors

Breast Cancer (*Algorithm 4.5-2*)

Initial systemic treatment of metastatic breast cancer usually involves antiestrogenic hormonal manipulation. After

TABLE 4.5-10 SURGICAL OPTIONS FOR PATHOLOGIC FRACTURES OF THE PROXIMAL TIBIA

Surgical Option	Immediate Stability?	Protects Entire Bone?	Unique Potential Complications	Indication
Curettage and cementing	Only for impending pathologic fractures	No	Fracture if lesion progresses	Small epiphyseal or metaphyseal eccentric defects
Curettage, cementing, and plate/screw fixation	Depends on bone quality, cement supplementation	No	Device failure if fracture nonunion	Adequate proximal bone to achieve fixation; no distal lesions
Tibial intramedullary nail	Depends on bone quality and continuity	Yes	Insertion site discomfort	Distal metaphyseal with adequate proximal bone to achieve fixation
Proximal tibial replacement megaprosthesis total knee arthroplasty	Yes	If long stems used	Embolization	Extensive destruction proximal tibia precluding other options

TABLE 4.5-11 MIRELS SCORING SYSTEM

Parameter	Points		
	1	2	3
Site	Upper extremity	Lower extremity[a]	Peritrochanteric
Nature	Blastic	Mixed[b]	Lytic
Size[c]	<1/3	1/3 to 2/3	>2/3
Pain	Mild	Moderate	Functional

[a]Non-peritrochanteric lower extremity
[b]Mixed lytic and blastic
[c]Relative proportion of bone width involved by tumor

TABLE 4.5-12 MIREL'S RECOMMENDATIONS FOR PROPHYLACTIC STABILIZATION BASED UPON TOTAL SCORE

	Mirel's Scale Point Total	Risk of Fracture	Mirel's Treatment Recommendations
Impending	≥9	≥33%	Prophylactic stabilization
Borderline	8	15%	Consider stabilization
Not impending	≤7	<15%	Nonoperative care

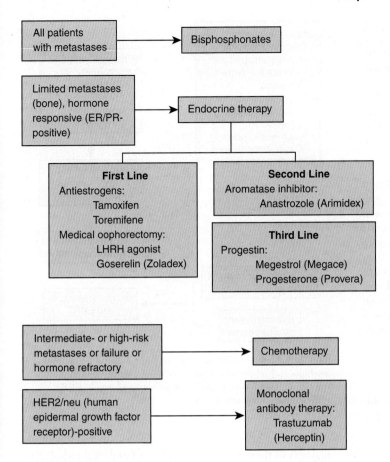

Algorithm 4.5-2. Systemic treatments for metastatic breast cancer.

the disease has become refractory to hormonal treatment, chemotherapy is usually employed. Monoclonal antibodies directed to the human epithelial growth factor receptor 2 (HER2/neu), which contributes to breast cancer tumorigenesis, may also be used for palliative care. Breast cancer metastases to bone are responsive to radiotherapy.

Prostate Cancer (Algorithm 4.5-3)
Specific antitumoral treatment for metastatic prostate cancer has consisted primarily of androgen suppression by hormonal manipulation. Chemotherapy combinations have shown some promise against hormone-refractory disease in recent years. Bisphosphonates are successful for decreasing bone pain associated with prostate metastases. Radiotherapy is very useful for prostate cancer. When there is a single predominant symptomatic site producing pain, external beam radiotherapy is useful. However, when patients have diffuse bone metastases with multiple symptomatic sites, or when tissue tolerance has been maximized by external beam therapy, systemic radionuclide therapy may be useful. Strontium-89 is the most common radionuclide used for systemic radiotherapy.

Lung Cancer
From a primary treatment viewpoint, lung cancer may be viewed as small cell lung cancer and non-small cell lung cancer. Small cell lung cancer is typically treated with chemotherapy, whereas until recently non-small cell has been viewed as poorly responsive to chemotherapy. Recent trials suggest some efficacy of chemotherapy in addition to radiotherapy for unresectable non-small cell lung carcinoma.

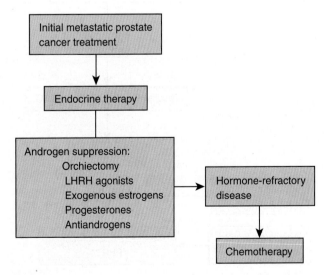

Algorithm 4.5-3. Systemic treatments for metastatic prostate cancer.

Metastases from lung cancer portend an extremely poor prognosis, and median survival is only 3 to 6 months. Systemic treatments are of limited usefulness except as research protocols to date. Radiotherapy provides effective palliation of bone metastases, although response is not as good as for breast or prostate cancer patients. Bisphosphonates play a similar role for lung cancer as for other metastatic tumors, reducing both pain and the number of skeletal events.

Renal Cancer

There are limited useful options for nonoperative treatment of metastatic renal carcinoma. Immunotherapy is the typical front-line treatment, although the efficacy of treatment has been called into question by a randomized phase III placebo-controlled trial that failed to show an advantage to treatment. Typical agents are interleukin-2, interferon 2-α, or combinations. The efficacy of chemotherapy has yet to be established. Pain relief from radiotherapy for renal metastases is seen in 50% of patients, less than those of breast, prostate, and lung cancers. Furthermore, radiation doses greater than 60 Gy are often required, and duration of radiotherapy response is frequently limited. Anti-angiogenics are beginning to play an increasing role as well.

Thyroid Cancer (Algorithm 4.5-4)

Thyroid cancers may be grouped according to degree of differentiation, which dictates treatment and prognosis. The

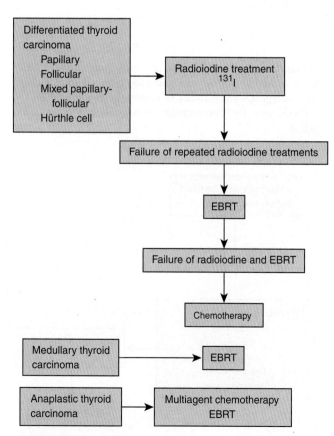

Algorithm 4.5-4. Nonoperative treatments for metastatic thyroid cancer according to subtype. EBRT, external beam radiation therapy.

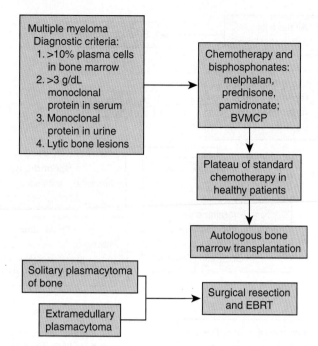

Algorithm 4.5-5. Standard nonoperative treatment for multiple myeloma and related conditions. BVMCP, carmustine (BCNU), vincristine, melphalan, cyclophosphamide, prednisone; EBRT, external beam radiation therapy.

majority of these tumors are differentiated, and radioiodine treatment for patients with increased uptake on radioiodide scans is the mainstay.

Multiple Myeloma (Algorithm 4.5-5)

Chemotherapy is the mainstay of treatment for patients with established multiple myeloma. Autologous stem cell transplantation using peripheral blood stem cells offers a survival advantage over standard chemotherapy maintenance. The opportunity for cure of multiple myeloma may only be afforded by allogeneic bone marrow transplants, but this comes with a price: the treatment-related mortality rate following allogeneic transplant approaches 30% and is highest in patients >60 years old.

Patients with solitary plasmacytoma of bone or extramedullary plasmacytoma, however, are treated by surgical resection (when feasible) and external beam radiotherapy. However, many of these patients will progress to full-blown myeloma over 10 to 15 years.

SUGGESTED READING

Bacci G, Ferrari S, Longhi A, et al. Nonmetastatic osteosarcoma of the extremity with pathologic fracture at presentation: local and systemic control by amputation or limb salvage after preoperative chemotherapy. *Acta Orthop Scand* 2003;74(4):449–454.

Enkaoua, E. A., L. Doursounian, et al. (1997). "Vertebral metastases: a critical appreciation of the preoperative prognostic tokuhashi score in a series of 71 cases." *Spine* 22(19):2293–8.

Frassica DA. General principles of external beam radiation therapy for skeletal metastases. *Clin Orthop Relat Res* 2003(Suppl):S158–164.

Fuchs B, Valenzuela RG, Sim FH. Pathologic fracture as a complication in the treatment of Ewing's sarcoma. *Clin Orthop Relat Res* 2003;(415):25–30.

Gainor BJ, Buchert P. Fracture healing in metastatic bone disease. *Clin Orthop Relat Res* 1983;178:297–302.

Mirels H. Metastatic disease in long bones: A proposed scoring system for diagnosing impending pathologic fractures. *Clin Orthop Relat Res* 1989;2003(415 Suppl):S4–13.

Ortiz EJ, Isler MH, Navia JE, et al. Pathologic fractures in children. *Clin Orthop Relat Res* 2005;(432):116–126.

Smith MR. Zoledronic acid to prevent skeletal complications in cancer: Corroborating the evidence. *Cancer Treat Rev* 2005 Oct 13 [Epub ahead of print]

Swanson KC, Pritchard DJ, Sim FH. Surgical treatment of metastatic disease of the femur. *J Am Acad Orthop Surg* 2000;8:56–65.

Tokuhashi, Y., H. Matsuzaki, et al. (1990). "Scoring system for the preoperative evaluation of metastatic spine tumor prognosis." *Spine* 15(11):1110–3.

Tomita, K., N. Kawahara, et al. (2001). "Surgical strategy for spinal metastases." *Spine* 26(3): 298–306.

Townsend PW, Smalley SR, Cozad SC, et al. Role of postoperative radiation therapy after stabilization of fractures caused by metastatic disease. *Int J Radiat Oncol Biol Phys* 1995;31:43–49.

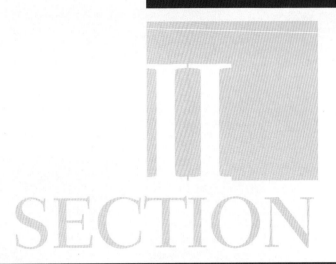

SECTION

SPECIFIC BONE NEOPLASMS AND SIMULATORS

5

BENIGN BONE TUMORS

5.1 BONE LESIONS

FELASFA M. WODAJO

OSTEOMA

Osteoma of bone is a densely mineralized endosteal lesion almost always seen in the head. The most common locations are in the ethmoid and frontal sinuses. The lesions are uniformly benign and usually discovered incidentally. In unusual cases, very large osteomas of the paranasal sinuses can cause obstruction of the nasal air ducts or other cranial symptoms. The radiographic hallmark is dense, ivory-like mineralization with smooth margins. Unless there are obstructive symptoms, observation is appropriate.

PATHOGENESIS

Etiology

- Unknown
- Component of Gardner's syndrome
  - Autosomal dominant disorder
    - Defect in adenomatosis polyposis coli gene (APC) on chromosome 5
  - Clinical manifestations
    - Intestinal polyps (familial polyposis coli)
    - Osteomas

117

■ Multiple cutaneous and subcutaneous skin lesions (sebaceous cysts, desmoids, Gardner fibromas)

Epidemiology

■ Estimated prevalence: 0.4%
■ Male:female ratio: 2:1
■ Location: ethmoid and frontal sinuses of the cranium most common

Pathophysiology

■ Osteomas are benign, indolent lesions.
■ Capacity for slow growth but no malignant potential

DIAGNOSIS (See Algorithm 5.1-1)

Clinical Features

■ Typically incidental findings on dental or other cranial radiography
■ Occasionally, very large osteomas cause sinus obstruction, loss of smell, or even in rare cases invasion into intracranial structures.

Radiographic Features

■ Plain radiographs and computed tomography (CT): smooth-contoured, densely mineralized lesion, within the medullary bone with no cortical invasion

Histologic Features

■ Mature lamellar bone with decreased marrow component
■ Sometimes haversian canals are seen within areas resembling cortical, compact bone.

Differential Diagnosis

Cemento-ossifying Fibroma (Ossifying Fibroma of Craniofacial Bones)

■ This is also another ossifying lesion of the cranium, but more often found in the mandible than the maxilla and cranial bones.
■ It must be distinguished from osteoma as it may have a more aggressive course and more often requires excision.
■ It appears as a well-circumscribed ossifying matrix, occasionally with expansile remodeling.
■ In contrast to dense ossification of osteoma, the periphery of these lesions is not always completely mineralized.
■ The histological appearance is also different, showing a mix of fibrous and fibromyxoid stroma in addition to combination of woven and lamellar bone and sometimes cementum.

Osteoid Osteoma

■ These have been described in the head and neck and also appear as small, densely mineralized lesions but with the important difference of a central radiolucent nidus and often nocturnal pain relieved by salicylates, in contrast to incidental, asymptomatic osteoma.

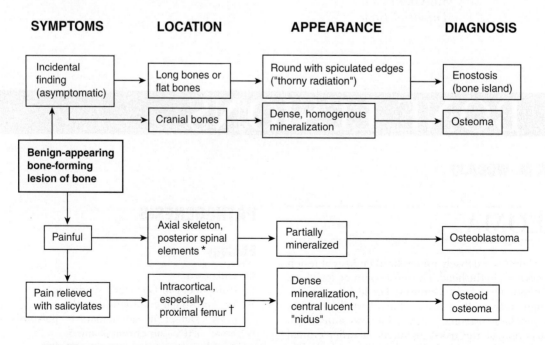

Algorithm 5.1-1. Diagnosis of benign-appearing bone-forming lesions of bone. *Most common; may also occur in long bones, but rarely. †Most common; may also occur in posterior spinal elements and flat bone.

Chronic Sclerosing Osteomyelitis

- Low-grade bone infections, presumably of oral origin, occur in the maxilla and mandible and appear as sclerotic lesions but are usually discovered due to symptoms.

Parosteal Osteosarcoma

- A rare juxta-cortical variant of osteoma, parosteal osteoma, is sometimes confused with parosteal osteosarcoma.
- The distinguishing feature of parosteal osteoma is the presence of dense, homogenous mineralization, whereas the mineralization in parosteal osteosarcoma may be incomplete and heterogeneous.

TREATMENT

Surgical Treatment

- Surgical intervention is rare as the vast majority of osteomas are asymptomatic, incidental findings.
- Excision has been occasionally reported for rare lesions with obstructive symptoms of the sinuses.

Results and Outcome (Prognosis)

- Observed lesions may progress very slowly.

ENOSTOSIS

Enostosis or "bone island" is a small, asymptomatic, densely mineralized lesion found within the cancellous bone. It is typically an incidental finding; the important diagnostic challenge often is ruling out the possibility of the lesion representing a small bone metastasis. The characteristic radiating thick trabeculae seen on imaging studies and absence of uptake on bone scan are distinguishing features.

PATHOGENESIS

- Etiology is unknown.

Epidemiology

- Most often found in adults undergoing testing for other reasons, although presumably develops at a younger age during skeletal maturation
- No gender predilection or inheritance pattern
- Distribution
    - Found within cancellous bone
    - Preference for pelvis, femur, and other long bones
    - Relatively rare in the spine

Pathophysiology

- Disorder of endochondral ossification
    - An error in resorption of the secondary spongiosum during bone formation leads to an island of heavily calcified matrix left within the spongy, cancellous bone.
- Enostoses do not change in size over time and have no malignant potential.

DIAGNOSIS (See Algorithm 5.1-1)

Clinical Features

- Asymptomatic, incidental findings, usually discovered during evaluation for other reasons

Radiologic Features

Radiographs

- Round or ovoid, homogeneously dense, sclerotic focus in cancellous bone
- Distinctive finding is the presence of radiating bony streaks ("thorny radiation") emanating from the sclerotic center.
- Almost always small, ranging from 1 mm to 2 cm
- "Giant" bone islands, measuring up to 6 cm, have been reported, but large lesions should raise suspicion for other diagnoses.

Computed Tomography/Magnetic Resonance Imaging

- Distinctive "brush borders" are more clearly seen on CT and are diagnostic.
- Appearance on magnetic resonance imaging (MRI) examination should emulate cortical bone.

Bone Scan

- Most important radiographic feature of enostosis is the usual absence of uptake on bone scan, which—when present—differentiates it from metastatic disease.
- Occasional scintigraphically active enostoses have been described, suggesting caution in using bone scan as the only modality for diagnosis, but bone scan remains very important in diagnosis.

Histologic Features

- Features include mature lamellar pattern with haversian canals within a focus of compact (cortical) bone.
- Thickened, radiating trabeculae merge with the surrounding trabeculae in the periphery of the lesion (Fig. 5.1-1).

Differential Diagnosis

Metastasis

- Differentiating enostosis from bone metastases is the most important diagnostic challenge.
- Small blastic lesions can be seen in breast cancer and prostate cancer metastases.
- Metastases usually show increased uptake on bone scan.
- Also helpful in men is serum prostate specific antigen

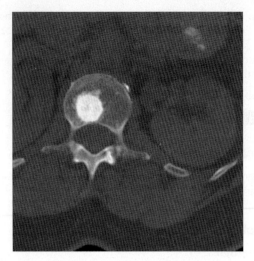

Figure 5.1-1   Enostosis in vertebral body. Note dense mineralization and thickened, radiating trabeculae.

(PSA), which is invariably elevated in metastatic prostate cancer.

Osteopoikilosis
- Osteopoikilosis is an inherited autosomal dominant disorder in which numerous enostoses are found, usually at the ends of long bones.
- Similar to isolated enostosis, no uptake is seen on bone scan.

Osteopetrosis (Albers-Schönberg Disease)
- This is typically a polyostotic disorder caused by an error in resorption of the primary spongiosum.
- The hallmark is dense osteosclerosis filling the entire medullary canal, as opposed to isolated bone islands.

Enchondroma
- A small enchondroma may be difficult to distinguish from an enostosis.
- CT imaging should help distinguish the pattern of mineralization.
- Enchondromas demonstrate incomplete mineralization with a speckled or whorled pattern in contrast to the dense, homogenous mineralization of enostoses.
- Enchondromas almost always demonstrate uptake on bone scan.

TREATMENT

Surgical Treatment
- No surgery is indicated; the main role of the consulting surgeon is to exclude other diagnostic possibilities.

Prognosis
- Observed lesions rarely progress.

OSTEOID OSTEOMA

Osteoid osteoma is a small, painful bone lesion that most commonly occurs in the cortices of long bones, with a prediction for the proximal femur. The pain pattern is usually distinctive, with nightly pain rapidly alleviated with salicylates (aspirin). The lesion has a characteristic small, radiolucent central nidus measuring up to 1 to 2 cm and thick, surrounding reactive bone. Standard treatment is percutaneous radiofrequency ablation.

PATHOGENESIS

Etiology
- Unknown
- Postulated developmental error or vascular malformation rather than a true neoplasm

Epidemiology
- Age of presentation: average 19 years (typical range 10 to 35 years)
- Youngest patient: age 2 years
- Male preponderance

Anatomic Location
- Most commonly found in the long bones, especially the femur and tibia
  - Predilection for the proximal femur
  - Less common, subperiosteal lesions have been described on the surface of long bones.
- Juxta-articular lesions: most common in the hip but have been described at many different articulations
- Spine lesions
  - Lumbar more than cervical
  - Most common in posterior elements, typically in laminae

Pathophysiology
- Presence of nerve fibers
  - Detected in the reactive zone and nidus of osteoid osteomas
  - Not seen in other bone tumors (osteoblastoma, osteosarcoma, etc.)
- Increased levels of prostaglandins also detected within nidus
  - Increased vascular pressure due to prostaglandins may stimulate afferent nerves in nidus, causing pain.
  - May explain why salicylates provide such dramatic pain relief

Natural History

The nidus does not increase in size over time, although reactive bone may become more prominent. Some authors have stated that some osteoid osteomas "burn out" over time. Infrequent painless cases have been described (1.6%

in one review of 860 patients). Nevertheless, the actual incidence of spontaneous regression is difficult to document.

DIAGNOSIS (Algorithm 5.1-1)

Clinical Features

- Clinical hallmark of osteoid osteoma is pain at rest and especially night pain.
  - The pain is dramatically relieved by salicylates (aspirin) typically within 20 to 25 minutes. While this is a reliable sign, the absence of immediate relief does not rule out the possibility of osteoid osteoma, as it occurs in only approximately 70% of patients.
- Symptoms typically occur for weeks to years before the patient seeks medical attention.
- The pain may be referred to remote anatomic locations (e.g., femur lesion presenting with leg or knee pain).
- Over time, symptoms gradually worsen, with an intermittent pain becoming a more constant ache.
- Lesions in special anatomic locations may have different presentations.
  - Juxta-articular lesions
    - May present with monoarticular arthropathy consisting of joint effusion and synovitis
    - In prolonged cases, degenerative articular changes
  - Spinal locations
    - Usually present with painful scoliosis caused by muscle spasm
    - Lesion found at the concavity of the curve

Radiologic Features

Radiography
- Small, sclerotic intracortical lesion with a central radiolucent nidus
- Intracortical lesions: easy to detect on plain radiography due to thick, dense reactive sclerosis. Often, the central, radiolucent nidus is visible on radiographs if the appropriate projection is obtained (Fig. 5.1-3).
  - Intramedullary or endosteal lesions: less reactive bone formation and more difficult to diagnose radiographically (see Fig. 5.1-3)
  - Subperiosteal lesions: may be extremely difficult to see on plain radiographs

CT
- CT is the definitive study modality, allowing for exact localization of nidus.
- Protocol: thin (2-mm) cuts
- Findings: The combination of thick, uniform reactive bone surrounding a central, 1- to 2-cm or less radiolucent nidus is highly suggestive of osteoid osteoma.
- Subperiosteal osteoid osteomas also have a radiolucent nidus but incite a less dense, nonconfluent ("shaggy") reactive bone formation.

Bone Scan
- Increased uptake is always identified in active osteoid osteomas.
- Scintigraphy is very sensitive for detecting the nidus and especially useful in subperiosteal and intra-articular le-

sions, which may be missed on plain radiography. Increased radiotracer activity is seen on immediate and delayed phases.
- "Double-density" sign: small focus of increased activity corresponding to nidus surrounded by larger, less intensely active region corresponding to the surrounding reactive bone

MRI
- MRI is of questionable value, as the large area of marrow and soft tissue edema can obscure diagnosis.
- It may be helpful in suspected cases of juxta-articular osteoid osteoma, where intense marrow edema in only one bone may be the initial clue.

Histologic Features

- The nidus of osteoid osteoma is a small, discrete lesion with disorganized seams of unmineralized or partially mineralized osteoid with prominent osteoblastic and osteoclastic activity.
- The spaces between the osteoid seams contain highly vascular, fibrous stroma.
- Toward the periphery, the osteoid is more mature and dense with smaller osteoblasts.

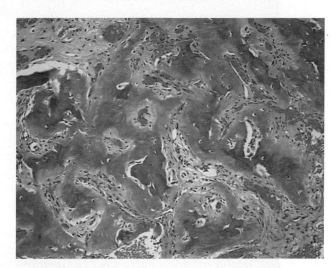

Figure 5.2-1 Histology for both osteoid osteoma and osteoblastoma show similar disorganized woven bone with intervening fibrovascular stroma.

Differential Diagnosis

Stress Reaction
- Differentiating stress reaction (stress fracture) from osteoid osteoma is not an uncommon dilemma in young patients.
- Both often present with unicortical periosteal reaction and pain.
- The pain pattern is typically diurnal and related to weight bearing on the affected extremity in stress reaction and nocturnal and nonmechanical in osteoid osteoma.
- Reactive bone formation runs transverse to long axis of bone in stress reaction rather than parallel to it in osteoid osteoma.

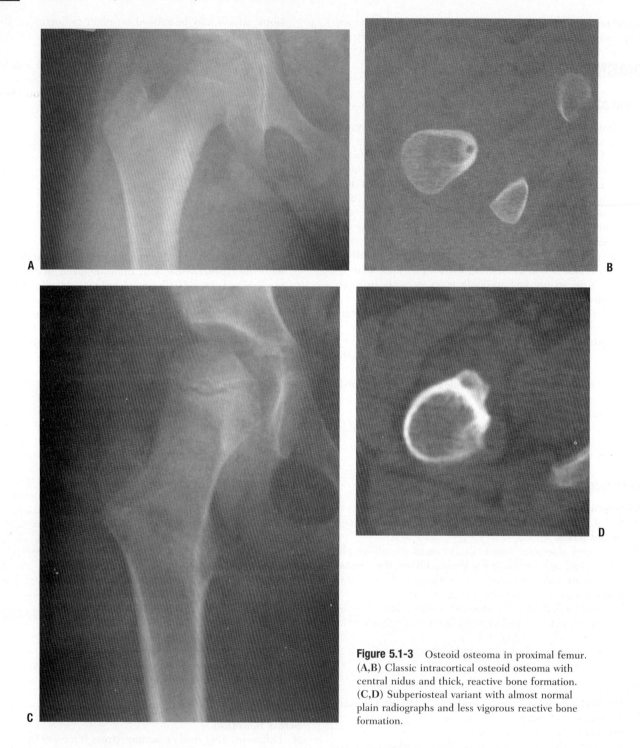

Figure 5.1-3 Osteoid osteoma in proximal femur. (A,B) Classic intracortical osteoid osteoma with central nidus and thick, reactive bone formation. (C,D) Subperiosteal variant with almost normal plain radiographs and less vigorous reactive bone formation.

Chronic Osteomyelitis (Brodie's Abscess)

- Chronic osteomyelitis in bone may present with thick reactive bone formation and central lucency.
- If there is a radiolucent central region, it is often larger than 2 cm.
- Bone scan should be beneficial, demonstrating center photopenia in infection, representing the necrotic sequestrum, versus intense central uptake representing the nidus in osteoid osteoma.
- MRI may not be helpful in distinguishing the two as both infection and osteoid osteoma may demonstrate extensive soft tissue and marrow edema.

Enostosis

- Enostosis also appears as a sclerotic intraosseous lesion but should be painless and lacking uptake on scintigraphy.
- Also helpful should be the brush borders of thickened trabeculae emanating from central, sclerotic core seen on CT in enostosis.

Osteoblastoma

- Although osteoblastoma is commonly grouped in the differential diagnosis of osteoid osteoma, it is a radiographically and histologically distinct entity.
- It is larger, with the nidus of osteoid osteomas rarely exceeding 2 cm in size, and comparatively only partially mineralized with a thin, expansile rim of sclerotic bone.

Intracortical Hemangioma

- Hemangioma of bone is most common in the vertebral bodies, where it presents with vertical, thickened trabeculae.
- It can also present as single or multiple sclerotic appendicular skeletal lesions.
- While some patients may experience pain, the nocturnal pattern and response to salicylates help distinguish the two.
- The lesions tend to be less well circumscribed, without the typical central lucent nidus.

TREATMENT

Surgical Management

- Although there may be some capacity for osteoid osteomas to spontaneously regress, in general definitive operative or medical treatment is indicated for all symptomatic osteoid osteomas.

Preferred Treatment

- Radiofrequency ablation (RFA) is performed as an outpatient procedure under CT guidance. Heat generated in the tissues near the tip of the probe necroses a small portion of bone and, presumably, the nidus.
- Contraindications include spinal lesions near cord or nerve root, subchondral lesions near articular surface, and inaccessible lesions.

Alternative Treatment

- Intralesional resection of the nidus (curettage)
- Indications include recurrent tumors not amenable to repeat RFA and lesions for which the diagnosis is in doubt.
- The main surgical challenge is locating the small nidus intraoperatively. Several techniques have been described:
  - Preoperative CT-guided localization via an implanted wire
  - Intraoperative nuclear scintigraphy (preoperative dye administration)
  - Preoperative fluorescent tetracycline labeling

Medical Treatment

- Salicylates or nonsteroidal anti-inflammatory agents (NSAIDs)
- Median duration of treatment before resolution of symptoms: 30 months

Results and Outcome

- The success rate of RFA is 80% to 90%. If initial treatment is unsuccessful, a second procedure is successful in most instances.
- Success rate for open curettage has been reported to be approximately 90%.
- Scoliosis induced by osteoid osteoma corrects after treatment of osteoid osteoma.
- The use of NSAIDs alone was reported to result in resolution of symptoms in approximately 70% of patients after a mean of 2.5 years in one study.

OSTEOBLASTOMA

Osteoblastoma is a benign, locally aggressive bone neoplasm in which abundant, plump osteoblasts produce disorganized and immature osteoid. It appears as a radiolucent, sometimes expansile, lesion with hazy mineralization and a thin sclerotic rim. It has a predilection for the spine and tends to recur if not completely excised.

PATHOGENESIS

- Etiology is unknown.

EPIDEMIOLOGY

- 1% of primary bone tumors and 3% of benign bone tumors
- Peak occurrence is in the first to third decades, with 80% of cases occurring in patients under 30 years old.
- Male:female ratio 2:1
- Distribution
  - Predilection for the spine (60% to 70% of cases)
  - Equally in cervical, thoracic, and lumbar regions
  - More commonly in the posterior elements (66% in one series)
  - Nonaxial tumors can be found in round or flat bones as well as cranial bones
    - Within the long bones, metaphyseal = diaphyseal, proximal femur > distal femur, proximal tibia
    - Also in juxtacortical or periosteal locations, with an appearance somewhat analogous to osteoid osteoma, except with a much larger, central lucent area

NATURAL HISTORY

Although histologically similar in some respects to osteoid osteoma, osteoblastoma is a distinct entity with a different natural history—one of progression rather than stasis or regression. A range of manifestations has been observed, from indolent growth to aggressive local growth.

In aggressive tumors, there is a tendency for multiple recurrences over a long period of time. Disease-free periods of up to 17 years have been reported. One patient had 11 surgeries over 30 years. However, even with multiple recurrences, the tumor typically remains benign. Nevertheless, rare cases of sarcomatous transformation have been described.

DIAGNOSIS (see Algorithm 5.1-1)

Clinical Features

- Pain is a typical symptom.
  - Often it is dull and aching.
  - Duration of 6 to 12 months before diagnosis
  - Rarely discovered incidentally
  - Nocturnal pain, like that seen in osteoid osteoma, is rare.
  - Not relieved by salicylates or NSAIDs
- Physical examination reveals tenderness over tumor site.
- Spinal osteoblastomas can cause painful scoliosis.
  - Objective neurologic findings in 29% of patients in one series
  - Deficits mostly minimal (e.g., muscle weakness, sensory disturbance, or abnormal reflexes), although two patients had neurogenic bladders and paraparesis

Radiologic Features

Radiographs

- Typical appearance is of radiolucent lesion with faint densities.

- A large range of radiographic appearances have been noted.
  - Cortical expansion is common, especially in the spine (Fig. 5.1-4), where there may be a significant aneurysmal component.
  - Dense mineralization may be seen in longstanding lesions or after radiotherapy.
  - Reactive bone formation is seen in lesions arising in cortex and less so with intramedullary lesions.

CT

- CT scanning shows more detail, outlining more clearly the sclerotic rim surrounding and separating the lesion from adjacent soft tissues or surrounding bone.
- CT is also better for showing the sometimes subtle hazy mineralization of the lesion itself (see Fig. 5.1-3).

Histologic Features (See Fig 5.1-2)

- Disorganized seams of abundant osteoid production in the form of woven bone
  - Similar to that of the central nidus in osteoid osteoma but without the tendency toward more organized, mature trabeculae seen toward the periphery
  - "Epithelioid" osteoblasts (rounded and larger than normal)
- Frequently seen: vascular spaces and giant cells, the latter of which are not normally seen in osteoid osteoma

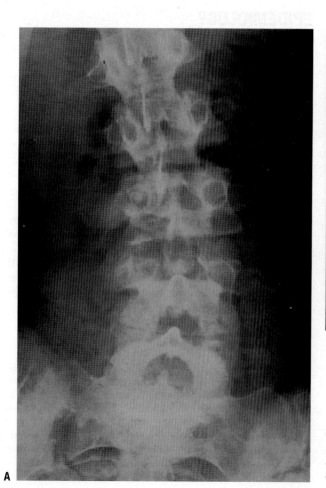

A

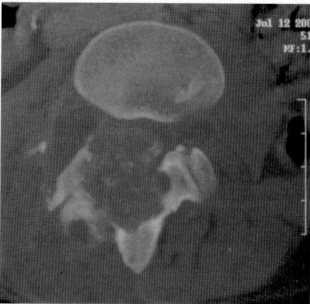

B

Figure 5.1-4   Osteoblastoma in lumbar spine. (**A**) Plain radiograph showing expansile, osteoblastic lesion with scoliosis. The lesion is in concavity. (**B**) CT scan showing expansile lesion in posterior spinal elements with faint calcifications and thin, incomplete sclerotic rim.

Differential Diagnosis

Osteoid Osteoma
- Clinically, the characteristic nocturnal pain of osteoid osteoma is not typical of osteoblastoma.
- No distinct small nidus is seen on imaging studies.
- Histologically, the large vascular spaces and giant cells seen in osteoblastoma are not common in osteoid osteoma.

Aneurysmal Bone Cyst
- These can resemble osteoblastoma radiographically and histologically.
- In particular, osteoblastomas have a known propensity for secondary aneurysmal cyst formation.
- If osteoblastoma is suspected in a resected aneurysmal bone cyst, thorough sampling of the tumor is necessary to locate what may be only a small, focal area of osteoblastoma.
- Disorganized osteoid seams and osteoblastic proliferation should be absent in primary aneurysmal bone cyst.

Giant Cell Tumor of Bone
- The similarity in the age of presentation of the two tumors and the presence of giant cells on histological examination of osteoblastoma may be a source of confusion.
- No mineralization is found in giant cell tumor.
- Further, giant cell tumor is less common in the spine and more common anteriorly, in the vertebral bodies, when it does occur.

Chondroblastoma
- Chondroblastoma may also present as an intraosseous lesion with stippled radiodensities.
- It is almost exclusively seen in the epiphyses of long bones.
- Histology also shows immature cartilage (chondroid), not seen in osteoblastoma.

Low-Grade Osteosarcoma
- Imaging studies should be distinctive, with conventional osteosarcoma rarely showing a sclerotic rim and dense, surrounding, reactive bone formation.
- Disorganized and immature osteoid is seen in osteosarcoma, but the hallmarks of malignancy (e.g., cellular and nuclear pleomorphism and mitoses) are absent in osteoblastoma.

TREATMENT

Surgical Treatment

Recommended Treatment
- Complete intralesional resection is recommended.
- The use of a physical adjuvant, such as phenol or liquid nitrogen, may help reduce the risk of recurrence.
- Wide resection may be considered in expendable bones such as rib, fibula, or metacarpals.

Indications
- All tumors undergo surgical resection due to natural history of progressive growth and worsening symptoms in untreated tumors.

Adjuvant Treatments
- Adjuvant radiation has been used but probably should be reserved for recurrent or inoperable lesions. Radiation may increase the risk of sarcomatous transformation.

Results and Outcome

Complete excision is typically curative. Local recurrence is higher in difficult anatomic locations, such as the spine. In one series of 23 patients across multiple institutions, two recurrences were reported, one patient with a disease-free interval of 17 years and one patient who had 11 operations over 27 years. In another series of 53 patients with more than 1 year of follow-up, 3 of 27 of spinal lesions recurred, 2 in patients who received adjuvant radiation, and 4 of 15 extremity lesions recurred, 1 in a patient who received postoperative radiation.

Cases of mortality and amputation have been reported due to aggressive and repeated local growth of the tumor in the spine and extremities.

Acknowledgments

I gratefully acknowledge research assistance by Brittany L. Rice, MLS, AHIP, and Smita Jhaveri at the Suburban Hospital Medical Library.

SUGGESTED READING

Beauchamp CP, Duncan CP, Dzus AK, et al. Osteoblastoma: experience with 23 patients. Can J Surg 1992;35:199–202.

Greenspan A. Benign bone-forming lesions: osteoma, osteoid osteoma, and osteoblastoma. Clinical, imaging, pathologic, and differential considerations. Skel Radiol 1993;22:485–500.

Greenspan A. Bone island (enostosis): current concept—a review. Skel Radiol 1995;24:111–115.

Ilyas I, Younge DA. Medical management of osteoid osteoma. Can J Surg 2002;45:435–437.

Marsh BW, Bonfiglio M, Brady LP, et al. Benign osteoblastoma: range of manifestations. J Bone Joint Surg [Am] 1975;57:1–9.

Nemoto O, Moser RP, Van Dam BE, et al. Osteoblastoma of the spine: a review of 75 cases. Spine 1990;15:1272–1280.

O'Connell JX, Nanthakumar SS, Nielsen GP, et al. Osteoid osteoma: the uniquely innervated bone tumor. Mod Pathol 1998;11:175–180.

Rimondi E, Bianchi G, Malaguti MC, et al. Radiofrequency thermoablation of primary non-spinal osteoid osteoma: optimization of the procedure. Eur Radiol 2005;15:1393–1399.

Sciubba JJ, Younai F. Ossifying fibroma of the mandible and maxilla: review of 18 cases. J Oral Pathol Med 1989;18:315–321.

Shankman S, Desai P, Beltran J. Subperiosteal osteoid osteoma: radiographic and pathologic manifestations. Skel Radiol 1997;26:457–462.

Torriani M, Rosenthal DI. Percutaneous radiofrequency treatment of osteoid osteoma. Pediatr Radiol 2002;32:615–618.

Vanhoenacker FM, De Beuckeleer LH, Van Hul W, et al. Sclerosing bone dysplasias: genetic and radioclinical features. Eur Radiol 2000;10:1423–1433.

5.2 CARTILAGE LESIONS

FELASFA M. WODAJO

CHONDROMAS

Chondromas, according to the latest World Health Organization classification, include enchondroma, periosteal chondroma, and enchondromatosis. The common thread is that all chondromas are tumors of hyaline cartilage. This distinguishes them from other cartilage tumors such as chondroblastomas and chondromyxoid fibromas, which are tumors of immature cartilage. The tumors of hyaline cartilage share a characteristic pattern of cartilage mineralization, evident radiographically, that allows them to be recognized with a great degree of certainty (Fig. 5.2-1). Enchondroma is the intramedullary variety, periosteal chondroma is the surface counterpart, and enchondromatosis is the congenital chondroma disorder. The latter is described in more detail in Chapter 7, Congenital and Inherited Bone Conditions.

ENCHONDROMA

Enchondromas are benign intramedullary lesions consisting of mature hyaline cartilage. They are common findings in the long bones and are generally asymptomatic.

PATHOGENESIS

Etiology

- Enchondromas are thought to arise from small rests of physeal cartilage entrapped in the metaphysis of growing bones.
- Chromosomal abnormalities of 6 and 12 noted in some.

Epidemiology

- Frequency: second most common benign chondroid lesion, after osteochondroma
  - 3% to 17% of all primary bone tumors
  - Autopsy studies: 1.7% of distal femoral metaphyses contain cartilage rests
  - Most lesions are asymptomatic, and therefore the true incidence is probably higher.
- No gender predilection has been noted.
- Distribution
  - Most common location: small bones of hand (40% to 65% of lesions)
    - Uncommon in distal phalanx
    - Less common in small bones of the feet
  - Common in the long bones (25%)
    - Femur > humerus
  - Solitary enchondromas of flat bones (rib, sternum, scapula): rare

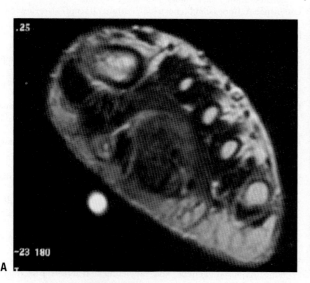
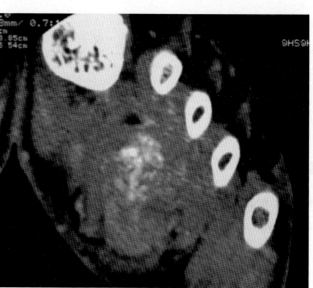

Figure 5.2-1   Soft tissue chondroma in the foot. Large, deep mass with areas of dark T1 signal on MRI (**A**) corresponding to mineralized portions well visualized on CT (**B**).

- Intramedullary cartilage lesion in these bones should lead to concern for chondrosarcoma.
  - In the ribs, chondrosarcoma usually at anterior costochondral junction
- Solitary enchondromas of the pelvis: very rare
  - Exception: enchondromatosis
  - Converse: Chondrosarcoma is relatively common in the pelvis.
- Solitary enchondromas of spine: rare
  - Converse: Chondrosarcoma is the second most common nonlymphoproliferative primary tumor of the spine after chordoma.

Natural History

In general, enchondromas are considered benign, indolent lesions. Slow or no growth is expected. Pathologic fracture through enchondromas in the hands and feet is not uncommon.

Malignant Transformation

- Transformation of enchondromas to malignant chondrosarcoma has been well described (Fig. 5.2-2).
- The actual incidence is controversial. Rates of transformation of up to 2% to 3% of large (3 to 7 cm) enchondromas have been suggested.

Atypical or Aggressive Enchondroma (Grade 1/2 Chondrosarcoma; Chondrosarcoma In Situ)

- More common than malignant transformation
- Painful intramedullary enchondroma that fills the marrow cavity and demonstrates deep (>50%) endosteal scalloping
- No significant metastatic potential has been described, but they nevertheless should undergo intralesional excision.

Ollier's Disease (also see Chapter 7.3)

- Nonhereditary congenital disease with multiple intramedullary foci of cartilage
- Ranges in presentation from asymptomatic enchondromatosis to significant growth disturbances, including bone shortening and deformity
- Often unilateral or even single limb in its distribution
- Significantly increased risk of secondary transformation to chondrosarcoma, with rates described as high as 5% to 30%

Maffucci's Syndrome (also see Chapter 7.3)

- Another disorder with multiple enchondromas but in association with soft tissue lesions, most commonly hemangiomas
- Predilection for hands and wrist
- Soft tissue lesions are usually in the same extremity.

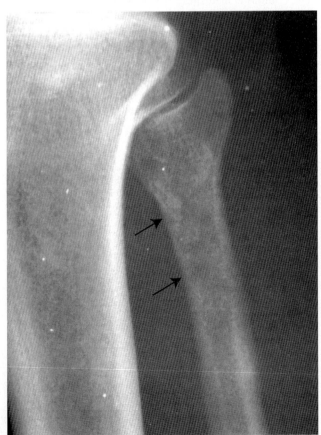

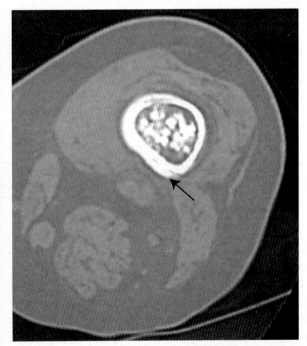

Figure 5.2-2   Transformed enchondroma. **(A)** Plain radiograph of a painful lesion in proximal fibula with extensive endosteal scalloping, consistent with an aggressive enchondroma or "carcinoma in situ." **(B)** CT scan of distal femur cartilage lesion with periosteal bone reaction indicative of grade 1 or higher chondrosarcoma.

■ Increased risk for developing chondrosarcoma, other sarcomas, and even other, nonskeletal malignancies

DIAGNOSIS (see Algorithm 5.2-1)

Clinical Features

Most common presentation is as an incidental finding, often in adults undergoing evaluation for other reasons. Often there is a history of knee or shoulder pain. In one series, magnetic resonance imaging (MRI) demonstrated that 81% of patients with proximal humerus enchondromas also had another shoulder disorder potentially causing pain.

Therefore, for patients with vague, nonlocalized pain and in the presence of an enchondroma, therapeutic measures such as steroid injections or physical therapy should be administered for both diagnostic and therapeutic reasons.

Radiologic Features

Radiographs
■ Long bones
 ■ Mineralized central or eccentric metaphyseal or diaphyseal lesion
  ■ Punctate rings and arcs mineralization pattern indicative of hyaline cartilage
 ■ Large majority (95%) of lesions demonstrate at least partial mineralization.
 ■ Typically <6 cm in size, but also sometimes extending for longer lengths (Fig. 5.2-3)
■ Short tubular bones of the hands and feet

■ Appearance may be somewhat different
 ■ Deep endosteal scalloping
 ■ Minimal radiographic mineralization
 ■ Well demarcated and sometimes extend to the ends of the bones (see Fig. 5.2-3)
 ■ Periosteal reaction and cortical disruption are seen in the setting of pathologic fracture.

Computed Tomography
■ Computed tomography (CT) is useful for detecting mineralization and extent of endosteal scalloping (see Fig. 5.2-3).
■ The depth and length of endosteal scalloping have been identified as helpful in distinguishing enchondroma versus chondrosarcoma (Box 5.2-1 and Fig. 5.2-2).

MRI
■ MRI is useful for determining marrow extent and the presence of soft tissue extension, if any.
■ The lobular nature of enchondromas is demonstrated well on T2-weighted images (see Fig. 5.2-3).
■ The dark areas on T1 and T2 represent mineralized portions. However, the value of MRI may be more in diagnosing the source of pain in the patient with a solitary enchondroma discovered incidentally during evaluation of knee or shoulder pain.

Bone Scan
■ Variable patterns of uptake can be seen on bone scintigraphy.
■ Some authors have proposed that uptake less than the anterior iliac spine is consistent with the diagnosis of enchondroma.

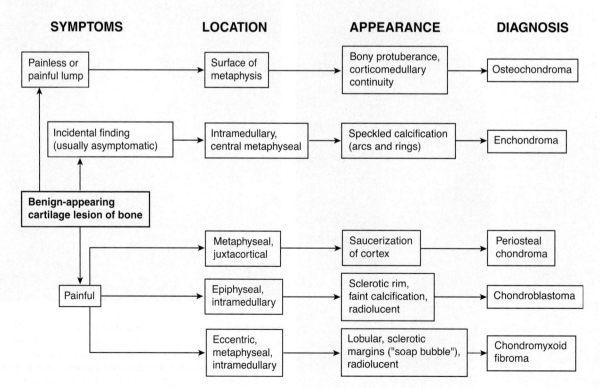

Algorithm 5.2-1.   Diagnosis of benign-appearing cartilage lesions of one.

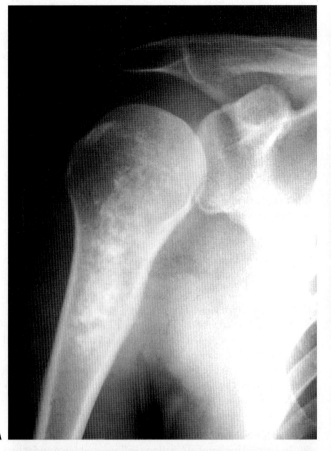

A

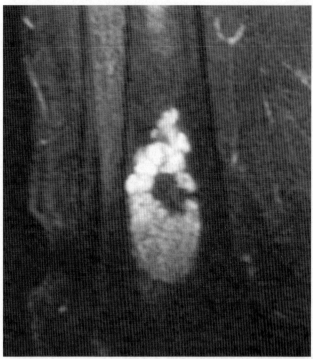

C

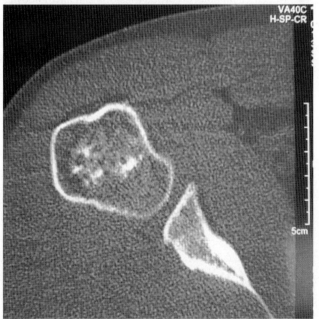

B

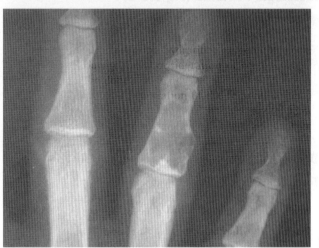

D

Figure 5.2-3   Enchondroma in various locations. Proximal
humerus, radiograph showing typical metaphyseal–diaphyseal
location (**A**) and CT scan showing speckles and whorls of cartilage
mineralization (**B**). (**C**) T2-weighted MRI of distal femur
enchondroma showing the lobular pattern of growth. (**D**) Plain
radiograph of phalangeal enchondroma showing lesion extending to
ends of bones and thinning and expanding the cortex.

BOX 5.2-1 OBJECTIVE SIGNS WORRISOME FOR MALIGNANT TRANSFORMATION OF ENCHONDROMAS

- Periosteal reaction, cortical destruction, and especially soft tissue extension
- Lysis within a previously mineralized area
- Deep cortical scalloping, especially greater than two thirds of thickness (see Fig. 5.2-2)
  - Chondrosarcomas have focal areas of greater than two-thirds scalloping in 90% of cases, enchondromas only 10% of cases
  - Longitudinal extent of scalloping is throughout the length of the lesion in 79% of chondrosarcomas, as opposed to a shorter extent in enchondromas.
- Large unmineralized areas or faint, amorphous calcification
- Medullary fill of >90%
- Large lesions: 50% of chondrosarcomas are >10 cm
- Bone scan radiotracer uptake greater than anterior superior iliac spine

Histologic Features (Fig 7.3-6)

- Mature lobules of hyaline cartilage, separated by hematopoietic marrow
- Focal myxoid change may be seen.
- Long bones: Cartilage should be relatively hypocellular, with only scattered binucleate cells.
- Lesions from the hands and feet: Hypercellularity is common, but the diagnosis of chondrosarcoma should almost never be made in those anatomic locations.

Differential Diagnosis

Intramedullary Infarct
- Also typically an incidental, asymptomatic finding, but mineralization appears more cloud-like or wispy, without typical arcs and rings calcification of cartilage
- It is more common with a history of steroid use or sickle cell disease.

Enostosis
- Enostoses or "bone islands" are also asymptomatic, incidental findings, but they have distinctive radiographic and CT findings.
- The lesions have dense, ivory-like mineralization and are rarely larger than 2 to 3 cm. The periphery demonstrates a brush-border pattern of trabeculation on CT, and no uptake is seen on bone scan.

Chondrosarcoma
- Differentiating between enchondroma and low-grade chondrosarcoma may be difficult (refer to text above and Box 5.2-1).
- Cortical disruption, periosteal reaction, and deep endosteal scalloping are associated with more aggressive cartilage lesions.

TREATMENT

Biopsy
- It is difficult to differentiate grade I chondrosarcoma from benign enchondroma by tissue examination alone.
- Radiologic and clinical correlation is essential, and therefore biopsy should be reserved for selected chondroid lesions with radiologically or clinically worrisome signs.

Surgical Indications/Contraindications

Observation
- Most lesions need no surgery.
- On careful search, the pain in the region of the lesion is found to be due to other causes.
- Simple follow-up of the lesion initially at 3- to 6-month intervals is indicated.

Pathologic Fracture Treatment
- For enchondromas of the short tubular bones that present with pathologic fracture, the phalanx is immobilized until the fracture heals.
- If the cortices are thinned such that future fractures are predicted, the enchondroma is curetted and the cavity packed with bone graft or bone cement.

Operative Management
- Indicated for painful cartilage lesions that have endosteal scalloping but not periosteal reaction or cortical disruption (i.e., "aggressive" enchondromas or "chondrosarcoma in situ"); intralesional excision is recommended. Some authors recommend the use of physical adjuvants such as phenol or liquid nitrogen to reduce the risk of recurrence.
- Intramedullary cartilage lesions of the pelvis are considered malignant and should be resected with wide margins.

Results and Outcome
- Recurrence is rare after intralesional excision of enchondromas in the long bones or short tubular bones.

PERIOSTEAL CHONDROMA

Periosteal or juxtacortical chondromas are small, mildly painful lesions of the metaphyseal long bones; the etiology is unknown. They are uncommon and have distinctive radiographic features consisting of a sclerotic saucerization of the cortex and small size. Cellular atypia and hypercellularity are common despite the benign nature of the lesion. Curettage of the lesion is usually curative.

PATHOGENESIS

Epidemiology

- Mean age: 23 years
- Gender: no gender predilection
- Distribution: By definition, the tumor occurs in a juxta-cortical location, often in the metaphyseal portion of long bones. The most common site in one series was the proximal humerus, but other reported cases have varied in location between small and large long bones.

Natural History

- Slow growth; no malignant potential

DIAGNOSIS (see Algorithm 5.2-1)

Clinical Features

- Patients present with mild pain of long duration, often present for 1 or more years.
- If the lesion is superficial, they may also note slowly growing mass.
- The lesion can also be discovered incidentally.

Radiologic Features

Radiographs
- Plain films are often diagnostic.
  - Well-defined "saucerization" of the cortex adjacent to a slightly mineralized soft tissue lesion
  - Thin rim of periosteal bone may extend over lesion (Fig. 5.2-4)
  - No intramedullary extension of the lesion

CT
- CT may demonstrate better the mineralization of the lesion.
- The mean size of periosteal chondromas is about 2.6 cm, with a round or oval shape, aligned to long axis of bone.

Histologic Features (Fig. 7.3-6)
- Lobules of mature hyaline cartilage
- Frequently, hypercellularity, binucleate chondrocytes, and focal, mild cytologic atypia
  - These do not have the same significance as with intramedullary cartilage lesions.
- Reactive bone formation is seen at the junction of tumor and periosteum.

Differential Diagnosis

Soft Tissue Tumor Pressing on Bone
- Extraosseous soft tissue tumors can also present with cortical scalloping and may be difficult to distinguish from periosteal chondroma.
- The absence of mineralization and size significantly

greater than a few centimeters would point toward another diagnosis.

Fibrous Cortical Defect
- This is also a metaphyseal lesion, sometimes contained entirely within the cortex.
- It is more commonly seen in skeletally immature subjects but is rarely symptomatic.
- The matrix is fibrous, without the speckled calcification of cartilage, and a surrounding rind of periosteal bone is not seen.

Periosteal Chondrosarcoma
- Chondrosarcoma arising from the periosteal surface has been described.
- It is rare and may be difficult to distinguish histologically from benign chondroma.
- The absence of a well-defined sclerotic rim of cortex and intramedullary extension of the lesion are worrisome signs.

TREATMENT

Surgical Indications/Contraindications

- Symptomatic lesions should undergo excision.
- Most lesions are small, and thus there is no need for separate biopsy if the radiological and clinical presentation is typical. Intralesional excision (curettage) is typically curative, but en bloc excision is better.

Results and Outcome

- Recurrence after intralesional or en bloc excision is rare.

OSTEOCHONDROMA

Osteochondromas are common benign bone lesions that occur as osteocartilaginous bony prominences arising from the metaphyses of growing bones. Their growth parallels the growth of the host bone. Asymptomatic, solitary osteochondromas require no treatment. There is a familial form presenting with many, even dozens of exostoses. These patients are at increased risk for mechanical and growth complications and secondary malignant transformation of the cartilage cap. The familial form is discussed in detail in Chapter 7.3.

PATHOGENESIS

Etiology

- Most are developmental lesions rather than true neoplasms, but inactivation of both copies of the EXT1 tumor suppressor gene is necessary for development.
  - Small herniation of physeal tissue into metaphysis,

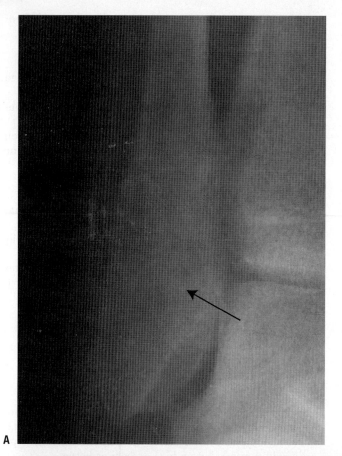

A

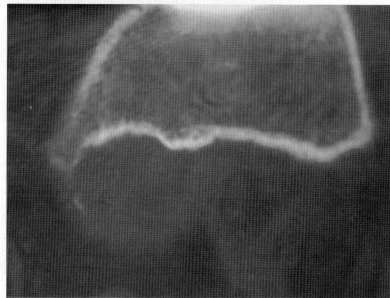

B

Figure 5.2-4 Periosteal chondroma. Plain radiograph of distal fibula showing a metaphyseal lesion with sclerotic rim (**A**). CT scan of distal femur showing scalloping of metaphyseal bone and minimally mineralized juxtacortical soft tissue lesion (**B**).

past the periosteal bone cuff (groove of Ranvier) during skeletal growth

- Growth of the exostosis parallels that of the growth plate.
- Growth ceases with skeletal maturity.

- The minority are the result of iatrogenic injury to the growth plate, such as following surgery or irradiation.

Epidemiology

- Frequency
    - Most common tumors of bone
    - 10% to 15% of all bone tumors
    - 20% to 50% of benign bone tumors
- Age: peak within second decade or earlier
- Male:female 1.6 to 3.4:1
- Distribution
    - 50% occur in lower extremity long bones (especially about the knee).
    - Less commonly in short tubular bones and flat bones (e.g., pelvis, scapula)

Natural History

- Growth continues until the host bone reaches skeletal maturity, then ceases.
- Secondary chondrosarcoma
    - Very small but documented risk of developing in the cartilage cap
    - Exact incidence unknown (probably <1%)
    - Worrisome signs for secondary malignancy: pain and continued or recurrent growth of exostosis after skeletal maturity

DIAGNOSIS (see Algorithm 5.2-1)

Clinical Features

- Typical clinical history: nontender, painless bony bump
- Bursal pain
    - Most common locations for large bursa formation: scapula (>50% of cases), lesser trochanter, shoulder
    - Bursal contents: inflammatory fluid, hemorrhage, metaplastic cartilage formation (secondary form of synovial chondromatosis)
    - Do not confuse secondary synovial chondromatosis within osteochondroma bursa for malignant degeneration to chondrosarcoma!
- Occasional associated symptoms: restricted joint motion, snapping of tendons, subscapular crepitus/snapping, fracture of pedunculated osteochondroma
- Neurovascular complications: rare
    - Pseudoaneurysm formation and compression neuropathies
    - Popliteal artery and peroneal nerve most commonly affected

Radiologic Features

Radiographs

- Plain film features characteristic and often diagnostic
    - Bony protrusion containing cortical and medullary bone with overlying cartilage cap

- Both cortical surface and medullary cavity of the host bone contiguous with those of the osteochondroma (Fig. 5.2-5)
- Mineralization of cartilage cap is not always visualized on plain radiography.
- Two general radiographic forms
    - "Sessile" osteochondromas: broad attachment to host bone
    - "Pedunculated" osteochondromas: narrow stalk connection to host bone

CT

- Very good modality for demonstrating cortical and medullary continuity, especially in areas of complex anatomy such as pelvis and spine
- Used to measure thickness of cartilage cap (not as good as MRI)
- Evaluate for worrisome signs of secondary malignancy
    - Focal regions of radiolucency
    - Destruction of adjacent bone
    - Contiguous soft tissue mass with scattered mineralization

MRI

- Test of choice to evaluate thickness of cartilage cap
    - Normal cartilage cap thickness: 1 to 3 cm in young patients (smaller in adults)
    - Abnormal cap thickness: >1.5 cm in adults should be viewed with suspicion
- Useful in demonstrating the presence of corticomedullary continuity, especially of the medullary marrow
- Contrast enhancement typically restricted to the septa between lobules and to peripheral perichondrium covering cartilage

Bone Scan

- Uptake on scintigraphy generally decreases as enchondral ossification slows toward skeletal maturity. This is, however, not reliable in distinguishing secondary malignancy.

Histologic Features

- Gross appearance: bony stalk with overlying cartilage cap
    - Cartilage cap of osteochondromas often irregular, with areas of invagination into the underlying bone (accounts for heterogeneity of large osteochondromas observed on imaging studies)
- Histology: Cartilage cap chondrocytes may be arranged in a columnar format, similar to physeal plate (Fig. 7.3-8)
    - Mild hypercellularity and some binucleate cells may be found.

Differential Diagnosis

Subungual Exostosis

- Subungual exostosis is a distinct pathological entity that is exclusively found on the dorsal aspect of the distal

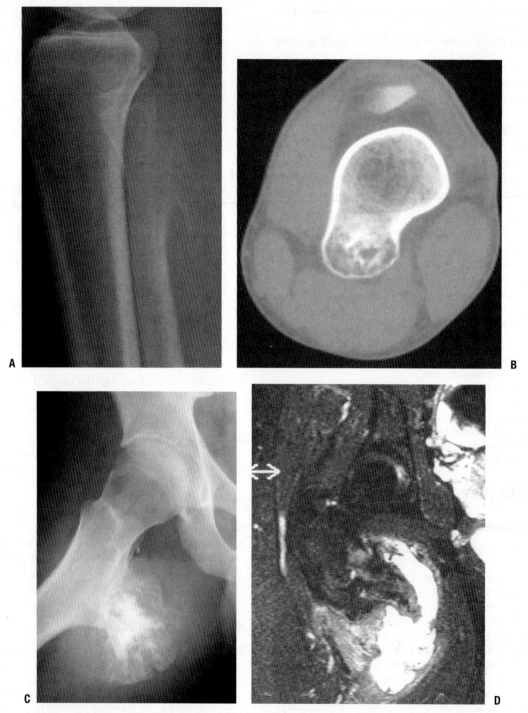

Figure 5.2-5 Solitary osteochondromas. Plain radiograph of pedunculated osteochondroma in proximal fibula (**A**) and CT scan of sessile osteochondroma in distal femur (**B**). Note corticomedullary continuity. Plain radiograph of large proximal femur osteochondroma with large, secondary bursa (**C**), which, when seen on T2-weighted MRI (**D**), could be mistaken for overgrown cartilage cap and malignancy.

phalanges, with the most common location being the big toe.

■ The overlying nail bed is usually deformed.
■ Radiologically, corticomedullary continuity is not seen; histologically, fibrous proliferation with cartilage metaplasia is seen.

Dysplasia Epiphysealis Hemimelica (Trevor's Disease)

■ This is a rare (1:1,000,000) variant of osteochondroma that arises from the epiphysis of one or more bones of a single lower extremity.
■ It has no hereditary component.

It may cause premature closure of physis or growth deformity but has no known malignant potential.

Periosteal (Juxtacortical) Chondroma
- This appears as a small soft tissue mass adjacent to bone with smooth scalloping of the underlying cortex.
- In contrast to an osteochondroma, only a thin shelf of mineralized periosteum covers a portion of the lesion.

Heterotopic Ossification
- Longstanding peri-articular heterotopic ossification, especially around the hip, may become confluent with adjacent bone and radiographically mimic osteochondroma.
- A history that includes known predisposing factors such as previous hip surgery or paraplegia and the absence of corticomedullary continuity should allow for distinction.

Parosteal Osteosarcoma
- This is a low-grade variant of osteosarcoma that grows adjacent to cortical bone, most commonly on the posterior distal femur.
- In contrast to osteochondroma, it does not recreate a central marrow cavity.
- The mineralization pattern is ivory-like and dense.

TREATMENT

- Observation is the most common treatment for solitary or multiple exostoses.
- Fractures of osteochondroma almost always heal spontaneously.
- Surgical excision is indicated for pain or occasionally for cosmesis.
- More commonly, large pedunculated lesions cause symptoms and undergo excision.
- Although unusual, repair of pseudoaneurysm and excision of the offending osteochondroma is indicated in those cases.

Results and Outcome
- Recurrence after resection of osteochondroma is related to incomplete excision of the cartilage cap and is estimated to occur 2% of the time.

CHONDROBLASTOMA

Chondroblastomas are distinctive benign bone tumors of immature cartilage cells arising within the epiphyses of long bones and are most commonly seen in patients with open physes. They commonly present with several months of peri-articular pain. The radiographic hallmarks include the epiphyseal location, sclerotic margins, and mineralized matrix, although subtle early findings often delay diagnosis. Curet-

tage is usually curative. Rare incidences of lung metastases have been described.

PATHOGENESIS

- Etiology is unknown.
- Chromosomal abnormalities on 5 and 8 have been identified.

Epidemiology
- Uncommon lesion
  - Only about 500 cases have been reported in the literature.
  - Represents 1% of bone tumors
- Peak age: Majority are discovered in the second decade, and most patients are under 20 years, but any age may be involved.
- Gender: slight male preponderance
- Distribution
  - Most common in the long bones (proximal humerus > distal femur > proximal tibia > proximal femur)
  - Almost exclusively within the epiphysis (may extend into epimetaphysis)
  - Flat bone sites: acetabulum, ilium
  - Other distinctive but less common locations
    - Talus, calcaneus, patella, craniofacial bones
    - Typically in older patients

Pathophysiology
- Tumor of immature cartilage cells (chondroblasts) rather than mature cartilage cells (chondrocytes)
- Without mature cells, does not produce hyaline cartilage, so lacks typical radiographic features of hyaline cartilage mineralization (arcs and rings)

Natural History

Typical course involves slow growth, with untreated lesions eventually eroding into the articular space. Invasion of adjacent joint, when it does occur, travels via the cruciate ligaments or ligamentum teres. Synovitis is especially seen when the tumor involves the joint.

The tumor has occasional aggressive behavior. Although considered a benign tumor, there are well-documented incidences of lung metastases. Only a handful of cases are documented, and in half of these cases, the tumor was originally in flat bones and most had experienced local recurrence. Unfortunately, no clear radiologic or histologic findings are known to be predictive of metastasis. The histological appearance of the metastases was similar to that of the original lesion, showing no malignant features. There appears to be a long interval to metastasis and a long survival time after metastasis, corresponding to the slow growth of the lesion in general.

DIAGNOSIS (see Algorithm 5.2-1)

Clinical Features

- Typical clinical presentation is aching pain in the proximity of the adjacent joint.

- Duration: Symptoms often present for 6 months or more.
- Physical examination reveals local tenderness and slight loss of motion.
- Up to 50% of the adjacent articulations have an effusion.

Radiologic Features

Radiographs

- Plain radiographs are often diagnostic, showing lytic, epiphyseal lesions with minimally sclerotic borders (Fig. 5.2-7).
- Sometimes faint speckled mineralization is seen.
- Not the characteristic arcs and rings of hyaline cartilage

CT

- Matrix calcification is best seen on CT, as is the otherwise faint sclerotic border.
- Secondary aneurysmal bone cyst formation is common.
- Presence of mineralization on CT scan may be helpful in predicting the presence of underlying chondroblastoma (see Fig. 5.2-7).

MRI

- Marrow edema, sometimes dramatic and extending into the metaphysis, is a hallmark of chondroblastoma (see Fig. 5.2-7).
- In some lesions, an adjacent joint effusion or synovitis can be seen on MRI (see Fig. 5.2-6).

Bone Scan

- Increased radiotracer uptake is seen.

Histologic Features

- Preponderance of round or polygonal cells, with indented or folded "coffee bean" nuclei
- Cells packed into "cobblestone" pseudolobulated pattern
- Foci of eosinophilic chondroid matrix and reactive multinucleate giant cells

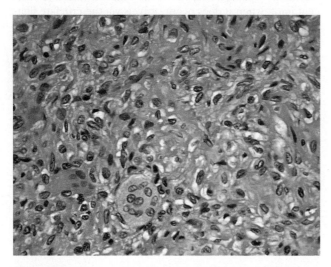

Figure 5.2-6 Tissue section from chondroblastoma shows plump polygonal cells with coffee-bean nuclei in cobblestone pattern separated by chicken-wire calcification. Scattered giant cells are also seen.

- Peripheral intercellular "chicken-wire calcification"
- Mitoses should be occasional and not atypical.

Differential Diagnosis

- A frequently employed mnemonic for the differential diagnosis of epiphyseal lesions is PGCAT (pigmented villonodular synovitis, giant cell tumor, chondroblastoma, clear cell chondrosarcoma, aneurysmal bone cyst, and tuberculosis).

Subchondral Cyst/Intraosseous Ganglion

- Because of the proximity to the subchondral surface of some chondroblastomas, the possibility of a subchondral cyst should be entertained.
- Both lesions may have a sclerotic rim and marrow edema on MRI, but subchondral cysts should not demonstrate any mineralized matrix and are more common in older patients with associated degenerative joint changes.
- Similar cysts may occur with pigmented villonodular synovitis in younger individuals.
- Marrow edema is usually less extensive with cysts.

Giant Cell Tumor

- Although most giant cell tumors occur in adults, they may occur in patients with an open growth plate.
- The epicenter of the rare pediatric giant cell tumor of bone is usually in the metaphysis, however, with occasional erosion into the epiphysis.
- In a typical chondroblastoma, the epicenter is within the epiphysis, with occasional erosion into the metaphysis.
- Giant cell tumor lacks any mineralization.

Clear Cell Chondrosarcoma

- This is a rare variant of chondrosarcoma with an epiphyseal predilection.
- It has been hypothesized that it is a malignant variant of chondroblastoma.
- The radiological differences usually include loss of geographic, sclerotic margins, and metaphyseal or extraosseous extension.
- Most occur in adults.

Aneurysmal Bone Cyst

- The epiphysis is an unusual location for an aneurysmal bone cyst, which is typified on plain radiographs by septations and absence of mineralization.
- On MRI, often numerous fluid–fluid levels are seen.
- Since one third of chondroblastomas have secondary aneurysmal bone cyst components, both may be present within a single lesion.

Osteomyelitis

- Infections are the most frequent cause of radiolucent lesions within the pediatric epiphysis.
- The clinical history is often shorter and may be accompanied by other clinical signs or laboratory evidence of infection.
- Similar to chondroblastoma, osteomyelitis usually shows extensive edema on MRI.
- Tuberculous osteomyelitis of the long bones is an infection that has a predilection for the epiphysis.

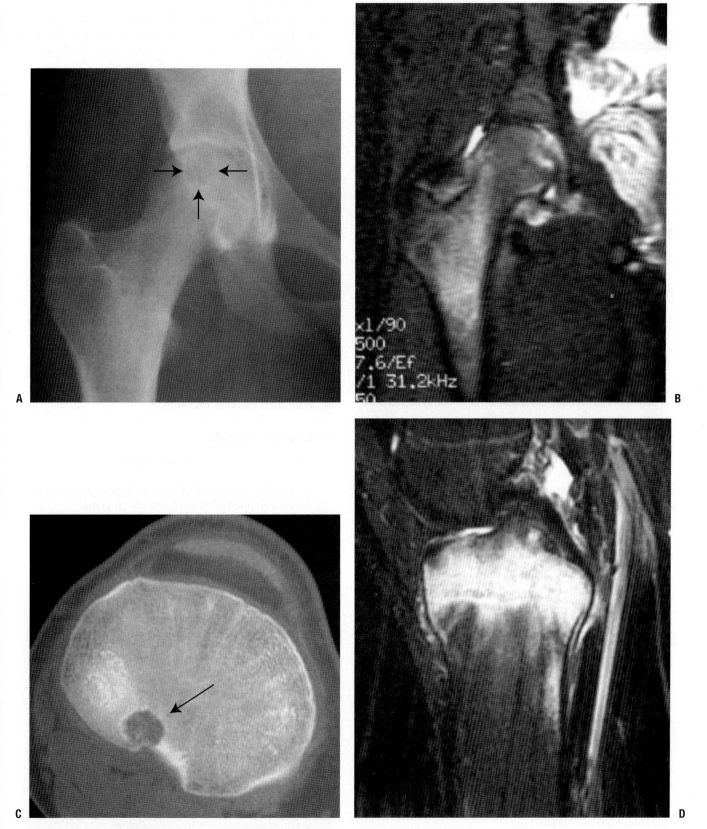

Figure 5.2-7   Chondroblastoma. (**A**) Plain radiograph of proximal femoral lesion showing epiphyseal location and sclerotic margins. (**B**) T2-weighted MRI demonstrates perilesional edema, and synovitis and effusion of adjacent joint. (**C**) CT scan is best modality for visualizing chondroid mineralization. (**D**) Often intense marrow edema is seen on MRI.

TREATMENT

Surgical Indications/Contraindications

- Primary tumor treatment
  - Because of the progressive nature of the lesion, curettage is indicated in all chondroblastomas.
  - Some authors have advocated the use of a physical adjuvant such as liquid nitrogen or phenol.
  - The rate of recurrence with simple curettage appears relatively low, and the role of physical adjuvant is not yet clear.
- Pulmonary metastases are typically nonprogressive lesions and may be observed or excised.

Results and Outcome

- Local recurrence rates: 14% to 18%, usually within 2 years
- Adjacent joint synovitis usually resolves with tumor excision.

CHONDROMYXOID FIBROMA

Chondromyxoid fibroma is a rare but distinctive bone tumor of immature cartilage origin that presents as an eccentric lytic lesion, usually immediately on the opposite side of the growth plate as its other immature cartilage tumor counterpart, chondroblastoma. Despite a high recorded incidence of local recurrence after curettage, no metastases have been reported.

PATHOGENESIS

- Etiology is unknown.
- Rearrangements of long arm of chromosome 6 described
- Distinctive matrix composition in chondroblastoma differs from that of other benign cartilage tumors (chondroblastoma, enchondroma, osteochondroma, chondrosarcoma): high expression of hydrated proteoglycans (myxoid component), type II cartilage (chondrocytic component), and types I, III, and VI cartilage

Epidemiology

- Exceedingly rare tumor
- <1% of bone tumors
- Age: mean 31 years (72% younger than 40)
- Slight male > female preponderance
- Distribution
  - Half of lesions occur in long bones.
    - Most commonly proximal tibia
    - Metaphyseal or metadiaphyseal region, sometimes eroding into epiphysis

- One third occur in flat bones.
  - Most commonly ilium (half)
- Bones of feet next most common (metatarsals usually)

Natural History

- Although the tumor appears to cause sometimes extensive bone destruction and may recur repeatedly after treatment, there are no reported cases of metastasis.

DIAGNOSIS (see Algorithm 5.2-1)

Clinical Features

- Pain, sometimes of long duration, is typically seen.
- Pathologic fracture is unusual.

Radiologic Features

- Radiolucent, sharply marginated eccentric metaphyseal lesion
- Lobulated, septated, or "soap bubble" appearance
- Usually elongated along the long axis of the bones
- Cortical thinning common
- Cortical destruction and soft tissue extension occasionally seen
- Periosteal reaction uncommon

Histologic Features

- Low-power histology: prominent lobular or zonation pattern
  - Lobules consist of a central, hypocellular myxoid area rimmed with more cellular regions.
- High-power histology: spindle or stellate-shaped cells with eosinophilic cytoplasm embedded within myxoid matrix

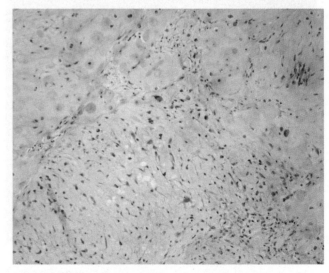

A

Figure 5.2-8   Chondromyxoid fibroma histopathology. **(A)** Low power view shows lobules of low cellularity myxoid areas separated by more cellular regions.

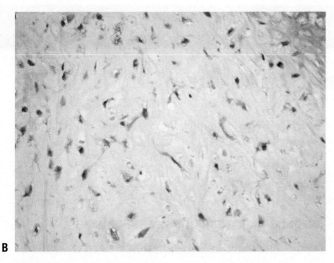

B

Figure 5.2-8   (B) Higher power view shows characteristic stellate cells.

- Areas of hyaline cartilage in 20%
- Aneurysmal bone cyst components in 10%
- Chondroblastoma-like cells as well as multinucleated giant cells occasionally seen

Differential Diagnosis

Chondrosarcoma
- Myxoid chondrosarcoma may have some of the same radiologic features of chondromyxoid fibroma.
- Chondrosarcoma will not have the typical sclerotic, well-defined margins of chondromyxoid fibroma.
- The presence of large, pleomorphic-appearing cells in chondromyxoid fibroma may also erroneously suggest a diagnosis of chondrosarcoma.
  - Mitoses are infrequent and atypical mitoses are not seen in chondromyxoid fibroma.
  - The center of the myxoid lobules in chondrosarcoma is hypercellular instead of hypocellular, as in chondromyxoid fibroma.

Giant Cell Tumor
- This also occurs in the metaphyses of young adults and presents as a lytic mass.
- The radiographic appearance, however, is not one of lobulation, and the margins are less sclerotic on plain radiographs.
- Histologically, the lesions are quite distinct.

Nonossifying Fibroma
- This also can appear as an eccentric, metaphyseal lesion.
- Typically, these are painless, incidental lesions and are often already partially ossified.

TREATMENT

- Because of the rarity of the tumor, no large study is available to compare different types of treatment.
- Most lesions have been treated with intralesional excision (curettage).

Results and Outcome

- Local recurrence rate: 15% to 25% recurrence (higher in younger patients in some series)

Acknowledgments

I gratefully acknowledge research assistance by Brittany L. Rice, MLS, AHIP, and Smita Jhaveri of the Suburban Hospital Medical Library.

SUGGESTED READING

Bauer TW, Dorfman HD, Latham JT. Periosteal chondroma. A clinicopathologic study of 23 cases. *Am J Surg Pathol* 1982;6:631–637.

Flemming DJ, Murphey MD. Enchondroma and chondrosarcoma. *Semin Musculoskelet Radiol* 2000;4:59–71.

Kransdorf M, Meis J. From the archives of the AFIP. Extraskeletal osseous and cartilaginous tumors of the extremities. *Radiographics* 1993;13:853–884.

Kunze E, Graewe T, Peitsch E. Histology and biology of metastatic chondroblastoma. Report of a case with a review of the literature. *Pathol Res Pract* 1987;182:113–123.

Lee KCY, Davies AM, Cassar-Pullicino VN. Imaging the complications of osteochondromas. *Clin Radiol* 2002;57:18–28.

Levy JC, Temple HT, Mollabashy A, et al. The causes of pain in benign solitary enchondromas of the proximal humerus. *Clin Orthop Relat Res* 2005;181–186.

Marcial-Seoane R, Marcial-Seoane M, Ramos E, et al. Extraskeletal chondromas. *Bol Asoc Med P R* 1990;82:394–402.

Marco RA, Gitelis S, Brebach GT, et al. Cartilage tumors: evaluation and treatment. *J Am Acad Orthop Surg* 2000;8:292–304.

Murphey MD, Choi JJ, Kransdorf MJ, et al. Imaging of osteochondroma: variants and complications with radiologic-pathologic correlation. *Radiographics* 2000;20:1407–1434.

Murphey MD, Walker E, Wilson A, et al. From the archives of the AFIP: imaging of primary chondrosarcoma: radiologic-pathologic correlation. *Radiographics* 2003;23:1245–1278.

Nojima T, Unni KK, McLeod RA, et al. Periosteal chondroma and periosteal chondrosarcoma. *Am J Surg Pathol* 1985;9:666–677.

Pierz KA, Stieber JR, Kusumi K, et al. Hereditary multiple exostoses: one center's experience and review of etiology. *Clin Orthop Relat Res* 2002:49–59.

Sandberg AA. Genetics of chondrosarcoma and related tumors. *Curr Opin Oncol* 2004;16:342–354.

Springfield DS, Capanna R, Gherlinzoni F, et al. Chondroblastoma. A review of seventy cases. *J Bone Joint Surg [Am]* 1985;67:748–755.

Vasseur MA, Fabre O. Vascular complications of osteochondromas. *J Vasc Surg* 2000;31:532–538.

Wilson AJ, Kyriakos M, Ackerman LV. Chondromyxoid fibroma: radiographic appearance in 38 cases and in a review of the literature. *Radiology* 1991;179:513–528.

Wu CT, Inwards CY, O'Laughlin S, et al. Chondromyxoid fibroma of bone: a clinicopathologic review of 278 cases. *Hum Pathol* 1998; 29:438–446.

5.3 CYSTIC LESIONS

SUNG WOOK SEO ■ YOUNG LAE MOON ■ FRANCIS YOUNG-IN LEE

This chapter includes cystic lesions which may occur in bone. Epidermal inclusion cysts and ganglions may also occur in soft-tissues, where the pathophysiology is similar. Simple bone cysts and aneurysmal bone cysts represent distinct clinical entities which occur within bone only.

EPIDERMAL INCLUSION CYST

Epidermal inclusion cysts are more commonly seen as soft-tissue lesions, but may involve bone, and present in either case as painful digital lesions which typically require surgical extirpation.

PATHOGENESIS

Etiology

■ For both soft-tissue and intraosseous epidermal inclusion cysts, penetrating trauma causes epidermal tissue to be deposited deep within the tissues

Pathophysiology

■ Epidermal tissue traumatically deposited within the deeper tissue grows and causes cyst formation
■ Cystic lesion filled with keratinous materials lined with flattened squamous epithelium

DIAGNOSIS

Physical Examination and History

Clinical Features
■ Painful, often swollen mass most often within distal digit
■ History of penetrating trauma in many cases

Radiologic Features
■ Intraosseous geographic radiolucent lesion
■ Distal phalanx of fingers common

Pathologic findings
■ Cystic cavity filled with keratinaceous debris

Diagnostic Workup Algorithm

■ Differential diagnosis includes intraosseous synovial or ganglion cyst

■ Diagnosis usually apparent radiographically, confirmed histologically

TREATMENT

Surgical Indications/Contraindications

■ Painful lesions bone can be curetted and grafted

DEGENERATIVE CYST (GEODES)

PATHOGENESIS

Etiology

■ Related to underlying degenerative arthritis

Pathophysiology

■ Damage to cartilage theorized to allow fluid intravasation within bone, leading to cyst formation
■ Pathology: Cystic lesion filled with fluid or gelatinous or proteinaceous material, demarcated by fibrocartilaginous tissues (Fig. 5.3-1)

DIAGNOSIS

Physical Examination and History

Clinical Features
■ Dictated by manifestations of underlying arthritis
■ Pain, local tenderness, variable stiffness, loss of motion

Radiologic Features
■ Plain x-ray
  ■ Cyst: geographic, smooth, often sclerotic borders with central radiolucency within epiphysis immediately adjacent to joint, often on both sides of joint
  ■ Variable associated arthritic changes:
    ■ loss of joint space, osteophytes, subchondral sclerosis, subluxation may be present
    ■ some joints show few or no degenerative changes
■ MRI
  ■ Fluid-filled well defined lesions adjacent to joint with communication to joint usually obvious

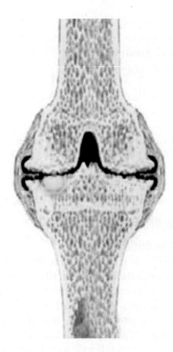

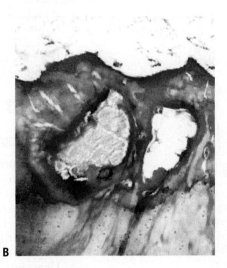

Figure 5.3-1 Histopathology of degenerative cyst. (**A**) Schematic shows white cyst below thinned (degenerative) cartilage, shown in black. (**B**) Intraosseous cysts within subchondral bone with overlying fibrillated cartilage.

A

B

- Typically homogenously dark on T1W, bright on T2W sequences
- Enhancement only peripherally

Pathologic findings
- Cystic cavity filled with serous fluid, proteinaceous, or gelatinous material and lined with flattened fibrocartilaginous tissues

Diagnostic Workup Algorithm

- Usually evident radiographically without the need for histological confirmation
  - In presence of established arthritis, plain radiographs often suffice
  - In absence of other radiographic signs of arthritis, MRI may be useful
- Differential diagnosis includes other epiphyseal lesions
  - PGCAT: Pigmented villonodular synovitis (PVNS), giant cell tumor of bone, chondroblastoma, clear cell chondrosarcoma aneurysmal bone cyst, tuberculosis (and other cause for Brodie's abscess)

TREATMENT

Surgical Indications/Contraindications

- If diagnosis is clear, direct treatment towards underlying joint arthritis
- If diagnosis not clear, biopsy may be necessary

SIMPLE BONE CYST (UNICAMERAL BONE CYST)

Unicameral bone cyst is a serous or serosanguineous fluid-filled cavity which typically behaves in an inactive fashion, not causing symptoms until pathological fracture occurs through the cyst. The clinical presentation, location, and radiographic features are classic enough that the diagnosis may usually be readily established. Treatment continues to evolve, and is site dependent, but often involves aspiration and injection.

PATHOGENESIS

Etiology:

Unknown but theories suggest epiphyseal plate defect or venous outflow obstruction

Epidemiology

- Ages
  - Peak incidence 4–10 years of age
  - 85% within first two decades
- Gender: Males > females 3:1
- Distribution
  - Proximal humerus most common
  - Proximal femur #2
  - Calcaneus #3
  - Other relatively common sites: proximal tibia, ilium
  - Most common sites in adults: calcaneus and ilium

Pathophysiology:

Unknown

Classification

- Active position: Immediately juxtaposed to growth plate
  - Not to be confused with Enneking stage 2 benign (active) classification
- Inactive position: Growth plate no longer adjacent to cyst
- Not to be confused with Enneking stage 1 benign (inactive) classification

DIAGNOSIS

Physical Examination and History

Clinical Features

- Well-defined fluid filled lesion in the metaphysis and diaphysis of the proximal humerus and proximal femur in children
- Large lesions may cause pathologic fractures, which is the most common clinical presentation
- Less commonly, they may cause pain and swelling

Radiologic Features

- Plain radiographs
  - Well-demarcated osteolytic lesion without much marginal sclerosis (Fig. 5.3-2)
  - Central location (occupies entire width of bone)
  - Metadiaphyseal location within long bones
    - Active position: juxtaposed to growth plate on metaphyseal side
    - Inactive position: growth plate no longer adjacent to cyst
  - Thinning of cortex
  - Intralesional fracture fragment (fallen leaf or fallen fragment sign)
    - Essentially pathognomonic for simple bone cyst, as it indicates that the cyst is comprised of fluid (fragment could not fall to bottom of a solid lesion)
- Magnetic resonance imaging
  - Homogenous fluid signal (dark on T1W, bright on T2W)
  - Peripheral rim enhancement only
  - Blood products may be identified if fracture has occurred (fluid-fluid level) but because the blood is usually mixed with serous fluid, the hematocrit sign (level of the horizontal delineation between serum and cells) is lower than that seen in an ABC

Pathologic findings

- A fibrous membrane-lined cavity containing a clear yellow fluid
- Fibrous membranes contain fibrous tissues, occasional multinucleated cells and CD 68 (+) foamy histiocytes

Diagnostic Workup Algorithm

- Plain radiographs
  - If radiographic diagnosis evident on XR, proceed with treatment
  - If diagnosis unclear, obtain MRI

- Magnetic resonance imaging
  - If radiographic diagnosis evident based on XR and MRI, proceed with treatment
  - If diagnosis unclear, aspirate
- Aspiration
  - If aspiration reveals clear fluid, diagnosis confirmed
  - If aspiration reveals blood, may be from fracture hematoma, but consider cytological examination
  - If aspiration fails due to solid tissue, proceed with open biopsy

TREATMENT

Surgical Indications/Contraindications

Surgical and Nonoperative Options

- Various treatment methods have been described. Treatment options include aspiration/injection therapies (steroid, bone marrow, demineralized bone matrix, or combinations), elastic intramedullary nailing, multiple drilling, curettage & bone grafting alone or with supplementary internal fixation (femoral neck lesion)
  - Upper extremity cysts: aspiration/injection preferred
    - Low morbidity of procedure (outpatient, minimal recovery)
    - Low morbidity of repeat fracture if treatment fails (usually extra-articular and most go on to heal with non-operative care)
  - Proximal femoral cysts: lower threshold for considering curettage & bone grafting alone or with supplementary internal fixation
    - Higher risk of fracture in proximal femur warrants consideration of open procedure
    - Proximal femoral fractures generally require ORIF
- Observation may be elected, particularly for humeral lesions and calcaneal lesions discovered incidentally
  - Calcaneal simple cysts
    - Often discovered due to pain
    - Need to distinguish source of pain (may be unrelated plantar fasciitis)
- Following pathological fracture through simple cyst, approximately 1/7 will show healing of cyst with healing of the fracture
  - For proximal humeral pathological fracture, allow fracture to heal and re-evaluate radiographically before considering operative treatment
  - For pathological proximal femoral fracture, ORIF should be combined with curettage and grafting of lesion

Results and Outcome

- Progressive lesional healing and resolution in 60% to 70% of lesions
- Partial lesional healing in 20% to 30%
- No lesional healing and/or cyst recurrence in 10% to 20%
- Deteriorating results with extended follow-up should dampen enthusiasm for short-term follow-up of newer techniques

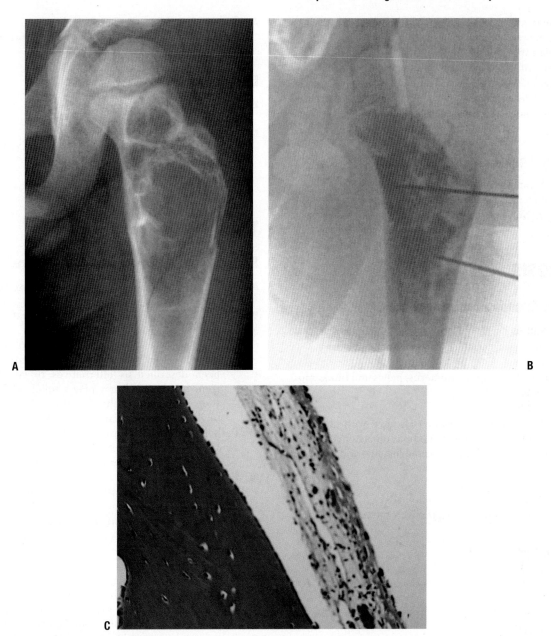

Figure 5.3-2 (**A**) Unicameral bone cyst in the proximal femur. (**B**) Cystography shows radioopaque dye filling throughout the lesion. (**C**) Photomicrography demonstrates cystic lesion lined with a fibrocellular membrane.

ANEURYSMAL BONE CYST

Aneurysmal bone cysts differ from other cystic bone lesions in having the potential for aggressive behavior and hence need to be distinguished from the other types of bone cysts. Furthermore, these benign lesions must be distinguished histologically from telangiectatic osteosarcoma. Treatment for aneurismal bone cyst is typically more aggressive than for other bone cysts.

PATHOGENESIS

Etiology

- Primary ABC likely neoplastic
  - Clonal chromosome band 17p13 translocations that place the USP6 (TRE2 or TRE17) oncogene under

the regulatory influence of the highly active CDH11 promoter

- Rearrangements of either USP6 or CDH11 in high percentage of primary ABCs
- Secondary ABC (associated with other primary bone lesions) likely reactive
    - Chromosomal rearrangements not seen

Epidemiology

- Ages: Mean 11 years (peak range 1 to 20)
- Frequency: 0.3 per 100,000
- Gender: No predilection

DIAGNOSIS

Physical Examination and History

Clinical Features

- May cause pain, swelling and pathologic fracture.
- Locations:
    - Femur, tibia, spine, humerus, pelvis and fibula most common
    - 2/3 in long bones
- Primary or secondary lesion associated with giant cell tumor, unicameral bone cyst, chondroblastoma, fibrous dysplasia, giant cell tumor, osteoblastoma and osteosarcoma
- Spontaneous regression
    - May occur in active primary ABC
    - Very uncommon in aggressive or secondary lesions

Radiologic Features

- Plain x-ray (Figs. 5.3-3 and 5.3-4)
    - Expansile, eccentric radiolucent lesion with septations
    - Classically, blown-out cortex with eggshell-thin rim of reactive bone
- Common sites: metaphysis of long bones and posterior elements of vertebrae, distal phalanx of fingers
- Fluid-fluid (blood/serum) levels can be seen on MRI or CT scans.
    - Not pathognomonic for primary ABC
    - Also seen in telangiectactic osteosarcoma and secondary ABCs
    - UBC fluid-fluid levels may be seen after fracture (usually solitary)

Pathologic Features

- Expansile, eccentric osteolytic blood-filled lesion containing multiple cysts separated by fibrous sept.
- Sponge like cavernous spaces filled with blood
- Cavities surrounded by gray or brownish tissue with an osseous component (reactive osteoblast-lined bone) and multinucleated cells

- Solid variant of ABC consists of fibrous or granular tissue with local hemorrhages and a layer of reactive bone

Diagnostic Workup Algorithm

- Differential diagnosis: giant cell tumor, telangiectatic osteosarcoma, osteoblastoma
- Workup
    - Radiographic evaluation with x-rays, MRI, BS suggests consideration of diagnosis
    - Biopsy confirms diagnosis

TREATMENT

Surgical Indications/Contraindications

- Inactive lesions (unusual): Intralesional excision (curettage)
- Active and aggressive lesions (usual): Intralesional excision (curettage) and bone grafting
    - Arterial embolization (Ethibloc), and injection with demineralized bone and/or bone marrow have also been described as alternatives to curettage with some success and may play a role in difficult locations such as the pelvis but they do not allow thorough histological examination of contents
- Pathologic fractures through ABCs
    - Usually require curettage and grafting +/− stabilization to allow fracture healing and control of lesion
- Pelvic ABCs
    - Spontaneous regression has been observed after biopsy
    - Consider observation after biopsy
        - If regression occurs, no need for further surgery
        - If progression occurs, proceed to curettage
- Spinal ABCs
    - Extended intralesional curettage with grafting (+/− limited fusion when necessary)
    - Embolization poses risks of vascular complications related to cord and of cerebral embolic phenomenon
- Incompletely resectable, aggressive, and/or recurrent ABCs:
    - Radiotherapy may cause secondary sarcoma and therefore should be avoided as primary treatment for this benign process but may play a role in isolated cases
        - Use low-dose (26 to 30 Gy) radiotherapy (RT)
        - Successful in 90% of cases

Results and Outcome

- Intralesional excision (curettage) and bone grafting
    - Recurrence is common: approximately 30% (20% to 70% in reported series)
        - Usually responds to repeat curettage
        - Some lesions stabilize and/or regress
        - Recurrences no more common in younger children

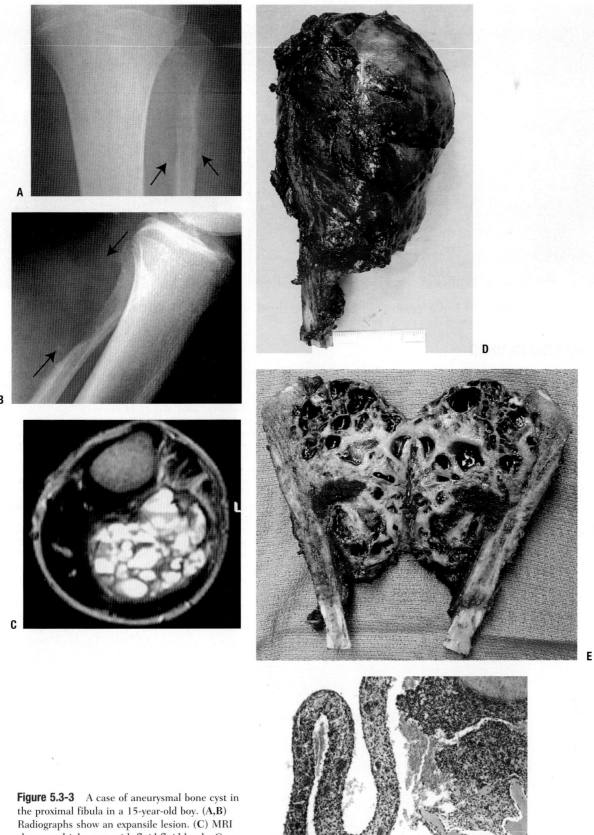

Figure 5.3-3   A case of aneurysmal bone cyst in the proximal fibula in a 15-year-old boy. (**A,B**) Radiographs show an expansile lesion. (**C**) MRI shows multiple cysts with fluid-fluid levels. Gross (**D,E**) and pathologic (**F**) specimens demonstrate multiloculated cysts filled with bloody fluid.

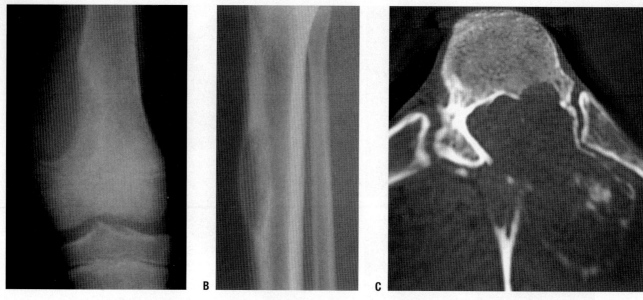

Figure 5.3-4   Radiographs of other cases of aneurysmal bone cyst in the distal femur (**A**), tibia (**B**), and vertebra (**C**).

SUGGESTED READING

Aho HJ, Aho AJ, and Einola S. Aneurysmal bone cyst, a study of ultrastructure and malignant transformation. *Virchows Arch A Pathol Anat Histol* 1982;395(2):169–179.

Biesecker JL, Marcove RC, Huvos AG, et al. Aneurysmal bone cysts. A clinicopathologic study of 66 cases. *Cancer* 1970;26(3):615–625.

Chang CH, Stanton RP, Glutting J. Unicameral bone cysts treated by injection of bone marrow or methylprednisolone. *J Bone Joint Surg* [Br] 2002;84(3):407–412.

Chigira M, Shimizu T, Arita S, et al. Radiological evidence of healing of a simple bone cyst after hole drilling. *Arch Orthop Trauma Surg* 1986;105(3):150–153.

Cole WG. Treatment of aneurysmal bone cysts in childhood. *J Pediatr Orthop* 1986;6(3):326–329.

Gokturk E, Kose N. Simple bone cysts treated by percutaneous autologous marrow grafting. *J Bone Joint Surg* [Br] 1997;79(4):695.

Green JA, Bellemore MC, Marsden FW. Embolization in the treatment of aneurysmal bone cysts. *J Pediatr Orthop* 1997;17(4):440–443.

Kyriakos, M., and Hardy, D.: Malignant transformation of aneurysmal bone cyst, with an analysis of the literature. *Cancer,* 68(8):1770–80, 1991.

Lichtenstein L. Aneurysmal bone cyst; observations on fifty cases. *J Bone Joint Surg* [Am] 1957;39(4):873–882.

Maclin TB, Jr. Posttraumatic epidermal inclusion cyst. A case report. *J Am Podiatry Assoc* 1965;55:209–210.

Oliveira AM, Perez-Atayde AR, Dal Cin P et al. Aneurysmal bone cyst variant translocations upregulate USP6 transcription by promoter swapping with the ZNF9, COL1A1, TRAP150, and OMD genes. *Oncogene.* 2005 May 12;24(21):3419–26.

Oliveira AM, Perez-Atayde AR, Inwards CY, et al. USP6 and CDH11 oncogenes identify the neoplastic cell in primary aneurysmal bone cysts and are absent in so-called secondary aneurysmal bone cysts. *Am J Pathol.* 2004 Nov;165(5):1773–8011.

Papagelopoulos PJ, Choudhury SN, Frassica FJ, et al. Treatment of aneurysmal bone cysts of the pelvis and sacrum. *J Bone Joint Surg* [Am] 2001;83(11):1674–1681.

Ramirez AR, Stanton RP. Aneurysmal bone cyst in 29 children. *J Pediatr Orthop* 2002;22(4):533–539.

Rougraff BT, Kling TJ. Treatment of active unicameral bone cysts with percutaneous injection of demineralized bone matrix and autogenous bone marrow. *J Bone Joint Surg* [Am] 2002;84(6):921–929.

Shinozaki T, Arita S, Watanabe H, et al. Simple bone cysts treated by multiple drill-holes. 23 cysts followed 2–10 years. *Acta Orthop Scand* 1996;67(3):288–290.

Yu CL, D'Astous J, Finnegan M. Simple bone cysts. The effects of methylprednisolone on synovial cells in culture. *Clin Orthop Relat Res* 1991;(262):34–41.

5.4 MYOGENIC, LIPOGENIC, AND NEURAL TUMORS

SEAN V. McGARRY ■ C. PARKER GIBBS

Myogenic, lipogenic, and neural tumors affecting bone are much less common than they are in soft tissues. The three most common benign bone lesions that fall into these categories are leiomyoma of bone, lipoma of bone, and schwannoma. Lipoma of bone, also commonly referred to as intraosseous lipoma, has both intramedullary and parosteal subtypes. Only the bone lesions will be discussed here; their soft tissue counterparts are discussed in Chapter 11, Benign Soft Tissue Tumors.

PATHOGENESIS

Etiology

The etiology for this group of rare tumors is unknown. Chromosomal abnormalities well described in soft tissue lipomas have been reported in some parosteal lipomas.

Epidemiology

- Leiomyoma of bone
  - Very rare
  - Age: Adults >30 (only exceptionally in children)
  - Gender: male = female
  - Common locations: facial bones (#1 = mandible) outweigh extragnathic bones (#1 tibia)
- Lipoma of bone (intraosseous lipoma)
  - Rare (<0.1% primary bone tumors)
  - Majority intramedullary; few parosteal
  - Intramedullary lipoma
    - Age: second to eighth decade, with median age in 40s
    - Male:female 1.6:1
    - Common locations
      - Metaphyseal in long bones: proximal femur > tibia > fibula
      - Calcaneus
- Parosteal lipoma
  - Age: peaks in fifth and sixth decades
  - Male > female (small difference)
  - Common locations
    - Diaphyseal in long bones: femur > humerus > tibia
- Schwannoma
  - Very uncommon (<1% primary bone tumors)
    - Only benign osseous neurogenic tumor
    - Neurofibromas do NOT arise within bone.
    - Bone lesions in patients with neurofibromatosis-1 are NOT usually neurogenic tumors.
  - Common locations
    - Mandible and sacrum or spine

Pathophysiology

- Same as for soft tissue counterparts (see Chapter 11)
- Histopathology
  - Leiomyoma of bone (see Fig. 11-30 in Chapter 11)
    - Interlacing bundles with uniform spindle cells
    - Immunohistochemistry: positive for smooth muscle actin, desmin
  - Lipoma of bone (see Fig. 11-3)
    - Fatty tissue surrounds normal trabeculae.
    - Some tumors have necrosis, foamy histiocytes, and fibrous tissue.
  - Schwannoma (see Fig. 11-26)
    - Spindle cells with wavy nuclei, often palisading within more hypercellular areas intermixed with hypocellular areas
    - Immunohistochemistry: positive for S100 diffusely

Classification

- All of these lesions are classified by Enneking's classification of benign tumors.
  - Latent (most) or active (few); generally none of these lesions are aggressive
- Lipoma of bone (intraosseous lipoma)
  - Intramedullary lipoma: central
  - Parosteal lipoma: surface lesion

DIAGNOSIS

Physical Examination and History

- Leiomyoma of bone
  - Pain
- Lipoma of bone
  - Intramedullary lipoma
    - Typically presents as a painless bone lesion discovered incidentally or during evaluation of pain from another cause
    - Occasionally may produce achy mild pain or, rarely, pathologic fracture
  - Parosteal lipoma
    - Asymptomatic bump
- Schwannoma
  - Usually asymptomatic incidental finding
  - Occasionally mildly to moderately painful bone lesion with slow growth

Radiologic Features

Radiography
- Leiomyoma of bone
  - Lucent, often multilocular, surrounded by sclerotic geographic rim
- Lipoma of bone
  - Geographic central radiolucency surrounded by thin sclerotic geographic rim
  - Cockade sign: central mineralized radiodensity with badge appearance (nearly diagnostic when present but not universal)
- Schwannoma
  - Nonspecific geographic radiolucency

Magnetic Resonance Imaging
- Leiomyoma of bone: nonspecific
- Lipoma of bone
  - Peripheral homogenous signal intensity that is the same as subcutaneous fat in all sequences often surrounding central mineralized region with characteristics of cortical bone (not universally present)
- Schwannoma: nonspecific

TREATMENT

Surgical Indications/Contraindications (also see Chapter 4.2, Treatment Principles)

Nonoperative Management
- Most of these lesions—leiomyoma of bone, lipoma of bone, and intraosseous schwannoma—should be treated with observation, particularly if they are incidental, asymptomatic findings.

- Lipoma of bone should usually be diagnosed by radiographic studies and does not require biopsy.

Surgical Management
- Biopsy may be necessary to establish the diagnosis, especially for leiomyoma of bone and intraosseous schwannoma.
- For symptomatic lesions, intralesional excision (curettage) suffices.

Results and Outcome

Observation
- There is essentially no risk of malignant degeneration of these lesions.
- Observation is an acceptable alternative to surgery, and many patients remain asymptomatic and never require surgery.

Surgery
- For each of these lesions, a simple curettage results in a negligible recurrence rate.

SUGGESTED READING

McCarthy E. Leiomyoma of bone. In: Fletcher CDM, Unni KK, Mertens F, eds. *Pathology & Genetics: Tumours of Soft Tissue and Bone.* World Health Organization of Tumours. Lyon: IARC Press, 2002: 326.

Rosenberg AE, Bridge JA. Lipoma of bone. In: Fletcher CDM, Unni KK, Mertens F, eds. *Pathology & Genetics: Tumours of Soft Tissue and Bone.* World Health Organization of Tumours. Lyon: IARC Press, 2002:328–329.

Unni KK. Schwannoma. In: Fletcher CDM, Unni KK, Mertens F, eds. *Pathology & Genetics: Tumours of Soft Tissue and Bone.* World Health Organization of Tumours. Lyon: IARC Press, 2002:331.

5.5 FIBROUS LESIONS OF BONE

SUNG WOOK SEO ■ YOUNG LAE MOON ■ FRANCIS YOUNG-IN LEE

Considerable controversy exists with respect to the terminology for fibrous lesions of bone. Although nonossifying fibromas (NOFs) and metaphyseal fibrous cortical defects (FCDs) are the most common lesions of bone, the current World Health Organization does not even include them in their classification, as they are not neoplastic (Box 5.5-1). Avulsive cortical irregularity has identical histology but is distinguished by a very specific location, the posteromedial distal femoral metaphysis. Benign fibrous histiocytoma, for which there are several synonyms, also has the same histol-ogy as NOF/FCD but is distinguished by its occurrence in older ages, in an atypical non–long bone location, with atypical radiographic appearance, or with unusual clinical presentation. Fibrous dysplasia and osteofibrous dysplasia have typical clinical presentations and radiographic appearances. Desmoplastic fibroma is a rare tumor that occurs most commonly in the mandible.

BOX 5.5-1 CURRENT TERMINOLOGY FOR FIBROUS LESIONS OF BONE

Non-neoplastic Lesions
Metaphyseal fibrous cortical defect
    Fibrous cortical defect
    Metaphyseal supracondylar cortical defect
    Developmental defect
Nonossifying fibroma
    Fibroxanthoma
Avulsive cortical irregularity
    Cortical avulsive irregularity
    Periosteal desmoid
    Subperiosteal desmoid
    Cortical desmoid
World Health Organization (WHO) Fibrogenic Tumors
Desmoplastic fibroma
    Desmoid tumor of bone
    Intraosseous counterpart of soft tissue fibromatosis
WHO Fibrohistiocytic Tumors
Benign fibrous histiocytoma
    Fibroxanthoma
    Fibrous xanthoma
    Xanthofibroma
    Xanthogranuloma
WHO Miscellaneous Lesions*
Fibrous dysplasia
    Fibrocartilaginous dysplasia
    Generalized fibrocystic disease of bone
Osteofibrous dysplasia
    Ossifying fibroma
    Kempson-Campanacci lesion
    Campanacci lesion
    Cortical fibrous dysplasia

---

*Other nonfibrous miscellaneous lesions in the WHO classification include aneurysmal bone cyst (see Chapter 5.3, Cystic Lesions), simple bone cyst (see Chapter 5.3), Langerhans cell histiocytosis (see Chapter 5.8, Other Tumors of Undefined Neoplastic Nature), Erdheim-Chester disease (see Chapter 5.8), and chest wall hamartoma.

NONOSSIFYING FIBROMA, METAPHYSEAL FIBROUS CORTICAL DEFECT, AND AVULSIVE CORTICAL IRREGULARITY

NOFs and their smaller counterparts, metaphyseal FCDs, are among the most common lesions of bones, particularly in children. Avulsive cortical irregularity (ACI) is a clinically distinct entity that shares the same histology but occurs only at the distal femoral posteromedial metaphysis. Each of these is most often discovered incidentally on radiographs obtained for other purposes, such as the evaluation of injuries about the knee. Their clinical presentations as incidental findings and their radiographic appearance of geographic, eccentric, radiolucent, partially intracortical lesions with a soap-bubble appearance are so characteristic that biopsy is usually unnecessary to establish the diagnosis. Their natural history of resolution over time strongly favors nonoperative treatment in most cases.

PATHOGENESIS

Etiology

■ NOF/FCD: focally defective periosteal cortical bone development leads to failure of ossification (developmental defect)
■ ACI: traumatic stress of avulsive microfracture, healing, and repeat avulsive fracture related to origin of medial head of gastrocnemius muscle and/or distal adductor magnus insertion on posteromedial cortical surface of distal femur only

Epidemiology

- Incidence: true incidence unknown
  - NOF/FCD
    - NOF/FCD most common bone lesion(s) overall
    - Up to 40% of children with knee radiographs have one or more.
  - ACI
    - On x-ray, 10% to 40%, but on MRI up to 60%
- Age: 3 to 20 for all three lesions (peak 10 to 15), with some NOFs and ACIs persisting into adulthood
- Male:female 2 to 3:1 (both NOF/FCD and ACI)
- Location
  - NOF/FCD
    - Long bone metaphyses predominate.
    - 55% around knee
    - Distal femur > proximal tibia > distal tibia
    - Diaphyseal lesions and flat bones less common
  - ACI: By definition, these occur only in the postero-medial distal femoral metaphysis and are frequently bilateral.

Pathophysiology

Pathology (Fig. 5.5-1)

- Fibrous tissues arranged in storiform or cartwheel pattern with foamy histiocytes (30% to 50%, more frequent in adults), hemosiderin (variable), occasional multinucleated giant cells

Natural History

- All of these lesions usually regress after skeletal maturity at the latest, sometimes sooner.
- Most FCDs resolve without residual radiographic evidence, but some progress to NOF size.
- Some lesions persisting into adulthood become latent or eventually ossify.
- Assessing fracture risk
  - >50% of diameter of bone on both anteroposterior and lateral radiographs
  - >33 mm vertical dimension in nonfibular lesions
  - Distal tibial lesions most common site with associated fracture

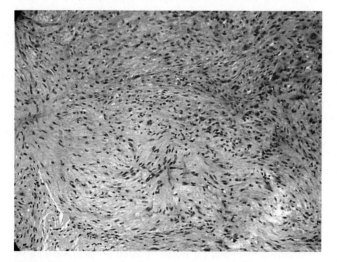

Figure 5.5-1 Histopathology of NOFs.

Classification

- NOF vs. FCD
  - FCD: typically small (<0.5 cm) radiolucency completely within the cortical bone
  - NOF: involves cortex but also extends into medullary bone
  - Some authors use a 3-cm size delineation.
- ACI: posteromedial distal femoral metaphyseal lesion
- Jaffe-Campanacci syndrome
  - *Forme fruste* of type I peripheral neurofibromatosis
  - Key components: multiple NOFs and café-au-lait spots
  - Variably associated: mental retardation, hypogonadism or cryptorchidism, ocular abnormality, cardiovascular malformations
- NOF in neurofibromatosis type I (NF-1)
  - Most common bone lesion of NF-1

DIAGNOSIS

Physical Examination and History

- Most common clinical presentation: incidental asymptomatic finding
- Other scenarios
  - Pathologic fracture with larger NOF
    - Usually not preceded by pain
  - Pain associated with lesions
    - Uncommon in FCD/NOF
    - Occurs more frequently with ACI but dissipates over time
    - Search for another source of pain.
    - Consider chondromyxoid fibroma, periosteal chondroma, and osteomyelitis in differential diagnosis for symptomatic lesions.

Radiographic Features

Plain Radiographs (Fig. 5.5-2)

- Usually diagnostic in vast majority of cases
  - Well-marginated (geographic), eccentric, partially intracortical, multiloculated, soap-bubble radiolucent lesion with a sclerotic rim
  - May be central within smaller bones such as fibula but still partially intracortical
  - Occasional cortical thinning and expansion
  - ACI best visualized on oblique radiographs; often bilateral

Magnetic Resonance Imaging

- Indicated for atypical plain film features, symptoms, or older patients
  - FCD: fibrous signal void within cortex, dark on T1-weighted but brighter on T2-weighted
  - NOF
    - Low-signal (dark) central region on both T1- and T2-weighted sequences due to hemosiderin and/or dense collagen
    - Typically no surrounding edema in absence of pathologic fracture

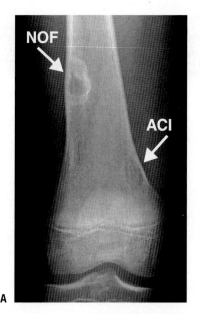
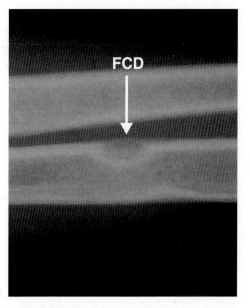
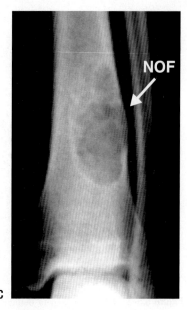

Figure 5.5-2   Various types of cortically based fibrous lesions: nonossifying fibroma (NOF), avulsive cortical irregularity (ACI), and fibrous cortical defect (FCD).

- ACI: variable manifestations, including discrete lesions and simple irregularity of the posteromedial cortex

Bone Scan
- Minimal to no uptake seen; bone scan usually not needed

TREATMENT

- Observation: treatment of choice for essentially all FCDs and ACIs and the vast majority of NOFs
- Open biopsy: atypical radiographic appearance, symptomatic lesions, and lesions in adults for which the diagnosis cannot be established by clinical and radiographic presentation (unusual)
- Curettage and grafting with or without internal fixation: usually reserved for larger lesions after fracture (see fracture risk above) or in very active patients

Results and Outcomes

- Local recurrence is nearly nonexistent for completely curetted NOF.
- Peripheral radiolucencies may indicate residual NOF tissue.

BENIGN FIBROUS HISTIOCYTOMA OF BONE

This rare neoplasm is the prototypical fibrohistiocytic benign tumor within the World Health Organization classification schema. Its importance lies in its distinction from the more common NOF, so this section will contrast the features of this lesion with NOF.

PATHOGENESIS

Etiology

- Unknown

Epidemiology

- Incidence: rare
- Age: 6 to 74 years (60% are above typical upper age limit for NOF)
- Unlike NOF, female > male preponderance (slight)
- Location
  - Any bone may be affected.
  - Like NOF, femur and tibia are most common, BUT diaphyseal or epiphyseal regions predominate in long bones (unlike metaphysis for NOF).
  - Higher frequency of pelvic bone involvement (25%) than in NOF (especially ilium)

Pathophysiology

- Histologically similar to that of NOF
- Storiform, whorled pattern of spindle cells with frequent foam (xanthoma) cells and variable benign multinucleated giant cells (Fig. 5.5-3)
- Variable hemorrhage, hemosiderin deposition

DIAGNOSIS

Physical Examination and History

- Clinical presentation varies from that of NOF.
  - Only one eighth of patients are asymptomatic.

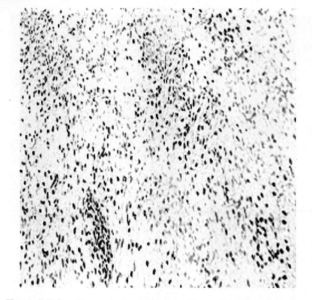

Figure 5.5-3 Histopathology of benign fibrous histiocytoma.

- Pain duration variable (days to years)
- Occasional pathologic fracture

Radiographic Features

Plain Radiographs
- Lytic medullary lesions with sharply defined margins and a sclerotic rim without matrix mineralization (Fig. 5.5-4)
- Trabeculation or pseudoseptations
- May lack well-defined margins
- Absent soft tissue extension or periosteal reaction
- Either central or eccentric in epiphyseal location
- Majority 3 cm or less (up to 7 cm)

TABLE 5.5-1 DISTINGUISHING FEATURES OF BENIGN FIBROUS HISTIOCYTOMA COMPARED WITH NONOSSIFYING FIBROMA

Nonossifying Fibroma	Benign Fibrous Histiocytoma of Bone
Metaphysis of long bones	Location in non–long bones Nonmetaphyseal in long bones
Usually <20 years old	Usually >20 years old
Painless unless fracture	Painful in absence of fracture
Geographic sclerotic soap-bubble margins	May lack typical margins

Differential Diagnosis
- Metaphyseal or diaphyseal lesion
  - NOF or metaphyseal FCD
- Epiphyseal lesion
  - Giant cell tumor of bone
  - Fibrosarcoma

Diagnostic Algorithm
Because benign fibrous histiocytoma of bone cannot be distinguished histologically from NOF, it must be distinguished based upon clinical and radiologic features (Table 5.5-1).

TREATMENT

- Extended curettage and grafting
- Wide excision

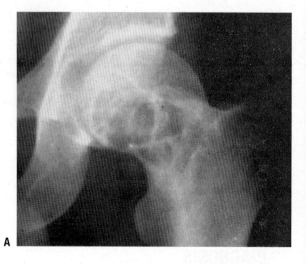

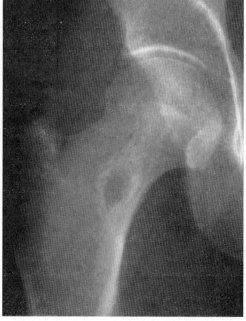

Figure 5.5-4 Benign fibrous histiocytomas of bone.

Results and Outcomes

- Excellent with appropriate surgical removal

FIBROUS DYSPLASIA

PATHOGENESIS

Etiology

- Developmental anomaly of bone formation caused by missense mutation in exon 8 of the GNAS gene (chromosome 20q13.2-13.3)
- Constitutive activation of the adenyl cyclase signaling pathway and synthesis of cyclic adenosine monophosphate (cAMP)

Epidemiology

- Incidence
  - Relatively common

- Monostotic six times more common than polyostotic form (Fig. 5.5-5)
- Age
  - Onset as children and adolescents (median onset 8 years)
  - Diagnosis in children and adults
- Male = female
- Location
  - Most common location in surgical series: jaw
  - Gender differences
  - Women: long bones most common
  - Men: ribs and skull most common
- Differences by type
  - Monostotic: skull > femur and tibia > ribs
  - Polyostotic: femur > pelvis > tibia
    - May be confined to one limb or one side of body

Pathophysiology

Pathology (Fig. 5.5-6)
- Bone replaced by firm, whitish fibrous stromal tissue of gritty consistency. It presents immature *woven bone* rather than lamellar bone without osteoblastic rimming

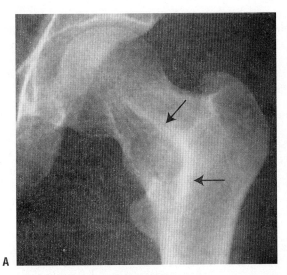

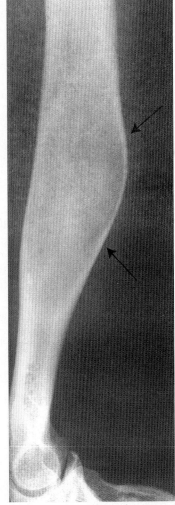

Figure 5.5-5 Radiographs of monostotic fibrous dysplasia showing typical ground glass matrix mineralization.

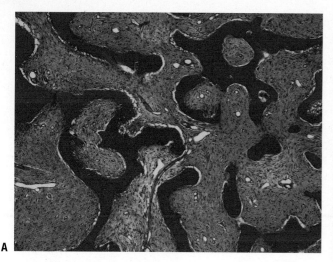

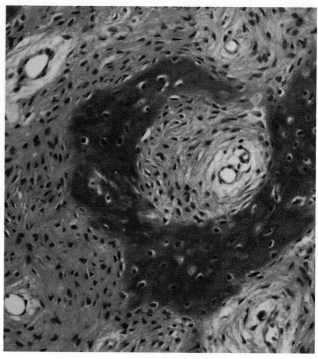

Figure 5.5-6   Histopathology of fibrous dysplasia. Photomicrographs show woven bone trabeculae without osteoblastic rimming.

of trabeculae (distinguishes from osteofibrous dysplasia, which exhibits osteoblastic rimming).

Natural History
- Normal medullary bone is replaced by variable amounts of fibrous/osseous tissues.
- More active lesions in children and adolescents; inactive more common in adults
- Malignant change rarely occurs.

Classification
- Monostotic: solitary lesion
- Polyostotic: multiple lesions
- McCune-Albright syndrome
  - Polyostotic disease, and usually presents earlier
  - Long bones, hands, feet, and pelvis often unilaterally involved (Fig. 5.5-7)
  - Café-au-lait spots with serrated borders (called "coast of Maine") that tend to stop abruptly at the midline of the body
  - Precocious puberty (endocrinopathy) may be present.
  - Malignant transformation (chondrosarcoma or osteosarcoma) about 4%
- Mazabraud's syndrome
  - Associated intramuscular myxomas

DIAGNOSIS

Physical Examination and History
- Clinical presentation: often asymptomatic, but may cause pain or fracture

- McCune-Albright syndrome: polyostotic form associated with endocrine abnormalities and skin lesions (see above)
- Mazabraud syndrome: associated intramuscular myxomas

Radiographic Features

Plain Radiographs
- Location: epiphysis, metaphysis, or diaphysis
- "Long lesion in long bone"
- Radiolucent lesion with fine, granular, ground glass matrix appearance
- Variable expansion of cortex
- No cortical disruption or periosteal reaction
- Extensive involvement of proximal femur results in a characteristic varus deformity that resembles a shepherd's crook (see Fig. 5.5-7).

Magnetic Resonance Imaging
- Dark on T1-weighted images, bright on T2-weighted images, enhancing
- Cystic degeneration may be seen.
- Defines extent of disease

Bone Scan
- Typically shows intense uptake on bone scan

Differential Diagnosis
- Paget's disease, fibrous cortical defect, hyperparathyroidism, osteoblastoma, osteosarcoma

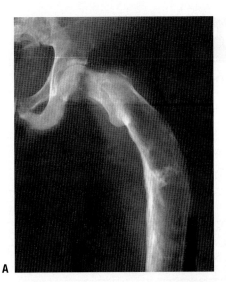

Figure 5.5-7   Radiographs (**A,B**) and bone scan (**C**) of polyostotic fibrous dysplasia. It usually involves unilateral bones. Note the shepherd's crook deformity of the proximal femur.

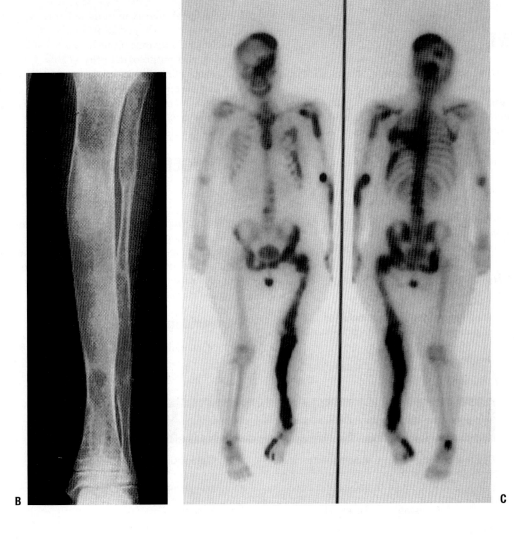

A

B

C

Table 5.5-2 DISTINGUISHING FEATURES OF FIBROUS AND OSTEOFIBROUS DYSPLASIAS

Characteristic	Fibrous Dysplasia	Osteofibrous Dysplasia
Location	Jaw, long bones	Middle third of tibia
Position within bone	Central	Eccentric (especially anterior aspect tibia)
Matrix	Ground glass	Lytic
Histology	No osteoblastic rimming	Typically some osteoblastic rimming

Diagnostic Workup Algorithm

■ Radiographic features are often diagnostic; if so, no need for biopsy.
■ If plain films are not diagnostic, additional imaging and biopsy needed

TREATMENT

■ Observation: diagnostic radiographic features with minimal or no symptoms
■ Curettage and bone grafting
  ■ Particulate graft material usually resorbed and replaced more rapidly, so not recommended
  ■ Structural graft material often resorbed more slowly, so recommended
■ Prophylactic stabilization: provides structural stability without concern for resorption of bone graft
■ Radiotherapy increases the risk of sarcomatous change and is generally avoided.
■ Bisphosphonate treatment has been used for symptomatic polyostotic fibrous dysplasia.

Results and Outcomes

■ Overall prognosis: good
■ Worst outcomes: higher local recurrence, pain, deformity in younger patients and those with polyostotic dysplasia
■ Malignant transformation: rare

OSTEOFIBROUS DYSPLASIA

Despite the similarity in nomenclature with fibrous dysplasia, osteofibrous dysplasia (formerly referred to as ossifying fibroma or Campanacci's lesion) is a distinct clinical, radiographic, and pathologic entity (Table 5.5-2). It should be recognized clinically and radiographically so that unnecessary and potentially damaging operations are avoided prior to skeletal maturity and so that it can be distinguished from adamantinoma, the low-grade malignancy with overlapping features (Table 5.5-3).

PATHOGENESIS

Etiology

■ Unknown; NOT related to GNAS gene mutations seen in fibrous dysplasia
■ Occurrence of areas with positive immunohistochemistry for epithelial elements has been termed "OFD-like adamantinoma" and suggests a relationship with adamantinoma.

Epidemiology

■ Age: usually <8 years old; rare after 15 (skeletal maturity)

TABLE 5.5-3 OVERLAPPING AND DISTINGUISHING FEATURES OF ADAMANTINOMA AND OSTEOFIBROUS DYSPLASIA

Characteristic	Adamantinoma	Osteofibrous Dysplasia
Location	Tibia	Middle third of tibia
Position within bone	Eccentric	Eccentric
Borders	Less well defined	Geographic
Cortical destruction	Frequent	Not present
Histology	Islands of epithelioid cells	Typically some osteoblastic rimming
Treatment	Wide resection	Observation until skeletal maturity

- Male > female
- Locations
  - Middle or proximal third of the tibia in vast majority; may be bilateral
  - Less commonly fibula, ulna, radius
  - May appear multifocal within single bone

Pathophysiology

Pathology (Fig. 5.5-8)

- Osteoblast-lined woven bone fragments separated by bland fibrous stroma
- Zonal architecture with loose fibrous tissue in the central zone, woven bone rimmed by osteoblasts in the fibro-osseous zone, and lamellar bone in loose, fibrous, vascular tissue in the peripheral zone

Natural History

- Benign fibrous tumor with potentially locally aggressive behavior
- Progresses during childhood but not after puberty
- Frequently recurs after curettage or subperiosteal resection
- Regression or resolution at skeletal maturity
- Rare cases may progress to adamantinoma.

DIAGNOSIS

Physical Examination and History

- Most common: swelling or painless anterior tibial bowing

- Occasionally: pathologic fractures (usually stress fractures) cause episodic pain
- Rarely: may exhibit aggressive behavior in terms of causing progressive deformity

Radiologic Features

Plain Radiographs (see Fig. 5.5-8)

- Anterior intracortical involvement of middle third of tibia is classic.
- Overlying cortex invariably thinned, expanded, or even missing
- Sclerotic, geographic intramedullary border
- Saw-toothed or soap-bubble, often multiple lucent areas anteriorly bordered by the deeper sclerotic border
- No soft tissue extension or periosteal reaction

Magnetic Resonance Imaging

- Lucent areas intermediate to dark on T1-weighted and bright on T2-weighted images
- Sclerotic surrounding reactive bone dark on all sequences

Bone Scan

- Increased uptake

TREATMENT

- Up to skeletal maturity
  - Typical radiographic features: observation, bracing
  - Atypical radiographic features: biopsy to confirm diagnosis, then observation with or without bracing

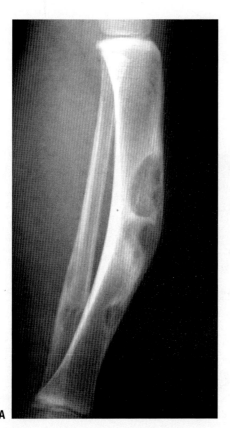

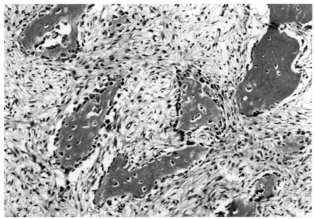

Figure 5.5-8   Radiograph (A) and histopathologic specimen (B) of osteofibrous dysplasia. Anterior intracortical tibial involvement is characteristic. Osteoblastic rimming is shown here as prominent, in contrast to fibrous dysplasia.

- Surgical excision and internal fixation occasionally indicated for progressive bowing or pathologic fracture
- After skeletal maturity
  - Curettage and grafting with or without stabilization

Results and Outcome

- High incidence of local recurrence and progression if operated on prior to skeletal maturity

DESMOPLASTIC FIBROMA

Among the benign fibrous lesions, desmoblastic fibroma is notable both for its rarity and its aggressive local behavior. Its histologic appearance mimics that of desmoid tumor of the soft tissue, but it may be confused with fibrosarcoma. Its radiographic appearance may also mimic bone sarcoma, but it does not metastasize.

PATHOGENESIS

Etiology

- Unknown, but trisomies of chromosomes 8 and 20 resemble those of soft tissue desmoids.

Epidemiology

- Incidence: rare
- Age: adolescents and young adults within first three decades of life
- Male = female
- Location: long bones (1/2) > mandible (1/4) > pelvis (1/8)

Pathophysiology

Pathology (Fig. 5.5-9)
- Identical finding to soft tissue fibromatosis
- Dense and irregularly arranged collagen bundles with infrequent fibroblasts
- Mitosis, vascularity, and necrosis are unusual.

Natural History
- Locally aggressive behavior except in rare instances
- No metastases

DIAGNOSIS

Physical Examination and History

- Pain, deformity, or loss of function

Radiologic Features (see Fig. 5.5-9)

Plain Radiographs
- Purely lytic, centrally located, and usually well circumscribed

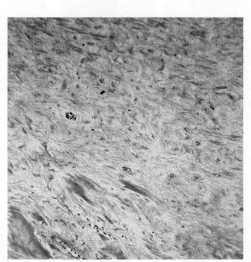

A   B

Figure 5.5-9   Radiograph and histopathology of desmoplastic fibroma.

- Intralesional trabeculation
- May be expansile or extend into soft tissues
- Differential diagnosis: giant cell tumor of bone, fibrosarcoma of bone, low-grade central osteosarcoma

Magnetic Resonance Imaging
- Dense fibrous tissue is low signal on T1-weighted and T2-weighted sequences.

TREATMENT

- *En bloc* wide resection: treatment of choice
- Extended intralesional curettage: recurrence rate unacceptably high
- Radiotherapy and chemotherapy (tamoxifen, indomethacin): reported anecdotally for inoperable tumors or locations

Results and Outcome

- Local recurrence rates
  - Extended intralesional curettage: 72%
  - *En bloc* wide resection: 17%

Postoperative Management

- Local recurrence may result years later.
- Long-term follow-up recommended

SUGGESTED READING

Bertoni F, Calderoni P, Bacchini P, et al. Benign fibrous histiocytoma of bone. *J Bone Joint Surg [Am]* 1986;68(8):1225–1230.
Gebhardt MC, Campbell CJ, Schiller AL, et al. Desmoplastic fibroma of bone. A report of eight cases and review of the literature. *J Bone Joint Surg [Am]* 1985;67(5):732–747.
Kumar S. Bisphosphonate therapy in polyostotic fibrous dysplasia. *Indian Pediatr* 2004;41(10):1069–1070.
Lane JM, Khan SN, O'Connor WJ, et al. Bisphosphonate therapy in fibrous dysplasia. *Clin Orthop Relat Res* 2001;(382):6–12.
Marks KE, Bauer TW. Fibrous tumors of bone. *Orthop Clin North Am* 1989;20(3):377–393.
O'Sullivan M, Zacharin M. Intramedullary rodding and bisphosphonate treatment of polyostotic fibrous dysplasia associated with the McCune-Albright syndrome. *J Pediatr Orthop* 2002;22(2):255–260.
Parisi MS, Oliveri MB, Mautalen CA. Bone mineral density response to long-term bisphosphonate therapy in fibrous dysplasia. *J Clin Densitom* 2001;4(2):167–172.
Pensak ML, Nestok BR, Van Loveren H, et al. Desmoplastic fibroma of the temporal bone. *Am J Otol* 1997;18(5):627–631.

5.6 GIANT CELL TUMOR OF BONE

SEAN V. McGARRY ■ C. PARKER GIBBS

Giant cell tumor (GCT) of bone is a benign but often aggressive tumor. It remains one of the most challenging of the benign bone tumors to treat. It is also unique from all other benign bone tumors except chondroblastoma in that it can metastasize. Metastases from GCT of bone almost always arise in the lung and rarely are fatal or cause significant morbidity at the site of metastasis.

PATHOGENESIS

Etiology

- Etiology is unclear.

Epidemiology

- 5% to 10% of all bone tumors
- Female:male 1.3 to 1.5:1
- Age distribution
  - Rare prior to skeletal maturity
  - Most (~75%) occur between 18 and 40 years.
- Skeletal distribution

- Nearly always involve epiphysis, but epicenter is in metaphysis
  - Rare pediatric giant cell tumors are metaphyseal but may erode across physis into epiphysis.
- Can occur in nearly any bone in the skeleton
- Most common sites of occurrence (half of all lesions occur about the knee)
  - Distal femur
  - Proximal tibia
  - Distal radius
  - Sacrum (anterior body)
  - Proximal humerus
  - Proximal femur
  - Distal tibia
- Rare in small bones of hands and feet

Pathophysiology

The cell of origin in GCT of bone is unknown, although immunohistochemical studies have suggested that the cells are of a histiocytic nature. More recently, the stromal cells have been suggested to be of osteoblastic lineage based on their expression of alkaline phosphatase, osteocalcin, and

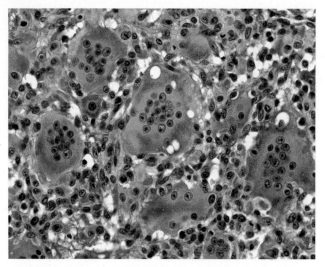

Figure 5.6-1 Photomicrograph of GCT. The nuclei of the giant cells and the monocytes appear similar, leading some to theorize that the giant cells occur from fusion of the monocytes. Currently this is not thought to be accurate.

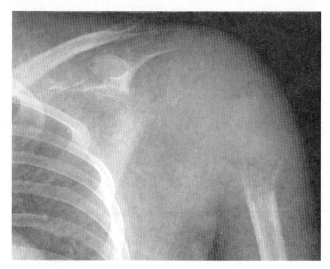

Figure 5.6-2 GCT in a 32-year-old man. The proximal humerus has been nearly completely destroyed by the lesion.

Cbfa1. The stromal cells are thought to produce RANKL, which leads to osteoclastogenesis, which in turn leads to osteolytic destruction of bone (Fig. 5.6-1). GCT of bone was at one time described as osteoclastoma. The destructive nature of GCT, in combination with its typical location in the epiphysis, explains the clinical course. The articular cartilage is initially spared. The lesion spreads across the epiphysis and eventually destroys the cortex and can form a soft tissue mass. Without the structural support of the underlying subchondral bone, pathologic fractures through the articular surface are not uncommon. Unchecked, this leads to severe secondary degenerative changes.

Histopathology (Fig. 5.6-1)

- Dense cellular pattern of monocytes admixed with numerous giant cells
- Nuclei of the monocytes appear identical to the nuclei in the giant cells.

Classification

- Following Enneking's classification of benign tumors, GCT of bone is most commonly active or aggressive.
  - Latent: rare in GCT
  - Active: any symptomatic or growing lesion
  - Aggressive (Fig. 5.6-2)
    - GCT is probably the most aggressive of the benign tumors.
    - Radiographically lesions can be extremely destructive of bone, resembling osteosarcoma.
    - Along with aneurysmal bone cyst and chondroblastoma, GCT is one of the three classically aggressive benign bone tumors.
- GCT defies the classic definition of benign tumors in that it can metastasize, although it does so rarely.
  - One of only two benign bone tumors that metastasize: GCT and chondroblastoma

DIAGNOSIS

- The radiographic findings associated with GCT are often strongly suggestive of the diagnosis.
- Other benign lesions in the differential would include chondroblastoma and aneurysmal bone cyst (ABC), although chondroblastomas are more common in the skeletally immature patient and are usually isolated to the epiphysis, and an epiphyseal location would be unusual for the ABC.
- Aggressive GCT can be mistaken for any of the primary or secondary bone malignancies that may extend into the epiphysis (telangiectatic or fibroblastic osteosarcoma, Ewing sarcoma, or metastatic disease).
- Clear cell chondrosarcoma is the one malignancy that classically occurs in an epiphyseal location and should be considered in the differential diagnosis.

Physical Examination and History

Clinical Features
- Generally relate to the extent of the joint involvement
- Patients initially present with dull achy pain of the involved joint.
- Extension of the lesion into the soft tissues and physical examination consistent with a soft tissue mass are relatively late findings.
- Extension of the lesion into the joint is unusual and is associated with complaints similar to osteoarthritis.

Radiologic Features (Fig. 5.6-3)
- Epiphyseal location: lesion is centered in the metaphysis of long bones but in skeletally mature patients uniformly involves the epiphysis and frequently extends to the subchondral bone
- Radiolucent: GCT is uniformly destructive of bone without matrix mineralization
- Eccentric: initially GCT is eccentric but spreads across the epiphysis with progression

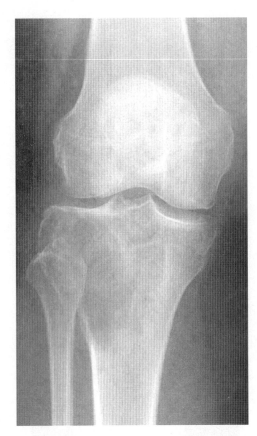

Figure 5.6-3 GCT of the proximal tibia. The lesion involves the epiphysis, is eccentric in location and destructive of bone, and extends to the articular cartilage.

- Extension to articular cartilage: extends to the subchondral bone, but initially preserves the joint
- Confined to bone: late spread breaks through the cortex

Initial Evaluation
- Orthogonal radiographs
- Magnetic resonance imaging (MRI) to assess local extent
- Chest radiograph and/or computed tomography (CT) scan of the chest as baseline for subsequent comparison in search of pulmonary metastases
- Bone scan to assess for multicentricity
- Biopsy to confirm diagnosis

Diagnostic Work-up Algorithm

GCT can rarely be multicentric. A bone scan should be performed as a staging study in all patients to evaluate for multicentricity. GCT has the potential to metastasize. Initial and follow-up evaluation should include chest radiographs or a CT scan of the chest.

TREATMENT

Indications and Contraindications

Surgery
GCT of bone is nearly always classified as active or aggressive. Because the differential diagnosis would include ma-

lignant lesions, including osteosarcoma, biopsy is usually required for diagnosis. Rarely does the lesion warrant nonoperative treatment. GCT is typically progressive and juxta-articular in location in young adults. Progression into the joint can cause irreversible damage to the joint necessitating joint replacement in a young patient. Occasionally, GCT of the axial skeleton is treated conservatively, either with radiation or observation.

Radiation Therapy
- Central inoperable lesions of the axial skeleton
- Lesions that would cause significant morbidity to operate on (i.e., sacrum or spine)

Observation
- Rarely indicated, except perhaps in the rare patient with an asymptomatic (latent) lesion

Surgical Management

- Simple curettage: high recurrence rate
- Extended intralesional curettage (with power bur and other adjuncts such as phenol, laser coagulation, or liquid nitrogen): lower, more acceptable recurrence rate
- Primary excision
  - Negligible recurrence rate
  - Overtreatment for most GCTs
  - May be indicated in expendable bones (e.g., fibula)

Preoperative Planning
- Consider surgical adjuvants to extend margin of curettage
  - Argon beam laser
  - Phenol
  - Liquid nitrogen
- Need to fill defect from curettage
  - Cement (Fig. 5.6-4)
    - Advantages
      - Immediate stability to allow weight bearing
      - Exothermic reaction during curing theoretically may provide additional antitumor effect.
      - Provides discrete radiological margin with bone that improves ability to discern local recurrence
    - Disadvantages
      - Nonbiological reconstruction
      - Cement against subchondral bone or cartilage alters biomechanics and may lead to premature degenerative arthritis.
  - Bone graft
    - Advantages
      - Biological reconstruction
    - Disadvantages
      - More difficult to distinguish local recurrence from resorption of bone graft
      - Large defects more often require prophylactic fixation and prolonged restricted weight bearing during graft incorporation.
  - Possible prophylactic fixation, depending on the extent of the lesion

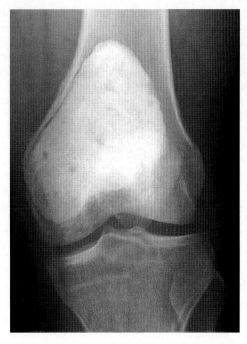

Figure 5.6-4 Postoperative radiograph of GCT in the distal femur. The lesion has been extensively curetted and the defect filled with cement. The subchondral space was packed with bone graft.

- Advisable for most large defects in long bones if bone graft used
- Advisable for poorly contained defects in long bones if cement used
  - Threaded Steinman pins within intramedullary canal and cement
  - Large screws within intramedullary canal and cement
- Joint-sacrificing procedures (*en bloc* excision) will require implants and instrumentation for reconstruction (Fig. 5.6-5).

Surgical Goals and Approaches
- Elimination of pain
- Preservation of joint (if possible)
- Restoration of function
- Low recurrence rate

Techniques
- Initially, GCT was treated with simple curettage.
- Unacceptably high recurrence rates led to more aggressive treatment (i.e., wide excision).
  - Wide excision of periarticular lesions requires sacrificing the joint.
  - This returned the patient's function to acceptable levels, but long-term results suffered in young patients undergoing reconstruction with megaprostheses.
- More recently GCT has been treated by a technique known as extended curettage.
  - The lesion is approached through a longitudinal incision.
  - The overlying cortex (intact or not) is exposed.

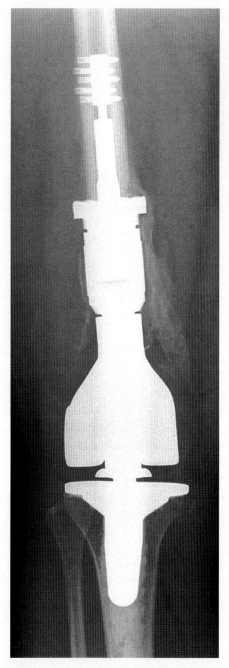

Figure 5.6-5 Postoperative radiograph of the patient with GCT of the distal femur that had progressed to destroy the joint surface. This patient underwent resection of the distal femur and reconstruction with a megaprosthesis.

- A wide cortical window is made in the bone.
- It is important that the window be sufficiently large to allow adequate visualization of the entire lesion; attempting to work around a corner or blindly curettage the lesion results in an unacceptable recurrence rate.
  - Windowing large enough to see all aspects of the defect is referred to as "exteriorization" of the defect.
- The lesion is then curetted to normal cortical or can-

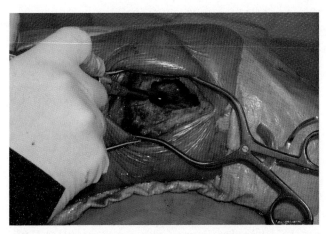

Figure 5.6-6   Intraoperative photograph of extended curettage of a GCT of bone. A bur can be seen within the lesion through the cortical window in the distal femur.

cellous bone. A high-speed bur is then used to extend the margin circumferentially around the entire lesion (Fig. 5.6-6).
- A water-pick is then used to irrigate and again visualize the lesion. The previous steps are repeated as necessary.
- An adjuvant, such as argon beam laser, phenol, or liquid nitrogen, is used to again extend the margin of the resection.
- The bony defect is then bone-grafted or cemented according to surgeon preference.
  - Cementation is most commonly used as it allows extensive curettage without concern for structural weakness.

Complications
- Oncologic complications
  - Recurrence: rate depends on technique used, as discussed in "Results and Outcome" section
  - Malignant degeneration: extremely rare, almost always related to treatment (secondary to radiation therapy)
  - Metastasis: rare, perhaps 3% (Fig. 5.6-7)
    - Most behave in a benign fashion.
    - Treatment options
      - Nonprogressive: observation
      - Progressive and limited: surgical resection
      - Progressive and extensive: chemotherapy
- Surgical complications
  - Pathologic fracture (Fig. 5.6-8)
  - Degenerative arthritis of adjacent joint

Results and Outcome

Surgery
- Simple curettage
  - Most studies have shown approximately 30% to 47% recurrence rate with simple curettage.
- Extended curettage
  - Approximately 0% to 25% recurrence rate with curettage, bur, and an adjuvant

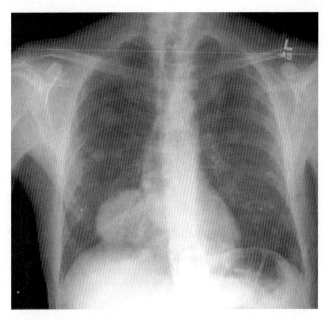

Figure 5.6-7   Chest radiograph of a patient with metastatic GCT of bone; note the multiple pulmonary lesions.

- *En bloc* excision
  - Essentially no recurrence with primary excision
  - Significant morbidity from reconstructive procedures

Radiation
- Feigenberg et al (2003) reported a recurrence rate of 23% with various combinations of surgery and radiation (many of which were in the pelvis, sacrum, or spine). One patient developed a radiation-induced sarcoma 22 years later.

Postoperative Management

Postoperative management of patients treated for GCT varies significantly based on the specific procedure performed.

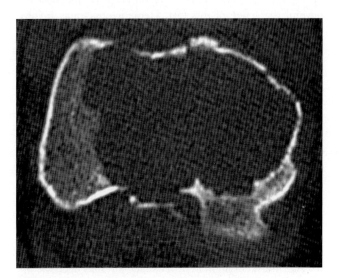

Figure 5.6-8   Axial-cut CT scan of the distal femur in a patient with GCT. A pathologic fracture in the sagittal plane is apparent.

Patients undergoing joint-replacement surgery will require extensive postoperative rehabilitation. Patients undergoing extensive curettage may require protected weight bearing if bone graft was used to fill the defect. Because of the low risk of metastases, these patients should be followed with periodic chest x-rays or chest CT scans. GCT has also been known to recur 20 years or more after the primary tumor, so these patients should be followed or at least made aware of the risk of late recurrence.

SUGGESTED READING

Campanacci M, Baldini N, Boriani S, et al. Giant-cell tumor of bone. *J Bone Joint Surg [Am]* 1987;69(1):106–114.

Capanna R, Fabbri N, Bettelli G. Curettage of giant cell tumor of bone. The effect of surgical technique and adjuvants on local recurrence rate. *Chir Organi Mov* 1990;75(1 Suppl):206.

Capanna R, Sudanese A, Baldini N, et al. Phenol as an adjuvant in the control of local recurrence of benign neoplasms of bone treated by curettage. *Ital J Orthop Traumatol* 1985;11(3):381–388.

Feigenberg SJ, Marcus Jr RB, Zlotecki RA, et al. Radiation therapy for giant cell tumors of bone. *Clin Orthop Relat Res* 2003;(411): 207–216.

Gitelis S, Mallin BA, Piasecki P, et al. Intralesional excision compared with en bloc resection for giant-cell tumors of bone. *J Bone Joint Surg [Am]* 1993;75(11):1648–1655.

Goldenberg RR, Campbell CJ, Bonfiglio M. Giant-cell tumor of bone. An analysis of two hundred and eighteen cases. *J Bone Joint Surg [Am]* 1970;52(4):619–664.

Larsson SE, Lorentzon R, Boquist L. Giant-cell tumor of bone. A demographic, clinical, and histopathological study of all cases recorded in the Swedish Cancer Registry for the years 1958 through 1968. *J Bone Joint Surg [Am]* 1975;57(2):167–173.

O'Donnell RJ, Springfield DS, Motwani HK, et al. Recurrence of giant-cell tumors of the long bones after curettage and packing with cement. *J Bone Joint Surg [Am]* 1994;76(12):1827–1833.

Simon MA, Springfield Dempsey S, eds. *Surgery for Bone and Soft-Tissue Tumors*. Philadelphia: Lippincott-Raven, 1998.

Unni KK. *Dahlin's Bone Tumors: General Aspects and Data on 11,087 Cases*, 5th ed. Philadelphia: Lippincott-Raven, 1996.

Vander Griend RA, Funderburk CH. The treatment of giant-cell tumors of the distal part of the radius. *J Bone Joint Surg [Am]* 1993; 75(6):899–908.

5.7 VASCULAR LESIONS

SEAN V. McGARRY ■ C. PARKER GIBBS

Hemangiomas are benign lesions originating from blood vessels. There is some controversy in the distinction between hemangiomas and vascular malformations. While histologically they appear identical under the microscope, vascular malformations are developmental irregularities that are usually latent and probably present at birth. Hemangiomas are true neoplasms that can be either active or latent. There are many histological subtypes of hemangiomas that have subtle microscopic differences, but these are beyond the scope of this text. Hemangiomas may involve one or more organs, including bone, the central nervous system, the liver, the skeleton, and skin and soft tissues. This chapter will discuss only lesions seen in bone. Bone hemangiomas usually occur as isolated lesions, although bone involvement may occur in conjunction with other organ systems when hemangiomas occur as part of a regional or systemic disease process, such as hemangiomatosis or skeletal/extraskeletal hemangiomatosis. Maffucci's syndrome is a combination of hemangiomas and multiple enchondromas.

PATHOGENESIS

Epidemiology

- Age: most common in fifth decade but may occur at any age
- Gender: slight female predominance

- Location: most frequently in the spine (vertebral body) and cranium
- Frequency: Asymptomatic hemangiomas of the spine are thought to occur in up to 10% of the population.

Pathophysiology (Also see Fig. 11-32)

Most simply stated, hemangiomas are capillary-sized proliferations of blood vessels occurring in bone. Hemangiomas of bone are generally asymptomatic. They are often found incidentally on radiographs taken in the work-up of other problems. When they occur in the spine they can rarely expand the vertebral body and cause neurological compromise. Pathologic fracture in the spine can also cause neurological symptoms by impinging on the cord. Hemangiomas have no potential for malignant degeneration.

Classification

- Solitary osseous hemangiomas follow Enneking's classification of benign tumors (see Chapter 4.2, Treatment Principles).
- There are numerous histologic subtypes of solitary hemangiomas, and the World Health Organization recognizes various forms of more disseminated hemangioma-related lesions as well as osseous glomus tumors and lymphangiomas (Box 5.7-1).

BOX 5.7-1 CLASSIFICATION OF HEMANGIOMAS AND HEMANGIOMA-RELATED LESIONS

Hemangiomas
Cavernous
Capillary
Epithelioid
Histiocytoid
Sclerosing
Papillary vegetant
  endothelial proliferation
  (Masson type)
Angiolymphoid hyperplasia
  with eosinophilia (Kimura
  disease)

Angiomatoses
Regional angiomatosis
Cystic angiomatosis
  (skeletal/extraskeletal
  angiomatosis)
Massive osteolysis (Gorham-
  Stout syndrome, Gorham's
  disease, disappearing
  bone disease)
Other related lesions
Osseous glomus tumor
  (glomangioma)
Lymphangioma
Lymphangiomatosis

Adapted from Adler CP, Wold L. Haemangioma and related lesions. In: Fletcher CDM, Unni KK, Mertens F, eds. *Tumours of Soft Tissue and Bone: Pathology and Genetics*. World Health Organization Classification of Tumours. Lyon: IARC Press, 2002:320–321.

DIAGNOSIS

Physical Examination and History

Clinical Features
- Asymptomatic or an incidental finding
- In a symptomatic patient, vague, achy pain
- In a subcutaneous bone, expansion of the bone may produce a mass or localized pain (Fig. 5.7-1)
- In the spine, hemangioma can cause pathologic fracture and neurological compromise with or without fracture

Radiologic Features
- Radiographs/computed tomography (CT) scans
  - Very characteristic "jail-cell striation" on sagittal or coronal imaging; axial imaging demonstrates the trabeculae as speckled areas ("polka-dot pattern") of ossification (Fig. 5.7-2)
- Magnetic resonance imaging (MRI)
  - Usually bright signal on T2 imaging (Fig. 5.7-3) and significantly enhanced by contrast

Diagnostic Work-up Algorithm

- Hemangioma of bone can usually be confirmed by radiographs or CT scan (Fig. 5.7-4).
- Serial examinations can confirm the benign nature of the lesion, although growth of the lesion can occur in the growing child.
- Any question of diagnosis can be confirmed with a biopsy.

TREATMENT

Surgical Indications/Contraindications

- Asymptomatic lesions: Surgical indications in the asymptomatic patient are extremely limited.

- Symptomatic lesions
  - Conservative treatment is offered initially for symptomatic lesions and includes anti-inflammatory medications, low-dose radiation, and sclerosing therapy.
  - In spinal lesions in which expansion of the bone is causing neurological symptoms, radiation therapy and surgical intervention are reasonable alternatives. (Any surgical intervention should probably include preoperative embolization.)
  - In acute pathologic fractures of the spine with neurological compromise, surgical intervention is generally required to stabilize the spine and decompress the cord.

Surgical and Nonoperative Options

- Surgical excision
  - Typically offered only for symptomatic spine lesions
  - Can be an option in symptomatic lesions of expendable bone (rare)
- Radiation therapy
  - Used for inaccessible symptomatic lesions
  - Symptomatic lesions in patients for whom excision would cause unacceptable morbidity
- Embolization
  - Typically used in combination with surgery to control intraoperative bleeding
  - Effect is usually only temporary.
- Sclerosing therapy
  - Multiple different agents used
  - Mixed results

Preoperative Planning

- Larger lesions considered for embolization therapy to prevent massive intraoperative blood loss
- Balance nonmalignant nature of lesion against the morbidity associated with excision.

Surgical Goals and Approaches

- The surgical goals for excision of a hemangioma are the same as any other tumor: removal of the mass, a low rate of recurrence, and acceptable perioperative and postoperative morbidity.
- Because hemangiomas have essentially no malignant potential, a higher recurrence rate is accepted to allow closer margins in the rare symptomatic case that requires operative intervention.

Techniques

- *En bloc* excision of smaller lesions can be used to decrease surgical bleeding.
- Radiation and/or embolization can be used in conjunction with surgical excision to decrease recurrence.

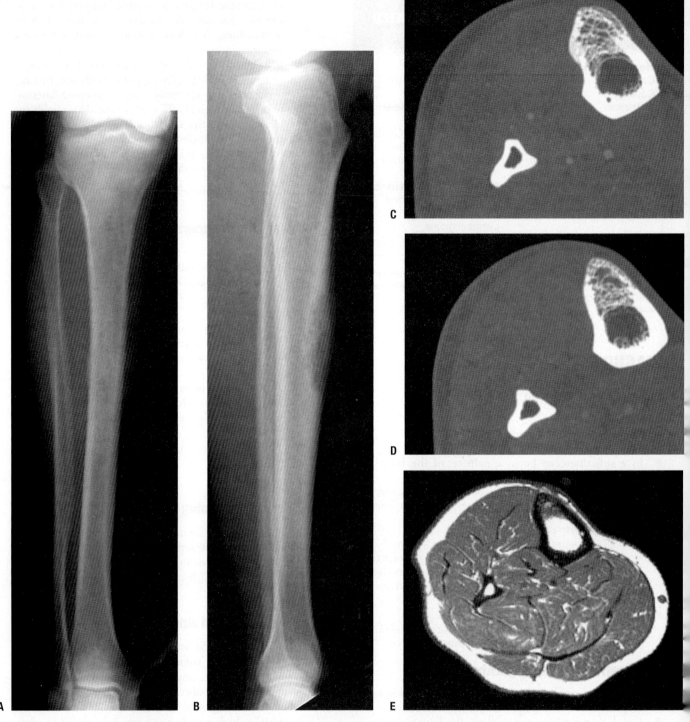

Figure 5.7-1   Rarely, osseous hemangiomas occur in the long bones, as in this case of a tibial hemangioma. The lesion is shown on plain anteroposterior (**A**) and lateral (**B**) radiographs, CT (**C,D**), and MRI (**E–G**). In a subcutaneous osseous site such as this, an osseous hemangioma may cause pain and local tenderness. (*continues*)

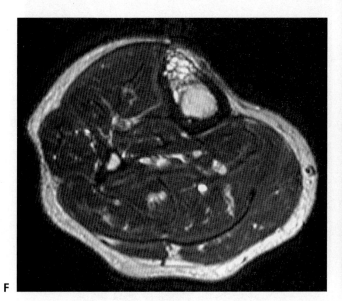

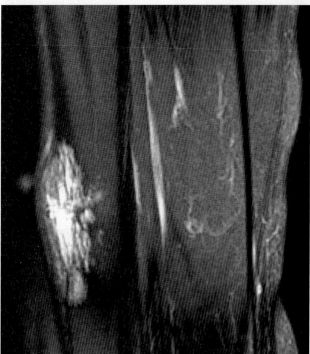

F   G

Figure 5.7-1 *(continued)*

Complications

- Oncologic complications
  - Recurrence
  - No risk of malignant degeneration
- Surgical complications
  - Massive hemorrhage

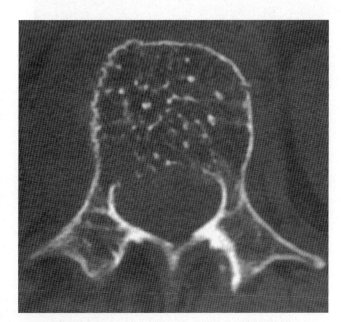

Figure 5.7-2 Axial-cut CT scan of L1 vertebrae demonstrates "speckled ossification" in the vertebral body, characteristic of hemangioma of bone.

- Neurovascular injury secondary to anatomic location of the lesion

Results and Outcome

Surgery
- Clean margins: very low recurrence rate
- Contaminated margins: often results in recurrence
  - Recurrence may or may not be symptomatic and require re-excision.

Radiation
- Radiation as sole treatment modality in vertebral hemangioma
  - Meta-analysis of 21 studies involving 63 patients
    - Complete remission 57%
    - Partial remission 32%
    - No response 11%
- Radiation in combination with other modalities in treatment of vertebral hemangioma
  - Meta-analysis of 55 studies involving 210 patients
    - Complete remission 54%
    - Partial remission 32%
    - No response 11%

Embolization
- Good as adjuvant to surgical excision to control bleeding
- Only temporary control as lone treatment

Sclerosing Therapy
- Mixed results

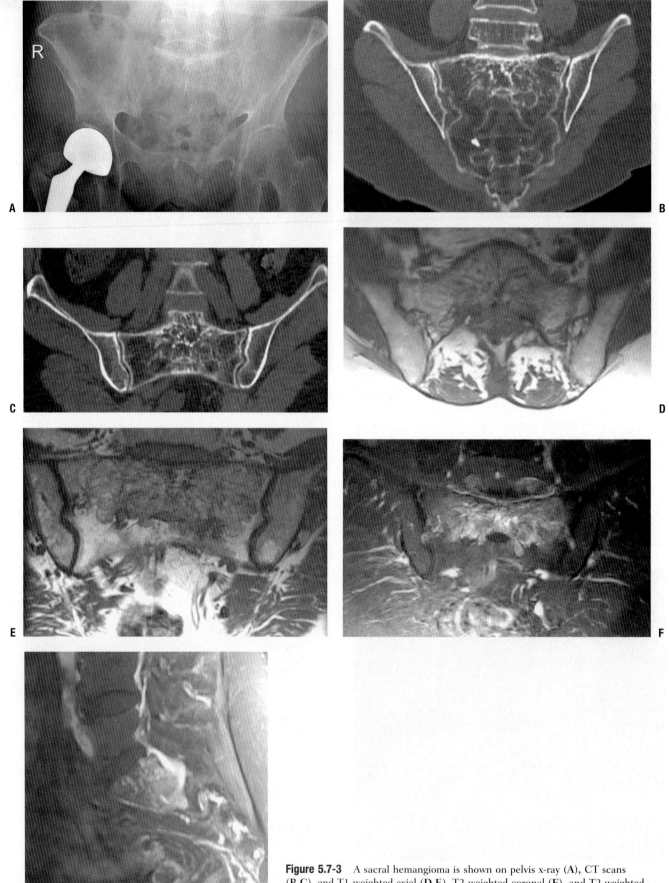

Figure 5.7-3 A sacral hemangioma is shown on pelvis x-ray (**A**), CT scans (**B,C**), and T1-weighted axial (**D,E**), T2-weighted coronal (**F**), and T2-weighted sagittal (**G**) MRIs.

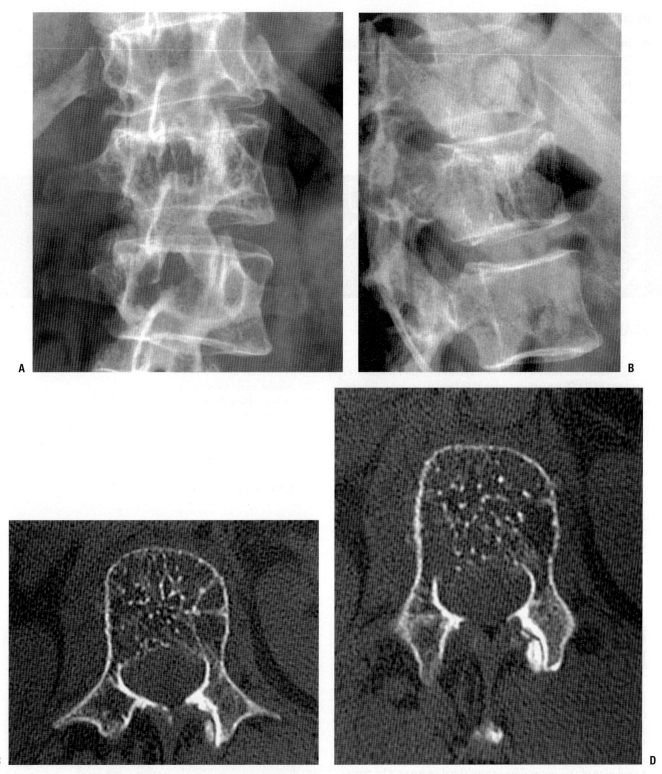

Figure 5.7-4   A typical vertebral hemangioma should be suspected based on the vertical striations often seen on plain radiographs (**A**) and shown best on the lateral view here (**B**). CT in this case confirms the diagnosis by showing the characteristic polka-dot pattern on axial imaging (**C,D**).

Postoperative Management

■ Immediate postoperative management following surgical excision should include surgical drains and compressive dressings to prevent seroma or hematoma.

■ Precautions vary considerably depending on the specific surgical intervention but may include protected weight bearing to allow healing of involved bone.

SUGGESTED READING

Adler CP, Wold L. Haemangioma and related lesions. In: Fletcher CDM, Unni KK, Mertens F, eds. *Tumours of Soft Tissue and Bone: Pathology and Genetics.* World Health Organization Classification of Tumours. Lyon: IARC Press, 2002:320–321.

Unni KK. *Dahlin's Bone Tumors: General Aspects and Data on 11,087 Cases,* 5th ed. Philadelphia: Lippincott-Raven, 1996.

5.8 OTHER TUMORS OF UNDEFINED NEOPLASTIC NATURE

SEAN V. McGARRY   ■   C. PARKER GIBBS

Langerhans cell histiocytosis (LCH) and Erdheim-Chester disease (ECD) are histiocytoses: rare benign lesions of bone in which the proliferating tumor cell of origin is a histiocyte. There are two types of histiocytes: (1) macrophages arising from monocytes and (2) dendritic cells arising from Langerhans cells. In LCH the involved cell is a Langerhans cell, in ECD a macrophage. Histiocytoses in general exist in multiple forms, ranging from a solitary lesion to a diffuse systemic disease, and they can affect any organ or tissue in the body. This section deals with the two histiocytoses involving bone: LCH and ECD. LCH is most commonly a solitary lesion occurring in children and young adults and often requires surgical intervention. ECD is often a systemic disease of older adults and very rarely involves surgical intervention.

ERDHEIM-CHESTER DISEASE

The original description of ECD was made by Chester in 1930. In 1972, Jaffe first used the eponym ECD to recognize that description. In 1983, a review of the literature by Alper found that 47 cases had been described up to that point. ECD remains an extremely rare entity; thus, our knowledge of the natural history of the disease and its treatment is somewhat limited. Its etiology is unknown.

PATHOGENESIS

Epidemiology

■ Typically a disease of older adults (Fig. 5.8-1)
  ■ Age range 7 to 84 years

  ■ Mean age 53 years
■ Slight male predominance
■ Affects long bones most commonly
  ■ Bilateral and symmetric
  ■ Classically affects diaphysis and metaphysis, sparing epiphysis (not always)
  ■ Lower extremity (femur, tibia, fibula) more common than upper extremity (humerus, radius, ulna)
■ Usually spares flat bones

Pathophysiology

■ Systemic lipid storage disorder affecting histiocytes
■ Lipid-laden histiocytes form granulomas in bones, other organs or tissues.

Prognosis and Natural History

■ Because of the infrequency of the disease, little is known about prognostic factors.

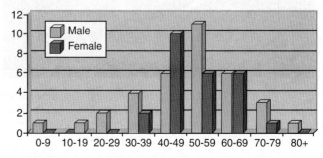

Figure 5.8-1   Sex and age at time of diagnosis for 59 patients with Erdheim-Chester disease. (After Veyssier-Belot C, Cacoub P, Caparros-Lefebvre D, et al. Erdheim-Chester disease: Clinical and radiologic characteristics of 59 cases. *Medicine* 1996;75:157–169.)

Prognosis is related to extent of visceral involvement.
- In some patients the disease is quiescent.
- In most patients the disease is progressive, and patients die of end-organ failure
  - Respiratory distress or pulmonary fibrosis
  - Heart failure
  - Renal failure

Classification

- There currently is no accepted classification scheme for ECD.

DIAGNOSIS

Physical Examination and History

- A definitive diagnosis requires the combination of history, physical examination findings, radiographs, and a tissue diagnosis.
- Classical radiographic findings with bilateral, symmetric osteosclerosis of the diaphysis and metaphysis with epiphyseal sparing can be considered pathognomonic.

Clinical Features
- Depends on the organ systems affected (Table 5.8-1 and Fig. 5.8-2)

Radiologic Features
- Densely sclerotic changes of the metaphysis and diaphysis, with coarsened trabeculae
  - Typically spares the epiphysis
  - Rarely, lesions are more lytic in nature.
- Long bones most commonly affected (Fig. 5.8-3)

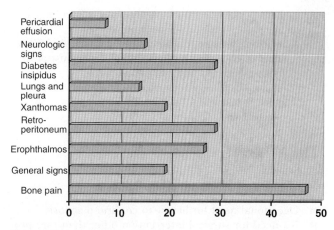

Figure 5.8-2 Prevalence of clinical signs in 59 patients with Erdheim-Chester disease. (After Veyssier-Belot C, Cacoub P, Caparros-Lefebvre D, et al. Erdheim-Chester disease: Clinical and radiologic characteristics of 59 cases. *Medicine* 1996;75:157–169.)

- Lower extremities more commonly affected than upper extremities

Diagnostic Workup Algorithm

- Radiographs are nearly always pathognomonic for ECD.
- When seen in concert with typical complaints of bone pain, exophthalmos, diabetes insipidus, or xanthomas, these patients are not a diagnostic challenge.
- They can show elevated erythrocyte sedimentation rate, alkaline phosphatase, or serum lipid profiles.
  - However, laboratory testing is unreliable and nonspecific.

TABLE 5.8-1 CLINICAL MANIFESTATIONS OF ERDHEIM-CHESTER DISEASE ACCORDING TO ORGAN OF INVOLVEMENT

Site of Involvement	Clinical Manifestation
Bone	Bone pain
Kidney	Hypertension Renal failure
Retrobulbar region	Exophthalmos
Pericardium	Pericarditis
Pituitary gland	Diabetes insipidus
Lungs	Pulmonary fibrosis
Skin	Xanthomas
Central nervous system	Confusion Ataxia

Adapted from Veyssier-Belot C, Cacoub P, Caparros-Lefebvre D, et al. Erdheim-Chester disease: Clinical and radiologic characteristics of 59 cases. *Medicine* 1996;75:157–169.

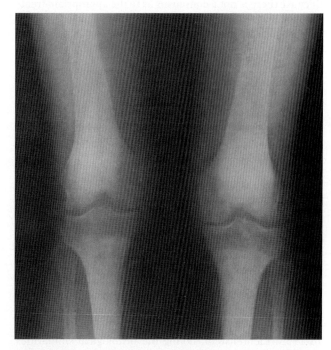

Figure 5.8-3 Radiograph of patient with Erdheim-Chester disease showing typical radiographic changes.

■ If there is any question as to the diagnosis, a biopsy of an accessible skeletal lesion is performed.
  ■ Histopathologic evaluation demonstrates infiltration of the bone by foamy, lipid-laden histiocytes, with giant cells and rare lymphocytes.
  ■ Immunostaining demonstrates negative staining for both S-100 and CD1a (which would suggest the diagnosis of LCH).

TREATMENT

Surgical and Nonoperative Options

■ Occasional need for biopsy to confirm diagnosis
■ No need for surgical intervention other than rare prophylactic fixation to prevent fracture
■ No good nonoperative treatment options, but historically patients are treated with any combination of the following:
  ■ Steroids
  ■ Chemotherapy
  ■ Radiation

Results and Outcome

Overall Outcome

With no good treatment options for ECD, overall survival is rather bleak. In a review of 37 patients followed for an average of 30 months, Veyssier-Belot reported a mortality rate of 59%. Other reports suggest a mortality rate of approximately 33%, but with limited follow-up. Patients die of end-organ failure (pulmonary fibrosis, heart failure, or renal failure most commonly).

Specific Treatment Outcome

Because there is not a consensus as to the appropriate treatment of ECD in combination with the rarity of the diagnosis, there are not sufficient numbers to assess specific treatment outcomes. In the review by Veyssier-Belot, the following results are presented:

■ Steroid therapy alone in 12 patients
  ■ Effective transiently in 4 patients
  ■ Ineffective in 8
■ Chemotherapy in combination with steroids in 8 patients
  ■ 4 patients improved
  ■ No effect in 4 patients
■ Radiation therapy in 6 patients
  ■ Transiently effective in 3 for bone pain
  ■ Not effective in 3 to treat exophthalmos

LANGERHANS CELL HISTIOCYTOSIS

In 1953, Lichtenstein, noting the histological similarities in eosinophilic granuloma, Hand-Christian-Schüller, and Letterer-Siwe, coined the term "histiocytosis X" as a general term to encompass all three diagnoses. We know today that all three diseases originate from a Langerhans cell and refer to the group of disorders as the Langerhans cell histiocytoses (LCH) or granulomatoses. The three share a common histopathology and are considered to be clinical variations of the same disease.

PATHOGENESIS

Etiology

■ Unknown
  ■ Possibly autoimmune
  ■ Possibly viral infection

Epidemiology

Eosinophilic Granuloma
■ Solitary or multiple lesions of bone, but most commonly solitary (80%)
■ Age and gender
  ■ Can occur at any age
  ■ Most patients are between 5 and 20.
  ■ Male:female ratio 2:1
■ Location
  ■ Flat bones > long bones
  ■ Skull, pelvis, ribs, spine (anterior column)
  ■ In long bones, occurs in diaphysis and metaphysis
  ■ Rare in hands, feet, posterior column of spine, epiphysis of long bones

Hand-Christian-Schüller
■ Disseminated, more severe
■ Three names (Hand-Christian-Schüller): think clinical triad:
  ■ Bone lesions (usually skull)
  ■ Exophthalmos
  ■ Diabetes insipidus
■ Age and gender
  ■ Most <5 years
  ■ Male:female closer to 1:1 than solitary eosinophilic granuloma
■ Location
  ■ Multifocal
  ■ Very common in skull and jawbones
  ■ Can occur in hands, feet

Letterer-Siwe
■ Disseminated, nearly always fatal
  ■ Extensive cutaneous lesions
  ■ Hepatosplenomegaly
  ■ Fevers/infections
■ Age/gender
  ■ Nearly all <2 years (two names [Letterer-Siwe]: think 2 years)
■ Location
  ■ Ends up involving nearly the entire skeleton

Pathophysiology

■ The reticuloendothelial system is a key component of the immune system involved in phagocytizing foreign material and debris.

- Langerhans cells are an important part of that system.
  - They originate in the bone marrow and then move to the lymph nodes, liver, lung, spleen, and skin.
  - LCH is a proliferation of these cells.

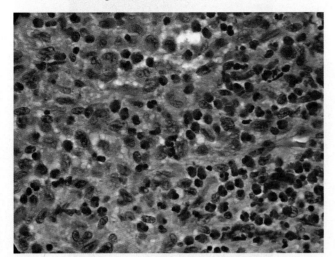

Figure 5.8-4   Typical histopathology section from bony LCH lesion shows the key langerhans histiocytes (large, basophilic, cleared, coffee-bean shaped nuclei) and eosinophils.

- This is followed by a granulomatous reaction by the body, with the characteristic eosinophilic cell population.

- It is the Langerhans cell that is required for the histological diagnosis, not the ubiquitous eosinophil, making the name "eosinophilic granuloma" a bit of a misnomer.

Classification

- Solitary lesions of eosinophilic granuloma are staged as benign bone tumors.
  - Latent
  - Active
  - Aggressive
- LCH defies most conventional bone tumor classification schemes (Table 5.8-2).

DIAGNOSIS

Physical Examination and History

- Physical examination and history can vary greatly with LCH, based on the subtype.
- Often in Hand-Christian-Schüller or Letterer-Siwe, the patient has already been given a diagnosis by the pediatrician before he or she is referred to the orthopaedic surgeon.
- A history of localized or referred pain often results from a solitary bone lesion.
- Patients may also be asymptomatic, the lesions being discovered incidentally on radiographs done for other reasons.

TABLE 5.8-2 STAGING SYSTEM FOR LANGERHANS' CELL HISTIOCYTOSIS

Stage	Description
I	
Ia	Single monostotic bone lesion
Ib	Multiple bone lesions
II	Age >2 years at diagnosis, having one or more of the following systems involved:
	Diabetes insipidus
	Teeth and gingivae
	Lymph nodes
	Skin
	Seborrhea
	Mild lung involvement
	Bone marrow focally positive
III	
IIIa	Age <2 years at diagnosis, having any of the above systems involved
IIIb	Age >2 years at diagnosis, with involvement of following:
	Liver and/or spleen
	Massive nodal involvement
	Major lung involvement (fibrosis)
	Bone marrow packed
IV	Spleen >6 cm palpable below costal margin and fever >1 month with or without any or all of the above systems involved
V	Monocytosis in peripheral blood >20% of differential cell count, in addition to stage III or IV findings

Adapted from Greenberger JS, Crocker AC, Vawter G, et al. Results of treatment of 127 patients with systemic histiocytosis. *Medicine (Baltimore)* 1981;60:311–338.

Clinical Features

Eosinophilic Granuloma
- Typically patients present with localized bone pain.
- Occasionally referred pain from a proximal site
  - Example: knee pain with normal x-ray, get hip x-ray
- Younger patients may present with limp or refusal to bear weight.

Hand-Christian-Schüller
- Classic triad is not all that classic (only 10% to 20%).
  - Bone lesions (typically skull)
  - Exophthalmos
  - Diabetes insipidus

Letterer-Siwe
- Bone lesions are not the typical initial presentation.
- Fevers/infections
- Exophthalmos
- Hepatosplenomegaly
- Lymphadenopathy
- Cutaneous lesions
  - Papular rash

Radiologic Features

Eosinophilic Granuloma
- Destructive, poorly marginated, lucent lesions (Fig. 5.8-5)
  - One of the "great mimickers," along with osteomyelitis (Fig. 5.8-6)
  - Usually based in the medullary canal
  - Later or healing lesions may have a cortical rim (Fig. 5.8-7).

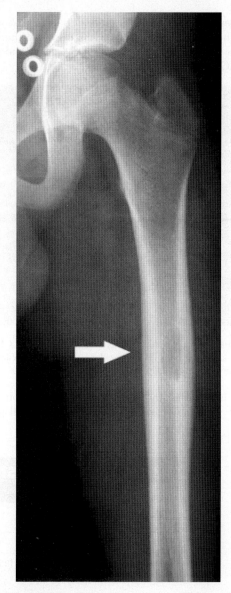

Figure 5.8-6   Note the radiolucent nature of eosinophilic granuloma in this femoral lesion found in a 12-year-old boy.

- When they occur in flat bones, they may resemble Ewing sarcoma.
- Vertebral body involvement
  - Vertebra plana (Fig. 5.8-8)
- Occasionally larger lesions show cortical destruction and periosteal reaction (resembling osteosarcoma, Ewing sarcoma, or osteomyelitis) (Fig. 5.8-9).

Hand-Christian-Schüller
- Radiographically similar to eosinophilic granuloma lesions
  - Multiple
  - Larger
  - May have a bubbly appearance as lesions overlay

Letterer-Siwe
- More subtle than eosinophilic granuloma or Hand-Christian-Schüller
- Lesions are smaller.

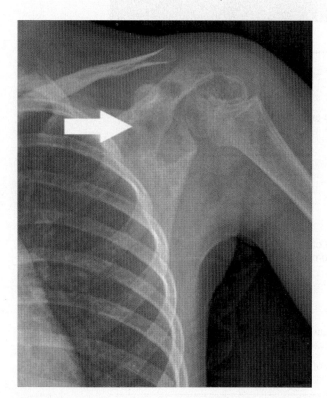

Figure 5.8-5   A destructive poorly marginated lesion in the scapula of a 5-year-old girl.

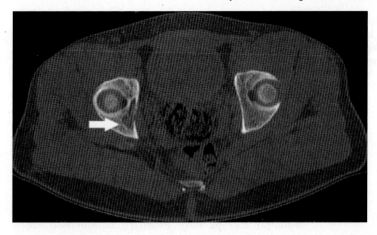

Figure 5.8-7   Axial CT of a well-corticated lesion in the posterior wall/column of an 18-year-old man.

Diagnostic Workup

- Work-up of a patient with lucent lesion suspicious for eosinophilic granuloma
  - Orthogonal radiographs
  - Possibly axial imaging (computed tomography [CT]/ magnetic resonance imaging [MRI])
  - Bone scan or skeletal survey to rule out polyostotic disease, based on other symptoms or clinical suspicion for polyostotic disease. However, approximately 30% of the lesions do not show increased uptake on bone scan, making bone scan less reliable than skeletal survey.
  - Biopsy

TREATMENT

Surgical Indications/Contraindications

- Usually biopsy is required to rule out other more serious diagnoses on the differential
  - Ewing sarcoma
  - Osteomyelitis
  - Osteosarcoma
  - Leukemia/lymphoma
- Once a diagnosis is made, surgical indications depend on symptoms, location, size, and number of lesions.
  - Painful solitary lesions may warrant a curettage and bone graft, particularly if able to be done coincident with an open biopsy.
  - Impending pathologic fractures should be considered for curettage and prophylactic stabilization.

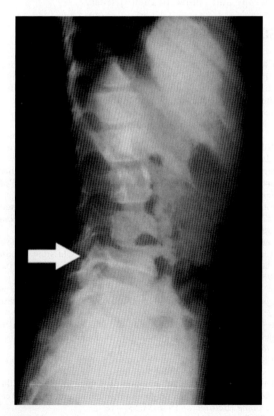

Figure 5.8-8   Radiographic findings of vertebra plana. Arrow indicates a flattened L4 vertebrae, secondary to eosinophilic granuloma.

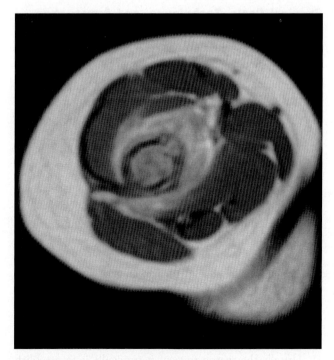

Figure 5.8-9   Axial cut of a T2-weighted MRI image showing extensive edema in the soft tissue of this distal humeral lesion.

- Numerous small lesions (Hand-Christian-Schüller or Letterer-Siwe) typically don't require surgery but will require chemotherapy and/or radiation therapy.
- Some authors have suggested the use of corticosteroid injection, but with mixed results.

Surgical and Nonoperative Options

- Surgical
  - Biopsy
  - Curettage/bone graft
  - Prophylactic stabilization
  - Aspiration and steroid injection
- Chemotherapy (for multiple or resistant lesions)
  - Vinblastine
  - Etoposide
  - Prednisone
  - Methotrexate
  - 6-mercaptopurine
- Radiation therapy
  - Consider for vertebral lesions at risk of collapse.
    - Establish diagnosis first (usually CT-guided needle biopsy) to avoid mistreatment of Ewing sarcoma or lymphoma.
    - Low dose (500 to 800 cGy)
  - Other inaccessible symptomatic lesions

Preoperative Planning

- Plan biopsy tract.
- Consider surgical adjuvant (phenol, liquid nitrogen, or argon-beam coagulation). This theoretically offers a lower recurrence rate, although most reports in the literature are small series or case reports.

Surgical Goals, Techniques, and Approaches

- Depend on location, size, symptoms
- Intralesional curettage with or without surgical adjuvant vs. aspiration and steroid injection

Complications

- Degenerative changes can occur in periarticular lesions that have been curettaged; consider an adjuvant.
- Neurologic symptoms in vertebral lesions
- Pathologic fracture

Results and Outcome

- Results and outcome vary significantly based on extent of systemic involvement.

Solitary Eosinophilic Granuloma
- Solitary eosinophilic granuloma will occasionally heal on its own.
- When it does not, simple curettage and bone graft is usually curative, with a low recurrence rate.
- Almost all solitary lesions ultimately heal.
- Usually the reason to treat it surgically is to establish the diagnosis and rule out a malignant diagnosis.

Systemic Disease
- Results and outcome for systemic disease not as good
- Because of the rarity of the disease and the lack of standardized protocols, there are not many reports in the literature on outcome other than case reports.
- Age of diagnosis is a significant prognostic indicator.
  - Diagnosis at 2 years of age or younger (typically Letterer-Siwe): 10-year survival 42%
  - Diagnosis in patients >2 years of age (usually Hand-Christian-Schüller): 85% 10-year survival
- Patients who survived had higher incidence of developmental delays, mental retardation, and secondary malignancies, though these data were from patients treated from 1941 to 1975, and chemotherapy and radiation therapy have improved considerably since that time.

Postoperative Management

- Anatomic location dictates the need for protected weight bearing.
- Patients with solitary lesions of eosinophilic granuloma should be followed closely until the lesion heals.
  - After the lesion heals, these patients are followed by routine surveillance to rule out recurrence.
- Patients treated with low-dose radiation are at an extremely low risk of radiation-induced sarcoma, but this should be kept in mind.
- Patients with Hand-Christian-Schüller or Letterer-Siwe will require pediatric oncology to manage their chemotherapy and course of their disease.

SUGGESTED READING

Alper MG, Zimmerman LE, Piana FG. Orbital manifestations of Erdheim-Chester disease. *Trans Am Ophthalmol Soc* 1983;81:64–85.

Azouz EM, Saigal G, Rodriguez MM, et al. Langerhans' cell histiocytosis: pathology, imaging and treatment of skeletal involvement. *Pediatr Radiol* 2005;35:103–115.

Cline MJ. Histiocytes and histiocytosis. *Blood* 1994;84:2840–2853.

Fernando Ugarriza L, Cabezudo JM, Porras LF, et al. Solitary eosinophilic granuloma of the cervicothoracic junction causing neurological deficit. *Br J Neurosurg* 2003;17:178–181.

Globerman H, Burstein S, Girardina PJ, et al. A xanthogranulomatous histiocytosis in a child presenting with short stature. *Am J Pediatr Hematol Oncol* 1991;13:42–46.

Greenberger JS, Crocker AC, Vawter G, et al. Results of treatment of 127 patients with systemic histiocytosis. *Medicine (Baltimore)* 1981;60:311–338.

Lichtenstein L. Histiocytosis X: integration of eosinophilic granuloma of bone, Letterer-Siwe disease, and Schuller-Christian disease as related manifestations of a single nosologic entity. *AMA Arch Pathol* 1953;56:84–102.

Miller RL, Sheeler LR, Bauer TW, et al. Erdheim-Chester disease. Case report and review of the literature. *Am J Med* 1986;80:1230–1236.

Mirra JM. *Bone Tumors,* 1st ed. Philadelphia: Lea & Febiger, 1989.

Resnick D, Greenway G, Genant H, et al. Erdheim-Chester disease. *Radiology* 1982;142:289–295.

Unni KK. *Dahlin's Bone Tumors: General Aspects and Data on 11,087 Cases,* 5th ed. Philadelphia: Lippincott-Raven, 1996.

Veyssier-Belot C, Cacoub P, Caparros-Lefebvre D, et al. Erdheim-Chester disease. Clinical and radiologic characteristics of 59 cases. *Medicine (Baltimore)* 1996;75:157–169.

Waite RJ, Doherty PW, Liepman M, et al. Langerhans cell histiocytosis with the radiographic findings of Erdheim-Chester disease. *AJR Am J Roentgenol* 1988;150:869–871.

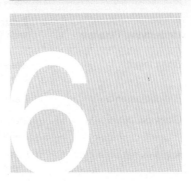

BONE SARCOMAS

6.1 OSTEOSARCOMA

FRANCIS R. PATTERSON

Osteosarcoma is the most common sarcoma of bone in young people. While relatively rare compared to other orthopaedic disorders, an appropriate level of suspicion must be maintained for osteosarcoma as a source of pain in this age group. When diagnosed early and treated appropriately, survival with a highly functional limb can often be achieved in this age group. Most osteosarcoma patients present with pain as the initial symptom, but some patients first notice this after an injury or falsely attribute their symptoms to a minor trauma. Therefore, pain that does not improve in the expected time period, or pain that is worsening despite treatment or rest, should raise a red flag, and an appropriate work-up, starting with plain radiographs, must be pursued. Osteosarcoma has a bimodal distribution with a second but smaller peak in late adulthood. Adult osteosarcomas are often secondary to conditions such as Paget's disease or prior radiation (Table 6.1-1). After biopsy, the standard treatment of osteosarcoma includes preoperative chemotherapy, followed by resection, and postoperative chemotherapy when appropriate.

PATHOGENESIS

Etiology

■ Osteosarcoma is a tumor composed of a malignant spindle cell stroma (background) with malignant osteoblasts

TABLE 6.1-1 DISEASE-ASSOCIATED OSTEOSARCOMAS

Underlying Disease	Evidence Supporting Association with Osteosarcoma	Caveats and Pearls
Bone infarct	Several case reports Small series	75% occur in patients with multiple infarcts
Retinoblastoma	Demonstrable increased risk of osteosarcoma	Rb gene germline defects
Giant cell tumor	Malignant transformation to osteosarcoma in small fraction of patients	More common after radiation and multiple recurrences
Aneurysmal bone cyst	Case reports of osteosarcoma within previously treated aneurysmal bone cysts	Consider telangiectatic osteosarcoma in differential diagnosis of any case of aneurysmal bone cyst due to radiologic similarity.
Fibrous dysplasia	Rare occurrence of osteosarcoma in some series Numerous case reports	Almost half of patients had prior history of irradiation.
Osteogenesis imperfecta	Case reports only	Need to distinguish from fracture callus
Chronic osteomyelitis	Case reports	Chronic osteomyelitis may mimic appearance of osteosarcoma radiologically and clinically.
Arthroplasty-associated	Case reports	

that produce tumor osteoid (collagenous immature bone that appears pink on hematoxylin-and-eosin [H& E] staining) or bone (Fig. 6.1-1).

- As is the case with most sporadic occurring malignancies, the factors that lead to the development of an osteosarcoma are largely unknown.
  - Most likely, a mutation or group of mutations occurs that leads to uncontrolled growth of the mutant cells.
  - Evidence exists to support the role of genetic abnormalities in patients with osteosarcoma, though these abnormalities are not identified in most patients.

- Two tumor suppressor genes may play a significant part in tumorigenesis in osteosarcoma: p53 (chromosome 17) and Rb (chromosome 13).
- Reported familial patterns of osteosarcoma
  - Chromosome 13:14 rearrangement in sisters
  - Deletion of part of chromosome 13 resulting in inactivation of the retinoblastoma (RB) gene in cousins
- Two genetic conditions that predispose to development of osteosarcoma
  - Retinoblastoma patients
    - May have germline mutation of Rb gene
    - Increased risk of osteosarcoma
  - Li-Fraumeni syndrome (a familial cancer syndrome; p53 gene abnormalities)
    - Increased risk of osteosarcomas and other malignancies
    - Mothers of children with sarcomas have up to a three times increased risk of breast carcinoma.

Epidemiology

Osteosarcoma is the most common type of bone sarcoma. It is neither the most common primary bone malignancy nor the most common malignancy affecting bone. The most common primary bone malignancy is multiple myeloma, and the most common malignancy affecting bone is metastatic carcinoma.

- Bimodal peak age incidence
  - Crude incidence: 0.3 per 100,000 per year in United States (roughly 900 per year)
  - Majority occur within the second decade (~60%)

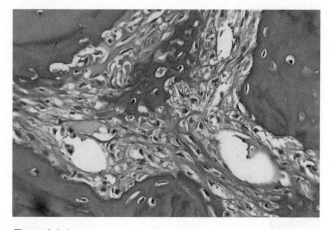

Figure 6.1-1 H&E stain shows a malignant spindle cell (osteoblast) stroma with lace-like (pink) osteoid and calcified (darker) osteoid in center, typical of a high-grade osteosarcoma.

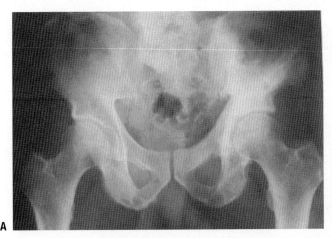
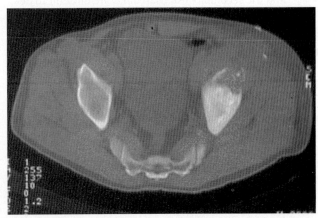

Figure 6.1-2   (A) Plain radiograph shows an area of bony destruction in the anterior left iliac wing and pagetic changes throughout the left hemipelvis. (B) Axial CT image shows lesion with soft tissue extension consistent with an osteosarcoma secondary to Paget's disease of the pelvis.

- Most occur at age <30 (~85%)
- Second peak age >55; often secondary osteosarcomas (e.g., Paget's sarcoma or postradiation sarcoma)
- Classic secondary osteosarcomas represent 5% to 7% of all osteosarcomas; usually with worse prognosis.
    - Definition: osteosarcomas that occur in relation to previous exposures or procedures as well as in the presence of other primary diseases
    - Paget's osteosarcoma (Fig. 6.1-2)
        - Most common of the "secondary osteosarcomas"
        - Estimated 1% of Paget's patients may develop osteosarcoma

- Majority in polyostotic Paget's, although they do occur in monostotic disease
- Reports as high as 5% of polyostotic symptomatic patients
- Postradiation osteosarcomas occur in bone that is in a previously irradiated field (Fig. 6.1-3).
    - Usually >3 years after exposure
    - May occur decades after treatment for other malignancies or after high-dose exposure
- Disease-associated osteosarcomas
    - Osteosarcomas have been reported in association with several other diseases, although the exact relationship between these underlying disease processes

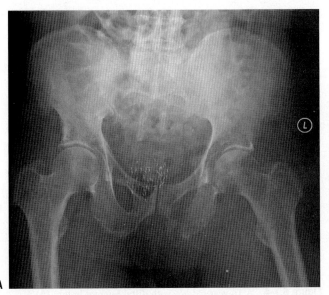
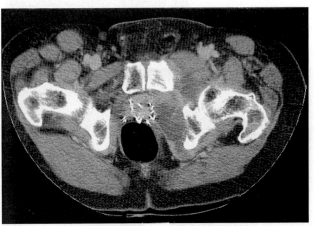

Figure 6.1-3   (A) Plain anteroposterior radiograph of the pelvis shows a destructive lesion of the left inferior pubic ramus. Note the metallic seeds previously placed for treatment of prostate cancer in combination with external-beam radiation 8 years prior. (B) Axial CT image shows bony destruction and soft tissue mass extending from pubic ramus. With the patient's history, biopsy confirmed the diagnosis of postradiation osteosarcoma.

and the secondary osteosarcomas are difficult to delineate.

Pathophysiology

Local Growth

Osteosarcomas usually arise within the metaphyseal region of long bones. They may be located within the bone or on the surface of the bone. If untreated, osteosarcomas will continue to grow, with local destruction of bone and extension outside the bone into the surrounding soft tissues. The physis and articular cartilage may act as a relative barrier to tumor extension, but epiphyseal or intra-articular extension is still seen frequently.

Metastases

- Osteosarcomas, as with all sarcomas, usually metastasize hematogenously.
- Lymph node metastases are not common and usually present only very late in the course of metastatic disease.
- 15% to 20% of patients present with metastases at time of diagnosis.
- Most common site of metastasis: lungs (Fig. 6.1-4)
  - Second most common: bone
- Skip lesions: distinct smaller areas apart from primary tumor within same bone

- Prognosis: same as or worse than distant metastases (lung or bone)

Death

- Occurs most commonly due to respiratory failure secondary to widespread pulmonary metastases, but also due to other sequelae of tumor burden
  - Superior vena cava obstruction
  - Pneumonia
  - Hemorrhage into tumor
  - Sepsis
  - Chemotoxicity (1% to 5%)

CLASSIFICATION

Osteosarcoma and Variants

"Classic" osteosarcoma, also referred to as conventional osteosarcoma, and central high-grade osteosarcoma represent the majority of osteosarcomas (up to 75% in some series). Variants of osteosarcomas exist that present differently, have unique radiographic and histologic characteristics, may be treated differently, and may convey a worse or better prognosis than conventional osteosarcoma. It is important that these differences are identified and understood so that correct diagnosis and treatment may be rendered.

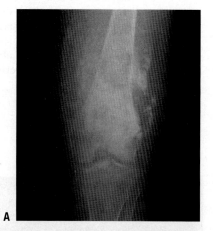
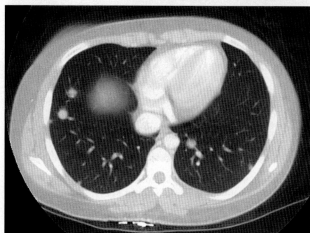
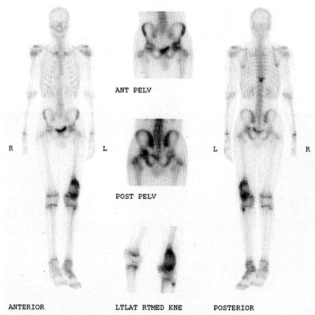

Figure 6.1-4 A 16-year-old boy with distal femoral lesion. **(A)** Plain radiograph shows abundant bone production and soft tissue extension strongly suggestive of an osteosarcoma. **(B)** Whole-body Tc-99 bone scan reveals a lesion of the ipsilateral acetabulum and thoracic spine. **(C)** CT axial image of the chest also reveals multiple pulmonary metastases.

Pathology

Osteosarcoma is classically described as a high-grade spindle cell sarcomatous stroma with malignant osteoblasts that produce malignant osteoid or bone. The tumor cells are typically anaplastic (less differentiated), may show marked atypia and pleomorphic (widely variable) nuclei, and may show many and/or bizarre mitoses. There may be areas of osteoblastic (osseous), fibroblastic (fibrous), or chondroblastic (cartilage) appearance, but if there is the presence of malignant osteoid (wavy, lace-like, uncalcified bone matrix produced by malignant osteoblasts), the diagnosis of osteosarcoma is made regardless of the associated areas.

Grade

- The grade of an osteosarcoma is used to:
  - Plan treatment: low-grade sarcomas are not treated with chemotherapy
  - Predict prognosis: low-grade osteosarcomas are less likely to develop metastases
- Most osteosarcomas are high-grade tumors.
- Low- and intermediate-grade osteosarcoma variants do exist (Box 6.1-1).

Stage

- Most osteosarcomas are stage IIB (high-grade and extra-compartmental Enneking/Musculoskeletal Tumor Society Staging System) at presentation.
- Patients with lung and/or bone metastases are considered MSTS stage III and have the worst prognosis.
  - 15% to 20% of osteosarcomas have metastases (stage III) at presentation.

DIAGNOSIS

Clinical Features

Pain is the most common complaint in patients seen by an orthopaedic surgeon. The important factors to consider in making the diagnosis of osteosarcoma follow.

Patient History

- Age
  - Most commonly occur in the second decade of life
  - Second peak in middle to late adulthood, usually from secondary osteosarcomas

BOX 6.1-1 OSTEOSARCOMA CLASSIFICATION

Low Grade	High Grade
Parosteal	Conventional
Low-grade central	Telangiectatic
Intermediate Grade	Small cell
Periosteal	Postradiation
	Pagetoid
	High-grade surface

- Location
  - Distal femur (most common) > proximal tibia > proximal humerus
    - Metaphysis > diaphysis
    - Proximally in limb more common than distally
    - Pelvis and other flat bones (e.g., scapula) less frequently
    - Can occur in any bone
- Symptoms
  - Pain is by far the most common complaint.
    - Pain gradually worsening, though may be intermittent or increase with activity
    - Pain is usually present for weeks to months, not acutely.
    - Red flags
      - Pain present or worse at night
      - Pain that is worsening despite treatment
      - Pain at rest
      - Pain without history of trauma
      - Antecedent pain, but worsened with minor injury

Physical Examination

- Most common presentation is a tender mass about the knee.
  - Mass is firm and fixed to bone, nonmobile.
  - Warmth may be present.
  - Fusiform swelling of extremity
  - Dilated (ectatic) subcutaneous veins (large tumors)
  - Tenderness is usually present to palpation, with range of motion, and with weight bearing.
- If pathologic fracture: antecedent pain is more worrisome for malignant pathologic fracture than if no prior pain.

Laboratory Studies

- There is no blood test for osteosarcoma.
- Erythrocyte sedimentation rate (ESR) and C-reactive protein (CRP) may be ordered to help distinguish from osteomyelitis/infection.
- Calcium and alkaline phosphatase are usually normal.
- Complete blood count usually normal, except with advancing disease
- Elevated white count unusual, may suggest infection
- Worse prognosis in osteosarcoma if elevated at time of diagnosis:
  - Serum lactate dehydrogenase (LDH)
  - Serum alkaline phosphatase

Radiologic Features

Plain Radiographs

- The typical findings seen on plain films of an osteosarcoma are usually destructive lesions within the metaphysis most common; surface osteosarcomas also occur.
- Evidence of malignant bone production, which appears as radiodensities within the lesion, adjacent to areas of lucency as well.
  - Usually cortical destruction with a soft tissue mass extending outside the normal contour of the cortex

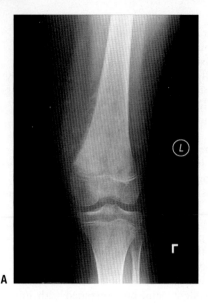

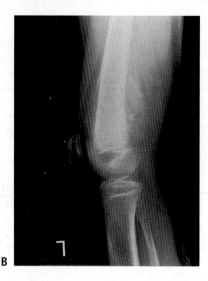

Figure 6.1-5 An 11-year-old girl with knee pain and distal femur mass. (**A**) Anteroposterior radiograph shows the classic signs of an osteosarcoma. Note the destructive, bone-forming lesion of the distal femoral metaphysis. A Codman's triangle is seen at the superior–medial periosteal border. (**B**) In a lateral radiograph of the distal femur lesion, the soft tissue extension is more clearly seen, as is the bone formation within the tumor.

- "Codman's triangle": elevation of the periosteum at the periphery of the soft tissue mass that forms a radiodense triangle along the outer surface of the cortex (Fig. 6.1-5)
- "Sunburst pattern" seen with some osteosarcomas
- Variants of osteosarcoma exist, each with typical plain radiographic findings.

Conventional Osteosarcoma
- Up to 75% of all osteosarcomas
- Most common distal femur, proximal tibia
- Typical findings of osteosarcoma
  - Malignant bone production within lesion
  - Destruction of cortex with soft tissue extension (extracompartmental) and Codman's triangle

Telangiectatic Osteosarcoma
- 0.4% to 12% of all osteosarcomas
- Typically a permeative, destructive radiolucent lesion with little if any bone production (see Fig. 6.1-6)
- Can be confused radiographically with aneurysmal bone cyst or giant cell tumor of bone
- Careful biopsy is important, as this variant consists of large blood pools within tumor with often scant cellular lining.
- Histologically may also be confused with aneurysmal bone cyst

Small Cell Osteosarcoma
- Rare; about 1% to 4% of all osteosarcomas
- Controversy: Are these "atypical Ewing sarcoma"?

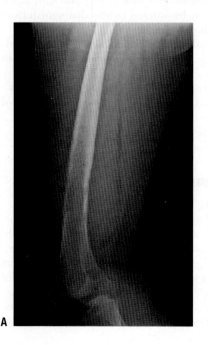

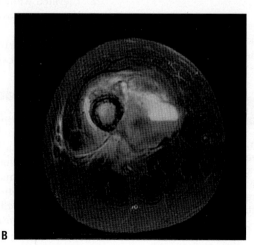

Figure 6.1-6 A 16-year-old girl with 5-month history of thigh pain. (**A**) Lateral radiograph shows a radiolucent, permeative lesion of the distal diaphysis of the femur. There is a Codman's triangle superiorly, and the large soft tissue extension can be seen posterior to the femur. Note the lack of ossification radiographically within the lesion and soft tissue extension. (**B**) T2-weighted, fat-suppressed axial image through the femur at the level of the lesion reveals a large soft tissue mass and fluid–fluid level within the mass. Biopsy of this lesion confirmed a telangiectatic osteosarcoma.

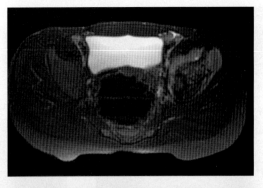

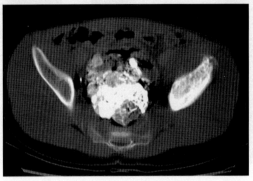

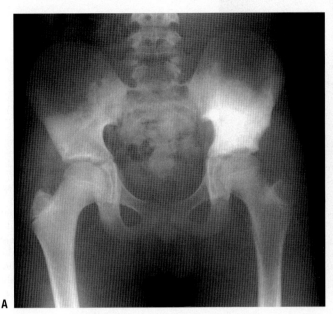

Figure 6.1-7   A 12-year-old boy with pain in the hip for 1 month. (**A**) Anteroposterior radiograph of the pelvis shows a radiodense supra-acetabular ilium on the left. (**B**) Axial T2-weighted, fat-suppressed MR image shows an infiltrative lesion with extension into the soft tissues. (**C**) A CT axial image at the same level reveals a radiodense lesion. Biopsy showed dense bone and nests of small, round blue cells. A diagnosis of a small cell osteosarcoma was made.

- Age, location, and radiographic picture similar to conventional osteosarcoma
- Typically has a destructive, permeative pattern, sometimes extends into diaphysis (Fig. 6.1-7)
- On biopsy, there is often difficulty in distinguishing this tumor from Ewing sarcoma and other small round cell tumors if no osteoid is seen on biopsy.
- Usually has areas of osteoblastic activity, which helps distinguish it from Ewing sarcoma

Low-Grade Central Osteosarcoma
- 1% to 2% of all osteosarcomas
- Usually presents with pain
- Older, typically third decade
- Radiographic picture is variable, often radiodense (Fig. 6.1-8).
- Often confused with fibrous dysplasia, or by progression or recurrence after treatment for suspected benign disease

Secondary Osteosarcomas
- Refers to osteosarcomas that occur in abnormal bone from other disease or after exposure to radiation
- 5% to 7% of all osteosarcomas
- Many osteosarcoma case reports associated with other disease

Paget's Sarcoma
- Most common secondary osteosarcoma
- Occurs in about 5% of patients with polyostotic Paget's

- Several thousand-fold increased risk of osteosarcoma in patients with Paget's disease compared to the general population
- Older patient population (55 to 85 years old)
- Increasingly painful mass is most common presentation.
- Flat bones; common, unlike conventional osteosarcoma due to frequent involvement of pelvis and scapula with Paget's disease
- Radiographs reveal destructive mass, usually with soft tissue extension in bone with Paget's disease.

Postradiation Osteosarcomas
- Usually 3 to 30 years after radiation exposure most commonly from previous malignancy (e.g., breast cancer, cervical cancer, Hodgkin's, Ewing)
- Usually >4,000 cGy, with risk increasing as total radiation dose increases
- Common in flat bones (scapula, pelvis, rib) as these more often exposed to radiation treatments for other malignancies
- Radiographically similar to conventional osteosarcoma in a prior radiated bone

Various Bone Diseases
- Multitude of case reports of osteosarcoma diagnosed in the presence of other bone diseases, even in fracture site or arthroplasty site. It is difficult to determine if these are sporadic incidences (coincidences).
  - Osteogenesis imperfecta
  - Fibrous dysplasia

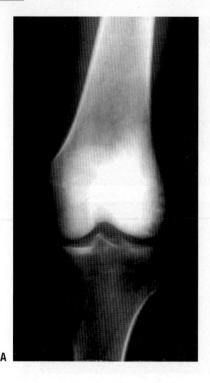 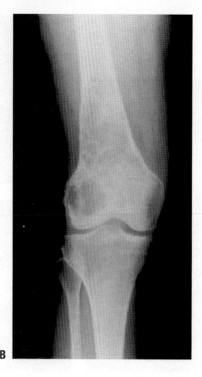

A   B

Figure 6.1-8 (A) Anteroposterior radiograph of a 34-year-old woman with knee pain shows a densely sclerotic lesion of the lateral femoral condyle. Biopsy showed a low-grade central osteosarcoma. (B) Anteroposterior radiograph of the distal femur of a 55-year-old woman with a 1-year history of knee pain reveals a radiolucent, slightly expansile, septated lesion. Biopsy also revealed a low-grade central osteosarcoma.

■ Chronic osteomyelitis
■ Osteopoikilosis

Surface Osteosarcomas

Osteosarcoma most commonly begins as an intramedullary tumor that destroys cortical bone as it grows and extends into the adjacent soft tissues. Osteosarcoma variants exist whose epicenter of growth occurs at the surface of long bones. These surface sarcomas have radiographic and clinical characteristics that can vary significantly from those of conventional osteosarcoma. It is necessary to be aware of these variants so that they are not confused with other bone tumors or abnormalities.

Parosteal Osteosarcoma

■ Approximately 5% of all osteosarcomas
■ Most common surface osteosarcoma
■ Presents later than conventional: late second and third decades
■ Dull ache or pain may be present, but painless mass also may be presenting complaint.
■ Typically appears as a dense bony mass adjacent to the metaphyseal cortex of long bones (Fig. 6.1-9)
  ■ Distal posterior femur most common; proximal humerus second most common
  ■ Usually a "cleavage plane" between the mass and the underlying cortex. Has a "stuck-on" appearance. It may wrap around cortex, with invasion into bone only later.
  ■ In contrast, the cortex of an osteochondroma is continuous with the cortex of the involved bone and the medullary canal of the bone is continuous with the medullary bone of the stalk (pedunculated) or base (sessile) of the osteochondroma.

■ Unlike conventional osteosarcoma, parosteal osteosarcomas are usually low grade, requiring surgery alone (no chemotherapy).
■ *Dedifferentiated parosteal osteosarcoma* occurs when there is dedifferentiation of a portion of this tumor to a high-grade sarcoma. In turn, the prognosis is worse if dedifferentiation occurs.

Periosteal Osteosarcoma

■ 1% to 2% of all osteosarcomas
■ Typically occurs on anterior surface of diaphysis of bone; tibia most common
■ Radiographically, a fusiform mass with lucency and ossification (Fig. 6.1-10)
■ "Sunburst pattern" of malignant bone can be seen.
■ Chondroblastic histology may predominate, but malignant osteoid is present.
■ Intermediate grade between parosteal and conventional

High-Grade Surface Osteosarcoma

■ Up to 1% of osteosarcomas
■ Located on surface of bone
■ Otherwise identical to conventional osteosarcoma in histology, treatment, and prognosis

Staging Work-Up

When plain radiographs reveal the possibility of an osteosarcoma, staging studies are required to determine the local and distant extent of disease, *prior* to biopsy. Biopsy of bone tumors without appropriate staging should not be done, as it may jeopardize the ability to properly stage the osteosarcoma.

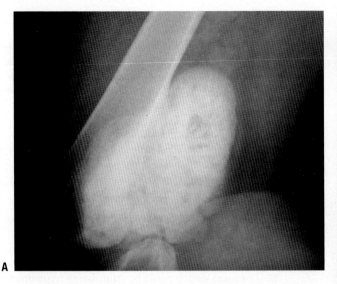

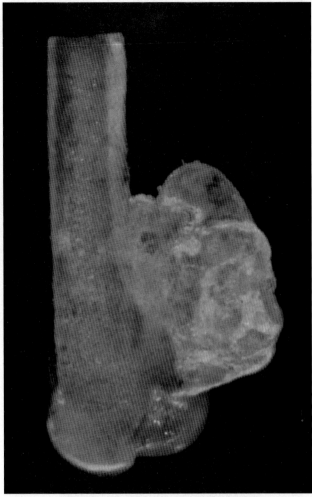

Figure 6.1-9 A 39-year-old woman with a several-year history of a slowly expanding mass in the popliteal fossa. (**A**) Lateral radiograph shows a large ossified lesion at the posterior aspect of the distal femur. This was thought to be consistent with a parosteal osteosarcoma and was confirmed by biopsy. Resection of the distal femur was performed. (**B**) This lesion is adjacent to an intact posterior cortex. This can usually be distinguished from an osteochondroma as the cortices of the stalk of the osteochondroma are in continuity with the cortices of the bone itself. The medullary bone appears to flow out into the osteochondroma.

- Appropriate staging work-up must include:
  - History and physical
  - Plain radiographs (of entire bone with joint above and below)
  - Laboratory evaluation should include alkaline phosphatase and LDH.
  - Magnetic resonance imaging of entire bone is required to:
    - Determine the extent of the tumor intraosseously
    - Determine the anatomic relationship to adjacent structures
      - Nerves
      - Vessels
      - Joints
      - Soft tissue (e.g., muscles, skin)
    - At least one sequence of entire bone (preferably coronal T1 images) to rule out skip lesion in same bone (metastasis)
  - Whole-body bone scan
    - Uptake on scan of primary lesion is almost always present, but scan is to rule out other sites of disease.
    - May detect other sites of disease
    - May also show skip lesion in same bone

- Computed tomographic (CT) scan of the chest
  - To evaluate for evidence of lung metastases
  - 15% to 20% present with lung metastases

TREATMENT

Chemotherapy and Surgery (Systemic and Local Therapy)

After biopsy, when the diagnosis of osteosarcoma is made, the grade and stage are determined. The grade and stage help to direct treatment of patients with osteosarcoma. Current standard of care involves the use of chemotherapy for high-grade osteosarcomas and wide resection of the sarcoma in all patients. This resection can be achieved by ablative surgery (amputation proximal to the extent of the tumor) or with limb-sparing (limb salvage) surgery. When limb salvage surgery is performed, skeletal defects must be reconstructed, unless the tumor involves an expandable bone (e.g. the fibula).

Chemotherapy

Prior to the use of chemotherapy, overall survival of osteosarcoma patients with nondetectable metastases by routine

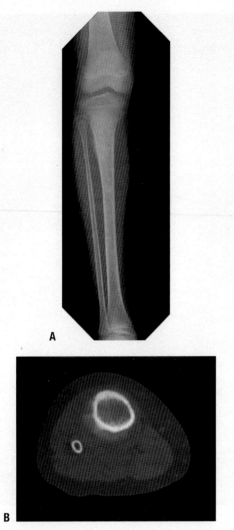

Figure 6.1-10 An 11-year-old boy with a 2-month history of pain. (A) Anteroposterior radiograph of the knee shows a lesion of the proximal metadiaphysis of the tibia. (B) CT scan shows this periosteal lesion and bone production within the lesion. A biopsy of the lesion revealed a periosteal osteosarcoma. Approximately 60% of the lesion pathologically was chondroid, but areas of malignant cells producing osteoid were seen and the diagnosis of osteosarcoma was made.

staging studies, even with radical amputations, was in the range of 15% to 20%. Without chemotherapy, it was likely that micrometastases not detectable on routine imaging (chest CT scan, bone scan) progressed and resulted in the later detection of disease despite the resection of the tumor. Chemotherapy is used for the systemic treatment of patients with osteosarcomas to eliminate these micrometastases. These patients are treated in protocols that use multiagent therapies, which alone may only slightly improve survival, but when used in combination have been shown to significantly improve overall survival.

Typically, neoadjuvant (preoperative or induction) chemotherapy is given, followed by surgical treatment and then postoperative chemotherapy to complete the protocol. The agents used most commonly in the treatment of osteo-

sarcomas and given in cycles include doxorubicin (Adriamycin), cisplatin, high-dose methotrexate, and ifosfamide.

Although standard treatment of osteosarcoma patients now usually involves preoperative chemotherapy, there has been no randomized study that shows an increase in survival with neoadjuvant chemotherapy followed by postoperative chemotherapy versus delivery of all chemotherapy postoperatively.

Side effects of these medications can be severe, and toxicities can occur. These include mucositis, cardiomyopathy (doxorubicin), alopecia, myelosuppression, nausea/vomiting, and relative immunocompromise, sepsis, and rarely even death.

- Medications used during chemotherapy treatment to minimize side effects
  - Granulocyte colony-stimulating factor (G-CSF; Neupogen)
    - Improves neutropenia by stimulating neutrophil production by marrow
    - Decreases infections and febrile neutropenias
  - Erythropoietin (Epogen) stimulates red blood cell production.
  - Dexrazoxane (Zinecard) protects against cardiomyopathy of doxorubicin.
  - Leucovorin rescues normal cells from effects of high-dose methotrexate and decreases myelosuppression and mucositis.

Radiation Therapy

While osteosarcoma is a relatively radiosensitive tumor, historical results of treatment of osteosarcoma by radiation therapy were dismal. Currently radiation therapy should be reserved for palliation only. Radiation therapy currently has no role in the standard management of patients with nonmetastatic osteosarcoma.

Surgery

Despite the advances in the use of chemotherapeutic agents in the treatment of osteosarcoma and its profound effect on survival, complete surgical resection of the sarcoma is still required for local control of the tumor. Historically, amputation was used for the treatment of osteosarcoma. Currently 85% to 90% of osteosarcomas are treated with limb salvage (limb-sparing) surgery. Current literature does not demonstrate a difference in overall survival between limb salvage versus amputation. However, an acceptable margin of resection must be obtained, as incomplete excision will most likely lead to recurrence, eventual metastasis, and death. The appropriate margin for resection of an osteosarcoma is a wide (cuff of normal tissue completely surrounds the tumor) margin. How thick the cuff of normal tissue should be or how close the margins should be has not been fully established. Tumor extending to the inked margin of resection (positive margin) is not an adequate resection. Amputation may be the safest oncologic treatment following initial resection with positive margins.

Limb Salvage Versus Amputation

Eighty-five to 90% of osteosarcomas can be treated with limb salvage procedures. The most important goal of the surgical treatment of osteosarcoma is complete (wide) resection of the tumor with a wide margin.

Results and Outcome

- For all nonmetastatic osteosarcomas, 60% to 70% 5-year survival rate
- Important prognostic factors
  - Metastatic disease
    - Single most important factor in predicting survival
    - Patients who present with metastatic disease, managed with chemotherapy and aggressive resection of distant disease (i.e., thoracotomies), may have up to a 30% to 40% 5-year survival rate.
    - Patients who develop metastatic disease after treatment also have a worse prognosis but with chemotherapy and metastasectomy may achieve up to 15% to 20% survival rates.
  - Response to chemotherapy
    - Patients who have a good response to chemo (>90% necrosis after examination of resected tumor) may have up to a 90% 5-year survival rate.
    - In high-grade osteosarcoma patients with no evidence of metastases, *response to chemotherapy is the single most important predictor of prognosis.*
  - Tumor grade
    - Patients with low-grade osteosarcomas (parosteal and low-grade central) have a better prognosis than those with high-grade osteosarcoma and approach a 90% survival rate with appropriate management.
- Subtypes of osteosarcomas also have a role in determining prognosis (Box 6.1-2).

BOX 6.1-2 RELATIVE PROGNOSIS OF OSTEOSARCOMA TYPES

Better Prognosis than Conventional Osteosarcoma
Parosteal
Low-grade central
Intermediate Prognosis (15% to 20% risk of metastases)
Periosteal
Equivalent Prognosis as Conventional Osteosarcoma
Telangiectatic
High-grade surface
Poorest Prognosis
Pagetoid
Postradiation
Small cell
Dedifferentiated

- Tumors with the poorest prognosis: chemotherapy is controversial as there is no documented benefit
- Tumors with intermediate prognosis: controversies regarding chemotherapy exist, but most patients get chemotherapy
- Better prognosis than conventional osteosarcoma: no chemotherapy used

SUGGESTED READING

Ruggieri P, Sim FH, Bond JR, Unni KK. Malignancies in fibrous dysplasia. *Cancer* 1994;73(5):1411–1424.
Sheppard DG, Libshitz HI. Post-radiation sarcomas: a review of the clinical and imaging features in 63 cases. *Clin Radiol* 2001;56(1):22–29.
Torres FX, Kyriakos M. Bone infarct-associated osteosarcoma. *Cancer* 1992;70(10):2418–2430.

6.2 EWING SARCOMA AND PRIMITIVE NEUROECTODERMAL TUMOR OF BONE

BRUCE ROUGRAFF

Ewing sarcoma was a feared cancer of childhood, with very few survivors, prior to the use of chemotherapy, surgical resection, and radiation. The disease manifests as chronic increasing pain in the area of a lytic, destructive bone lesion of flat bones and the diaphysis of long bones.

The initial presentation is frequently confused with osteomyelitis, and it can be mistakenly treated as that for a period of time before the diagnosis is established. Ewing sarcoma and a less virulent related disease, primitive neuroectodermal tumor of bone (PNET), metastasize to lung, bone, and bone marrow most frequently. Current management includes biopsy, staging, neoadjuvant chemotherapy, surgical resection and/or radiation, and further chemotherapy. The 5-year survival rate is 60% to 65% for nonmetastatic disease and 25% to 30% for metastatic disease.

PATHOGENESIS

Etiology

- Unknown; associated with reciprocal translocation of chromosomes 11 and 22 (90% of cases), which involves bands q24 and q12 of both chromosomes respectively
- This results in a new chimeric EWS/FLI-1 fusion product, which produces the EWS/FLI-1 or MIC2 protein, stained for by the CD99 immunohistochemistry marker.

Epidemiology

- Third most common primary bone sarcoma (after osteosarcoma and chondrosarcoma, respectively)
- Three times less common than osteosarcoma
- Rare in African-Americans (0.5% of Ewing cases); peak incidence in the second decade of life
- Male:female ratio 1.3:1

Pathophysiology

- Sheets of monotonous, small, round blue cells with indistinct cytoplasm (Fig. 6.2-1)
- Glycogen granules in the cytoplasm can be seen after periodic acid Schiff (PAS) staining or with electron microscopy.
- PAS-positive granules sensitive to digestion with diastase

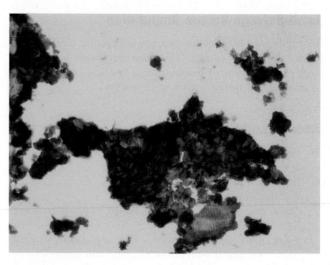

Figure 6.2-2   This CD-99 immunohistochemical staining shows positivity that is consistent with Ewing sarcoma. Cytogenetics is used to confirm Ewing/PNET (t11:22).

- The nuclear chromatin is finely granular, with one to three small nucleoli per nuclei.
- CD99 immunohistochemistry marker stains for EWS/ FLI1 fusion or MIC2 protein, which is present in 90% of cases. (Fig. 6.2-2)

CLASSIFICATION

- Ewing sarcoma: most common, least differentiated, worst prognosis
- PNET: more neural differentiation, better prognosis
- Askin's tumor: primary in thoracopulmonary region, best prognosis

DIAGNOSIS

Clinical Features

- Typical age at diagnosis: 5 to 30 years
- Rare in patients <5 years old; this distinguishes it from metastatic neuroblastoma
- Usually presents as a painful mass
- May be accompanied by fever and weight loss, which are poor prognostic signs

Radiographic Features

- Location
  - Typically originates in flat bones (pelvis, rib, clavicle) or the diaphysis of long bones (femur, tibia, humerus)
  - Pelvis > femur > tibia > humerus

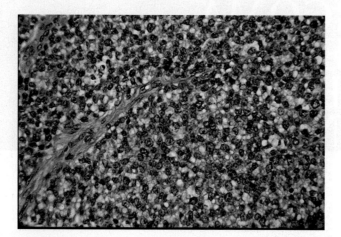

Figure 6.2-1   This hematoxylin-and-eosin (H&E) staining shows typical Ewing sarcoma features of monotonous sheets of small, round blue cells with indistinct cytoplasm.

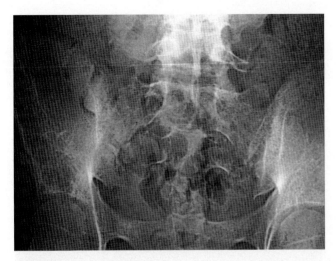

Figure 6.2-3   Anteroposterior pelvis radiograph of a 14-year-old with a lytic destructive iliac lesion.

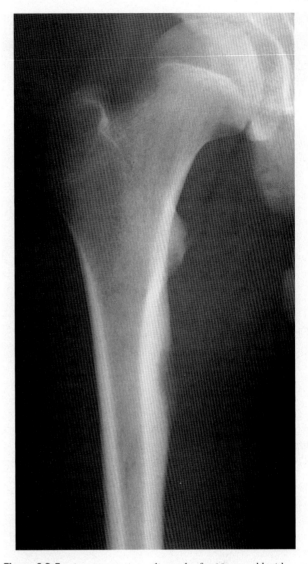

- Mostly, lytic destructive lesion with "onion-skinning" periosteal reaction (Figs. 6.2-3 to 6.2-8)
- 90% of patients have soft tissue mass.
- A destructive, lytic, diaphyseal lesion in a child is two times more likely to be a Ewing sarcoma than an osteosarcoma.
- A destructive, lytic, metaphyseal lesion in a child is 12 times more likely to be an osteosarcoma than a Ewing sarcoma.

TREATMENT

Surgical Indications/Contraindications

- Traditionally surgery for Ewing sarcoma was reserved for expendable bones.

Figure 6.2-5   Anteroposterior radiograph of a 19-year-old with chronic hip pain. Note the cortical destruction and periosteal changes.

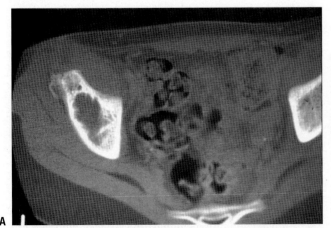
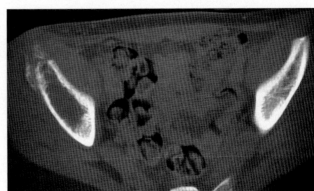

Figure 6.2-4   Computed tomographic scans demonstrating the lytic destructive changes of the ilium.

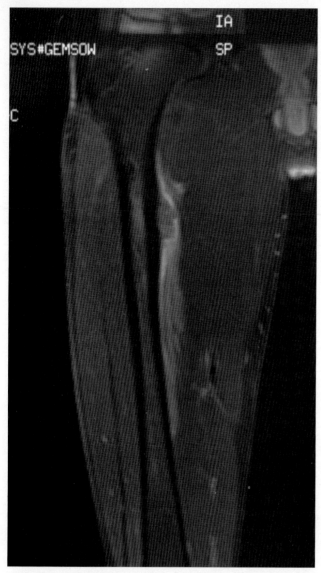

Figure 6.2-6 Magnetic resonance imaging shows large area of soft tissue involvement without a stress fracture. This was diagnosed as a Ewing sarcoma of bone and was treated with chemotherapy, wide resection, and bone grafting.

- Because of improved local control with surgery compared to radiation alone, most Ewing sarcoma patients have surgical resection if adequate margins are attainable and the defect is reconstructable (Fig. 6.2-9).
- Spine and acetabulum are sites that pose difficulties with resection and reconstruction.
- Most resections are reconstructed with bone-grafting procedures.
  - Frequent diaphyseal location lends itself to intercalary allograft reconstruction.
  - Young age (small skeletal size) often requires expandable prostheses if growth plate has to be resected.

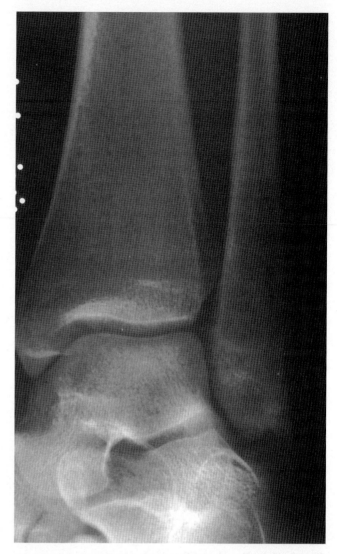

Figure 6.2-7 Subtle distal fibula lytic lesion without periosteal signs.

Results and Outcome

- Local relapse rate with radiation alone is 25%; with surgery and radiation it is 8%.
- It is unclear whether this difference affects survival.
- Five-year disease-free survival rate for non-metastatic Ewing sarcoma is 60% to 65%.
  - Recurrent disease after 5 years for patients with non-metastatic disease is very unusual.
- Five-year survival rate for patients with metastatic disease at the time of diagnosis is 25% to 30%.

Postoperative Management

- Early postoperative pain control is very important.
  - Patient-controlled analgesia
  - Regional and epidural pain management
- Early rehabilitation emphasizing range of motion is critical.

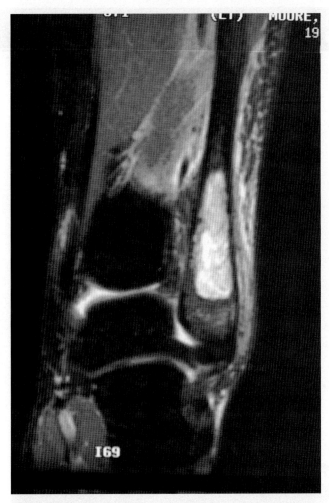

Figure 6.2-8 Magnetic resonance imaging shows marrow replacement with tumor. This was diagnosed as a Ewing sarcoma.

- Avoid weight bearing until after bony union.
- Long-term antibiotics for segmental allografts

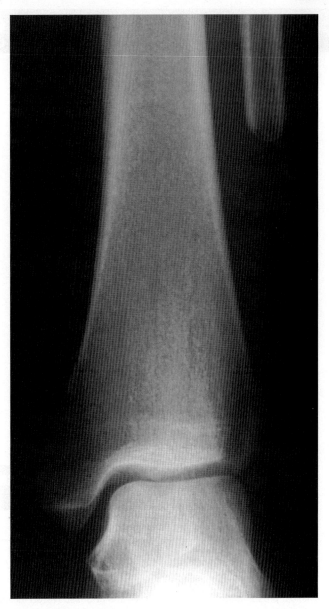

Figure 6.2-9 The patient was treated with wide resection and chemotherapy. No reconstruction was performed, and no instability of the ankle was noted on follow-up examinations.

SUGGESTED READING

Bacci G, Ferrari S, Longhi A, et al. Local and systemic control in Ewing's sarcoma of the femur treated with chemotherapy, and locally by radiotherapy and or surgery. *J Bone Joint Surg [Br]* 2003; 85:107–114.

Nesbit ME, Gehan EA, Burgert EO, et al. Multimodal therapy for the management of primary, nonmetastatic Ewing sarcoma of bone: A long-term follow-up of the first intergroup study. *J Clin Oncol* 1990; 8:1664–1674.

Picci P, Rougraff BT, Bacci G, et al. Prognostic significance of histopathologic response to chemotherapy in nonmetastatic Ewing's sarcoma of the extremities. *J Clin Oncol* 1993;11: 1763–1769.

Sluga M, Windhager R, Lang S, et al. The role of surgery and resection margins in the treatment of Ewing's sarcoma. *Clin Orthop* 2001; 392:394–399.

Sucato DJ, Rougraff BT, McGrath BE, et al. Ewing's sarcoma of the pelvis. *Clin Orthop* 2000;373:193–201.

Toni A, Neff JR, Sudanese A, et al. The role of surgical therapy in patients with nonmetastatic Ewing's sarcoma of the limbs. *Clin Orthop* 1993;286:225–240.

Vlasak R, Sim FH. Ewing's sarcoma. *Pediatr Orthop Oncol* 1996;27: 591–603.

Wilkins RM, Pritchard DJ, Burgert O, Unni KK. Ewing's sarcoma of bone. *Cancer* 1986;58:2551–2555.

Yang RS, Eckhardt JJ, Eilber FR, et al. Surgical indications for Ewing's sarcoma of the pelvis. *Cancer* 1995;76:1388–1397.

6.3 CHONDROSARCOMA

R. LOR RANDALL ■ KENNETH J. HUNT

Chondrosarcomas of bone can be found in any bone in the human body and include a spectrum of lesions that range from low grade to dangerously aggressive. Although cartilage bone lesions in general have a characteristic radiographic appearance, differentiating between benign and low-grade malignant cartilage lesions often presents a diagnostic challenge (Table 6.3-1). Since treatment and outcome are based in large part upon an accurate diagnosis, this distinction is important (Fig. 6.3-1).

PATHOGENESIS

Etiology

- Unknown
- Current speculation: may arise from monoclonal expansion of single chondrocyte

Epidemiology

- Peak age: third to sixth decades (Fig. 6.3-2)
- Frequency of chondrosarcomas in the United States

- ~10% to 25% of primary bone tumors are chondrosarcomas.
- Approximately 250 to 625 cases/year in United States
- Second to osteosarcoma among bone sarcomas

Pathophysiology

Histopathology (Fig. 6.3-3)
- *Macroscopic appearance*
  - Heterogeneous gross properties, including lobulated areas of chalky calcific admixture
  - Regions of firm translucent unmineralized gray cartilage with relatively low vascularity
  - Intermixed areas of necrosis and degeneration
- *Low-grade chondrosarcomas*
  - Relatively acellular, heavily calcified areas
  - Regions of increased activity exhibiting immature cartilage cells with multiple nucleated lacunae
  - Permeation pattern of cartilage surrounding pre-existing bony trabeculae

TABLE 6.3-1 DIFFERENTIATION BETWEEN BENIGN AND LOW-GRADE MALIGNANT CARTILAGE LESIONS

Parameter	Enchondromas	Chondrosarcomas
Definition	Benign cartilage tumors	Malignant cartilage tumors
Metastatic potential	None	Increases with grade
Clinical presentation	Often painless and discovered incidentally	Often painful
Location	Metacarpals and phalanges > long bones Metaphyseal > diaphyseal	Pelvis > femur > ribs > humerus > scapula > tibia
Plain radiographs	Variably mineralized central lesions with arcs, smoke rings, or popcorn patterns No or <50% cortical width endosteal scalloping	Variably mineralized with same patterns or more punctate calcifications Often radiolucencies with sparse mineralization Endosteal scalloping >50% cortical width Cortical breech with soft tissue mass in advanced cases
MRI	Multilobular Dark T1, bright T2	Soft tissue extension and surrounding edema more common Dark T1, bright T2
Histopathology	Hyaline cartilage encased by rim of reactive bone ("enchondroma encasement" pattern) Lobular growth Bland chondrocytes with pyknotic nuclei Variably cellular Lesions of digits and those in Ollier's disease often more worrisome in appearance (e.g., cytologic atypia and binucleation)	Cartilage permeates around pre-existing bone trabecula ("permeation pattern") Invasion of haversian canals Lobular growth Cytologic atypia Binucleation more prominent Increased cellularity

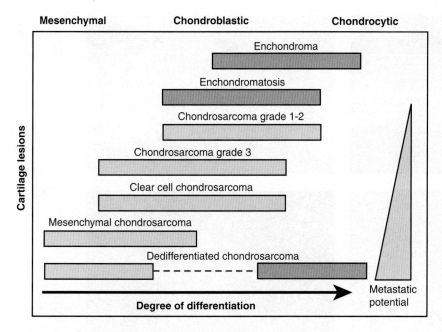

Figure 6.3-1 Degree of differentiation in cartilage tumors. (Adapted from Dorfman HD, Czerniak B. Malignant cartilage tumors. In: Dorfman HD, Czerniak B, eds. *Bone Tumors*. St. Louis: Mosby, 1998.)

- *High-grade chondrosarcomas*
  - Densely packed, hyperchromatic, malignant-looking cells
  - May be difficult to determine that these cells are truly of cartilaginous origin
  - Myxomatous changes and highly degenerative areas common

Classification

- Several classification schemes
  - Histologic grade (I, II, III, dedifferentiated)
    - The most important factor in the malignant potential of a chondrosarcoma is its histologic grade. Most (~85%) chondrosarcomas are low-grade lesions.
  - Location within the bone and body
    - Peripheral (periosteal or juxtacortical chondro-sarcoma and secondary chondrosarcoma arising from osteochondroma) versus central (intramedullary)
    - Axial versus appendicular skeleton
  - Primary versus secondary
    - Primary: arises de novo
    - Secondary central: arises from enchondroma
    - Secondary peripheral: arises from osteochondroma
  - Specific histologic subtype
    - Conventional
    - Clear cell chondrosarcoma
    - Mesenchymal chondrosarcoma
    - Dedifferentiated chondrosarcoma
- Histologic grades of conventional chondrosarcomas (Table 6.3-2)
  - Grade I ("low-grade") tumors
    - Slow-growing and locally aggressive

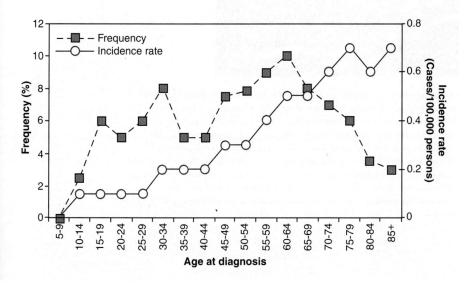

Figure 6.3-2 Age-specific frequency and distribution of chondrosarcoma, based on SEER 1973–1987 data. (After Dorfman HD, Czerniak B. Bone cancers. *Cancer* 1995;75: 223–227.)

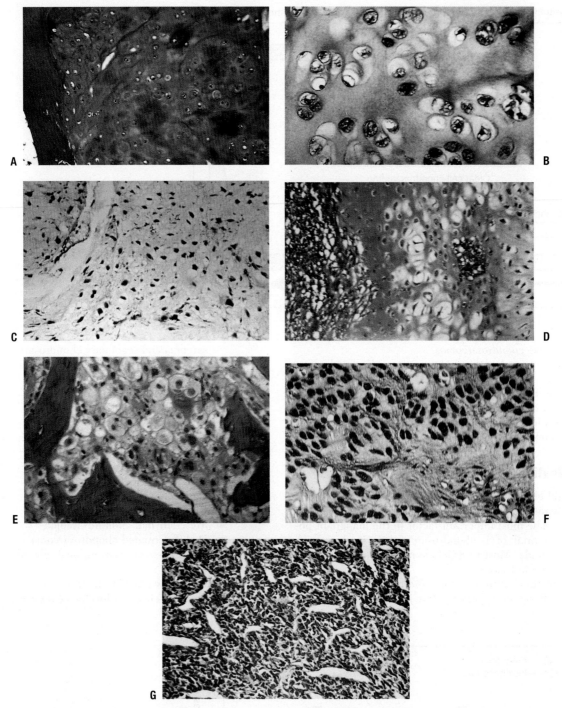

Figure 6.3-3 Representative histopathology specimens from typical chondrosarcomas. (**A**) Grade I chondrosarcoma demonstrates increased cellularity, perhaps some hyperchromatism but not necessarily atypia. (**B**) Grade II chondrosarcoma demonstrates increased cellularity and atypia. (**C**) Grade III chondrosarcoma demonstrates markedly increased cellularity and pleomorphism. (**D**) Dedifferentiated chondrosarcoma demonstrates area of low-grade chondrosarcoma with abrupt transitions into a spindle cell sarcoma. (**E**) Clear cell chondrosarcoma demonstrates bony trabeculae-intertwined tumor cells containing clear cytoplasm with central atypical nuclei admixed with benign giant cells. (**F**) Myxoid chondrosarcoma demonstrates round cells with myxoid features. (**G**) Mesenchymal chondrosarcoma demonstrates nodules of chondroid tissue surrounding vascular spaces, resembling a hemangiopericytoma.

TABLE 6.3-2 CLINICOPATHOLOGIC FEATURES OF CARTILAGINOUS TUMORS

Lesion	Clinical	Radiology	Histopathology	Treatment
Enchondroma	Mostly asymptomatic and incidentally recognized	9% have endosteal scalloping	Enchondroma encasement pattern	Surveillance, intralesional excision if symptomatic
Chondrosarcoma				
Grade I	60% are painful	Endosteal scalloping, calcifications in rings or spicules, uniform calcifications, eccentric lobular growth	Chondrosarcomatous permeative pattern	*Controversial:* Extended intralesional excision versus wide resection
Grade II	Up to 80% painful	Endosteal scalloping, potentially more aggressive and adaptive changes	Mixture of grade I and grade III characteristics	Wide resection
Grade III	Up to 80% painful	Endosteal scalloping, faint amorphous calcifications, large lucent areas, growing soft tissue mass	Densely packed hyperchromatic malignant-looking cells, cells of questionable cartilaginous origin, myxomatous changes, highly degenerative areas	Wide resection Possible adjunct radiation therapy and chemotherapy in selected cases

- Recurrence common, but very low metastatic potential
- Histologically resemble normal hyaline cartilage, may surround or permeate through areas of lamellar bone (a feature not seen in benign lesions, which are more typically encased by bone)
- Radiographically may show bone expansion, cortical thinning, endosteal scalloping, periosteal reaction, lytic areas
- Grade II ("intermediate-grade") tumors
  - Locally aggressive with higher potential for recurrence
  - ~10% to 15% metastasize (lung > bone)
  - Histologically show increased cellularity and cytological atypia (enlarged nuclei and often multinucleated cells) with foci of myxoid changes
  - Radiographically, grade II lesions show endosteal scalloping.
- Grade III ("high-grade") tumors
  - Highly aggressive and rapidly growing, with significant metastatic potential
  - More than 50% will metastasize.
  - Grade II lesions may recur as grade III.
  - Histologically: high cellularity, marked pleomorphism, and necrosis
  - Radiographically, these lesions show aggressive cortical destruction and a destructive pattern of growth.
- Special histologic subtypes of chondrosarcoma
  - Clear cell chondrosarcoma
    - <5% of all chondrosarcomas

- Low-grade malignant tumor with significant amounts of glycogen
- Produces lytic defects in epiphysis that imitate chondroblastoma
- Frequently extends to joint surface
- Typically involves proximal portion of femur, tibia, or humerus
- Histologically, displays tumor cells with abundant clear cytoplasm embedded in a loose cartilaginous matrix and infiltrative growth pattern
- Radiographically, produces lytic defect at end of long bones that is sharply demarcated with sclerotic margins
- Peak age range 20 to 40
- Mesenchymal chondrosarcoma
  - 2% of all chondrosarcomas
  - Highly aggressive tumor that is radiographically and histologically distinct from conventional and dedifferentiated chondrosarcoma
  - Noncartilaginous elements usually predominate.
  - Eccentrically located in bone
  - Prominent extension into soft tissues is common.
  - Usually affects young adults and teenagers
  - Usually affects axial skeleton; maxilla and mandible are frequent sites
  - Surgical excision is mainstay of treatment.
  - Ten-year survival rate ~28%
- Dedifferentiated chondrosarcomas
  - ~10% of all chondrosarcomas
  - Thought to represent the transformation of a

low-grade (I or II) chondrosarcoma into a high-grade malignant sarcoma
- Distribution in femur > pelvis > humerus > ribs > scapula
- Two components on histologic analysis with clear demarcation
  - The dedifferentiated component likely arises from one of the other three histologic subtypes or from a benign precursor.
  - High-grade sarcoma with or without heterologous elements
- Low-grade cartilaginous lesion
  - Radiographically, displays area of punctuate opacities surrounded by lytic area with complete cortical disruption and extension into the soft tissues

Genetics

There is considerable complexity and heterogeneity in the histopathology and clinical behavior of chondrosarcomas. This is reflected in the diversity of cytogenetic and molecular genetic characteristics that have been described in these tumors. Chondrosarcoma karyotypes may range from a few simple numerical changes to complex numerical and structural abnormalities. A number of genes have been investigated in chondrosarcoma. Table 6.3-3 offers a basic summary of current research on the genetics of chondrosarcoma.

The genetic changes specific to chondrosarcoma continue to be investigated extensively. The understanding of these genetic alterations will have profound implications on prognosis and may serve as a foundation for the development of therapy unique to these tumors.

Staging

Chondrosarcomas are staged using either the method of the American Joint Committee on Cancer (AJCC) or Enneking (see Chapter 1, Evaluation of Bone Tumors).

DIAGNOSIS

Physical Examination and History

Clinical Features

Distribution
- Pelvis > femur > ribs > humerus > scapula > tibia (Fig. 6.3-4)
- Metaphysis > diaphysis

Pain
- Most patients with a chondrosarcoma will have dull, aching pain.
- Benign cartilage tumors less frequently produce pain.
- Grade II or III chondrosarcomas present with pain in up to 80% of cases.
- Rest pain and night pain are common in chondrosarcomas.

TABLE 6.3-3 TUMOR SUPPRESSOR GENES AND ONCOGENES IN CHONDROSARCOMA

Gene	Significance
TP53	Altered patterns of p53 expression and mutations in TP53 have been detected in high-grade chondrosarcoma tumors.
HRAS	Mutations in HRAS occur during the course of dedifferentiation and may affect malignant potential.
ABL	Expression of the ABL gene has been detected in grade I and II chondrosacoma and is likely associated with inhibition of apoptosis.
MET	MET (hepatocyte growth factor receptor) expression has been detected in benign and malignant cartilage tumors.
MMPs	Increased expression of several MMPs (1, 2, 9, 13) and decreased expression of others (3, 8) has corresponded with malignancy in chondrosarcoma.
MDR1	Multiple drug resistance gene 1 (MDR1) has been seen in chondrosarcoma and may be related to chemotherapy response.
EXT1,2	Germline mutations and functional loss of *EXT1* or *EXT2* are often found in multiple osteochondromas and predispose to the development of chondrosarcoma (about 2% to 3%).
Sox9	The transcription factor Sox9, which plays an essential role in the early phases of chondrocyte differentiation and is a key regulator of chondrogenesis, has been shown to be expressed almost exclusively in the small cell component of mesenchymal chondrosarcoma.
PDGF-α	High expression of PDGF-α has been shown in aggressive chondrosarcoma. This may have a role in therapeutic strategies.

Pathologic Fracture
- Occurs in a relatively small number of cases (3% to 8%) of low-grade chondrosarcoma
- Incidence much higher in high-grade tumors (36% of dedifferentiated chondrosarcomas in one series)

Physical Examination Findings
- Local swelling and tenderness
- Antalgic gait for lower extremity tumors (variable)
- Decreased range of motion at adjacent joints (variable)
- Palpable mass in tumors with associated soft tissue extension

Radiologic Features

It is frequently a challenge to differentiate between enchondromas and grade I chondrosarcomas based on radio-

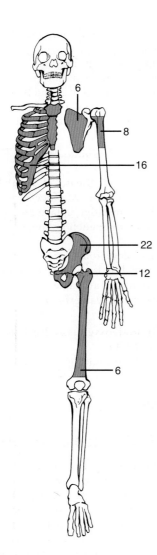

Figure 6.3-4   Distribution of chondrosarcoma by site of lesion (numbers represent percentage frequency).

graphic features. Both can demonstrate the classic discrete stippled calcified opacities indicative of hyaline cartilage matrix within the intramedullary region(s) of typical long bones.

Plain Radiography (Fig. 6.3-5)
- Radiolucent area with varying numbers of punctate opacities
- Endosteal scalloping can indicate malignant potential but is not confirmatory (Box 6.3-1).
- Adaptive changes include cortical expansion or thickening.
- Aggressive features include cortical disruption and soft tissue expansion.
- Change in radiographic appearance with time. Radiographs taken at different points in time (usually 3 months apart) illustrating increases in endosteal scalloping and cortical destruction or fewer intralesional calcifications suggest a malignant lesion.

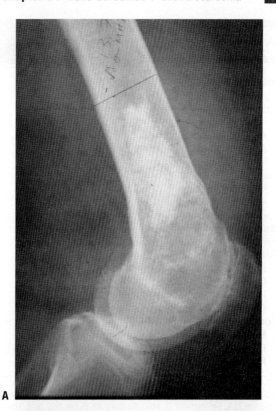

A

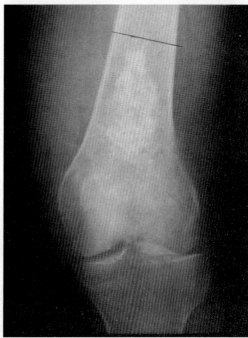

B

Figure 6.3-5   Plain radiographs of a low-grade cartilage lesion.

Computed Tomography (Fig. 6.3-6)
- Axial computed tomography (CT) can assist in determining extent of endosteal scalloping and bony destruction.
- Change in the nature of calcifications with sequential scanning can suggest malignancy.

BOX 6.3-1 INDICATORS FAVORING MALIGNANCY IN CARTILAGE TUMORS

Clinical Features

Age >40

Pain

   Insidious onset

   At night, waking from sleep

   At rest, unrelated to activity

   Persistent over 6 months

Mass

   Firm and fixed

   Nodular surface

   Enlargement after skeletal maturity

Radiographic Findings

>6 cm in greatest diameter

Calcifications

   Faint, hazy windblown densities

   Overall intramedullary radiolucency

   High ratio of lucent to calcified matrix

   Discrete densities beyond outer bone margin

Cortex

   Endosteal erosions

   Expansion, thickening, destruction

   Periosteal new bone formation

Adapted from Weis L. Common malignant bone tumors: osteosarcoma. In: Simon MA, Springfield D, eds. *Surgery for Bone and Soft Tissue Tumors.* Philadelphia: Lippincott-Raven, 1998.

Magnetic Resonance Imaging (Fig. 6.3-7)

- Degree of medullary fill
  - Involvement of >90% of the medullary canal suggests chondrosarcoma.
  - <90% medullary involvement and noncontiguous foci of cartilage suggest a benign cartilage tumor.

- Low-signal T1-weighted images, high-signal T2-weighted images
- Septal enhancements on magnetic resonance imaging (MRI) suggest intralesional fibrotic bands, a histologic finding associated with grade I and II chondrosarcomas.
- Gadolinium enhancement delineates extent of tumor and proximity to neurovascular structures.

Technetium-99m Diphosphonate Bone Scan (Fig. 6.3-8)

- Identifies multifocal disease of multiple enchondromatosis (Ollier's disease, Maffucci's syndrome)
- Lesions with radioisotope uptake are more likely to be chondrosarcoma than enchondroma, especially in long bones.
- Bone scan may play a role in screening malignant transformation of enchondroma into chondrosarcoma if serial examinations are available.
- Some enchondromas can exhibit uptake of radioisotope.

Fluorine-18 Fluorodeoxyglucose Positron Emission Tomography (FDG PET)

- May have a role in tumor grading in chondrosarcoma

TREATMENT

Surgical Indications and Contraindications

Surgical resection remains the primary and most successful means of treating chondrosarcomas. The decision regarding the extent of surgical resection and adjuvant therapy depends on the clinical and histologic characteristics of the lesion. This remains somewhat controversial. To date, studies have not shown adjuvant treatments such as chemotherapy or radiation to have any significant impact on patient

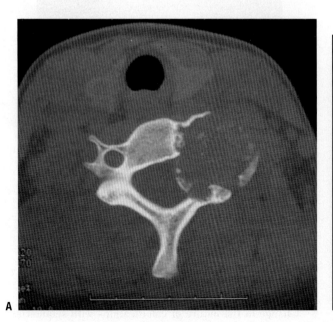
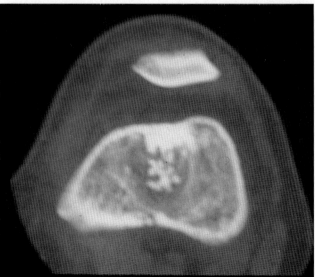

A   B

Figure 6.3-6   Axial CT of chondrosarcoma of vertebral elements (*left*) and distal femur (*right*).

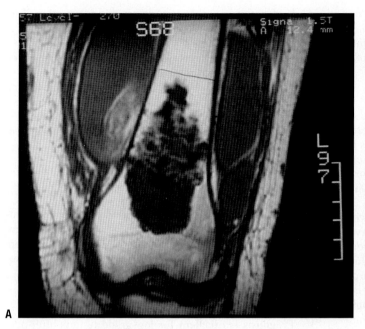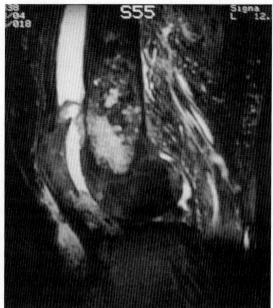

Figure 6.3-7   MRI images of distal femoral chondrosarcoma.

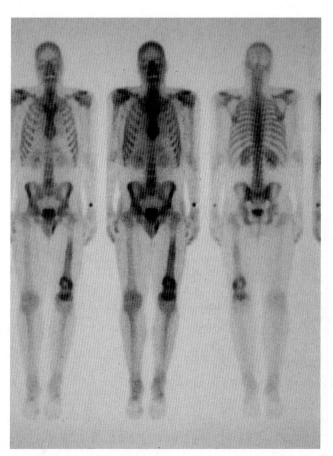

Figure 6.3-8   Bone scan of patient with left distal femoral chondrosarcoma.

morbidity or mortality in most isolated primary lesions. Possible exceptions are younger patients with a dedifferentiated subtype and those with metastatic disease. As these adjunctive modalities are of no proven benefit, the burden of a cure falls upon adequate initial surgical resection.

Surgical and Nonoperative Options

Historically, wide resection was considered the method of choice for all chondrosarcomas. Unfortunately, these tumors are frequently found in regions such as the pelvis or proximal long bones, where aggressive surgical management may endanger adjacent vital organs and structures or compromise limb function. For low-grade tumors with minimal metastatic potential, less aggressive approaches such as marginal excision and extended intralesional excision with margin expansion using adjuncts such as phenol or cryotherapy have received increasing attention. While rigorous evidence-based criteria are lacking at present, individual centers may have their own criteria and algorithms for surgical decision making (see Algorithm 6.3-1). In general, benign lesions should be treated conservatively, while high-grade malignancies should be treated aggressively with complete resection. Optimal treatment for low-grade chondrosarcoma remains a diagnostic and therapeutic dilemma.

- Primary indications for surgical treatment of cartilaginous tumors are for:
  - Symptomatic lesions
  - Aggressive appearance on radiographic studies

- Change over time in radiographic appearance of lesion without initial aggressive appearance
- Specific treatments
  - Low-grade lesions: wide resection versus extended intralesional curettage
    - Phenol and liquid nitrogen are commonly used adjuvants for extended intralesional curettage.
  - Intermediate grade: wide resection necessary
  - High-grade, aggressive tumors: wide resection necessary

Results and Outcome

- In general, the prognosis for chondrosarcoma depends on the histologic grade of the lesion and the attainment of complete excision of the tumor (Table 6.3-4). There is a limited role for adjuvant therapies (i.e., chemotherapy and irradiation).

Conventional Chondrosarcoma

- Prognosis is excellent for low-grade tumors after adequate excision.
- Low incidence of pulmonary metastasis in low- and intermediate-grade tumors if the primary lesion is widely resected
- Recurrences can occur, even up to 15 years after treatment.

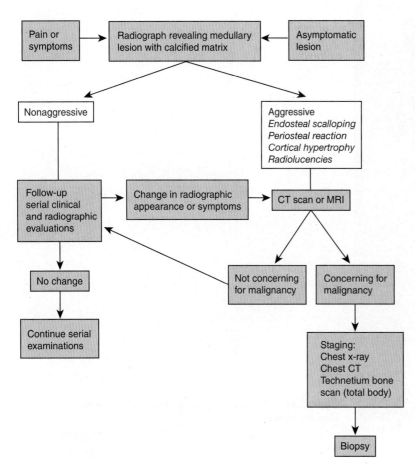

Algorithm 6.3-1. Diagnostic work-up of chondrosarcoma.

TABLE 6.3-4 SURVIVAL FEATURES OF CHONDROSARCOMA

Type	5-Year Survival	Metastatic Potential	Recurrence Rate
Grade I	90%	0%	Low
Grade II	81%	10% to 15%	Intermediate
Grade III	29%	>50%	High
Dedifferentiated	<10% (1-year)	Most	High

- Secondary and peripheral chondrosarcomas have better prognosis than primary/central.

Dedifferentiated Chondrosarcoma
- Uniformly poor prognosis

Clear Cell Chondrosarcoma
- Fair prognosis with wide resection and reconstruction
- Overall recurrence rate 16%
- Poor prognosis if treated with simple curettage and allografting
- Often mistaken for chondroblastoma

Mesenchymal Chondrosarcoma
- Prognosis very poor despite aggressive treatment
- High incidence of pulmonary metastatic disease
- High mortality

Postoperative Management

- Patients should be followed for serial surveillance radiographic and clinical examinations to assess for recurrence and/or metastatic disease.

SUGGESTED READING

Aoki J, Watanabe H, Shinozaki T, et al. FDG-PET in differential diagnosis and grading of chondrosarcomas. *J Comput Assist Tomogr* 1999;23:603–608.

Colyer RA, Sallay P, Buckwalter K. MRI assessment of chondroid matrix tumors. In *Limb Salvage: Current Trends—Proceedings of the 7th International Symposium.* Singapore: International Symposium on Limb Salvage, 1993:89–93.

Dickey ID, Rose PS, Fuchs B, et al. Dedifferentiated chondrosarcoma: the role of chemotherapy with updated outcomes. *J Bone Joint Surg [Am]* 2004;86:2412–2418.

Dorfman HD, Czerniak B. Bone cancers. *Cancer* 1995;75:223–227.

Dorfman HD, Czerniak B. Malignant cartilage tumors. In: Dorfman HD, Czerniak B, eds. *Bone Tumors.* St. Louis: Mosby, 1998.

Geirnaerdt MJ, Hogendoorn PC, Bloem JL, et al. Cartilaginous tumors: fast contrast-enhanced MR imaging. *Radiology* 2000;214:539–546.

Mirra JM, Gold R, Downs J, et al. A new histologic approach to the differentiation of enchondroma and chondrosarcoma of the bones. A clinicopathologic analysis of 51 cases. *Clin Orthop Relat Res* 1985;201:214–237.

Murphey MD, Andrews CL, Flemming DJ, et al. From the archives of the AFIP. Primary tumors of the spine: radiologic pathologic correlation. *Radiographics* 1996;16:1131–1158.

Sandberg AA, Bridge JA. Updates on the cytogenetics and molecular genetics of bone and soft tissue tumors: chondrosarcoma and other cartilaginous neoplasms. *Cancer Genet Cytogenet* 2003;143:1–31.

Unni KK. *Dahlin's Bone Tumors,* 5th ed. Philadelphia: Lippincott-Raven, 1996.

6.4 FIBROUS, FIBROHISTIOCYTIC, AND GIANT CELL TUMOR MALIGNANCIES

HANNAH D. MORGAN

Fibrosarcoma, malignant fibrous histiocytoma (MFH) of bone, and malignancy in giant cell tumor (GCT) are three relatively rare bone sarcomas that tend to be of high grade. All are found primarily around the knee. MFH and malignancy in GCT of bone may be primary or secondary malig-

nancies. Malignancy in GCT is the current World Health Organization (WHO) terminology for what has also been referred to as malignant giant cell tumor or dedifferentiated giant cell tumor. MFH is now referred to as pleomorphic sarcoma not otherwise specified (NOS) as it is thought to represent a final common pathway toward dedifferentiation for many sarcomas.

PATHOGENESIS

Etiology

- Fibrosarcoma
  - Malignant spindle cell tumor with fibroblastic differentiation and a collagenous intercellular background
- MFH
  - Malignant mesenchymal neoplasm of histiocytic origin
  - 72% primary; 28% secondary
  - Conditions associated with secondary form: bone infarction, fibrous dysplasia, intraosseous lipoma, Paget's disease, prolonged steroid use, hematopoietic malignancy, history of radiation therapy, and possibly presence of metallic orthopaedic implant (controversial)
- Malignancy in GCT
  - Primary malignancy in GCT: high-grade sarcoma arising beside or within a conventional GCT of bone
  - Secondary malignancy in GCT: high-grade sarcoma arising at the site of a previously treated conventional GCT (either with surgery alone or with radiation therapy); tumors often multiply recurrent prior to diagnosis of malignancy

Epidemiology

- Fibrosarcoma
  - <5% of malignant bone tumors; may be lower as more cases are diagnosed as fibroblastic osteosarcoma or MFH
  - Male:female 1:1
  - Most patients second through seventh decade
  - Arises in metaphysis, most commonly around the knee
- MFH
  - <2% of malignant bone tumors
  - Male:female 3:2
  - All ages affected, but majority >40 years old
  - 75% affect ends of long tubular bones; 50% about the knee
- Malignant GCT
  - Very rare: 1% to 2% of all GCT of bone
  - Primary malignant GCT: male > female
  - Secondary malignant GCT: male:female 1:1
  - Average age: 45 to 50 years
  - Secondary malignant GCTs
    - Typically occur >3 years after treatment of original tumor
    - Average latent period: 9 years
  - Majority of tumors occur about knee, as for benign GCT of bone.

Pathophysiology

- Fibrosarcoma
  - Uniform fibroblast-like spindle cells arranged in par-

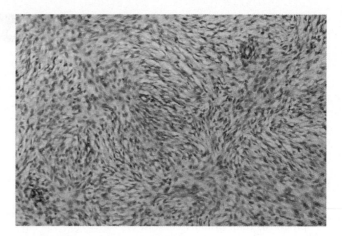

Figure 6.4-1 Fibrosarcoma of bone.

allel bundles with intercellular collagen in herringbone pattern (Fig 6.4-1)
- One study found 22q aberration leading to increased platelet-derived growth factor beta (PDGF-β).
- MFH
  - Plump malignant spindle-shaped cells in sheets and storiform patterns with granular eosinophilic cytoplasm; may have cytoplasmic vacuoles; marked nuclear atypia and numerous atypical mitoses (Fig. 6.4-2)
- Malignant GCT
  - High-grade lesions that usually exhibit a continuum of microscopic change between areas of conventional benign GCT of bone (multinucleated giant cells with benign spindle cell stroma) and areas of high-grade sarcoma (usually pleomorphic sarcoma or osteosarcoma)
  - May have p53 or H-ras molecular abnormality

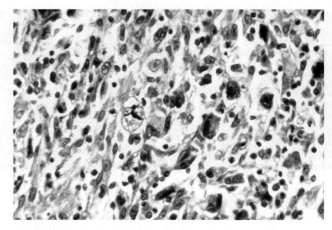

Figure 6.4-2 Malignant fibrous histiocytoma. An anaplastic tumor exhibits spindle cells, plump lipid-laden histiocytes, tumor giant cells, an abnormal mitosis (center), and a mild chronic inflammatory infiltrate. (From Rubin E, Farber JL. *Pathology*, 3rd ed. Philadelphia: Lippincott Williams & Wilkins, 1999.)

Classification

- Fibrosarcoma
  - May be low- or high-grade malignancy
- MFH
  - Aggressive high-grade tumor
  - Pleomorphic, histiocytic, giant cell, myxoid, and inflammatory variants described
- Malignant GCT
  - High-grade lesions
  - Primary malignant GCT: occurs *de novo*
  - Secondary malignant GCT: occurs following latent period after treatment of benign GCT of bone with surgery and/or radiation

DIAGNOSIS

Physical Examination and History

Clinical Features

Pain and swelling are most common; all may present with pathologic fracture.

- Fibrosarcoma
  - Nothing unique
- MFH
  - Palpable tender mass
  - Symptoms develop over months to years.
  - Pathologic fracture in 30% to 50% of patients
- Malignant GCT
  - Primary malignant GCT: symptoms present for an average of 12 months
  - Secondary malignant GCT: symptoms present for an average of 7 months

Radiologic Features

- Radiographs
  - Show destructive lytic lesion, often in metaphyseal area; may have diaphyseal or epiphyseal extension; with or without pathologic fracture
- Computed tomography (CT) scan
  - Bone involvement
    - Assess intraosseous and extraosseous extent of tumor
    - Best test for demonstrating cortical involvement
  - Chest CT
    - Used to look for pulmonary metastases in high-grade lesions
- Magnetic resonance imaging (MRI)
  - Best test for evaluating marrow involvement and associated soft tissue mass, which is frequently present with all of these
  - Can also demonstrate cortical involvement
  - Evaluate relationship of tumor to adjacent neurovascular structures
- Bone scan
  - Look for osseous metastasis; determine extent of bony involvement of tumor
- Positron emission tomography: investigational

TREATMENT

Surgical Indications and Contraindications

Surgical and Nonoperative Options

All high-grade fibrosarcomas, MFH, and malignant GCT of bone should be treated surgically with the intent of achieving a wide surgical resection, either by way of limb-sparing surgery or amputation. Neoadjuvant and adjuvant chemotherapy (often doxorubicin [Adriamycin]-based) and radiation therapy may enhance tumor control and are supported by univariate analysis of retrospective multi-institutional survey data.

Preoperative Planning (also see Chapter 4, Treatment Principles)

Appropriate imaging studies should be obtained to determine the extent of resection that is necessary. Any allograft or orthopaedic implants that will be used for reconstruction should be ordered. The patient should have a preoperative medical work-up when appropriate, and blood products should be ordered if significant intraoperative blood loss is anticipated. Surgical goals and approaches, techniques, and complications are covered in Chapter 4.

Results and Outcome (Prognosis)

- *Fibrosarcoma*
  - True prognosis difficult to determine, as many tumors once labeled fibrosarcoma are actually MFH of bone
  - Low grade: 10-year survival estimated to be 80%; metastasis in 5% to 20% of patients
  - High grade: 10-year survival 40% or less; metastasis in 55% to 65% of patients
- *MFH*
  - Estimated 50% to 60% 5-year survival
  - Younger patients and those receiving chemotherapy have better prognosis.
- *Malignancy in GCT*
  - Approximately 50% 5-year survival
  - Chemotherapy may offer increased survival in some patients, but no randomized prospective trials have been done.
  - Postradiation secondary malignant GCT has worse prognosis.

Postoperative Management

Same as for all bone sarcomas (see Chapter 4).

SUGGESTED READING

Bertoni F, Bacchini P, Staals EL. Malignancy in giant cell tumor of bone. *Cancer* 2003;97:2520–2529.

Bielack SS, Schroeders A, Fuchs N, et al. Malignant fibrous histiocytoma of bone: a retrospective EMSOS study of 125 cases. European Musculo-Skeletal Oncology Society. *Acta Orthop Scand* 1999; 70(4):353–360.

Dorfman HD, Czerniak B. *Bone Tumors.* St. Louis: Mosby, 1998: 530–555.

Hattinger CM, Tarkkanen M, Benini S, et al. Genetic analysis of fibrosarcoma of bone, a rare tumour entity closely related to osteosarcoma and malignant fibrous histiocytoma of bone. *Eur J Cell Biol* 2004;83:483–491.

Papagelopoulos PJ, Galanis EC, Sim FH, et al. Clinicopathologic features, diagnosis, and treatment of malignant fibrous histiocytoma of bone. *Orthopedics* 2000;23:59–65.

Smith SE, IKransdorf MJ. Primary musculoskeletal tumors of fibrous origin. *Semin Musculoskelet Radiol* 2000;4:73–88.

6.5 NOTOCHORDAL TUMORS

HANNAH D. MORGAN

In human embryos, the notochord is a rod of cells on the ventral aspect of the neural tube. It is the foundation of the spinal column, as the vertebral segments are formed around it. In the adult, notochord remnants form the nucleus pulposus of vertebral disks. Chordomas are slow-growing malignant tumors of bone arising from the remains of notochordal tissue almost exclusively in the axial skeleton and exhibiting notochordal differentiation. There is frequently an associated soft tissue mass, which most commonly extends anteriorly but may have intraspinal extension as well. Chordomas are typically only locally aggressive, but occasionally they do metastasize. Prompt diagnosis of the tumor followed by complete surgical resection with or without adjuvant radiation therapy offers the best clinical outcome.

PATHOGENESIS

Etiology

Chordomas are low-grade malignant neoplasms of bone arising from vestigial notochordal remnants that are almost exclusively found in the midline of the sacrococcygeal, spheno-occipital (cranial), and mobile spine regions.

Epidemiology

- 3% to 4% of primary bone tumors
- Incidence rate in United States: 0.08 per 100,000
- Male > female (male:female incidence rate 0.1–0.06 per 100,000)
- Median age: 58 years; rare <40 years; extremely rare in first decade
- Race: 91% Caucasian, 2% African-American, 7% other
- Anatomic distribution: 30% to 50% sacral, 30% cranial, 15% to 30% spinal
- Younger patients and females have propensity for cranial tumors.
- Older patients more likely to have sacral site

Pathophysiology

Chordomas are soft, grayish, lobular masses. They may have gelatinous portions. They may cause expansion of the cortical bone, and many have associated soft tissue masses. Histologically, the tumors are composed of cords or nests of cells with vacuolated cytoplasm. Mitoses are infrequent. The hallmark cells are physaliferous cells (cells with bubbly cytoplasm surrounding the nucleus), although they may be sparse or absent altogether. Occasionally there is chondroid differentiation (Fig. 6.5-1).

Classification

- Grade and stage: most chordomas are low grade and localized
  - Rarely patients present with metastatic disease.
- Variants: dedifferentiated and chondroid (skull base) described

DIAGNOSIS

Physical Examination and History

Clinical Features
- Pain and neurologic deficits are usual symptoms.
  - Sacral: bowel, bladder, and sexual dysfunction
  - Clival: cranial nerve dysfunction (facial weakness, double vision)

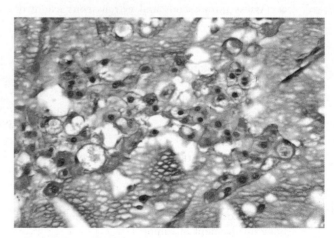

Figure 6.5-1   Chordoma.

- Mobile spine: back pain, leg pain, autonomic dysfunction
- Delay in diagnosis of months to years common, due to chordoma's slow growth and deep locations
- Physical examination: thorough neurologic examination and rectal examination (for sacrococcygeal chordomas)

Radiologic Features
- Plain radiographs
  - May show bony destruction but do not often characterize soft tissue extension
  - False-negative studies common
- Computed tomography (CT)
  - Shows bony detail well; may demonstrate associated soft tissue mass
- Magnetic resonance imaging (MRI)
  - Tumors demonstrate low signal intensity on T1-weighted and high signal intensity on T2-weighted images; associated anterior soft tissue masses are well demonstrated.
  - Shows lobular nature and midline location of tumor—aids in accurate diagnosis
  - Helpful in defining extent of tumor for adequate surgical planning
- Bone scan
  - Sacral chordomas may show decreased tracer uptake, in contrast to many other sacral tumors.
- Positron emission tomography (PET)
  - Metabolic imaging of tumor
  - (11)C-methionine (MET) PET imaging reported in literature; may help gauge effectiveness of treatment
  - Investigational

Diagnostic Work-up Algorithm
- Same as for all aggressive bone lesions (see Chapter 1, Evaluation of Bone Tumors)
- Avoid transrectal biopsies of sacrococcygeal masses!

TREATMENT

Surgical and Nonoperative Options
- Wide surgical resection leads to a longer disease-free survival than nonoperative treatment or subtotal resection.
- Radiation therapy improves disease-free interval in patients with marginal or contaminated margins; can typically be used only once.
  - Intensity-modulated radiation therapy (IMRT) and particle beam therapy offer promising alternatives to conventional external-beam radiation therapy.
- Chemotherapy ineffective

Preoperative Planning
- Preoperative planning is essential to properly counsel patient on risks of surgery (e.g., loss of bowel and bladder function in high-level sacral chordomas) and to en-

sure that all operative and reconstructive tools are available at the time of surgery.
- CT and/or MRI essential to determine extent of tumor

Surgical Goals and Approaches
- Wide resection of tumor is the most successful treatment.
- Surgical approach depends on tumor location.
  - Anteroposterior approach necessary for many chordomas of the mobile spine and sacrum
  - Some sacral tumors below S2 may be treated with posterior approach alone.

Techniques
- Anterior approach, if needed, to free external iliac arteries from mass and begin tumor resection
  - Rarely colostomy needed
- Posterior approach can be performed through three-limbed incision from lower back to both buttocks so wide exposure obtained (Fig. 6.5-2).
- Ligation of dural sac above level of resection
- If 50% or more of sacroiliac joint is intact, reconstruction is not needed.

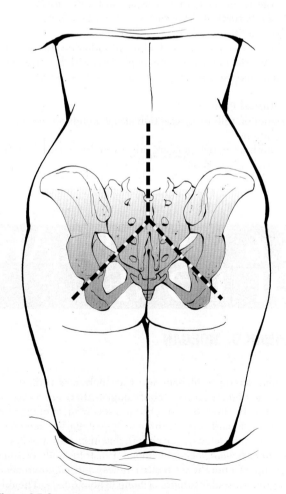

Figure 6.5-2 Sacrectomy incision.

- If >50% of sacroiliac joint is resected, stabilization of sacrospinal junction and pelvic ring is recommended with instrumentation and bone grafting.
- Gluteal or rectus abdominis flaps or synthetic material may be needed to fill sacral defect.
- Consider intraoperative or postoperative radiation therapy if resection margins are minimal or contaminated.

Complications

- The rates of occurrence and types of complications depend on the extent and location of tumor resection. The most common complications are:
  - Wound breakdown or deep infection
  - Bowel or urinary disturbance
  - Sexual dysfunction
  - Mobility impairment, especially with higher-level sacral tumors
  - Intraoperative blood loss
  - Oncologic problems (local recurrence or metastasis)

Results and Outcome

Oncologic Outcome

- Depends on the location, size, and stage of the tumor, as well as the potential for complete resection
- Local recurrence after surgery: up to 60% to 70%
- Overall survival: 75% to 85% at 5 years, but drops to 40% to 50% at 10 years
- Tumor-free margins and adjuvant radiation therapy following the initial resection in patients with positive margins increase the length of disease-free survival.

Functional Outcome

- Function following resection also depends on the tumor location.
- If both S3 nerve roots are preserved, bowel and bladder function is normal.

- If both S2 nerve roots are resected, however, there is complete urinary and bowel incontinence.
- Unilateral resection of S1, S2, S3 nerve roots typically allows preservation of at least partial sphincter function; however, unilateral sensory and motor deficits result.

Postoperative Management

The initial postoperative management is wound-related. Drains are often left in the wound for over a week, and antibiotics are continued while the drains remain. Dressings are changed frequently, and if there is persistent wound drainage, the patient may require an early incisional irrigation and débridement procedure. Patients who undergo a resection that destabilizes the spine or spinosacral junction may require postoperative bracing. If nerve roots above the level of S3 are resected with the tumor, early consultation with the physical medicine and rehabilitation service for training in urinary catheterization and bowel care protocol is recommended. Patients with chordoma should undergo tumor surveillance with CT or MRI scanning of the primary site as well as imaging of the lungs at routine intervals. Radiographs of any spinal or pelvic instrumentation should also be obtained.

SUGGESTED READING

Cheng EY, Ozerdemoglu RA, Transfeldt EE, et al. Lumbosacral chordoma: prognostic factors and treatment. *Spine* 1999;24(16): 1639–1645.

McMaster ML, Goldstein AM, Bromley CM, et al. Chordoma: incidence and survival patterns in the United States, 1973–1995. *Cancer Causes Control* 2001;12:1–11.

Ozaki T, Hillmann A, Winkelmann W. Surgical treatment of sacrococcygeal chordoma. *J Surg Oncol* 1997;64:274–279.

Sung MS, Lee GK, Kang HS, et al. Sacrococcygeal chordoma: MR imaging in 30 patients. *Skeletal Radiol* 2005;34:87–94.

York JE, Kaczaraj A, Abi-Said D, et al. Sacral chordoma: 40-year experience at a major cancer center. *Neurosurgery* 1999;44(1):74–79.

6.6 VASCULAR SARCOMAS OF BONE

HANNAH D. MORGAN

Vascular sarcomas of bone are extremely rare tumors for which the nomenclature is confusing, as there are a myriad of terms in the literature describing a spectrum of malignant vascular lesions. There are three major categories: *hemangioendothelioma*, a low-grade endothelial malignancy of bone; *epithelioid hemangioendothelioma*, a histologically distinct subgroup of endothelial malignancies; and *angiosarcoma*, high-grade vascular tumors of bone (Table 6.6-1). The differential diagnosis, treatment, and prognosis of these lesions vary according to the age of the patient, anatomic location(s) of disease, and histologic grade of each tumor.

PATHOGENESIS

Etiology

A potential predisposing factor is external-beam radiotherapy.

TABLE 6.6-1 COMPARISON OF VASCULAR SARCOMAS OF BONE

Sarcoma Type	Age	Gender	Anatomic Distribution	Gross Appearance	Histologic Features	Other Details
Hemangioendothelioma	First through ninth decades	M > F (slightly)	Half involve lower extremity; any bone affected	Firm, friable, bloody	Well-formed vascular spaces ("staghorn spaces") lined by plump endothelial cells. Intermixed with corded pattern mimicking carcinoma.	Multicentricity common; one third of cases multifocal
Epithelioid hemangioendothelioma	Second through eighth decades; peaks in second and third decades	M > F (slightly)	Femur most common; any bone affected	Firm, lobulated, tan	Corded, nested, or stranded pattern of plump endothelial cells with eosinophilic cytoplasm within hyalinized stroma (see Fig. 6.6-1). May form narrow vascular channels. Occasional cytoplasmic vacuoles (represent primitive blood vessel lumina). Signet ring–like appearance.	
Angiosarcoma	Peaks in fourth decade	M > F (slightly)	Long tubular bones and spine most common; any bone affected	Firm, bloody	Less vasoformative than hemangioendotheliomas. Regions with vascular differentiation and plump malignant endothelial cells. Some areas may show epithelioid appearance.	

Epidemiology

- Extremely rare
  - <1% of primary bone sarcomas
  - Epithelioid sarcomas: <100 cases reported
- If the tumor occurs after radiotherapy, the onset is typically several years following completion of the therapy.

Classification

- Hemangioendothelioma: low-grade endothelial malignancy of bone
- Epithelioid hemangioendothelioma: low- to intermediate-grade endothelial malignancy of bone (Fig. 6.6-1)
- Angiosarcoma: high-grade endothelial malignancy of bone

DIAGNOSIS

Clinical Features

- Localized pain and occasionally soft tissue swelling
  - Angiosarcomas are more likely than others to present with pathologic fracture.
- 25% to 30% of patients with bony vascular malignancies present with multicentric disease, either clustered in one limb or other anatomic location ("skipping joints") or spread throughout the skeleton.
  - Patient must be questioned about additional sites of bone pain.

Radiologic Features

- Lesions may be single or multiple—look for multifocal disease with skeletal survey or bone scan.
- Tumors are typically lytic but may be mixed lytic and sclerotic.
- May see bony expansion, cortical thinning, or endosteal

erosion on plain radiographs or computed tomography (CT) scan
- Soft tissue mass is not usually a prominent feature of vascular bony malignancies.
- Magnetic resonance imaging (MRI) shows marrow involvement and proximity of lesion to neurovascular structures.

TREATMENT

Surgical Indications and Contraindications

Surgical treatment of vascular bony malignancies depends on the grade of the lesion (low, intermediate, or high), the anatomic location of the tumor (whether it is surgically accessible or not), the size of the lesion, and whether the lesion is solitary or multifocal.

- Hemangioendothelioma
  - Solitary and accessible: may be cured with surgical resection, with or without adjuvant therapy
  - Multifocal: typically treated with radiation therapy
  - Bisphosphonates may play a role when bone loss is significant.
- Epithelioid hemangioendothelioma
  - Unifocal or localized multifocal lesions: should undergo wide resection when possible
  - If wide excision is not possible because of patient factors or multifocal disease, chemotherapy, radiation therapy, and radiofrequency ablation therapy have all been employed.
- Angiosarcoma
  - Should be resected with a wide or radical surgical margin when disease and patient factors permit
  - Surgically inaccessible or multicentric lesions: radiotherapy has been employed
  - Effectiveness of chemotherapy has not been proved, although it is commonly used.

Preoperative Planning

Preoperative planning is as for other bone sarcomas (see Chapter 4, Treatment Principles).

Surgical Goals and Approaches

- Ideally, lesion should be resected with wide margins.
- Bony defect reconstruction (see Chapter 4)

Techniques

- Resect and reconstruct according to principles of bone sarcoma surgery (see Chapter 4).
- Amputation may be necessary for extensive multifocal disease or for tumors involving major neurovascular structures.

Complications

- Same as for all bone sarcomas (see Chapter 4)
- Recurrence of tumor

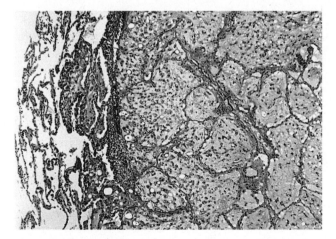

Figure 6.6-1   Metastatic epithelioid hemangioendothelioma. A nodule of tumor has spread within alveolar spaces. (From Rubin E, Farber JL. *Pathology*, 3rd ed. Philadelphia: Lippincott Williams & Wilkins, 1999.)

- Consider adjuvant radiotherapy for close margins.
- Rule out multifocal disease before surgery.

Results and Outcome

- Hemangioendothelioma
  - Important prognostic variables: degree of tumor differentiation (grade) and multifocality (extent)
    - Multifocal tumors tend to be lower grade with better prognosis.
  - Overall the prognosis is good
    - Risk of recurrence: as much as 15%
    - In rare instances, tumor may metastasize.
- Epithelioid hemangioendothelioma
  - Important prognostic variables: grade and extent (as above)
  - Intermediate risk of both local recurrence and metastasis, somewhat greater than that in patients with hemangioendothelioma
- Angiosarcoma
  - High risk of local recurrence and metastasis
  - Long-term survival: 20%

Postoperative Management

The postoperative management of these tumors depends on the type of bony reconstruction performed after surgical resection (see Chapter 4). Radiation therapy, when indicated, should be started when the wound is healing satisfactorily, typically about 2 weeks following surgery.

SUGGESTED READING

Aflatoon K, Staals D, Bertoni F, et al. Hemangioendothelioma of the spine. *Clin Orthop* 2004;418:191–197.
Evans HL, Raymond AK, Ayala AG. Vascular tumors of bone: a study of 17 cases other than ordinary hemangioma, with an evaluation of the relationship of hemangioendothelioma of bone to epithelioid hemangioma, epithelioid hemangioendothelioma, and high-grade angiosarcoma. *Hum Pathol* 2003;34:680–689.
Lezama-del Valle P, Gerald WL, Tsai J, et al. Malignant vascular tumors in young patients. *Cancer* 1998;83(8):1634–1639.
O'Connell JX, Nielsen GP, Rosenberg AE. Epithelioid vascular tumors of bone: a review and proposal of a classification scheme. *Adv Anat Path* 2001;8:74–82.
Wenger DE, Wold LE. Malignant vascular lesions of bone: radiographic and pathologic features. *Skeletal Radiol* 2000;29:619–631.

6.7 MYOGENIC, LIPOGENIC, AND EPITHELIAL BONE SARCOMAS

HANNAH D. MORGAN

Leiomyosarcoma and liposarcoma of bone and adamantinoma are all rare osseous malignancies, each constituting less than 1% all bone sarcomas. Patients with leiomyosarcoma and liposarcoma of bone should be carefully examined to ensure that the bony lesion is a primary tumor and not a metastasis from a soft tissue malignancy. Adamantinoma should be always be considered in the differential diagnosis of a tibial aggressive lesion.

PATHOGENESIS

Etiology

- Leiomyosarcoma: arises from smooth muscle cells of intraosseous blood vessels
- Liposarcoma: etiology unknown; immature adipose tissue
- Adamantinoma: presumed ectopic epithelial cell residues

Epidemiology

- Leiomyosarcoma
  - Extremely rare; <0.1% of all bone sarcomas
  - Male = female
  - First through ninth decades; mean age 45 to 50 years
  - Femur/tibia > humerus > ilium in extragnathic sites
- Liposarcoma
  - One of the rarest primary bone tumors
  - Second through sixth decades; typically third and fourth decades
  - Major long tubular bones affected
- Adamantinoma
  - ~0.4% of bone sarcomas
  - Male:female 3:2
  - Young adults and children (mean age 30 years); typically older than osteofibrous dysplasia
  - 85% involve tibia (especially anterior aspect); 10% tibia and fibula

Pathophysiology

- Leiomyosarcoma
  - Spindle-shaped cells with eosinophilic cytoplasm and cigar-shaped nuclei arranged in bundles intersecting at right angles (Fig. 6.7-1)
  - Immunohistochemistry: positive vimentin (as for all sarcomas), positive smooth muscle actin

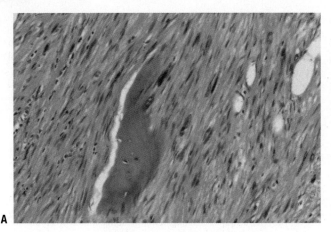 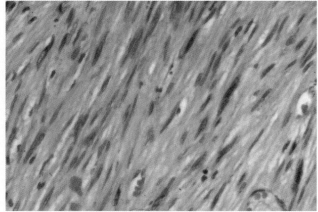

A   B

Figure 6.7-1   Leiomyosarcoma of bone. Note pleomorphic elongated cells with cigar-shaped nuclei.

- Liposarcoma
  - Either pleomorphic or round cell–rich high-grade lesion
  - Signet-ring lipoblasts may be seen.
- Adamantinoma
  - Epithelial cells surrounded by spindle-shaped fibrous tissue; little pleomorphism (Fig. 6.7-2)

Classification

- Leiomyosarcoma: 80% of tumors are high-grade malignancies of smooth muscle origin
- Liposarcoma: high-grade lesions of immature adipose tissue
- Adamantinoma: low-grade malignant epithelial lesions with strong predilection for the tibia

DIAGNOSIS

Physical Examination and History

Clinical Features
- Leiomyosarcoma
  - Pain, palpable mass; pain usually present >6 months

- 20% of patients present with pathologic fracture.
- Liposarcoma
  - Patient typically presents with pain.
- Adamantinoma
  - Pain, swelling, with or without pathologic fracture, with or without bowing
  - Symptoms are often present for months to years.

Radiologic Features
- Leiomyosarcoma
  - Radiographs: aggressive osteolytic lesion with indistinct margins
  - Computed tomographic (CT) scan: bony destruction and extraosseous extension
    - Abdomen/pelvis scan to look for primary uterine/gastrointestinal tumor
  - Magnetic resonance imaging (MRI): typically low intensity on T1, high intensity on T2 images
    - Soft tissue mass often much larger than expected on x-ray
- Liposarcoma
  - Radiographs show bone-destructive process.
  - MRI shows lesion bright on T2-weighted images.
- Adamantinoma
  - Radiographs: lesion of mid-tibia (diaphyseal or me-

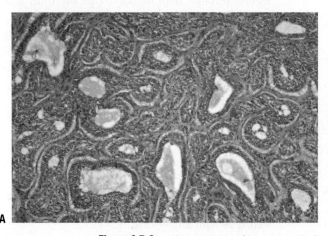 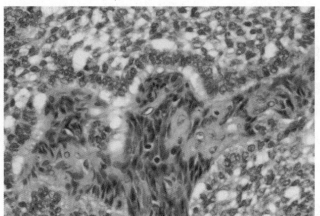

A   B

Figure 6.7-2   Adamantinoma of bone. Note biphasic pattern of epithelioid component within fibrous background.

taphyseal) especially involving anterior subcutaneous region with well-defined margins and sclerotic areas; "soap-bubble" radiolucencies within lesion
- CT scan: shows cortical involvement
- MRI: high signal on T2-weighted images, possible soft tissue extension, may see multifocal disease and bone marrow extension

TREATMENT

Surgical and Nonoperative Options

All three of these tumors are usually amenable to limb salvage and are treated most successfully with wide resection of the involved bone followed by a reconstructive procedure. Leiomyosarcoma and liposarcoma of bone, both of which tend to be high-grade, aggressive tumors, may respond to adjuvant and/or neoadjuvant chemotherapy and radiotherapy.

Preoperative Planning

- Essentially the same as for all bone sarcomas (also see Chapter 4, Treatment Principles)
- CT scans of chest/abdomen/pelvis
  - Determine whether bony lesion is truly primary tumor.
  - Rule out pulmonary or other metastatic disease.

Surgical Goals and Approaches (also see Chapter 4)

- Remove all tumor with margin of surrounding normal tissue.

Techniques

- Same as for all bone sarcomas (see Chapter 4)

Complications

- Same as for all bone sarcomas (see Chapter 4)

Results and Outcome (Prognosis)

- Leiomyosarcoma
  - Estimated 5-year survival 68% (100% if low grade)
  - Local recurrence 25%, lung metastases 25%
- Liposarcoma
  - Difficult to determine due to small number of patients
  - Approximately 50% will develop metastases.
- Adamantinoma
  - 10-year survival approximately 85%
  - Time to local recurrence 5 to 15 years
  - Time to metastases up to 27 years
    - Patients need long-term follow-up.

Postoperative Management

- Same as for all bone sarcomas (see Chapter 4).

SUGGESTED READING

Antonescu CR, Erlandson RA, Huvos AG. Primary leiomyosarcoma of bone: a clinicopathologic, immunohistochemical, and ultrastructural study of 33 patients and a literature review. *Am J Surg Pathol* 1997;21(11):1281–1294.
Bouaziz MC, Chaabane S, Mrad K, et al. Primary leiomyosarcoma of bone: report of 4 cases. *J Comput Assist Tomog* 2005;29(2):254–259.
Goto T, Ishida T, Motoi N, et al. Primary leiomyosarcoma of the femur. *J Orthop Sci* 2002;7:267–273.
Kahn LB. Adamantinoma, osteofibrous dysplasia and differentiated adamantinoma. *Skeletal Radiol* 2003;32:245–258.
Qureshi AA, Shott S, Mallin BA, et al. Current trends in the management of adamantinoma of long bones: an international study. *J Bone Joint Surg [Am]* 2000;82(8):1122–1131.

CONGENITAL AND INHERITED BONE CONDITIONS

7.1 FAMILIAL ADENOMATOUS POLYPOSIS

KATHRYN PALOMINO

Familial adenomatous polyposis (FAP) is characterized by early onset of multiple colorectal polyps. These polyps are premalignant lesions that are highly likely to progress into carcinomas. Its orthopaedic importance lies in the association of osteomas with FAP and in the fact that Gardner syndrome, previously considered a distinctly different entity, is now considered to be a subset of FAP in which patients, in addition to having polyps, may develop osteomas, epidermoid cysts, desmoid tumors, and dental abnormalities.

PATHOGENESIS
Etiology

- Genetic defect for both FAP and Gardner syndrome: mutation of the adenomatous polyposis coli (APC) gene (5q21-22 region)
  - Creates premature stop codon resulting in production of a truncated nonfunctioning protein

- Inheritance: autosomal dominant with high but variable penetrance
- *De novo* mutations: 10% to 20% of cases
- Phenotype varies by mutation site.

Epidemiology

- Incidence: 1 in 8,000 to 1 in 10,000 people
- Accounts for 1% of all cases of colorectal cancer

Pathophysiology

- Gene for FAP has been cloned, but function is unknown, as is the biological basis of the syndrome.
- Abnormalities in colonic epithelium and skin fibroblasts are present.

CLASSIFICATION

- Classic FAP
  - Polyps (Fig. 7.1-1)
    - Colonic and duodenal adenomas
    - Gastric fundic hyperplasia

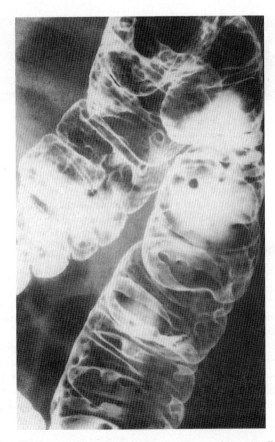

Figure 7.1-1 Familial polyposis. Small uniform polyps virtually carpet the colon. This patient had familial adenomatous polyposis. (From Swischuk LE. *Imaging of the Newborn, Infant and Young Child*, 4th ed. Philadelphia: Lippincott Williams & Wilkins, 1997: 486.)

- Jejunal and ileal adenomas
- Ileal lymphoid polyps
  - Extraintestinal lesions
    - Mandibular osteomas
    - Dental abnormalities
- Gardner variant
  - Polyps
    - Same as FAP
  - Extraintestinal lesions
    - Osteomas of long bones, mandible, and skull
    - Epidermoid and sebaceous cysts
    - Lipomas
    - Fibromas
    - Desmoid tumors

CLINICAL FEATURES

- Endoscopically detectable lesions develop in the second decade.
- Natural history in untreated patients: symptoms at average age of 33 years; cancer at 39 years; death at average age of 42 years
- Extraintestinal features (Table 7.1-1)
  - Osteomas
    - Do not evolve into malignant lesions
  - Impacted or supernumerary teeth
  - Epidermoid lesions (Gardner)
  - Lipomas (Gardner)
  - Fibromas (Gardner)
  - Desmoid tumors (Gardner)
    - Occur in 8% to 13% of cases
    - Most lethal complication of syndrome after carcinoma
- Extraintestinal manifestations are frequently detectible before adenomas and may enable early diagnosis of FAP.

TABLE 7.1-1 BONE AND SOFT TISSUE LESIONS MOST COMMONLY SEEN IN GARDNER SYNDROME

Bone	Soft Tissue
Common lesions	
Osteomas	Epidermoid cysts
Cortical thickening of bone	Desmoid-type fibromatoses
Associated lesions	Ill-defined connective tissue masses
	Lipomas
	Fibrous dysplastic lesions
	Familial infiltrative fibromatosis
	Fibromatous mesenteric plaques
	Juvenile nasopharyngeal angiofibroma
	Gardner fibroma
	Rhabdomyosarcoma

DIAGNOSIS

- FAP diagnosis: must meet one of the following criteria
  - At least 100 colorectal adenomas
  - Gene mutation of APC gene
  - Family history of FAP with one of the following:
    - Epidermoid cyst
    - Osteoma
    - Desmoid tumor

TREATMENT

- Polyposis
  - Annual endoscopic screening beginning at age 10
  - Antioxidants and nonsteroidal anti-inflammatory drugs may reverse small lesions and are in trial.
  - Only reasonable option for colon in FAP
    - Prophylactic colectomy is performed.
      - Timing and extent decided on an individual basis
- Orthopaedic manifestations
  - Desmoid tumors

- Surgical wide excision is first-line treatment for resectable desmoid tumors.
- Nonoperative options
  - Nonsteroidal anti-inflammatory agents: sulindac may reduce size of desmoid tumors and is under investigation
  - Hormones (tamoxifen)
  - Steroids (prednisone)
- Osteomas
  - Nonoperative care indicated except in rare cases

SUGGESTED READING

Boland CR, Kim YS. Gastrointestinal polyposis syndromes. In: Sleisenger JS, Fordtran JS, eds. *Gastrointestinal Disease: Pathophysiology, Diagnosis, Management*. Philadelphia: WB Saunders, 1993: 1430–1438.

DeVita Jr V, Hellman S, Rosenberg S, eds. *Cancer: Principles and Practice of Oncology,* 6th ed. Philadelphia: Lippincott Williams & Wilkins, 2001:1221.

Nilbert M, Coffin CM. Familial adenomatous polyposis. In: Fletcher CDM, Unni KK, Mertens F, eds. *Tumours of Soft Tissue and Bone: Pathology and Genetics*. World Health Organization Classification of Tumours. Lyon: International Agency for Research on Cancer Press, 2002:352–354.

7.2 BECKWITH-WIEDEMANN SYNDROME

DANIELLE A. KATZ

Beckwith-Wiedemann syndrome is defined by the presence of macroglossia, omphalocele, and visceromegaly. Typically these children are seen by an orthopaedic surgeon for hemihypertrophy and/or cerebral palsy. It is thought that the cerebral palsy is the result of hypoglycemia and seizures in the neonatal period.

PATHOGENESIS

Etiology

- Mapped to a mutation at 11p15, which is near the gene for insulin-like growth factor (11p15.5) and the gene for Wilms tumor (11p13)
- Most mutations are sporadic.
- Inheritance is autosomal dominant with evidence of paternal imprinting.

Epidemiology

- Affects approximately 1:14,000
- Associations with Beckwith-Wiedemann syndrome

- Most babies are >90th percentile weight at birth.
- Most are at the 97th percentile by 1 year of age.
- 15% of babies born with an omphalocele have Beckwith-Wiedemann syndrome.

Pathophysiology

Leg-length discrepancy results from hemihypertrophy. Hyperplasia of pancreatic islet cells leads to hypoglycemia, which in the neonatal period can lead to seizures and later spasticity. There is increased risk of tumor development, probably related to the impaired regulation of growth (e.g., visceromegaly, macroglossia, hemihypertrophy). Approximately 7% to 9% of patients with Beckwith-Wiedemann syndrome develop tumors. Most common is Wilms tumor, followed by hepatoblastoma and adrenal carcinoma. The risk of tumor development is higher in those with hemihypertrophy (~25%).

DIAGNOSIS

- Diagnosis typically is made at birth based on the classic clinical findings.

■ Genetic testing may be performed to confirm the diagnosis.

TREATMENT

Nonorthopaedic Care

Primary treatment concerns are nonorthopaedic.

■ Management of hypoglycemia, particularly in infancy, is crucial.
■ Macroglossia can interfere with breathing and feeding, and tongue reduction surgery sometimes is performed.
■ Routine abdominal ultrasounds to screen for Wilms tumor (or other intra-abdominal tumors) are essential. Protocols vary, but scans are typically recommended every 4 to 6 months until the child is 6 to 8 years old.

Orthopaedic Care

■ Treatments of spasticity and leg-length discrepancy are similar to treatment of these findings in other children.
■ Epiphysiodesis is the most common surgical technique for equalizing leg lengths.

SUGGESTED READING

Beckwith JB. Macroglossia, omphalocele, adrenal cytomegaly, gigantism, and hyperplastic visceromegaly. *Birth Defects* 1969;V(2): 188–196.

Cohen MM. Beckwith-Wiedemann syndrome: Historical, clinicopathological, and etiopathogenetic perspectives. *Pediatr Dev Pathol* 2005;8:287–304.

Herring JA, ed. *Tachdjian's Pediatric Orthopaedics*, 3rd ed. Philadelphia: WB Saunders, 2002.

Weng EY, Mortier GR, Graham JM. Beckwith-Wiedemann syndrome: An update and review for the primary pediatrician. *Clin Pediatr* 1995;34(6):317–326.

7.3 SKELETAL DYSPLASIAS

DANIELLE A. KATZ

POLYOSTOTIC FIBROUS DYSPLASIA AND ALBRIGHT'S SYNDROME

Fibrous dysplasia is a condition in which there is fibro-osseous tissue in place of normal lamellar bone. Most often (85%) this process is monostotic (affecting a single bone), but it may be polyostotic (involving multiple bones). Cutaneous markings and endocrinopathies may accompany the polyostotic form, which usually has more severe skeletal involvement. This section will focus on the polyostotic form.

PATHOGENESIS

Etiology

■ Not inherited
■ May be due to failure of woven bone to mature to lamellar bone
■ G-protein gene mutations in both monostotic and polyostotic fibrous dysplasia, Albright's syndrome, and solitary pituitary adenoma
■ Activating (gain of function) mutations in GNAS1 (encodes alpha subunit of stimulatory G protein)

Epidemiology

■ Female predominance
■ Diagnosis usually made in late childhood or early adolescence
■ 30% to 50% of patients with polyostotic fibrous dysplasia have Albright's syndrome.

Pathophysiology

■ Fibro-osseous tissue within bone, most often metaphyseal
■ One side more involved than other

CLASSIFICATION

■ Monostotic or polyostotic
■ McCune-Albright (Albright's) syndrome is:
    ■ Polyostotic fibrous dysplasia
    ■ Café-au-lait spots ("coast of Maine" irregular border)
    ■ Precocious puberty or other endocrine abnormalities (Box 7.3-1)
■ Mazabraud's syndrome

BOX 7.3-1 CONDITIONS ASSOCIATED WITH MCCUNE-ALBRIGHT SYNDROME

Sexual precocity	Metabolic acidosis
Pituitary adenoma	Abnormalities in serum
Hyperthyroidism	electrolytes, glucose, or
Gastrointestinal polyps	insulin levels
Thymus hyperplasia	Hyperphosphaturic
Splenic hyperplasia	hypophosphatemia
Pancreatic islet cell	Osteosarcoma
hyperplasia	Developmental delay
Hepatobiliary disease	Microcephaly
Cardiac disease	Sudden or premature
Failure to thrive	death

- Fibrous dysplasia
- Soft tissue myxomas

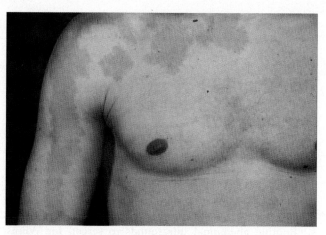

Figure 7.3-1 Irregular "coast of Maine" border in the pigmented skin lesion associated with polyostotic fibrous dysplasia. This differs from the smooth "coast of California" border seen typically in type I peripheral neurofibromatosis and in Jaffe-Campanacci syndrome (multiple nonossifying fibromas and café-au-lait spots).

DIAGNOSIS

Clinical Features

Polyostotic Fibrous Dysplasia
- May be asymptomatic, although that is less common in polyostotic form
- Pain
- Limp (can be from pain, leg-length discrepancy, or Trendelenburg gait from "shepherd's crook" deformity of proximal femur)
- Swelling (if bone in subcutaneous location)
- Angular deformity
- Leg-length discrepancy
- 50% with craniofacial manifestations

McCune-Albright Syndrome (features in addition to the above)
- Cutaneous macular pigmentation similar to café-au-lait spots of neurofibromatosis
  - Irregular "coast of Maine" border (unlike smooth "coast of California" border seen in neurofibromatosis) (Fig. 7.3-1)
  - Tend to cluster centrally, especially on the back
  - Most frequent extraskeletal manifestation (approximately one third)
  - Unusual in monostotic fibrous dysplasia
- Precocious puberty or endocrinopathy
  - Precocious puberty more common (20%)
    - Females > males
    - Female presentation: vaginal bleeding, premature development of sexual organs, premature secondary sex characteristics
    - Male presentation: enlarged genitals, premature secondary sex characteristics
  - Endocrinopathy may include hyperparathyroidism, hyperthyroidism, Cushing syndrome, acromegaly, diabetes, rickets, osteomalacia, hyperprolactinemia.

Mazabraud's Syndrome
- Myxomas with fibrous dysplasia bone lesions
- Usually polyostotic (86%) over solitary fibrous dysplasia, rarely with McCune-Albright's

Radiologic Features

- Diaphyseal or metaphyseal
  - Epiphyseal involvement rare
  - Involvement of flat bones (skull, jaw, ribs) common
  - Spinal involvement uncommon
- Lucent or "ground glass" appearance (Fig. 7.3-2)
- May have calcifications
- Sclerotic rim typical
- May expand cortex (usually does not break cortex)
- May have angular deformities (e.g., "shepherd's crook" deformity) (Fig. 7.3-3)
- Increased uptake on bone scan

Histologic Features

- Fibrous stroma with spindle cells
- Spicules of osteoid or woven bone that have the appearance of "alphabet soup" (often described as resembling the letters C, O, J, and Y) or "Chinese characters" (Fig. 7.3-4)
- Few osteoblasts (lacking osteoblastic rimming)
  - Lack of osteoblastic rimming distinguishes fibrous dysplasia from osteofibrous dysplasia, more common in the tibia, which is characterized by osteoblastic rimming.
- Cartilaginous foci may be present.

TREATMENT

Observe if asymptomatic. Endocrinologist should manage precocious puberty or other endocrinopathies.

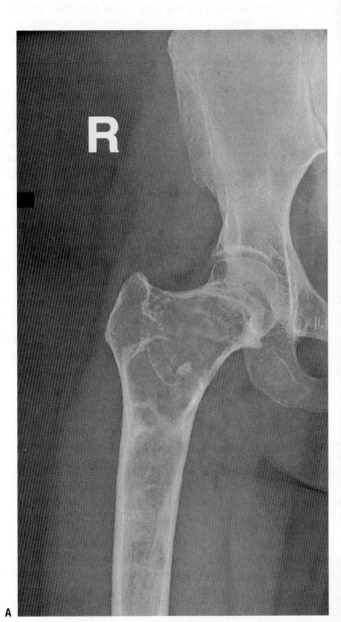

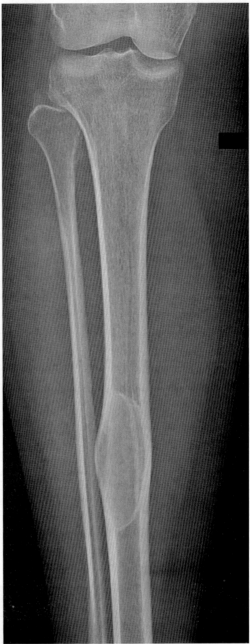

Figure 7.3-2   Radiographs from a patient with polyostotic fibrous dysplasia show extensive involvement of the proximal femur (**A**) and a single lesion in the ipsilateral tibia (**B**). Note the characteristic loss of normal trabeculation within the lesion in the tibia, which has been referred to as a "ground glass" mineralization pattern. This less organized appearance reflects the histology, which shows a more random "Chinese character" pattern of mineralization.

Indications for Surgery

- Biopsy indicated if diagnosis in question
- Fracture through lesion
    - If alignment unacceptable or high-risk location (e.g., proximal femur)
    - In children may be able to treat pathologic fractures with casting
- Progressive deformity

- If causing functional disability, unacceptable disfigurement, significantly increased risk of pathologic fracture
- Pain

Surgical Technique

- In children, simple curettage or curettage and bone grafting typically are followed by recurrence of the le-

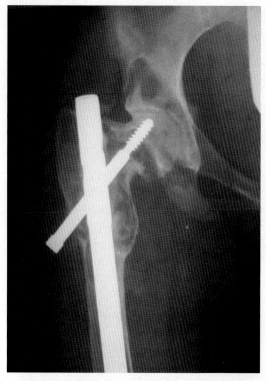

Figure 7.3-3 A classic "shepherd's crook" deformity of the proximal femur consisting of coxa vara due to fibrous dysplasia is shown on this hip radiograph. In this case, the patient has undergone previous internal fixation.

sion. Prophylactic intramedullary nails may be useful in the setting of progressive deformity (see Fig. 7.3-3).

- In adults, curettage and bone grafting has better success.
- If open reduction and internal fixation (ORIF) is performed:

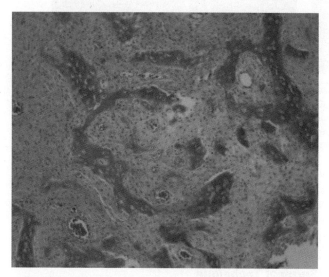

Figure 7.3-4 Typical histology of fibrous dysplasia, with multiple "alphabet soup" or "Chinese character" bone formation surrounded by a fibrous tissue background and lacking osteoblastic rimming.

- Must have good alignment of bones (may need osteotomies to accomplish this)
- Screws may not have good purchase in abnormal bone.
- Allograft cortical struts may provide additional stability and be less likely to be resorbed.

Results and Outcome

Surgical treatment may be challenging because of tendency for recurrence and pathological nature of bone. Malignant transformation of lesions is rare and usually is associated with a history of radiation therapy. For this reason radiation therapy is *not* indicated for this disease. When malignancy develops, the prognosis is poor.

OLLIER'S DISEASE AND MAFFUCCI'S SYNDROME

Solitary enchondromas are relatively common benign tumors of bone. Multiple enchondromatosis is far less common and has been given the eponym "Ollier's disease." Maffucci's syndrome consists of multiple soft tissue hemangiomas in the presence of multiple enchondromatosis. This section will focus on Ollier's disease and Maffucci's syndrome.

PATHOGENESIS

Etiology

- Unknown
- Mutations in parathyroid hormone receptor 1 (PTHR1), the receptor for parathyroid hormone (PTH) and parathyroid hormone-related protein (PTHRP), identified in some patients with Ollier's disease
- Ollier's disease usually sporadic but affected families reported
- Maffucci's syndrome sporadic

Epidemiology

- Uncommon
- Typically diagnosed in childhood

Pathophysiology

Cartilaginous rests remain within normal bone, possibly due to delay in differentiation resulting from constitutive activation of Ihh (Indian Hedgehog) signaling secondary to mutant PTHR1. In Ollier's disease there is up to a 20% to 33% chance of malignant degeneration to chondrosarcoma. In Maffucci's syndrome the risk is higher; some authors report 100%. Patients with Maffucci's syndrome are also at increased risk for the development of acute lymphocytic leukemia (ALL), astrocytoma, and malignancies of the gastrointestinal system.

CLASSIFICATION

- Ollier's disease: multiple enchondromatosis
- Maffucci's syndrome: multiple enchondromatosis with multiple soft tissue hemangiomas

DIAGNOSIS

Clinical Features

- Multiple enchondromas (Fig. 7.3-5), frequently unilateral predominance
- Enlargement of affected bones
- Deformity (bowing)
  - Especially genu valgum in lower extremities
  - May lead to decreased forearm rotation
- Leg-length discrepancy possible (may be 10 to 25 cm at maturity)
- In Maffucci's syndrome, can also see:
  - Cutaneous hemangiomas
  - Pigmented nevi (may be multiple)
  - Vitiligo

Radiologic Features (see Fig. 7.3-5)

- Typically metaphyseal (may extend into diaphysis) (see Fig. 7.3-5D)
- Thinning of cortex
- Endosteal scalloping
- May have longitudinal radiolucent "streaks"; "fan-like" septation of metaphyses
- Usually have hyaline cartilage matrix calcifications ("stippled," "popcorn," "rings and arcs") (see Fig. 7.3-5A)
  - May be completely lytic
- Increased uptake on bone scan
- May use computed tomography (CT) to better define bony anatomy and assess endosteal scalloping (see Fig. 7.3-5C)

Histologic Features (see Fig. 7.3-6)

- Hyaline cartilage
- Relatively hypocellular with small cells with single nucleus
- Proteoglycan matrix (pale blue staining with hematoxylin and eosin)
- May be more aggressive-looking, especially in hands, and still be benign
- This appearance can mimic low-grade chondrosarcoma.
  - Nuclei more pleomorphic, hyperchromatic, and anaplastic
  - Chondrosarcoma more likely in pelvis, proximal femur, proximal humerus
  - Chondrosarcoma much less likely in hand

- More likely if symptomatic (pain) or increasing in size

TREATMENT

Nonoperative Management

Mainstay of nonoperative treatment is monitoring. X-rays of known lesions and of pelvis should be obtained on a yearly basis, more often if symptomatic. It has been recommended that patients with Maffucci's syndrome also have periodic imaging of the abdomen and brain to screen for gastrointestinal malignancies and astrocytoma.

Surgical Management

Indications for Surgery

- Biopsy is indicated for lesions that are painful or increasing in size or that have worrisome radiologic features (e.g., rapid growth, excessive thinning, or breakthrough of cortex).
- If a lesion is symptomatic but not malignant, curettage and bone grafting may be successful.
- Angular deformities may be treated with osteotomies
- Leg-length discrepancy may be treated with epiphysiodesis or lengthening (distraction osteogenesis).
- Lesions that transform into chondrosarcoma require wide resection.

Results and Outcome

Multiple enchondromatosis (Ollier's disease) may be disfiguring and impair function. Surgery may be beneficial in that setting. Surveillance for malignant degeneration of lesions is required. Risk of malignant degeneration (usually chondrosarcoma) is approximately 25%.

Patients with Maffucci's syndrome have soft tissue hemangiomas as well as multiple enchondromas. Risk of malignancy (which may include visceral malignancies such as brain, ovary, or soft tissue primaries in addition to chondrosarcoma) may approach 100%. Early detection is key to survival.

MULTIPLE OSTEOCHONDROMAS (HEREDITARY MULTIPLE EXOSTOSES)

Solitary osteochondromas (exostoses) are the most common benign bone tumors. Hereditary multiple exostoses (HME) are far less common. Affected individuals may have dozens or even hundreds of osteochondromas. HME is inherited in an autosomal dominant pattern with 96% to 100% penetrance. Approximately 10% of cases have no family history (presumed to be new, sporadic mutation).

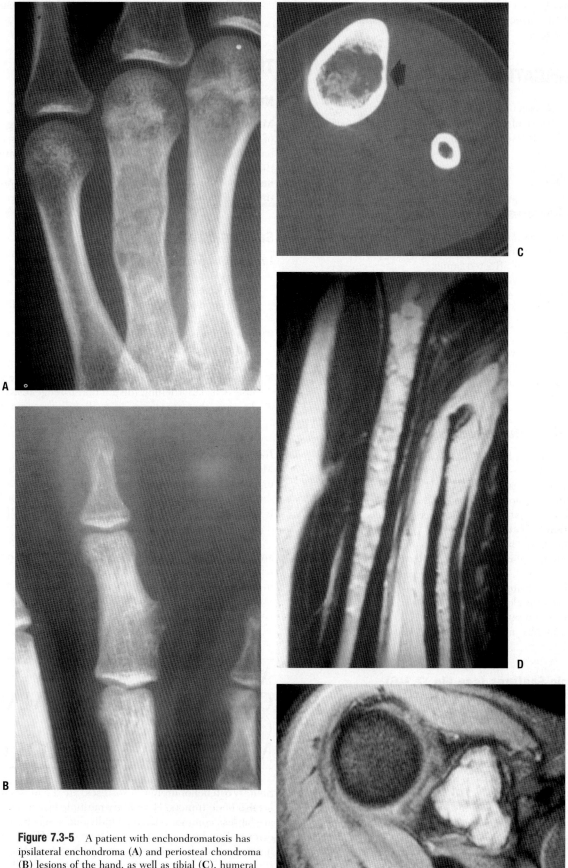

Figure 7.3-5   A patient with enchondromatosis has ipsilateral enchondroma (**A**) and periosteal chondroma (**B**) lesions of the hand, as well as tibial (**C**), humeral (**D**), and scapular (**E**) lesions.

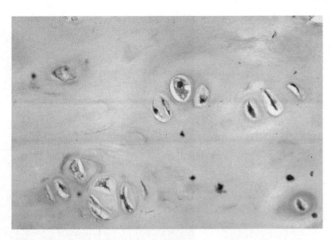

Figure 7.3-6   Bland histology of an enchondroma from a patient with enchondromatosis.

PATHOGENESIS

Etiology

- Genetic defect linked to loci EXT1 (chromosome 8p24.1), EXT2 (11p11-12), and EXT3 (19p)
    - EXT1 and EXT2 encode proteins involved in cartilage metabolism.
    - Thought to act as tumor suppressor genes whose inactivation leads to exostosis formation and whose multiple inactivations lead to malignancy
- Autosomal dominant inheritance pattern
    - Variable penetrance in females, possibly due to an X-linked modifying gene
- 10% sporadic

Epidemiology

- 1 in 50,000 to 100,000
- Slight male predominance (1.5:1)
- Diagnosis of HME often made early in childhood (mean age 3 years) but rare before 2 years of age

Pathophysiology

- Ectopic foci from physes that then grow independently
- Mechanical complications and growth disturbances are more common with HME than with solitary osteochondroma.
- Risk of malignant transformation higher for HME, estimated at around 3%, than for solitary exostoses. When it occurs, however, it is usually of low grade.
- Central locations (i.e., pelvis, hips, and shoulders) are more likely to undergo malignant transformation.

DIAGNOSIS

Clinical Features

- HME is diagnosed at an earlier age than solitary enchondromas, usually within first decade.

- 80% of those with HME will have noticeable exostoses by 10 years of age, and nearly 100% by 12 years.
- "Knobby" prominences near joints, with the distal femur and proximal tibia being the most common sites
    - Other common sites (in decreasing order of frequency) include proximal humerus, scapula and ribs, proximal fibula, distal radius and/or ulna, distal fibula, distal tibia, and foot.
- Afflicted individuals within a single family can have greatly varying amounts of disease.
- Shortened stature is seen in more severely affected individuals.
- With severe involvement, the limbs may appear short relative to the trunk.
- Genu valgum may be seen, as may radial head dislocation if the radius develops a marked bow because of a severely shortened ulna.
- Pain may develop from trauma (exostoses may fracture), pressure on muscles or nerves, or inflammation of an overlying bursa (common), or malignant degeneration (rare).
- Rarely, a pseudoaneurysm may develop from irritation of an adjacent blood vessel.

Radiologic Features

- In HME, 90% of the exostoses are sessile (broad-based) and only 10% are pedunculated (narrow base with longer stalk) (Fig. 7.3-7).
    - Pedunculated lesions typically grow away from the adjacent physis.
- Radiographs are diagnostic!
    - Key findings are the continuity of the cortex of the bone with the cortex of the lesion and the appearance that the medullary contents of the bone "flow into" and are continuous with the inside of the lesion.
- Magnetic resonance imaging (MRI) is used to evaluate the cartilaginous cap.
    - In childhood, the cap normally may be up to 2 to 3 cm thick. In adults, the cap is usually 2 to 3 mm thick, although up to 1.5 cm is occasionally seen.

Histologic Features

The lesion itself looks like normal bone, and the cartilage cap resembles the histology of a physis (Fig. 7.3-8). This histology does not differ from solitary osteochondroma.

TREATMENT

Nonoperative Management

Observation is the most common treatment for solitary or multiple exostoses. Fractures of osteochondromas almost always heal spontaneously. For patients with multiple exostoses, imaging of the pelvis and scapulae should be obtained at the initial examination as large lesions in these regions may go clinically undetected. Thereafter, patients should

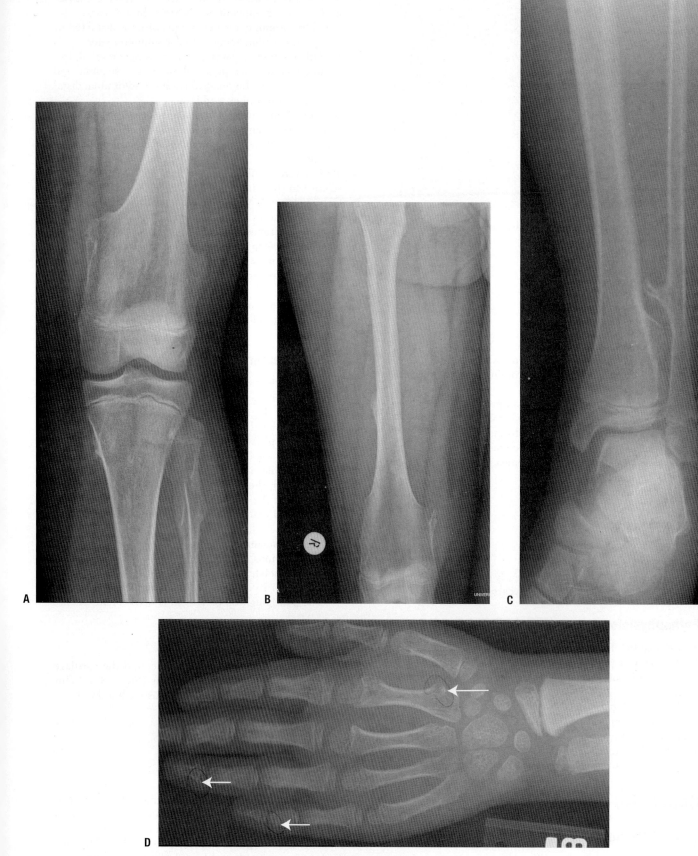

Figure 7.3-7 Radiographs from a patient with hereditary multiple exostoses show numerous typical osteochondromas about the knees (**A,B**), ankle (**C**), and hand (**D**).

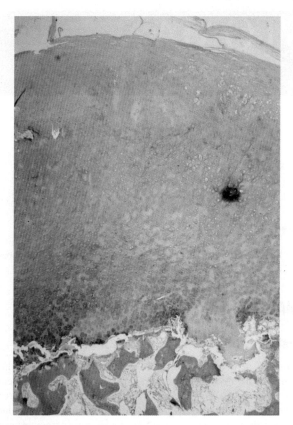

Figure 7.3-8 Histology section through the cartilage cap of an osteochondroma shows the blue-staining cartilage cap with underlying trabecular bone.

be followed at yearly intervals. Parents and siblings should also be screened.

If an exostosis is painful or enlarging, an MRI should be obtained to assess the cartilage cap. It is normal for osteochondromas to grow in children, and malignant degeneration in children is rare. A cartilage cap of more than 1 cm in an adult is concerning for chondrosarcoma.

Surgical Management

Indications for Surgery

- Pain (from lesion; most often repetitive trauma, bursa)
- Deformity (angular or leg-length discrepancy)

- Functional limitation (e.g., decreased range of motion because of impingement, muscle irritation or tethering)
- Spinal cord compression (uncommon)
- Presence of pseudoaneurysm (uncommon)
- Cosmesis (rare)
- Rapid enlargement or other signs of malignant change

Surgical Technique

- In children it is imperative to excise the entire lesion, including the cap with its perichondrium and the base and surrounding periosteum, or it will recur.
- In adults, intralesional excision may be adequate.
- If transformation to chondrosarcoma has occurred, wide excision is required to prevent recurrence. If there are no metastases, prognosis is excellent.

Results and Outcome

Recurrence after resection of osteochondroma is related to incomplete excision of the cartilage cap and is estimated to occur 2% of the time. Secondary chondrosarcomas are typically grade 1 with good long-term survival and metastatic rates of 3% to 7%. Complication rates as high as 13% have been reported with excision of benign osteochondromas.

SUGGESTED READING

DiCaprio MR, Enneking WF. Fibrous dysplasia: Pathophysiology, evaluation, and treatment. *J Bone Joint Surg [Am]* 2005;87(8): 1848–1864.

Herring JA, ed. *Tachdjian's Pediatric Orthopaedics,* 3rd ed. Philadelphia: WB Saunders, 2002.

Lewis RJ, Ketchum AS. Maffucci's syndrome: Functional and neoplastic significance. *J Bone Joint Surg [Am]* 1973;55:1465–1479.

Parekh SG, Donthineni-Rao R, Ricchetti E, et al. Fibrous dysplasia. *J Am Acad Orthop Surg* 2004;12:305–313.

Porter DE, Lonie L, Fraser M, et al. Severity of disease and risk of malignant change in hereditary multiple exostoses: A genotype-phenotype study. *J Bone Joint Surg [Br]* 2004;86(7):1041–1046.

Schmale GA, Conrad EU, Raskind WH. The natural history of hereditary multiple exostoses. *J Bone Joint Surg [Am]* 1994;76(7): 986–992.

Shapiro F, Simon S, Glimcher MJ. Hereditary multiple exostoses: Anthropometric, roentgenographic, and clinical aspects. *J Bone Joint Surg [Am]* 1979;61(6):815–824.

Stieber JR, Dormans JP. Manifestations of hereditary multiple exostoses. *J Am Acad Orthop Surg* 2005;13:110–120.

Unni KK. *Dahlin's Bone Tumors: General Aspects and Data on 11,087 cases,* 5th ed. Philadelphia: Lippincott-Raven, 1996.

7.4 RETINOBLASTOMA SYNDROME

TIMOTHY A. DAMRON

Retinoblastoma syndrome encompasses familial retinoblastoma and a number of secondary malignancies that may develop as a result of a "second hit" at the site of the RB1 gene, where a somatic mutation added to the germline RB1 mutation inactivates the tumor suppressor gene function. The synonym "retinoblastoma/osteogenic sarcoma syndrome" reflects the fact that osteosarcoma is the most common secondary tumor in these patients. Retinoblastoma is a malignancy of the embryonic neural retina.

PATHOGENESIS

Etiology

- Prototypical example of "two-hit" theory for genetic predisposition to cancer
    - First hit: germline (familial form) or somatic (nonfamilial form) mutation of RB1 gene at 13q14.1
    - Second hit: somatic mutation in all cases at RB1 locus
        - Radiation increases the risk in a dose-dependent fashion above 5 Gy.
        - Resultant inactivation of RB1 tumor suppressor gene function is associated with retinoblastoma, post-retinoblastoma osteosarcomas, and other sarcomas (Box 7.4-1), and in some sarcomas not associated with retinoblastoma syndrome (breast and non–small-cell lung carcinoma).
- Inheritance: autosomal dominant (AD) with almost full penetrance in familial form

Epidemiology

- Retinoblastoma
    - Frequency: 1/3,500 to 1/25,000 (Fig. 7.4-1)
    - Male:female equal
- Secondary sarcoma
    - Relative risk compared to normal population: 30

BOX 7.4-1 SECONDARY TUMORS ASSOCIATED WITH RETINOBLASTOMA SYNDROME

Osteosarcoma	Leukemia
Fibrosarcoma	Lymphoma
Chondrosarcoma	Melanoma
Ewing sarcoma	Brain tumors, including
Epithelial tumors	pinealoblastoma

- Cumulative incidence over 50 years
    - Hereditary retinoblastoma: 51%
    - Nonhereditary retinoblastoma: 5%

Pathophysiology

- Known genetic defect (RB1) inactivates tumor suppressor gene, resulting in tumor formation (Fig. 7.4-2)

DIAGNOSIS

History and Physical Examination

From an orthopaedic standpoint, patients with retinoblastoma syndrome will have had retinoblastoma diagnosed earlier in their life, so the key is to recognize that the history of retinoblastoma predisposes to development of secondary tumors that may either be musculoskeletal (osteosarcoma, chondrosarcoma, Ewing) or present with musculoskeletal complaints (see Box 7.4-1).

History
- Age at diagnosis of retinoblastoma: 90% at <3 years
    - Unilateral: 18 months
    - Bilateral: 12 months
- Previous treatment for retinoblastoma: chemotherapy and/or radiotherapy

Physical Examination
- Evidence of previous retinoblastoma: characteristic narrow facies, sometimes blindness
- Secondary tumor: manifestations depend upon type of secondary tumor
    - Classification of secondary tumors

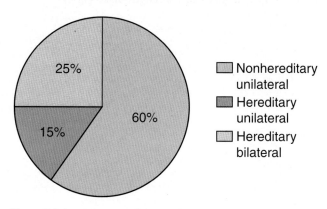

Figure 7.4-1   Frequency of various forms of retinoblastoma.

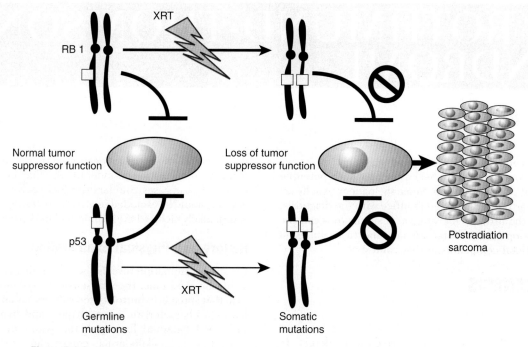

Figure 7.4-2   Two-hit theory for retinoblastoma and p53 tumor suppressor genes.

- Tumors within radiation field
- Tumors outside radiation field
- Tumors in patients without radiotherapy

Diagnostic Work-up

With the history of retinoblastoma, a high index of suspicion for sarcoma must be maintained in any patient with pain and/or a mass. The diagnostic work-up is the same as that for any other bone or soft tissue mass, as discussed in earlier chapters.

TREATMENT

Treatment of the secondary tumors is the primary concern for the orthopedic surgeon. This treatment depends upon the specific type of tumor, as discussed in each of the individual sections. Aggressive treatment is indicated for most patients, although the prognosis classically has been considered to be poor.

Results and Outcome

Classically considered to have a dismal prognosis, the latest results for aggressive treatment of postradiation osteosarcoma, in particular, are encouraging.

- Postradiation osteosarcoma treated with chemotherapy and surgery
  - 5-year disease-specific survival: 71%
  - 5-year overall survival: 68.3%

SUGGESTED READING

Aerts I, Pacquement H, Doz F, et al. Outcome of second malignancies after retinoblastoma: a retrospective analysis of 25 patients treated at the Institut Curie. *Eur J Cancer* 2004;40(10):1522–1529.

Cavenee WK, Bogler O, Hadjistilianou T, et al. Retinoblastoma syndrome. In: Fletcher CDM, Unni KK, Mertens F, eds. *Tumours of Soft Tissue and Bone: Pathology and Genetics*. World Health Organization Classification of Tumours. Lyon: International Agency for Research on Cancer Press, 2002:363–364.

Koshy M, Paulino AC, Mai WY, et al. Radiation-induced osteosarcomas in the pediatric population. *Int J Radiat Oncol Biol Phys* 2005; 63(4):1169–1174.

Smith LM, Donaldson SS. Incidence and management of secondary malignancies in patients with retinoblastoma and Ewing's sarcoma. *Oncology (Williston Park)* 1991;5(5):135–141.

Wong FL, Boice JD Jr, Abramson DH, et al. Cancer incidence after retinoblastoma. Radiation dose and sarcoma risk. *JAMA* 1997; 278(15):1262–1267.

7.5 ROTHMUND-THOMSON SYNDROME

KATHRYN PALOMINO

Rothmund-Thomson syndrome is an autosomal recessive congenital syndrome (Box 7.5-1) associated with potential development of osteosarcoma. Since the patient usually arrives in the orthopaedic surgeon's office with the diagnosis, the key for the orthopaedic surgeon is simply to recall the risk of development of osteosarcoma and to evaluate all musculoskeletal complaints in that context.

PATHOGENESIS

Etiology

- Genetic defect: subset associated with defect in RECQL4 helicase gene at locus 8q24
- Inheritance: autosomal recessive (AR)

Epidemiology

- Rare
  - Incidence unknown
- Male:female 2:1

Pathophysiology

- Known genetic defect (RECQL4) present in 40% of cases
  - Normal expression highest in thymus and testes
  - Homology with genes that cause syndromes with some clinical overlap
    - Bloom syndrome: BLM gene defect on 15q26 with AR inheritance and increased incidence of osteosarcomas
    - Werner syndrome: WRN gene defect on 8p11-12 with AR inheritance and increased risk of various bone and soft tissue tumors

DIAGNOSIS

Although no specific criteria have been established, generally the diagnosis is first suspected in the neonate based upon the characteristic rash that occurs within the first 6 months of life. Genetic testing may identify the characteristic defect in up to 40% of cases. Similar disorders, such as Werner syndrome, should be excluded (e.g., urinary testing for the characteristically elevated hyaluronic acid in Werner syndrome).

History and Physical Examination

Physical examination reveals the key finding in Rothmund-Thomson syndrome, the sun-sensitive erythematous facial rash that spreads to buttocks and extremities and eventually leaves a characteristic mixed hyper- and hypopigmented rash (poikiloderma) for which the syndrome received its other name, poikiloderma congenitale. Other nonorthopedic and orthopaedic manifestations may be present.

- Nonorthopaedic clinical features
  - Poikilodermatous skin changes
    - Develop in first 6 months of life
    - Usually appear in sun-exposed areas and around buttocks (Fig. 7.5-1)
    - Photosensitivity and blister formation
  - Thin hair and/or alopecia
  - Short stature
  - Juvenile cataracts
  - Malignancies, particularly of the skin
- Orthopaedic clinical features
  - Osteoporosis

BOX 7.5-1 COMPONENTS OF ROTHMUND-THOMSON SYNDROME

Various skin abnormalities	Predisposition to tumors
Skeletal defects	Osteosarcoma
Juvenile cataracts	Skin cancer
Premature aging	Others

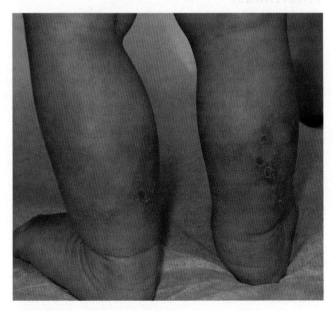

Figure 7.5-1   Rothmund-Thomson syndrome: posterior leg poikiloderma. (Image provided by Stedman's.)

- Clavicular hypoplasia
- Syndactyly
- Patella aplasia
- Genu valgum
- Benign osseous defects
  - Osteosclerosis
  - Bone cysts
  - Metaphyseal chondrodysplasia
- Sarcomas
  - Second most frequently occurring malignancy

Differential Diagnosis

- Werner syndrome
- Bloom syndrome

TREATMENT

- No specific treatment for Rothmund-Thomson syndrome exists.

- Symptomatic management of conditions as they arise
- Surgical treatment not advised for height, alignment, or nonmalignant osseous abnormalities due to poor bone and wound healing
- Hypervigilance in investigating bone pain and or soft tissue swelling is mandatory due to increased risk of malignancy, including multiple primary malignancies.

SUGGESTED READING

Anbari KK, Ierardi-Curto LA, Silber JS, et al. Two primary osteosarcomas in a patient with Rothmund-Thomson syndrome. *Clin Orthop Rel Res* 2000;(378):213–223.

Behrman RE, Kliegman RM, Arvin AM, et al, eds. *Nelson Textbook of Pediatrics*, 15th ed. Philadelphia: WB Saunders, 1996:1862.

Lindor NM. Rothmund-Thomson syndrome. In: Fletcher CDM, Unni KK, Mertens F, eds. *Tumours of Soft Tissue and Bone: Pathology and Genetics*. World Health Organization Classification of Tumours. Lyon: International Agency for Research on Cancer Press, 2002:365.

7.6 WERNER SYNDROME

KATHRYN PALOMINO

Werner syndrome is a rare hereditary systemic disease, also known as adult progeria. It is characterized by signs of premature aging (gray hair, skin changes, and cataracts) in patients after the onset of puberty. Atherosclerosis, diabetes, and neoplastic diseases are also associated with the syndrome. Life expectancy is around 50 years, with cardiovascular, atherosclerotic disease and cancers being the most common causes of death.

ETIOLOGY

- Werner syndrome gene (WRN) is located on chromosome 8 (8p11-12).
- WRN protein encodes DNA helicase and exonuclease activities and is involved in response to DNA damage.
- Inheritance: autosomal recessive

EPIDEMIOLOGY

- Prevalence: ranges from 1/22,000 to $1/10^6$
- More common in Japanese and Caucasian populations but has been described throughout the world
- Frequency is higher in populations with consanguineous marriage.
- Male:female equal
- Age: diagnosis is usually not made until adulthood

PATHOPHYSIOLOGY

- Precise mechanism for the phenotype of Werner syndrome is unknown.
  - Defective DNA metabolism is involved, leading to altered bioavailability of growth factors.
- RecQ helicase deficiency syndrome leads to heritable cancer predisposition (10% to 30% increased risk).
  - Numerous types of tumors are seen (Fig. 7.6-1).

DIAGNOSIS

Nonorthopaedic Clinical Features

- Develop at onset of puberty
- Dermatologic changes resembling scleroderma
- Short stature (mean height: male 157 cm; female 147 cm)
- Premature graying and alopecia
- Nonsenile cataracts
- Weak, high-pitched voice
- Calcific deposits on heart valves
- Atherosclerosis
- Diabetes mellitus
- Hypogonadism
- Neoplasm (nonorthopaedic)
  - Thyroid carcinomas
  - Melanoma

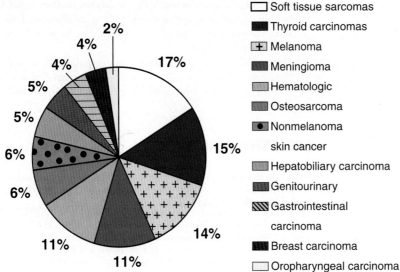

☐ Soft tissue sarcomas
▓ Thyroid carcinomas
⊞ Melanoma
▓ Meningioma
▒ Hematologic
▒ Osteosarcoma
⬤ Nonmelanoma
 skin cancer
▒ Hepatobiliary carcinoma
▓ Genitourinary
▨ Gastrointestinal
 carcinoma
▓ Breast carcinoma
☐ Oropharyngeal carcinoma

Figure 7.6-1   Tumors associated with Werner syndrome.

■ Meningioma
■ Hematological disorders

Orthopedic Clinical Features

■ Osteoporosis, usually presenting with vertebral abnormalities or insufficiency fractures
■ Muscle wasting
■ Calcific deposits in ligaments and tendons
■ Pes planus
■ Neoplasms (orthopedic)
 ■ Soft tissue sarcomas: most common malignancy
 ■ Osteosarcoma

Diagnostic Algorithm

■ Presence of all consistent clinical features with at least two of the following:
 ■ Loss of WRN protein from peripheral lymphocytes or fibroblasts
 ■ Elevated 24-hour urinary hyaluronic acid level
 ■ Detection of mutation of WRN gene on chromosome 8 by Western blot

TREATMENT

■ There is no specific therapy for Werner syndrome.
■ Management involves symptomatic medical management of conditions as they arise.

■ Management of orthopedic conditions
 ■ Osteoporosis: human insulin-like growth factor has been used
 ■ Fractures: heal poorly regardless of method of treatment
 ■ Pes planus: best managed with orthotics
 ■ Surgical incisions heal poorly.
■ Tumor management
 ■ Early diagnosis of Werner syndrome and subsequent hypervigilance in investigating skin of soft tissue abnormalities or bone pain are paramount in decreasing death rate from malignancy in the Werner syndrome patient.
 ■ Unique features of malignancy in Werner syndrome patients
  ■ Develop at early age
  ■ Develop in unusual sites
  ■ May develop multiple primaries (synchronously or metachronously)
  ■ One of most common causes of death

SUGGESTED READING

Monnat RJ Jr. Werner syndrome. In: Fletcher CDM, Unni KK, Mertens F, eds. *Tumours of Soft Tissue and Bone: Pathology and Genetics.* Lyon: World Health Organization Classification of Tumours. International Agency for Research on Cancer Press, 2002: 366–367.

Walton NP, Brammer TJ, Coleman NP. The musculoskeletal manifestations of Werner's syndrome. *J Bone Joint Surg [Br]* 2000;(82): 885–888.

METASTATIC DISEASE

TIMOTHY A. DAMRON

Metastatic disease to bone accounts for the largest number of bone lesions in patients greater than 40 years of age. In fact, the differential diagnosis for an aggressive bone lesion in an adult is "mets, mets, mets, myeloma, lymphoma, and sarcoma," in decreasing order of frequency. Even solitary bone lesions in this age group are most commonly due to metastatic carcinoma. The role of the orthopaedist is to establish or confirm the diagnosis, evaluate for risk of fracture, and stabilize or otherwise surgically treat pathological fractures and impending fractures. Pathologic fractures are discussed in Chapter 4, Treatment Principles.

Despite the prevalence of metastatic carcinoma as a cause of bone lesions in this age group, bone lesions should never be assumed to be due to metastatic disease without compelling evidence. One of the most important pitfalls in the evaluation and treatment of bone lesions in adults is the erroneous treatment of a sarcoma under the mistaken assumption that the lesion is due to metastatic carcinoma. Because the principles for treatment differ so greatly between sarcomas and metastatic carcinomas, the specific diagnosis must be established before initiation of care. Hence, an aggressive bone lesion in an adult, while frequently due to metastatic disease, should be considered a sarcoma until proven otherwise.

PATHOGENESIS

Etiology

- Common sources of bone carcinomas metastasizing to bone in adults
  - Most common "osteophilic" carcinomas
    - Breast, prostate, lung, kidney, thyroid (the "big 5")
    - Melanoma: emerging osteophilic tumor
    - Common sources of metastatic carcinoma (Fig. 8-1)
  - Most common when there is an established history of cancer:
    - Breast and prostate
  - Most common when there is no established history of cancer
    - Lung and kidney, respectively
- Common sources of metastases to bone in pediatric patients
  - Neuroblastoma (<5 years old) > rhabdomyosarcoma > retinoblastoma
- Common sources for unusual patterns of distribution (any primary may)
  - Most common metastases distal to the elbows and knees ("acral" mets)
    - Lung and kidney, respectively
    - 50% of acral mets due to lung carcinomas
  - Most common metastases to soft tissue
    - Lung and kidney, respectively

Epidemiology

- Frequency of common sources of bone carcinoma metastases (Table 8-1)
- New cases: prostate > breast > lung > kidney > thyroid

■ Frequency of metastases and survival according to primary source (Table 8-2)

Pathophysiology

While the local "soil" in which the metastases deposit is very important to allowing the establishment of a tumor growth, the distribution of metastases is intimately related to the route that metastases take from their site of origin to get to their ultimate destination (Fig. 8-2 and Table 8-3). Most metastases escape the circulation by traversing thin-walled venous structures, so they follow the distribution of the systemic (caval), portal, or vertebral venous circulation (Batson's plexus; Box 8-1) to arrive within the lung, liver, or bone, respectively (see Table 8-3). The axial pattern of distribution of the vertebral venous circulation is reflected in the predominance of axial locations for the most common sites of bone metastases (see Fig. 8-2). Lung carcinomas, given their location, have a relatively greater frequency of accessing the arterial circulation by means of eroding the pulmonary venous vasculature within the lungs. Hence, lung carcinomas are the most common source of bone metastases to the acral skeleton (distal to the elbow and knee).

Distribution of Metastases Overall
■ Common sites
   ■ Thoracolumbar spine > sacrum > proximal femur > pelvis > ribs > sternum > proximal humerus > skull
■ "Soil and seed" versus circulation controversy
   ■ Classic argument: idea that certain tissues are better "soil" for cancer cells versus idea that the circulation determines the patterns of metastases
   ■ "Soil hypothesis" from Paget (1889) with modern considerations
      ■ Metastatic tumors have a predilection for red marrow (proximal sites) over yellow marrow.
      ■ Adhesion molecules favor recruitment of tumor cells.
         ■ For example, stromal cell–derived factor-1 (SDF-1) recruits prostate cancer cells via interaction with chemokine receptor (CXCR4) on tumor cells.

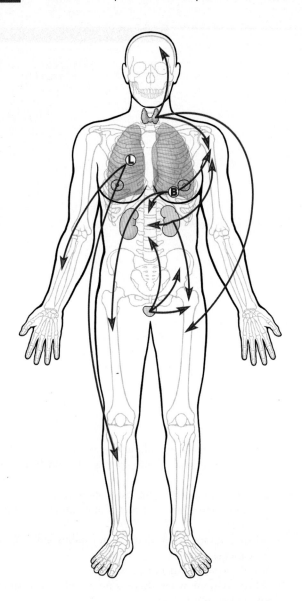

Figure 8-1   Body diagram showing breast, prostate, lung, kidney, and thyroid with arrows to bone.

TABLE 8-1 EPIDEMIOLOGY OF THE "BIG FIVE" MOST COMMON PRIMARY SOURCES OF METASTASES TO BONE

Site	% New Cases (Rank in Top 10)		Number Annual Cases
	Female	**Male**	
Prostate	—	33 (1)	230,110
Breast	32 (1)	<1 (−)	215,990
Lung	12 (2)	13 (2)	173,770
Kidney	1 (−)	3 (7)	35,710
Thyroid	3 (8)	2 (−)	23,600

Data from Jemal A, Tiwari RC, Murray T, et al. Cancer statistics, 2004. *CA Cancer J Clin* 2004;54:8–29.

TABLE 8-2 FRACTION OF PATIENTS WITH EACH PRIMARY SOURCE WHO WILL DEVELOP METASTASES, FRACTION OF THOSE THAT WILL INVOLVE BONE, AND SURVIVAL WITH METASTASES

Primary Tumor	Pts. with Metastatic Disease (%)	Pts. with Metastases who Have Bone Involvement Clinically (%)	Median Survival After Diagnosis of Metastases (mo)	Mean 5-year Survival Rate (%)
Breast carcinoma	65–75		24	20
Prostate carcinoma	65–75	30–40	40	25
Lung carcinoma	30–40	20–40	<6	<5
Renal carcinoma	20–25	15–25	6	10
Thyroid carcinoma	60	20–40	48	40
Multiple myeloma	95–100	100	20	10

Data from Coleman RE. Skeletal complications of malignancy. *Cancer* 1997;80:1588–1594.

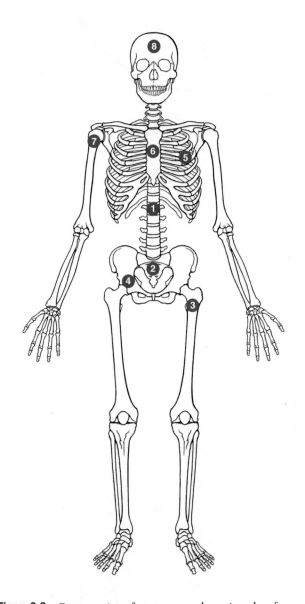

Figure 8-2 Common sites of metastases to bone, in order of relative frequency.

TABLE 8-3 CIRCULATION THEORY OF METASTATIC DISTRIBUTION

Circulatory Component	Consequent Site of Metastases
Systemic (caval) venous circulation	Lung
Portal venous circulation	Liver
Batson's vertebral venous plexus	Bone
Pulmonary venous circulation	All organs, bones

BOX 8-1 FEATURES OF BATSON'S PLEXUS

- Network of interconnected veins with thin, low-pressure walls
- Extends longitudinally from skull to sacrum, supplying segmental vertebra
- Location outside thoracoabdominal cavity: unaffected by Valsalva maneuvers
- Retrograde movement possible via valveless veins
- Connections to common osteophilic primaries (breast, prostate, lung, kidney, thyroid)

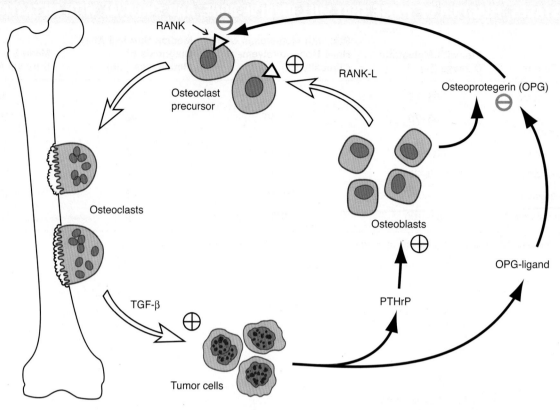

Figure 8-3   Disruption by tumor cells of normal osteoblast–osteoclast interaction via OPG-ligand.

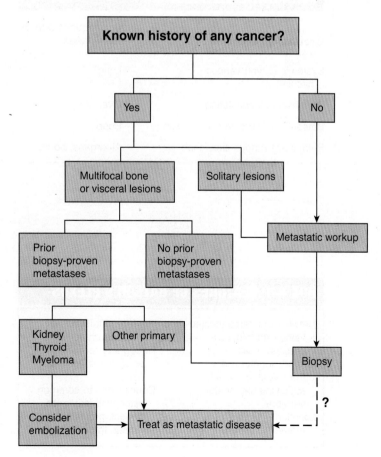

Algorithm 8-1   Diagnostic work-up of metastatic tumors.

- Growth factors capable of stimulating tumor proliferation are replete in bone.
  - Insulin-derived growth factor (IGF)
  - Bone morphogenic proteins (BMP)
  - Transforming growth factor-beta (TGF-β)
- "Circulation theory" from Ewing (1928) (see Table 8-3)

Source of Destruction: Role of the Osteoclast

- Osteoclasts, not tumor cells, destroy bone.
- Osteoclasts mediate tumor cell attachment to bone.
- Breast cancer cells recruit osteoclasts via parathyroid hormone–related protein (PTHrP) (Fig. 8-3).
  - Tumor cells produce PTHrP and osteoprotegerin ligand (OPG-L).
  - PTHrP stimulates osteoblasts to release osteoprotegerin (OPG) and receptor activator of nuclear factor kappa ligand (RANK-L).
  - RANK-L stimulates the RANK receptor on osteoclast precursors to cause differentiation into osteoclasts, which leads to resorption.
  - Osteoprotegerin inhibits the interaction of RANK-L with RANK, decreasing the bone resorption.

- Myeloma cells stimulated by interleukin-6 (IL-6) released by osteoclasts

CLASSIFICATION

Metastatic disease to bone represents the most advanced stage of any primary malignancy and carries a similar weight in staging systems for these cancers as metastases to other distant sites. While the TLM (tumor, lymph node, metastasis) classification systems differ in their details between sarcomas and the common carcinomas that metastasize to bone, spread to bone in all cases shifts the disease to the highest level.

DIAGNOSIS

The diagnosis of metastatic disease to bone relies on assimilation of data from numerous sources (Algorithms 8-1 and 8-2). In some cases, the diagnosis is apparent on review of only the history, physical examination, and radiographs.

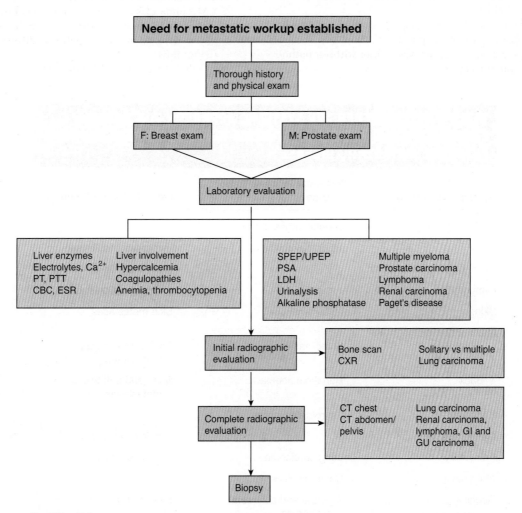

Algorithm 8-2　Evaluation for metastatic disease of unknown primary site. (Adapted from Rougraff BT, Kneisl JS, Simon MA. Skeletal metastases of unknown origin: A prospective study of a diagnostic strategy. *J Bone Joint Surg [Am]* 1993;75:1276–1281.)

However, in many cases in which the orthopaedic surgeon will be involved, the diagnosis will require a more comprehensive evaluation and biopsy for confirmation.

Physical Examination

- Key examinations search for common sources of bone metastases:
    - Breast, prostate, lungs, flank (kidney), thyroid
- Comprehensive evaluation for other less common sources of bone metastases and sites of concurrent metastases (Table 8-4):
    - Skin (melanoma), lymphatics (lymphoma), guaiac examination (colon)

History

- Pain
    - The most common presenting clinical symptom of bone metastases
    - Night pain characteristic
- Less common presentations of metastases
    - Soft tissue mass (from soft tissue extension or soft tissue metastasis)
    - Incidental findings on staging studies coincident with primary tumor diagnosis
    - Paraplegia (spine metastases with or without pathologic spinal fracture)

- Pathological fracture (usually preceded by pain, even of short duration)
- Soft tissue metastases: more frequently painful rather than painless, whereas most soft tissue sarcomas are painless

Radiologic Features

- Most common radiographic appearance: aggressive features (Box 8-2)
    - Typical margins: moth-eaten to permeative
    - Typical effects on bone: cortical destruction, soft tissue extension (variable)
    - Typical bone reactions: nonlaminar periosteal reaction (variable), Codman's triangle (unusual) (Fig. 8-4, onion-skinning (rare), sunburst (rare)
    - Matrix: lytic (Fig. 8-5), sclerotic (Fig. 8-6), or mixed (Fig. 8-7)
    - Bone scan: increased uptake (see Fig. 8-4), except in very aggressive lytic tumors (e.g., renal, thyroid, myeloma)
    - Radioiodide nuclear medicine study: increased uptake for thyroid carcinoma
- Differentiation from myeloma
    - Myeloma classic features not typical in metastases
    - Myeloma classic features: multiple punched-out lytic defects, raindrop pattern, diffuse osteopenia (Fig. 8-8)
    - Only 20% to 30% of lesions "hot" on bone scan

TABLE 8-4 COMPREHENSIVE SYSTEMIC APPROACH FOR PHYSICAL EXAMINATION AND REVIEW OF SYSTEMS RELATIVE TO PATIENTS WITH POTENTIAL METASTATIC DISEASE

System Examination	Potential Primary Tumor Source	Other Potential Findings
HEENT	Oropharyngeal tumors	
Neck	Thyroid carcinoma	Lymphatic metastases
Neurologic		Brain metastases
Lymphatic	Lymphoma	Lymphatic metastases
Skin	Melanoma	Skin metastases
Musculoskeletal Extremities	Sarcomas	Bone and soft tissue metastases
Back	Renal carcinoma	Bone and soft tissue metastases
Endocrine	Thyroid carcinoma	
Cardiovascular		Cardiovascular fitness
Pulmonary	Lung carcinoma	Lung metastases
Abdominal	Colon carcinoma	
Rectal	Prostate and colorectal carcinoma	Stool guaiac
Psychiatric	Brain tumors	Brain metastases

BOX 8-2 TYPICAL RADIOLOGIC APPEARANCE OF COMMON METASTATIC CARCINOMAS AND THEIR DIFFERENTIAL DIAGNOSES

LYTIC	MIXED (MAINLY LYTIC)
*Lung**	
Kidney	*Lung*
Thyroid	*Breast*
Adrenal	Cervix
Gastrointestinal tract	Ovary
Melanoma	Testicles
Head and neck	Neuroblastoma
Chordoma	Chondrosarcoma
Mesothelioma	**Differential diagnosis**
Fibrosarcoma	Paget's disease
Malignant fibrous	**OSTEOBLASTIC**[†]
histiocytoma	**B**reast
Ewing sarcoma	**B**ronchial carcinoid
Hepatoma	**B**owel (stomach)
Pheochromocytoma	**B**ladder
Differential diagnosis	**B**rain (medulloblastoma)
Myeloma	**B**one (osteosarcoma)
Lymphoma	**L**ymphoma
Paget's disease (lytic	**P**rostate
phase)	**Differential diagnosis**
Hyperparathyroidism	Paget's disease

*Classic, most common osteophilic tumors are shown in *italics*.
[†]Mnemonic: "Six bees lick pollen."
Data from Tuite MJ. Radiologic evaluation. In: Heiner JP, Kinsella TJ, Zdeblick TA, eds. *Management of Metastatic Disease to the Musculoskeletal System.* St. Louis: Quality Medical Publishing, 2002: 55–81.

- Differentiation from lymphoma
  - Paucity of radiographic changes typical for lymphoma
  - Magnetic resonance imaging (MRI) marrow replacement with subtle plain radiographic findings
  - Predilection for ends of long bones
  - Confluent epiphyseal/metaphyseal/adjacent diaphyseal uptake on bone scan (Fig. 8-9)
- Differentiation from Paget's disease
  - Paget's disease shows classic features of expansion with coarsening of trabeculae and cortical thickening in blastic phase (Fig. 8-10), which are atypical for metastases.
  - Paget's disease lytic phase classic features: blade-of-grass advancing edge sharply delineated from normal bone
  - Predilection: ends of long bones, pelvis, spine
  - Bone scan: increased uptake on bone scan if untreated

Laboratory Features

Laboratory tests play a role in the initial evaluation of any patient suspected to have a metastatic bone lesion (Table 8-5). A limited number of specific laboratory tests are helpful in seeking a specific diagnosis, while others seek information that may be related to visceral involvement and potential complications of the malignancy.

- Role of specific serum tumor markers in primary workup: unclear
  - Examples: prostate specific antigen (PSA) for prostate cancer, carcinoembryonic antigen (CEA) for colon carcinoma
- Tests to seek potential visceral involvement and/or complications
  - Complete blood count (CBC) and platelets: marrow replacement by tumor or the adverse effects of tumor treatment (radiation, chemotherapy) may result in anemia, thrombocytopenia, or neutropenia
  - Metabolic panel: either visceral involvement or the toxicities of treatment may result in electrolyte disturbances such as hypercalcemia and/or alterations in renal or hepatic function
  - Erythrocyte sedimentation rate (ESR): elevations in ESR are frequently seen in lymphoma and myeloma, but only uncommonly in metastatic carcinoma

Hypercalcemia of Malignancy

- Hypercalcemia is common in patients with bone metastases.
- It is important to recognize for treatment and as a prognostic factor.
- Hypercalcemia can be seen in primary or secondary hyperparathyroidism, which can create multifocal bone lesions that may be confused with metastatic carcinoma.
- Two types of hypercalcemia of malignancy
  - Local osteolytic hypercalcemia: effect of bone metastases
  - Humoral hypercalcemia: systemically mediated effect without bone metastases
  - Common tumors: squamous cell carcinoma of lung, head and neck carcinoma, kidney cancer, ovarian cancer
- Mediators of hypercalcemia of malignancy
  - PTHrP, IL6, TNF-β, vitamin D
- Interpreting serum calcium levels
  - Ionized calcium is the portion of the total ("uncorrected") calcium not bound to albumin.
  - Serum calcium reflects calcium both bound and not bound to albumin.
  - If serum albumin is low, an elevated ionized calcium level may be masked by a normal total uncorrected calcium level.
- Symptoms of hypercalcemia: weakness, urinary frequency, thirst, nausea, constipation
- Treatment of hypercalcemia of malignancy: hydration, bisphosphonates
- Prognostic importance: hypercalcemia in metastatic cancer is a poor prognosticator, especially for metastatic lung cancer

Hematologic Complications of Malignancy

- Hypercoagulable states are much more common in malignancy than are coagulopathies.
  - Hypercoagulability may be due to paraneoplastic erythrocytosis or thrombocytosis from tumor-produced circulating erythropoietin and thrombopoietin, respectively.

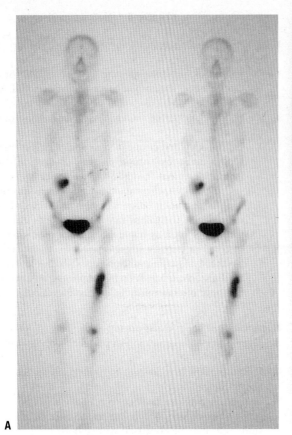

A

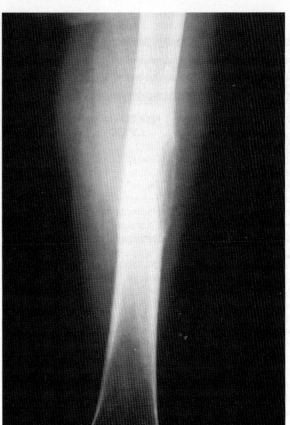

B

Figure 8-4 (A) An isolated left distal femoral bone lesion in an elderly woman without a history of cancer demonstrates increased uptake on bone scan, permeative borders, Codman's triangle, and soft tissue extension. Biopsy showed metastatic adenocarcinoma. (B) Computed tomography scan of the lung revealed a mediastinal mass consistent with a lung carcinoma primary.

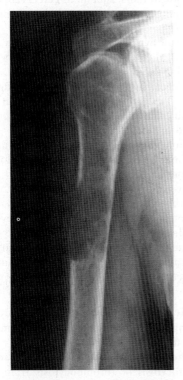

Figure 8-5 A lytic, relatively well-defined metastatic lesion of the right humerus in a patient with renal cell carcinoma.

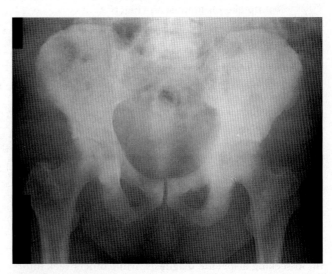

Figure 8-6 A pelvic radiograph shows typical blastic metastases from prostate cancer.

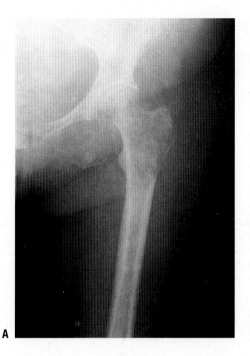
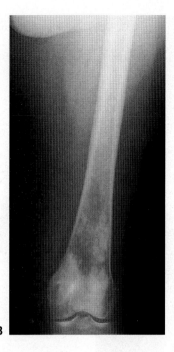

A   B

Figure 8-7   Multiple bone lesions in a woman with breast cancer show the wide variation in appearance of breast cancer metastases to bone, from the predominately lytic appearance in the ischium, the mixed lytic and blastic proximal femur metastases, and the sclerotic distal femur metastases.

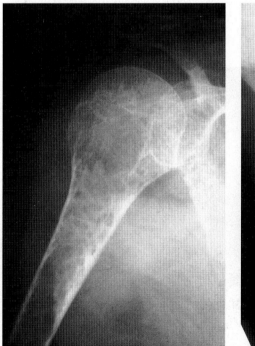
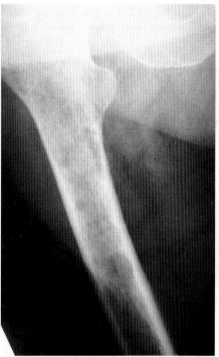

A   B

Figure 8-8   Radiographs from humerus and femur of a patient with multiple myeloma show classic raindrop pattern of punched-out lytic defects throughout the bones.

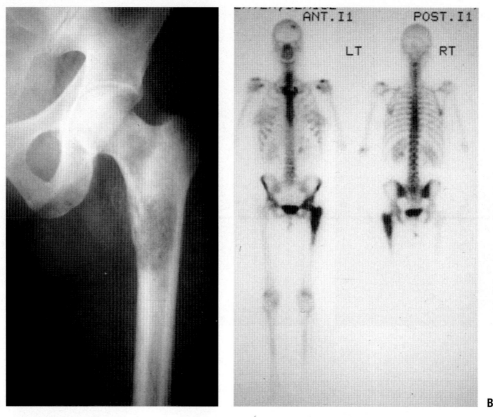

Figure 8-9 An isolated left proximal femoral bone lesion shows a permeative lytic process involving the proximal femur with confluent uptake on bone scan involving the femoral epiphysis, metaphysis, and proximal diaphysis. Biopsy showed lymphoma.

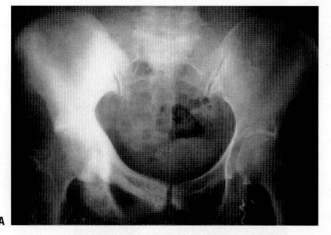

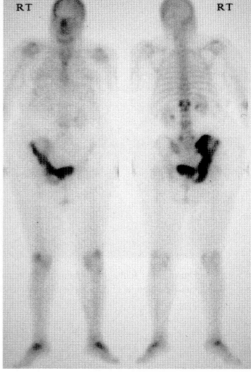

Figure 8-10 Paget's disease of bone in its sclerotic phase can be confused with prostate cancer. This patient with Paget's disease of the entire right hemipelvis shows the typical coarsening of trabeculae and bony expansion (both best seen in the pubic rami) as well as confluent uptake on the bone scan.

TABLE 8-5 LABORATORY TESTS IMPORTANT IN THE EVALUATION OF METASTATIC DISEASE

Laboratory Test	Positive Finding	Disease Association
Serum protein electrophoresis	Monoclonal spike (monoclonal gammopathy)	Multiple myeloma
Urine protein electrophoresis	Bence Jones proteins	Multiple myeloma
Lactate dehydrogenase	Elevated	Lymphoma (nonspecific; depends on disease load; also with osteogenic sarcoma, Ewing sarcoma)
Prostate specific antigen	Elevated	Prostate carcinoma
Urinalysis	Hematuria	Renal cell carcinoma
Alkaline phosphatase	Elevated	Paget's disease of bone (nonspecific; also with osteogenic sarcoma)

- Common tumors: adenocarcinomas, especially lung, pancreas, and stomach
- Diagnosis: no helpful screening laboratory tests available

Biopsy of Lesions Suspected to be Metastatic (also see Chapter 3, Biopsy of Musculoskeletal Tumors)

Biopsy of bone and soft tissue lesions suspected to be metastatic in origin should follow the same principles as those for a sarcoma. If a biopsy is to be done prior to the stabilization of an impending or actual pathologic fracture, care should be taken to avoid contaminating tissue or bone regions not already involved by the tumor. *Do not* send reamings from the femur or humerus as a biopsy specimen to establish the diagnosis; in addition to being histologically inferior to a standard biopsy, if the patient has a sarcoma, the lesion will then have been unnecessarily spread throughout the reamed region of bone and possibly disseminated into the caval venous system as well. The best solution in the case of an impending or pathologic fracture is to establish the diagnosis first by way of a direct approach to the tumor for an incisional biopsy, contaminating the fewest tissue planes and compartments possible. In the proximal femur, this is done through a lateral approach at or near the ridge between the gluteus maximus insertion and the vastus lateralis origin. In the proximal humerus, a proximal biopsy should be performed through the anterior aspect of the deltoid but not exposing the cephalic vein.

Pathology Features

The histology of metastatic carcinoma usually does not reveal the specific site of origin. There are a limited number of exceptions to that rule (Table 8-6 and Fig. 8-11). More importantly, when an appropriate metastatic work-up has been done in advance, the pathology only needs to confirm the presence of metastatic carcinoma consistent with the identified probable source to allow surgical treatment to

TABLE 8-6 METASTATIC TUMORS WITH HISTOPATHOLOGY OF SPECIFIC ORIGIN

Tumor	Source	Histopathology
Clear cell carcinoma	Kidney	Groups of clear cells separated by delicate arborizing vasculature
Well-differentiated follicular carcinoma	Thyroid	Colloid-filled follicles
Metastatic pigmented malignant melanoma	Skin	Intracytoplasmic melanin

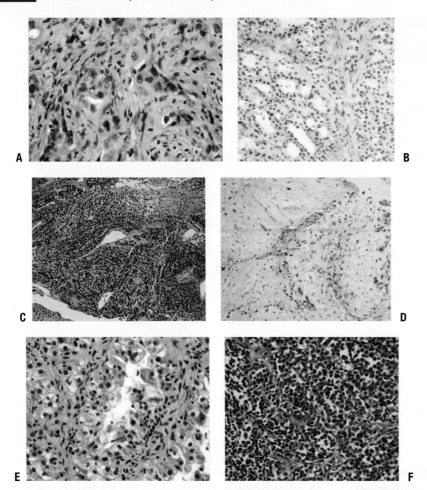

Figure 8-11   Representative pathology sections from typical metastatic lesions. Metastatic adenocarcinoma of lung (**A**), follicular thyroid carcinoma (**B**), malignant melanoma (low power) (**C**), squamous cell carcinoma (**D**), clear cell renal carcinoma (**E**), and melanoma (high power) (**F**).

proceed. Since many of these cases rely upon frozen section for diagnosis, the pathologist does not have the luxury of waiting for immunohistochemistry staining results, which can be very helpful (Table 8-7).

■ Histopathology that identifies the specific source of origin (see Table 8-6)
■ Histopathology suggestive of source of origin
    ■ Adenocarcinoma of breast

■ Adenocarcinoma of colon
■ Histopathology of nonspecific origin (Table 8-8)
    ■ Differential pathology diagnoses
    ■ Anaplastic large cell lymphoma
    ■ Poorly differentiated angiosarcoma
    ■ Primary and metastatic sarcoma

TABLE 8-7 IMMUNOHISTOCHEMISTRY FOR METASTATIC CARCINOMAS AND TUMORS IN THEIR DIFFERENTIAL

Primary Tumor	Immunohistochemistry Marker
Carcinomas in general	Cytokeratins, epithelial membrane antigen (EMA)
Prostate carcinoma	Prostate specific antigen
Lung carcinoma	Thyroid transcription factor (TTF-1)
Malignant melanoma	HMB45
Lymphoma	Leukocyte common antigen

TABLE 8-8 TUMORS WITH HISTOPATHOLOGY OF NONSPECIFIC ORIGIN

Tumor	Potential Sources
Metastatic squamous cell carcinoma	Lung, head and neck, esophagus, cervix
Metastatic adenocarcinoma without differentiating features	Breast, colon, prostate, ovary, endometrium, stomach, lung
Metastatic clear cell adenocarcinoma	Ovary, endometrium, lung
Poorly differentiated carcinomas	Lung, prostate, pancreas, thyroid, breast, colon, ovary, endometrium, stomach, etc.

TREATMENT

Surgical and Nonoperative Options

The three main indications for surgical treatment of patients with metastases are for diagnosis, prophylactic fixation of impending fractures, and stabilization of pathologic fractures. Many patients with bone involvement by metastatic disease or myeloma can be treated nonoperatively. Both surgical and nonsurgical options are discussed in more detail in the chapter on pathologic fractures (Chapter 4).

Indications for Biopsy of Suspected Metastatic Disease
- Solitary new destructive lesion with or without history of cancer
  - Biopsy first before proceeding with treatment!
  - Other processes seen in adults that should not be treated the same as a metastatic lesion and therefore must be considered in the differential diagnosis
    - Bone sarcomas: chondrosarcomas, malignant fibrous histiocytoma, fibrosarcoma, postradiation sarcoma, Paget's sarcoma
    - Most common mistake: placement of an intramedullary nail through a bone sarcoma without biopsy
    - Most common result: unnecessary amputation
  - Other processes seen in adults that may require medical intervention prior to surgical procedure
    - Hyperparathyroidism
    - Paget's disease
- Multiple bone lesions without biopsy-proven metastatic bone disease (even with history of cancer)
  - Biopsy first before proceeding with treatment!
  - Multiple other scenarios mimic metastatic carcinoma! (Box 8-3)
- Situation that does not require biopsy of new bone lesion
  - Established histologically proven mets to bone and/or viscera

Indications for Stabilization of Pathologic Fracture
- The site and type of pathologic fracture determine to a large extent the need for surgical stabilization, and those specific details are discussed in Chapter 4.5, Pathologic Fractures.
  - Sites that frequently require stabilization
    - Upper extremity: humerus
    - Lower extremity: femur, tibia
- Patient factors should be considered as well.
  - Moribund, immediately preterminal patients are a contraindication to surgery.
  - Minimum expected survival: 6 to 12 weeks

Indications for Prophylactic Fixation of Impending Fractures
- These factors are discussed in detail in Chapter 4.5.

Preoperative Planning

Search for Concomitant Lesions Requiring Prevention or Intervention
Other coexisting metastatic lesions may require modification of the technique for anesthesia and/or difficulty with postoperative care. These lesions and the potential problems they may create should be investigated. Review of the most recent bone scan is useful in this regard.

- Cervical spine disease: an anesthesia concern
  - History and examination: Does patient have neck pain or tenderness?
  - Radiologic investigation: Review most recent bone scan, consider new plain cervical spine radiographs.
- Impending upper extremity pathologic fractures: may cause postoperative pain and/or fracture if recovery period requires ambulatory aids for weight bearing.
  - History and examination: Does patient have shoulder or arm pain and/or tenderness?
  - Radiologic investigation: Review most recent bone scan; consider new shoulder or humeral radiographs.

Search for Hematologic Abnormalities
Hematologic abnormalities may result from marrow replacement by tumor, chemotherapy, and/or radiotherapy.

- Anemia management guidelines
  - Consider preoperative transfusion if hemoglobin is <10.0 mg/dL or large amount of blood loss anticipated.
  - Use leukodepleted, irradiated red blood cells if patient has been on chemotherapy.
- Thrombocytopenia management guidelines
  - Preoperative platelet transfusion if platelet count is <50,000/mm^3
- Leukopenia management guidelines
  - Consider canceling major operation if absolute neutrophil count (ANC) is <1,000/mm^3.
  - Avoid major operations at time of typical nadir in white blood cell count following chemotherapy.

Search for Hypercalcemia
- Most common primary malignancies: lung carcinoma, head and neck, kidney, ovarian
- Early symptoms are flu-like: fatigue, lethargy, anorexia, constipation, nausea, polyuria

---

BOX 8-3 MULTIFOCAL BONE LESIONS IN ADULTS OTHER THAN METASTATIC DISEASE OR MYELOMA

Paget's disease	Multiple hereditary
Hyperparathyroidism	exostoses
Vascular bone sarcomas:	Ollier's disease
hemangiopericytoma,	Polyostotic fibrous
hemangioendothelioma,	dysplasia
angiosarcoma	Angiomatosis
Multicentric	(lymphangiomatosis)
chondrosarcomas	

- Late symptoms of stupor and dysrhythmias
- Treatment: hydration, bisphosphonates

Does the Patient Need Preoperative Embolization?
- Highest risk of bleeding during intralesional procedures: renal carcinoma metastases
- Increased risk of bleeding (others): myeloma and thyroid carcinoma metastases
- Consider embolization.
    - Especially for renal carcinoma intralesional procedures
    - Also myeloma and thyroid carcinoma of spine, pelvis

Surgical Goals and Approaches

Patients with metastatic disease to bone or myeloma have limited ability to heal fractures, shortened life spans, and the potential to develop other sites of bone involvement, which may compromise prior surgery. Therefore, these patients cannot be treated the same as those with routine fractures. The specific approaches to achieving these goals are discussed in Chapter 4.5.
Goals of surgical intervention:

- Achieve immediately rigid fixation to allow early use.
- Achieve durable fixation to last the patient's expected shortened lifetime.
- Protect the entire bone when feasible.

Techniques

Internal Fixation
- Intramedullary fixation
    - Diaphyseal fractures and impending fractures
    - Metaphyseal fractures with adequate epiphyseal bone
    - Consider bone cement supplementation.
- Plate fixation
    - Metaphyseal and diaphyseal fractures
    - Supplement with bone cement in most cases.

Prosthetic Replacement
- Indications
    - Failure of or inability to achieve goals by internal fixation (e.g., extensive peritrochanteric destruction not necessarily involving femoral head)
    - Joint surface destruction (e.g., femoral head, femoral condyles, humeral head)
    - Need for resection and reconstruction, such as sometimes indicated for the solitary renal carcinoma metastasis

Complications

Orthopaedic operative intervention for patients with metastatic disease and myeloma entails all of the usual risks. Only those with specifically increased or unique risks are detailed below.

- Infection
    - Administer prophylactic cephalosporin antibiotics in all cases.

- Consider adding aminoglycoside for patients with neutropenia or large prosthetic reconstructions.
- Failure of internal fixation
    - Avoid by achieving goals of surgical intervention in operating room.
    - Administer postoperative radiotherapy to avoid disease progression that may compromise result.
- Cardiovascular collapse from cementing
    - Especially with long-stem cemented femoral stems
    - Communicate with anesthesia prior to cementing.

Results and Outcome (Prognosis)

The recovery period for any operative intervention in a patient with metastatic disease should not be longer than the patient's expected survival. However, prediction of survival is difficult at best.

Prognostication for Surgical Candidates
- Nonspinal sites postoperative survival (patients undergoing surgical intervention for metastatic bone disease of any site other than spine)
    - Postoperative survival rates over time
        - 1 year: 40%
        - 2 years: 30%
        - 3 years 20%
    - 1-year survival rates (Table 8-9)
    - Negative prognostic factors (multivariate analysis)
        - Pathologic fracture
        - Visceral metastases
        - Hemoglobin <7 mmol/L
        - Lung cancer
    - Positive prognostic factors (multivariate analysis)
        - Myeloma
- Proximal femur (patients undergoing hip arthroplasty for femoral and/or acetabular metastatic bone disease)
    - Survival rates over time following hip arthroplasty for metastatic disease
        - 1 year: 40%

TABLE 8-9 POSTOPERATIVE 1-YEAR SURVIVAL RATES

Primary Tumor with Metastases	Survival Rate (%)
Myeloma	65
Lymphoma	50
Breast	50
Kidney	43
Prostate	26
Lung	24
Unknown primary	20

Data from Hansen BH, Keller J, Laitinen M, et al. The Scandinavian Sarcoma Group Skeletal Metastasis Register. Survival after surgery for bone metastases in the pelvis and extremities. *Acta Orthop Scand Suppl* 2004;311:11–15.

- 2 years: 20%
- 3 years: 15%
  - Negative prognostic factors (multivariate analysis)
    - Time from diagnosis of primary to hip surgery (shorter interval = poorer prognosis)

Disease-Specific Prognostication
- Metastatic breast cancer
  - Poor prognostic factors
    - Caudal metastases: 5-year survival rate is 16% for those with bone mets below lumbosacral junction versus 36% for those above lumbosacral junction
    - Extraosseous metastases: median survival 5 months after identified
    - Lytic metastases: 5-year survival 23% versus 42% with blastic metastases
    - Hypercalcemia: harbinger of subsequent visceral metastases
  - Good prognostic factors
    - Cranial metastases (above lumbosacral junction)
    - No extraosseous metastases
    - Blastic metastases
    - No hypercalcemia
- Metastatic prostate cancer
  - Number of metastatic sites inversely proportional to expected survival duration
  - Best prognoses: (1) pelvis only, (2) thoracic vertebra only
  - Worst prognoses: (1) skull combined with other sites, (2) sternum combined with other sites

Postoperative Management (Guidelines)

- Antibiotics
  - Routine cases: 24 to 48 hours intravenous cephalosporin coverage or until drain discontinued

- Mobilization
  - Strive for goal of early mobilization with full weight bearing when feasible.
- External-beam radiotherapy
  - Radiotherapy as an adjunct to operative treatment
    - There are documented benefits in metastatic disease patients treated surgically for bone disease.
      - Reduces need for subsequent surgical procedures (3% versus 15%)
      - Improves postoperative functional status
    - Postoperative timing
      - After wound healing completed
      - Typically 2 to 4 weeks postoperatively
    - Doses
      - 3,000 cGy in 10 fractions or 2,000 cGy in 5 fractions
      - 4,500 cGy in 180-cGy fractions for patients with renal and thyroid carcinoma and life expectancy of 12 months or more

SUGGESTED READING

Coleman RE. Skeletal complications of malignancy. *Cancer* 1997;80:1588–1594.

Jemal A, Tiwari RC, Murray T, et al. Cancer statistics, 2004. *CA Cancer J Clin* 2004;54:8–29.

Rougraff BT, Kneisl JS, Simon MA. Skeletal metastases of unknown origin. A prospective study of a diagnostic strategy. *J Bone Joint Surg [Am]* 1993;75:1276–1281.

Townsend PW, Rosenthal HG, Smalley SR, et al. Impact of postoperative radiation therapy and other perioperative factors on outcome after orthopedic stabilization of impending or pathologic fractures due to metastatic disease. *J Clin Oncol* 1994;12:2345–2350.

Tuite M. Radiologic evaluation. In: Heiner J, Kinsella T, Zdeblick T, eds. *Management of Metastatic Disease to the Musculoskeletal System.* St. Louis: Quality Medical Publishing, 2002:55–70.

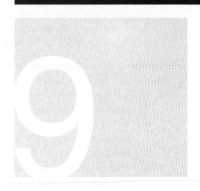

HEMATOLOGIC MALIGNANCIES

VALERAE O. LEWIS

Hematologic malignancies such as lymphoma and myeloma can manifest in bone, and these osseous manifestations can often be the first presentation of the systemic disease. After metastatic disease, myeloma and lymphoma are the second and third major categories in the differential diagnosis of an aggressive bone lesion in an adult. To avoid unnecessary surgery and to create a definitive treatment plan, it is important to become familiar with the presentation and the work-up of these lesions. Often the orthopaedic surgeon is the first to diagnose these diseases; however, surgical intervention may not be required. In addition, because the principles for treatment of hematologic malignancies differ so greatly from sarcomas, the diagnosis must be established before initiation of treatment.

LYMPHOMA

The vast majority of cases of lymphoma involving bone are non-Hodgkin's lymphoma (NHL). Non-Hodgkin's lymphoma is not a single disease, but a group of closely related B- and T-cell cancers of the lymphatic system. B-cell lymphomas represent 85% of NHL cases. Non-Hodgkin's lymphoma can start in the lymph nodes or lymphatic tissue such as the spleen, stomach, or skin, and because lymphocytes circulate throughout the lymphatic vessels and bloodstream, abnormal lymphocytes can reach any organ. Thus, lymphoma can manifest in any organ. In fact, along with lung carcinoma, lymphoma is one of the most common malignancies that may manifest as soft tissue metastases.

EPIDEMIOLOGY

- Incidence of NHL is increasing.
    - Worldwide incidence has risen steeply from the 1970s to the 2000s.
    - From a relatively rare disease to the fifth most common cancer in the United States
- Purported reasons for rise
    - Increasing exposure to chemicals
    - Increasing incidence of viral infections
    - Increasing incidence of organ transplantation
    - Increasing number of blood transfusions

CLASSIFICATION

- Revised European-American Classification of Lymphoid Neoplasms (REAL) (Table 9-1)
    - Most common types: diffuse large B-cell lymphoma (45%) and follicular (25%) lymphomas
- Clinical classification
    - Low grade (indolent), intermediate, or aggressive (high grade)
    - Based on the natural history of the disease
- Modified Ann Arbor Staging System (Table 9-2)
    - Describes extent of disease
        - International Prognostic Index (IPI: an excellent prognostic tool)

B-cell Lymphoma	T-cell Lymphoma
Precursor B-cell lymphomas	**Precursor T-cell lymphomas**
B-lymphoblast	T-lymphoblast
Mature B-cell lymphomas	**Mature T-cell lymphomas**
Follicular	Mycosis fungoides/Sezary
Marginal zone nodal	syndrome
Extranodal marginal zone	Peripheral T-cell
(MALT)	Anaplastic large T/null cell
Splenic marginal zone	Adult T-cell leukemia/lymphoma
Lymphoplasmacytic	
Mantle cell	
Diffuse large B-cell	
Primary mediastinal large	
B-cell	
Burkitt-like	
Burkitt's	

- Clinical stage (I/II versus III/IV)
- Number of extranodal sites (0 or 1 versus >1)
- Lactic dehydrogenase (LDH) (normal versus >1)
- Age at diagnosis
- Performance status (Eastern Cooperative Oncology Group [ECOG])
  - The IPI can identify prognostic groups, and for patients with IPI >2 peripheral stem cell or bone marrow transplantation should be considered.

Stage	Characteristics
I	Single lymph node region (I) *or* Single extralymphatic site (IE)
II	Two or more lymph node regions on the same side of the diaphragm (II) May include localized involvement of extralymphatic site (IIE)
III	Two or more lymph node regions on both sides of the diaphragm (III) May include localized involvement of extralymphatic site (IIIE) or spleen (IIIS) or both (IIISE)
IV	Diffuse or disseminated involvement of extralymphatic organ, with or without associated lymph node involvement

DIAGNOSIS

Clinical Findings

- Painless swelling of lymph nodes
- Chills
- Fever
- Night sweats
- Malaise
- Unexplained weight loss

Staging Studies

- Biopsy of lesion/lymph nodes
- Computed tomography (CT) scan
- Positron emission tomography (PET) scan
- Bone marrow biopsy

TREATMENT

- Depends on stage of disease
- Multimodality
- Combination of chemotherapy and radiation
  - CHOP with rituximab
    - CHOP: cyclophosphamide, doxorubicin, vincristine, and prednisone
    - Rituximab: works by targeting the CD20 antigen on normal and malignant B cells
- Peripheral stem cell transplantation
- Bone marrow transplantation

PRIMARY LYMPHOMA OF BONE

Primary lymphoma of bone (PLB) is a distinct clinical entity. Although it was first identified by Oberlin in 1928, it was not until 1939, when Parker and Jackson reported on their series of "reticulum cell sarcoma," that lymphoma of bone was classified distinct from systemic lymphoma.

- Definition: malignant lymphoid infiltrate within bone with or without cortical invasion or soft tissue extension but <u>without</u> concurrent involvement of regional lymph nodes or distant viscera
- Synonyms
  - Reticulum cell sarcoma (misnomer; not a sarcoma)
  - Malignant lymphoma of bone
  - Primary skeletal lymphoma
  - Osteolymphoma

EPIDEMIOLOGY

- 0.2% of all bone tumors and 5% of all extranodal lymphomas
- Large B-cell lymphoma represents 90% of the cases of PLB.

- Age: broad range
- Male:female 1.8:1
- Location
  - Femur
  - Ilium
  - Ribs

DIAGNOSIS

Clinical Findings

- Localized bone pain
- Mass
- Pathologic fracture in 20% to 30%
- Generally not systemically ill

Radiologic Findings (Fig. 9-1)

Plain Radiographs
- Diaphyseal
- Permeative/mottled
- Poorly marginated
- Associated soft tissue mass

Magnetic Resonance Imaging (MRI)
- Large soft tissue mass
- Enhances with gadolinium

Histologic Findings

- Sheet-like proliferation of round blue cells without significant matrix (Fig. 9-2)
- Pleomorphic
- Nuclear heterogeneity
- Special stains
  - Reticulum stains
  - Leukocyte common antigen (LCA)
    - CD45
  - B-cell marker
    - CD19, CD20

TREATMENT

- Multidisciplinary: combination of systemic chemotherapy and local radiation is thought to be the most effective treatment in decreasing the local recurrence and systemic relapse
  - Chemotherapy: CHOP (cyclophosphamide, doxorubicin, vincristine and prednisone)
  - Rituximab (monoclonal antibody to CD20)
- Radiation: to the local site
- Surgery: limited to diagnostic biopsy and to prevent impending pathologic fractures or to repair actual pathologic fractures

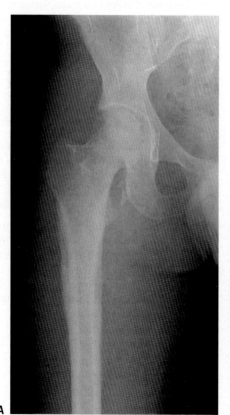
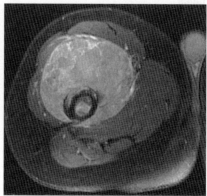

A   B

Figure 9-1   Anteroposterior radiograph of the proximal femur and MRI (axial T1 with contrast) of a 20-year-old man with primary lymphoma of bone. Note permeative changes in the diaphysis of the femur on the radiograph and large enhancing soft tissue mass demonstrated on the MRI.

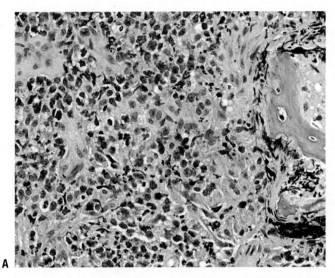 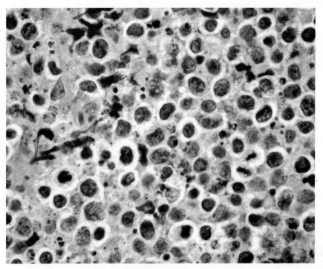

Figure 9-2   Diffuse large B-cell lymphoma of bone: (**A**) 20× magnification, (**B**) 40× magnification.

Prognosis

- 60% to 80% 5-year survival rate
- Worsens with age

MULTIPLE MYELOMA

Multiple myeloma is a plasma cell dyscrasia, but it is not the only such entity. Other plasma cell dyscrasias sometimes encountered in orthopaedic oncology include monoclonal gammopathy of uncertain significance (MGUS) and solitary plasmacytoma. Both MGUS and plasmacytoma may progress, and often do, to the disseminated form, multiple myeloma.

- Definition: disseminated malignancy of monoclonal plasma cells
  - Monoclonal proteins
    - IgG: 60%
    - IgA: 20%
    - IgD: 2%
    - IgE: 0.1%
    - Light-chain kappa or lambda: 18%
    - Biclonal: <1%
    - Nonsecretory: <5%

PATHOPHYSIOLOGY

- Increased expression by osteoblasts of the receptor activator of nuclear factor KB (NF–KB) ligand (RANKL) and a reduction in the level of its decoy receptor osteoprotegerin
- The increase in the ratio of RANKL to osteoprotegerin results in activation of osteoclasts and bone resorption.

EPIDEMIOLOGY

- 1% of all malignancies
- 14,400 new cases/year
- Male:female 1.8:1
- Age: 50s to 70s
  - Median 65 years
- Race propensity
  - African Americans > Caucasians (2:1)
- Risk factors: obesity, genetics (HLA), immunological challenges

DIAGNOSIS

Clinical Findings

- Pain
- Pathologic fracture
- Bone marrow failure
  - Anemia: fatigue and weakness
  - Thrombocytopenia: bruising, bleeding
  - Neutropenia: recurrent infections (gram-negative infections)
- Renal insufficiency (50%): multifactorial
  - Bence Jones protein precipitation
  - Interstitial nephritis
  - Hypercalciuria
- Hypercalcemia (25%)
  - Manifestations
    - Nausea
    - Muscle weakness
    - Confusion
    - Polyuria
    - Constipation
  - Treatment
    - Bisphosphonates
      - Pamidronate (Aredia) 90 mg IV
      - Zolendronate (Zometa) 4 mg IV

- Hydration: normal saline + Lasix
    - The combination of the hypercalcemia and renal insufficiency leads to the need to hydrate the patient well before surgical intervention.
- Diagnostic criteria
    - 10% plasma cells in the bone marrow
    - Monoclonal protein in the serum (serum protein electrophoresis) or urine (urine protein electrophoresis)
    - Evidence of end-organ failure (CRAB)
        - <u>H</u>ypercalcemia
        - <u>R</u>enal insufficiency
        - <u>A</u>nemia
        - <u>B</u>one lesions

Diagnostic Work-Up

- Serum protein electrophoresis
    - Monoclonal gammopathy does not automatically signify multiple myeloma.
    - MGUS
        - IgG peak slightly elevated
            - IgG $\leq$3.5 g/dL, IgA $\leq$2 g/dL, urine light chain $\leq$1 g/dL
        - Normal radiographs
        - < 10% plasmacytosis
        - No symptoms
- Urine protein electrophoresis
    - Monoclonal gamma globulin spike
    - Quantitative Ig levels
- Serum chemistries
    - Complete blood count (may show anemia)
    - Electrolytes
        - Blood urea nitrogen (BUN), creatinine, calcium (may show azotemia, hypercalcemia)
    - β_2-microglobulin
- Bone marrow aspiration
    - Plasmacytosis >10%
- Bone survey
    - Bone scan can underestimate extent of disease.
        - 80% of lesions are "cold."
    - Spine MRI
        - Vertebral lesions difficult to visualize on plain film
- Biopsy: need for biopsy can be alleviated in the face of multiple osseous lesions on bone survey and a positive serum/urine protein electrophoresis.

Radiologic Findings

- Punched-out lytic lesions (Fig. 9-3): single or multiple

Histologic Findings

- Uniform plasma cells (Fig. 9-4)
- Large round nuclei
    - Clockface
    - Eccentric
- Distinct cell borders
- Abundant cytoplasm, perinuclear clearing

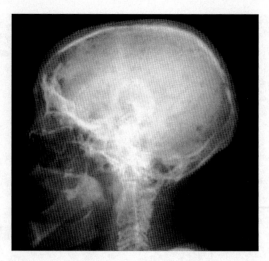

Figure 9-3 Lateral radiograph of skull displaying "salt-and-pepper" punched-out lesions of multiple myeloma.

TREATMENT

Local Treatment

- Radiation (very sensitive)
    - Surgical adjuvant (postoperative): 30 Gy
    - Radiation alone
        - Moderate, symptomatic lesions without impending or actual fracture
        - <50% cortex, <2.5 cm
- Surgery
    - Large lesions
        - Impending pathological fracture
        - Actual pathological fracture
    - Protect the whole bone
        - Intramedullary rod fixation
- Perioperative management
    - Highly vascular
    - Preoperative embolization of lesion important to consider
    - Type and cross-match
        - Even for closed nailing
- Acute renal failure
    - Hydrate the patient well!

Systemic Treatment

- Chemotherapy and corticosteroids: If patient is eligible for stem cell transplantation, alkylating agents for induction chemotherapy should be avoided.
    - Pulsed steroids alone
    - Melphalan + prednisone (MP)
    - Vincristine + doxorubicin (Adriamycin) + dexamethasone (VAD)
    - Thalidomide and dexamethasone: anti-angiogenic
    - Bortezomib (Velcade, PS-341): proteasome inhibitor
- Stem cell transplantation
    - Autologous stem cell transplantation
        - Can prolong disease-free survival and overall survival

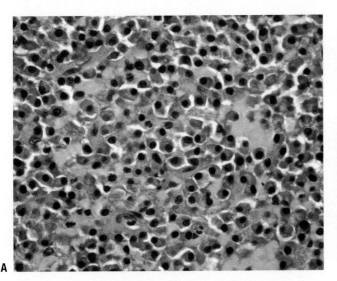
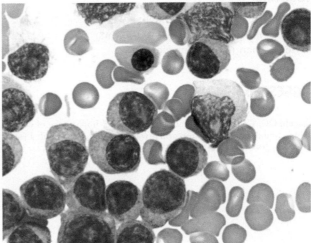

Figure 9-4   Representative pathology sections from a multiple myeloma specimen. Note eccentric nuclei, abundant cytoplasm, and distinct cell borders. (**A**) Tissue section (20×). (**B**) Cytology on touch prep (80×).

■ Can be done in tandem
■ Can be used as salvage therapy
■ Induction chemotherapy before stem cell harvest reduces the tumor burden.
■ Allogenic stem cell transplantation
  ■ Transplant not contaminated with tumor cells
  ■ Only 5% to 10% of patients are candidates.
  ■ High mortality rate

Prognosis

■ Median survival 3 years
■ Overall survival depends on stage.
■ International Staging System (Table 9-3): based on serum β_2-microglobulin and albumin levels

SOLITARY PLASMACYTOMA OF BONE

PATHOPHYSIOLOGY

■ Rare presentation of a plasma cell dyscrasia
  ■ 3% of patients with myeloma
  ■ Early manifestation of multiple myeloma: 70% progress to multiple myeloma

EPIDEMIOLOGY

■ Male:female 3:1
■ Age of presentation younger than multiple myeloma

■ Most common locations
  ■ Long bones
  ■ Pelvis
  ■ Spine

DIAGNOSIS

■ Solitary bone lesion
■ Skeletal survey: normal
■ MRI skull/spine/pelvis: normal
■ Bone marrow: normal plasma cell count
■ No anemia, hypercalcemia, or renal disease
■ Normal serum/urine protein electrophoresis or serum protein electrophoresis that becomes normal after treatment of the lesion

TREATMENT

■ Radiation only (45 Gy)
  ■ Exquisitely sensitive
  ■ Rapid response

TABLE 9-3 INTERNATIONAL STAGING SYSTEM FOR MULTIPLE MYELOMA WITH CORRESPONDING MEDIAN SURVIVAL

Stage	Serum Albumin and Serum β_2-Microglobulin	Median Survival (months)
I	Serum albumin ≥3.5 g/dL and serum β_2-microglobulin <3.5 µg/mL	62
II	Neither stage I nor III	44
III	Serum β_2-microglobulin ≥5.5 µg/mL	29

Prognosis

- Relatively good
- 20% remain free of disease >10 years.
- Better than multiple myeloma

SUGGESTED READING

Baiocchi OC, Colleoni GW, Rodrigues CA, et al. Importance of combined-modality therapy for primary bone lymphoma. *Leuk Lymphoma* 2003;44(10):1837–1839.

Kilborn TN, Teh J, Goodman TR. Paediatric manifestations of Langerhans cell histiocytosis: a review of the clinical and radiological findings. *Clin Radiol* 2003;58(4):269–278.

Kyle RA, Rajkumar SV. Multiple myeloma. *N Engl J Med* 2004; 351(18):1860–1873.

Lewis VO, Primus G, Anastisi J, et al. Oncologic outcomes of primary lymphoma of bone in adults. *Clin Orthop Relat Res* 2003;(415): 90–97.

Yasko AW, Fanning CV, Ayala AG, et al. Percutaneous techniques for the diagnosis and treatment of localized Langerhans-cell histiocytosis (eosinophilic granuloma of bone). *J Bone Joint Surg [Am]* 1998;80(2):219–228.

Zinzani PL. Lymphoma: diagnosis, staging, natural history, and treatment strategies. *Semin Oncol* 2005;32(1 Suppl 1):S4–10.

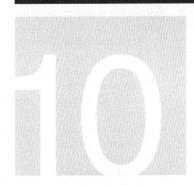

METABOLIC BONE DISEASES

SUSAN V. BUKATA

Metabolic bone diseases include a variety of diseases that affect the strength and overall quality of bones. Some of these diseases affect a huge proportion of the population. Osteoporosis alone affects 45% of women over age 50. Other diseases are extremely rare and usually result from a genetic anomaly that affects normal bone metabolism. In every metabolic bone disease there is an imbalance in the cells and pathways that allow for the skeleton to be continually remodeled throughout one's lifetime.

PATHOPHYSIOLOGY FUNDAMENTALS

- Bone metabolism is an integral part of the endocrine system.
- Three cell types are involved:
  - Osteoblasts
    - Originate from mesenchymal cells
    - Synthesize organic bone matrix
    - Bear receptors for parathyroid hormone and hormones, including estrogen
    - Produce osteoprotegerin (OPG) and receptor activator of nuclear factor (NF)-kappa B (RANK) ligand
    - Produce alkaline phosphatase (marker for bone formation)
  - Osteoclasts
    - Originate from monocyte precursors
    - Recruitment/development/activity signals through RANK ligand and macrophage colony-stimulating factor (M-CSF)
    - Resorb bone at ruffled membrane
    - Secrete protons/lysosomal enzymes
  - Osteocytes
    - Derived from osteoblasts encased in matrix
    - Interconnected through cytoplasmic processes
    - No longer form bone
    - Respond to mechanical signals and influence remodeling

RANK/RANK-Ligand Signaling

- Responsible for the coordination between osteoblasts and osteoclasts; plays an important role in bone metabolism. The osteoblast is the cell controlling this pathway.
  - RANK-ligand (RANK-L) signal on surface of osteoblasts and secreted by them
  - RANK receptor on osteoclast
  - OPG is inhibitor of RANK-L (blocks binding to RANK).

Bone Metabolic Unit

- Osteoclastic bone resorption and osteoblastic bone formation
- Concept of coupling
  - Resorption > formation leads to bone loss.
  - Resorption < formation leads to bone gain.
  - Resorption = formation leaves bone mass balanced.
- Peak bone mass reached at age 25 to 30. After that, resorption is slightly greater than formation, leading to slow bone mass loss.

Calcium

- Regulation is extremely important in bone mass maintenance.
  - Intestines/kidneys/bone involved in calcium metabolism
  - Bone first source for calcium when needed (99% of body store is there)
  - Active absorption in duodenum (calcium binding protein)
  - Passive absorption in jejunum
  - Calcium balanced when renal excretion = intestinal absorption
  - Renal reabsorption
    - Actively in distal convoluted tubule
    - Passively in proximal tubule and loop of Henle
- Dietary intake requirement varies with age.
  - Adolescents age 9 to 18 need >1,300 mg daily.
  - Age 19 to 49 need >1,000 mg daily.
  - Older adults >50 need >1,200 mg daily.
- Drugs that decrease calcium retention (thus increase calcium loss)
  - Furosemide (Lasix)
  - Heparin
  - Corticosteroids
  - Tetracycline
- Drugs that increase calcium retention
  - Hydrochlorothiazide (HCTZ): can be used to help retain calcium through renal channels in patients with high urinary loss

Vitamin D

- Important for calcium regulation and bone health
  - Fat-soluble steroid hormone
  - Sources
    - Diet (vitamin D_2)
    - Endogenous production in skin (vitamin D_3)
  - Hydroxylated in liver (at 25th carbon), then kidney (at 1st carbon) to create 1,25-dihydroxyvitamin D
  - 25-hydroxyvitamin D also recognized as important in maintaining bone health
    - Levels >30 ng/dL desired
  - Targets
    - Kidney: increases resorption in proximal tubule
    - Intestines: regulates production of calcium binding protein
    - Bone: major target enhancing mobilization of calcium stores
  - Receptors on osteoblasts stimulate RANK ligand production and therefore osteoclast development and activity.
  - Recommended daily intake: 400 to 800 IU daily for adults

Parathyroid Hormone

- Controls regulation of serum calcium levels
- Calcium-sensing receptor on parathyroid cells initiates hormone release with low serum calcium levels.
- Bone: PTH binds to osteoblast receptors
  - Neutral protease release initiates bone remodeling.

- Stimulates production of factors that signal osteoclasts to resorb bone
- Kidney
  - Proximal tubule: PTH decreases PO_4 resorption
  - Distal tubule: PTH increases calcium resorption
- Stimulates 1α hydroxylase to increase 1,25-vitamin D levels
- Intestine
  - Increases calcium binding protein production to increase calcium absorption
  - Greatest quantitative effect on calcium
- PTHrP production by some cancers with similar effects

OSTEOPOROSIS

Osteoporosis is a metabolic bone disease characterized by low bone mass and a microarchitectural deterioration of bone tissue that results in enhanced bone fragility and a consequent increase in fracture risk.

PATHOPHYSIOLOGY

- Imbalance in bone metabolic unit between osteoclastic bone resorption and osteoblastic bone formation
  - Resorption > formation leads to bone loss.
- Peak bone mass reached at age 25 to 30
- After age 30, resorption is slightly greater than formation.
- Can see rapid increase in bone resorption during menopause
  - Can see 30% bone mass loss over perimenopausal period

Epidemiology

- Etiology is unknown.
- Affects 45% of women and 25% of men aged 50 and older
- Osteoporotic fractures
  - 4 times more common than stroke
  - Having one is a major risk factor for subsequent fractures.
    - 10% have another fragility fracture in <1 year.
    - 17% to 21% have another fragility fracture in <2 years.
  - Pose a lifetime risk of death comparable to breast cancer
- 1 in 3 women and 1 in 6 men will suffer a hip fracture.
  - Annual hip fractures
    - United States: >300,000
    - Europe: >400,000
    - Incidence expected to double over the next 50 years.
- Surgeon General's report in 2004 recognizes poor bone health as an epidemic and major health crisis.
  - Personal cost of fracture
  - Quality of life
  - Economic costs of fracture

- Risk factors for osteoporosis
  - Genetic
    - Female > male
    - Caucasian or Asian > Hispanic or African American
  - Environmental
    - Smoking
    - Alcohol
    - Sedentary lifestyle
    - Low body weight (<85% ideal body weight or <120 lbs)
    - History of eating disorder
  - Other
    - Personal/family history of fragility fracture
    - Age >50

Classification

- High-turnover osteoporosis
  - Primary form at menopause, but can be seen at any age and in men
  - Enhanced osteoclastic bone resorption with more and deeper lacunae
  - Osteoblasts unable to fully replace resorbed bone
  - Elevated bone turnover markers
  - Bone loss rate can be 2% to 3% per year, lasting 6 to 10 years.
- Low-turnover osteoporosis
  - Most commonly seen with aging, but can be seen at any age
  - Failure of osteoblasts to form bone
  - Bone formation markers show decreased levels (not good bone formers); osteoclastic bone resorption is normal or slightly decreased.
  - Bone turnover markers at premenopausal level or lower
  - Can also be seen in individuals with underlying genetic collagen disorder

DIAGNOSIS

Clinical Features

- Biochemical markers
  - Collagen cross-link products measured for bone loss rate
    - Urine N-telopeptide
      - Measure in any urine except the first of the day
      - Generally want to have value <30 nM BCE/mM creatinine, definitely <40 nM BCE/mM in postmenopausal women and older men
      - Expect marker level to go down with bisphosphonate treatment by at least 30% to 40% from baseline.
    - Serum cross laps
      - Diurnal variation for each individual
      - More commonly used in Europe
  - Markers for bone formation (low levels = poor bone formation)
    - Osteocalcin
    - Alkaline phosphatase
      - Get bone-specific alkaline phosphatase (BSAP), or also need liver function enzymes to evaluate if liver activity is elevated.
  - All biochemical markers are elevated in the setting of a healing fracture and then return to baseline.

Radiologic Features

Dual-Energy X-Ray Absorptiometry {DXA}
- Currently gold standard
- Low radiation doses (1 to 3 mrem), short scanning times
- Error range from 3% to 5% between serial scans on same machine, can be greater between scans on different machines
- DXA scan scoring (matching race and gender)
  - T-score
    - Compares density relative to peak bone mass (normal healthy 25-year-old)
    - Score used to determine level of disease over age 25
  - Z-score
    - Compares density to peers of same age
    - Measurement used for children and adults up to age 25

Quantitative Computed Tomography (CT)
- More radiation exposure, more operator-dependent
- Assesses both trabecular and cortical areas separately
- Use hydroxyapatite phantom for calculating density.

Ultrasound
- May be a good tool for preliminary screening
- Can evaluate only subcutaneous bones (calcaneus/tibia)
- Fracture risk at hip/spine not highly correlated (only 70%)

World Health Organization Definitions of Osteoporosis and Osteopenic
- Bone mass measured at hip and spine for adults
  - Defined from lower of two levels
  - Total body and spine measured for children
- 1 to 2.4 standard deviations below peak bone mass (T = −1.0 to −2.4)
  - Osteopenic with range of mild to moderate bone deficiency
- >2.5 standard deviations below peak mass (T = −2.5 or lower)
  - Osteoporotic
- Fragility fracture defines as osteoporotic regardless of T-score

Diagnostic Work-up Algorithm
- DXA scan for bone density
- Laboratory tests
  - Intact parathyroid hormone (PTH)
  - 25-vitamin D level
  - 1,25-vitamin D level
  - Serum calcium

- Serum alkaline phosphatase
- 24-hour urinary calcium
- Urine N-telopeptide

TREATMENT

Prevention

- Attainment of peak bone mass (age 20 to 30)
- Prevention of postmenopausal resorption and age-related bone loss (Table 10-1)

- Calcium and vitamin D
- Bisphosphonates
- Selective estrogen receptor modulators (SERM)
- Calcitonin
- PTH treatment
- Estrogen
- Fall prevention: hip protectors
  - Decrease hip fracture risk up to 93%
  - Poor compliance with wear (31%)
- Balance training: Tai Chi, dancing
- Exercise

TABLE 10-1 PREVENTION OF POSTMENOPAUSAL RESORPTION AND AGE-RELATED BONE LOSS

Treatment	Dose	Side Effects	Issues with Treatment	Mechanism of Action
Oral Bisphosphonates				
Fosamax (alendronate)	70 mg/wk	Reflux	GI bleeding and esophageal erosions	Affects osteoclast function and number
Actonel (risedronate)	35 mg/wk	GI distress	Poor absorption	Stops bone loss
Boniva (ibandronate)	150 mg/mo	Myalgias and bone pain in early doses	Renal clearance of intact drug (need good renal function or drug accumulates)	
IV Bisphosphonates				
Aredia (pamidronate)	90 mg q 3 mo	Myalgias and bone pain with initial doses	Rare cases of osteonecrosis of the jaw	Affects osteoclast function and number
Zometa (zoledronic acid)	4 mg/yr			Stops bone loss
Boniva (ibandronate)	3 mg q 3 mo			
SERM (selective estrogen receptor modulator)				
Evista (Raloxifene)	60 mg/day	Leg cramps	Increased risk of deep vein thrombosis in first 4 months of dosing	Returns bone dynamics to premenopausal pattern
		Hot flashes	Cardiovascular neutral	Stops bone loss
			Breast cancer protective	
			Use only in postmenopausal women	
Estrogen (with progesterone)				
Prempro	0.625 mg/2.5 mg	Persistent menstrual bleeding	Use lowest effective dose to manage postmenopausal symptoms.	Return to premenopausal bone dynamics
	0.45 mg/1.5 mg	Increased risk heart attack, stroke, pulmonary embolus, invasive breast cancer		Protection against hip and vertebral fracture
	0.3 mg/1.5 mg			
Estrogen				
Premarin	0.625 mg	Increased risk of stroke	Increased risk of endometrial cancer in women with intact uterus	Return to premenopausal bone dynamics
	0.45 mg		No increased risk of breast cancer	Protection against hip and vertebral fracture
	0.3 mg		Bone benefits equal at all doses; use lowest effective dose for other symptoms	
	1.25 mg			
	0.9 mg			
1-34 PTH				
Forteo (teriparatide)	20 mcg/day SC for maximum of 2 yr	Dizziness and myalgias in first 4 to 6 weeks of use in some patients	Black Box Warning with increased rate of osteosarcoma in rats	Stimulates osteoblastic bone formation greater than osteoclastic bone resorption

- Strength
- Weight bearing
  - Especially important in children and young adults (can see gains with increased activity)
  - In older adults it helps to slow bone loss (no gains, but maintenance or slower loss).
- Endurance
- Avoid abdominal crunches and limit weight lifting to low weights (<10 lbs).

Pharmacologic

- Calcium and vitamin D supplementation
  - Necessary for all patients
  - Not sufficient alone to treat osteoporosis in adults
  - Useful alone in prevention and in children
  - Given in divided doses of 500 to 600 mg calcium per dose
  - Two types of calcium supplements available
    - Calcium carbonate (Oscal, Caltrate, Tums)
      - Needs acid environment to dissolve completely
        - Beware use in elderly (many people over age 70 are achloridic).
        - Beware H$_2$ blockers.
    - Calcium citrate (Citrical)
      - Dissolves in absence of acid
      - Increased risk of kidney stones in the small percentage of patients who get citrate-based stones (most get oxalate stones)
      - Clinical significance of difference not completely clear
- Bisphosphonates (Table 10-2)
  - Analogues of pyrophosphate
  - Mode of action
    - Bind to surface of hydroxyapatite crystals
    - Inhibit crystal resorption
    - Inhibit mevalonate pathway and protein prenylation
    - Reduce production of protons and lysosomal enzymes by osteoclasts
    - First-generation forms also inhibit bone formation (not used clinically anymore).
    - Second and third generations inhibit resorption 1,000 times greater than they inhibit formation.
    - Recent data show importance of cumulative dose.

- Allows for weekly, monthly, quarterly, or yearly dosing for effect
- Not metabolized; excreted in urine intact
- Long half-life (estimated 6 to 10 years)
- Cessation of treatment does not lead to rapid bone loss
- Fracture rates decline 50% at spine/hip/wrist after 1 year
- Side effects include esophagus irritation (10% to 15%) and osteonecrosis of jaw occuring at a rate of 1 per 100,000 patient years of drug intake
- Used as treatment for men
- Used to prevent losses during steroid treatment
- Bone mass gains can sometimes be seen in the first 4 years of treatment, but not seen in all patients
  - 2% to 4% per year for vertebral body
  - 1% to 2% per year for hip
- SERM: raloxifene (Evista)
  - Antagonist to breast cancer but agonist to bone formation
  - Antiestrogens with bone augmentation effects
  - Very effective in improving bone mass, preventing vertebral fractures
  - Can augment treatment with bisphosphonates (additive effects of both drugs)
  - Reduces incidence of breast cancer 50%
  - No cardiovascular effects, no increase in cardiovascular complications
  - No added risk of uterine cancer
  - Not as potent as estrogen therapy
  - Dose 60 mg daily
- Calcitonin (Miacalcin Nasal Spray)
  - Non-sex/non-steroid hormone
  - Binds to osteoclasts to decrease activity/number
  - Dose 200 units/day sprayed in alternate nostrils
  - Analgesic effect with painful vertebral fractures
    - Mechanism unknown; no deleterious effects on healing
  - Effective in stabilizing spinal bone mass and decreasing vertebral fractures, but no effect on hip fractures
- PTH (Forteo)
  - First approved therapy that actually builds significant bone (anabolic agent)
  - Daily low-dose injections increase bone mass in animals and humans.
  - Increase life span of osteoblasts
  - Forteo is amino acids 1–34 of PTH.
    - Dose is 20 mcg daily for 2 years.
    - Spine bone mineral density increases at 6 to 12 months.
    - Hip bone mineral density increases delayed as much as 18 to 24 months
    - Overall bone mass gains of 8% to 15% per year of therapy
  - Follow therapy with agents to maintain bone mass (usually bisphosphonates).
  - Conflicting evidence about concurrent use with bisphosphonates
    - Some studies show decreased gains with PTH with simultaneous bisphosphonate therapy.

TABLE 10-2 BISPHOSPHONATES

Brand Name	Generic Name	Dosage
Fosamax	Alendronate	70 mg once weekly
Actonel	Risedronate	35 mg once weekly
Boniva	Ibandronate	150 mg once monthly
Zometa*	Zoledronic acid	4 mg IV once yearly

*Not currently approved by the U.S. Food and Drug Administration for this indication

- Sequential use does not appear to decrease effect.
- Common side effects
    - Myalgias in back and thigh muscles in first month of therapy
        - Not common
        - Resolve after this time frame
    - Dizziness in first 4 to 6 weeks
        - More common in elderly
        - Take before going to bed to decrease fall risk.
        - Generally not a problem after this time frame
- Black Box Warning
    - Contraindications include previous radiation therapy, Paget's disease, and very young patients
    - In animal studies at higher dosing levels, osteosarcoma developed before death from drug.
        - Significance related to human osteosarcoma unclear
- Estrogen
    - While not a part of the black box warning, as a part of the general warnings from the manufacturer this drug should not be used if
        - Bone metastases or a history of skeletal malignancies
        - Metabolic bone diseases other than osteoporosis
        - Pre-existing hypercalcemia
        - Pregnancy and lactation
    - Formerly the gold standard for therapy
    - Receptors on both osteoblast and osteoclast
    - Patients with intact uterus should take progestin/estrogen combination.
        - Unopposed estrogen increases endometrial cancer risk.
    - Women's Health Initiative
        - 16,608 postmenopausal women age 50 to 79 randomized to estrogen 0.625 mg and medroxyprogesterone 2.5 mg/day or placebo
        - Terminated trial 3 years early because threshold for breast cancer events reached and global index showed risk > benefit
        - Unequivocal benefit for reducing hip fractures (hazard ratio [HR] = 0.66)
        - Overall increase in breast cancer (HR = 1.26), cardiovascular events (HR = 1.29), strokes (HR = 1.41), and PE (HR = 2.13)
    - Still used in some women, often at patient's request due to severe perimenopausal symptoms
        - Lower doses available

OSTEOMALACIA AND RICKETS

PATHOGENESIS

Etiology

- Nutritional deficiency of vitamin D
    - Results in inadequate intestinal calcium absorption

- Genetic anomalies
    - 1α-hydroxylase deficiency from mutation
    - Vitamin D receptor (VDR) mutation
    - PHEX gene mutation in X-linked hypophosphatemic rickets

Pathophysiology

- Total amount of bone normal; mineralization inadequate

Histology

- Bone biopsy
    - Widened osteoid seams
    - Smudging of tetracycline labels from slow mineralization rate
- Growth plate
    - Widened growth plate with lack of mineralization in provisional zone of calcification

Epidemiology

- Children get rickets (bone and growth plate effected).
- Adults get osteomalacia.
- Accounts for at least 8% of hip fractures in United States

Classification

- Nutritional deficiency more common (calcium/vitamin D)
    - Inadequate vitamin D intake/inadequate sun exposure
    - Calcium chelators, phosphate binders
    - Elderly need more sun exposure for enough vitamin D (impaired hepatic/renal hydroxylation).
    - Intestinal malabsorption most common cause
- PO$_4$ disorders
    - Renal disease with leakage
    - Oncogenic osteomalacia (or tumor-induced osteomalacias)
    - X-linked hypophosphatemic rickets
    - Renal osteodystrophy

DIAGNOSIS

Clinical Features

Physical Findings
- Rickets
    - Frontal skull bossing
    - Enlarged costochondral junction (rachitic rosary)
    - Bowing of long bones
    - Delay in eruption of permanent teeth
    - Minimal-trauma fractures
- Osteomalacia
    - Minimal-trauma fractures
    - Proximal muscle weakness
    - Gait instability

Laboratory Findings
- High PTH
- High alkaline phosphatase
- Low to normal calcium
- Low 25-hydroxy vitamin D
- Often normal 1,25-dihydroxy vitamin D

Radiologic Features

- Rickets
  - Metaphyseal flaring, widened growth plates
  - Best seen in distal radius/ulna or around knee
  - Loss of provisional zone of calcification
- Osteomalacia
  - Long bones appear osteopenic.
  - Looser lines
    - Stress fractures result in radiodense lines.
    - Prominent on concave side of extremity bows
    - Can see adjacent areas of radiolucency as healing produces unmineralized osteoid (looser zones)

TREATMENT

- Nutritional deficiency
  - Short-course, high-dose therapy with vitamin D
    - 50,000 IU vitamin D_2 once weekly or 1,000 IU vitamin D_3 daily for 3 to 6 months
    - Modulate vitamin D dosing depending upon severity.
    - May require chronic higher dosing of vitamin D
    - Recent data show vitamin D_3 supplements are better at maintaining levels than vitamin D_2.
- X-linked hypophosphatemic rickets
  - Renal tubular defect from mutation in PHEX
  - Phosphate loss leaves insufficient levels for mineralization.
  - Treat with large doses of phosphate.

PRIMARY HYPERPARATHYROIDISM

PATHOGENESIS

Etiology

- Excessive PTH secretion from one or more parathyroid glands

Epidemiology

- Female predilection 3:1
- Incidence 1 per 500 to 1,000

Pathophysiology

- Cells have higher "set point" for sensing elevated serum calcium levels and stopping PTH production.
- Oversecretion of PTH
  - Affects bones, kidneys, intestine (indirectly by stimulating vitamin D production in kidney)
  - Results in hypercalcemia

Genetics

- Several possibilities
  - Gene rearrangement in PRAD-1 oncogene
  - Overexpression of cyclin D1
  - Loss of one copy MEN-I tumor suppressor gene on chromosome 11

Classification

- Solitary adenoma (80% to 85%)
- Four-gland hyperplasia (15% to 20%)
- Parathyroid carcinoma (<0.5%)

DIAGNOSIS

Clinical Features

- Renal
  - Nephrolithiasis
  - Nephrocalcinosis (calcium deposition in the renal parenchyma)
  - Hypercalciuria
    - >250 mg for women, >300 mg for men
- Skeletal
  - Bone density losses
  - Osteitis fibrosa cystica (brown tumors of long bones)
- Laboratory findings
  - Diagnosis is made by elevated PTH and elevated calcium
  - Other laboratory anomalies include hypophosphatemia, hyperphosphaturia, elevated uric acid levels, and increased alkaline phosphatase levels.

Radiologic Features

- X-ray changes
  - Tufts distal phalanges affected first (subperiosteal resorption)
  - Radial border of middle phalanges
  - More advanced cases show erosion of distal clavicles.
  - Brown tumors rare in primary hyperparathyroidism
  - Densitometry more sensitive early measurement
  - 50% of patients show demineralization, mostly cortical.

TREATMENT

- Surgical excision of adenoma
- Excise 3.5 glands with general hypertrophy.

- Medical management
  - Patients mildly symptomatic, poor surgical candidates
  - Hydration, low calcium intake, osteoclast-inhibiting drugs like bisphosphonates
- With treatment, improved bone mass in 2 to 4 years

RENAL OSTEODYSTROPHY (SECONDARY HYPERPARATHYROIDISM)

PATHOPHYSIOLOGY

- High PO_4, low 1α hydroxylase leads to low calcium levels.
- Hyperplasia of parathyroid glands results in response to chronic low calcium.
- Skeletal resistance to the ability of PTH to liberate calcium from the skeleton
- Osteomalacia from aluminum toxicity
  - From aluminum-based phosphate binders
  - Not used since mid-1980s, rarely an issue now
  - Most aluminum seen now from environmental exposure
  - Disrupts formation of hydroxyapatite crystals and inhibits osteoblasts
- Adynamic bone with little bone formation
  - Generally also see poor osteoblast function and poor bone formation

Etiology

- Combination of secondary hyperparathyroidism and osteomalacia as a complication of the metabolism anomalies associated with chronic renal disease

Epidemiology

- Rate of end-stage renal disease in United States: 334 per million

DIAGNOSIS

Clinical Features

- Begin to appear only with advanced kidney disease
- Fragility fractures, especially vertebrae and ribs
- Proximal muscle weakness
- Spontaneous rupture of tendons with severe hyperparathyroidism can be seen.
- β-2 microglobulin amyloidosis can be associated.
- Laboratory findings
  - Low calcium

- High phosphate
- High PTH
- High creatinine and blood urea nitrogen (BUN)
- Increased urinary phosphate
- Commonly low hydroxy vitamin D and 1,25 dihydroxy vitamin D levels

Radiologic Features

- Osteopenia
- Fragility fractures
- Extraskeletal calcifications
  - Vascular
  - Periarticular

TREATMENT

- Management of the mineral metabolism
  - Administer phosphate binders.
  - Treat acidosis.
  - Ensure adequate calcium intake.
  - Monitor PTH levels.
  - Replace vitamins as needed: supplement if 25-hydroxy vitamin D is <30 ng/mL.
- Parathyroidectomy for severe hyperparathyroidism.
- Surgical treatment of fragility fractures may also require supplementation with 1,25 dihydroxy Vitamin D in severe renal failure and dialysis patients.

OSTEOPETROSIS

PATHOPHYSIOLOGY

- Normal new bone formation, but deficiency of bone/cartilage resorption in one of two ways
  - Decreased or absent osteoclasts
  - Large numbers of defective osteoclasts present
- Diffuse increased skeletal density/marrow space obliteration
  - New bone formed is immature, woven bone: bones more fragile and susceptible to fractures

Etiology

- Disorder of osteoclast function that interferes with normal skeletal remodeling and leads to trabecular and cortical bone thickening

Classification

- Four phenotypes
  - Adult (tarda) form
    - Majority of patients, normal life span, mild anemia, autosomal dominant
  - Congenital (infantile/malignant) form
    - Autosomal recessive, most severe form, death in childhood

- Anemia, thrombocytopenia, hepatosplenomegaly, immune system compromise, cranial/optic nerve palsies
- Intermediate form
  - Severity between adult/congenital
- Carbonic anhydrase II gene mutation form
  - Autosomal recessive
  - Associated with renal tubular acidosis, cerebral calcifications, and mental retardation
- OL-EDA-ID
  - X-linked trait affecting boys
  - Newly defined
  - Associated osteopetrosis, lymphedema, anhydrotic ectodermal dysplasia
- One case report of drug-induced osteopetrosis with large doses of pamidronate

DIAGNOSIS

Clinical Features

- Adult form
  - Long bone fractures
  - Hearing loss
  - Carpal tunnel
  - Slipped capital femoral epiphysis (SCFE)
  - Osteomyelitis of mandible
- Infantile form: manifestations in first year
  - Nasal stuffiness
  - Hearing loss
  - Delayed tooth eruption
  - Failure to thrive
  - Recurrent infections
  - Short stature

Radiologic Features

- Generalized increase in bone mass
- Dense, sclerotic bone
  - Thickening of both trabecular and cortical bone
  - Can see alternating bands of density in iliac wings
- Widened, club-shaped metaphyses ("Ehrlenmeyer flask deformity")
- Vertebrae can have sclerotic bands underlying end plates for "rugger jersey" appearance.

Diagnostic Work-up

- Laboratory findings
  - Adult form: usually normal laboratory test results
  - Infantile form: presence of brain isoenzyme of creatine kinase (BB-CK), secondary hyperparathyroidism, and hypocalcemia

- Biopsy findings
  - Remnants of primary spongiosa: calcified bars of cartilage within trabeculae

TREATMENT

- Depends on type of disease
- Bone marrow transplant
  - Infantile form
- Gamma interferon can be used for severe forms.
- Interest in using PTH and 1,25-dihydroxy vitamin D

SUGGESTED READING

Avenell A, Gillespie WJ, Gillespie LD, et al. Vitamin D and vitamin D analogues for preventing fractures associated with involutional and post-menopausal osteoporosis. *Cochrane Database Syst Rev* 2005; (3):CD000227.

Bilezikian JP, Potts JT, El-Hajj Fuleihan G, et al. Summary statement from a workshop on asymptomatic primary hyperparathyroidism: A perspective for the 21st century. *J Bone Miner Res* 2002;17(S2): N2–N11.

Cranney A, Guyatt G, Griffith L, et al. Summary of meta-analyses of therapies for postmenopausal osteoporosis. *Endocrine Rev* 2002; 23:570–578.

Cummings SR, Melton LJ. Epidemiology and outcomes of osteoporotic fractures. *Lancet* 2002;359:1761–1767.

Fauvus MJ, ed. *Primer on the Metabolic Bone Diseases and Disorders of Mineral Metabolism*, ed 6. Washington DC: American Society for Bone and Mineral Research, 2006.

Freedman KB, Kaplan FS, Bilker WB, et al. Treatment of osteoporosis: are physicians missing an opportunity? *J Bone Joint Surg [Am]* 2000;82(8):1063–1070.

Goodman WG. Renal osteodystrophy for nonnephrologists. *J Bone Miner Metab* 2006;24(2):161–163.

Kado DM, Browner WS, Palermo L, et al. Vertebral fractures and mortality in older women: A prospective study. *Arch Intern Med* 1999;159:1215–1220.

Mankin HJ, Mankin CJ. Metabolic bone disease: an update. *AAOS Instr Course Lect* 2003;52:769–784.

Physician's Guide to Prevention and Treatment of Osteoporosis. Washington DC: National Osteoporosis Foundation, 2003.

Rossouw JE, Anderson GL, Prentice RL, et al. Risks and benefits of estrogen plus progestin in healthy postmenopausal women: Principal results from Women's Health Initiative randomized controlled trial. *JAMA* 2002;288:321–333.

Silverberg SJ, Shane E, de la Cruz L, et al. Skeletal disease in primary hyperparathyroidism. *J Bone Miner Res* 1989;4:283–291.

Siris ES. Paget's disease of bone. *J Bone Miner Res* 1998;13: 1061–1165.

Tejwani NC, Schachter AK, Immerman I, et al. Renal osteodystrophy. *J Am Acad Orthop Surg* 2006;14:303–311.

Tolar J, Teitelbaum SL, Orchard PJ. Osteopetrosis. *N Engl J Med* 2004; 351:2839–2849.

U.S. Department of Health and Human Services. *Bone Health and Osteoporosis: A Report of the Surgeon General.* U.S. Department of Health and Human Services, Rockville, MD, 2004.

Whyte MP. Clinical practice. Paget's disease of bone. *N Engl J Med* 2006;355(6):593–600.

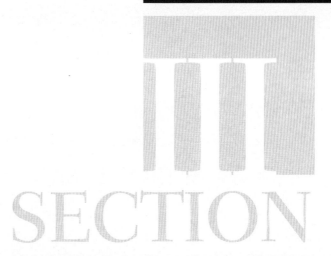

SECTION III

SPECIFIC SOFT TISSUE NEOPLASMS AND SIMULATORS

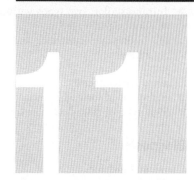

BENIGN SOFT TISSUE TUMORS

TIMOTHY A. DAMRON
GUSTAVO DE LA ROZA

Benign soft tissue tumors outnumber soft tissue sarcomas by approximately 100:1. In adults, lipomas are the most common soft tissue tumor; in children, hemangiomas are the most common. Recognition of these relatively more common benign tumors is important not only to avoid over-treatment but also to allow distinction from their malignant counterparts. Soft tissue tumors, both benign and malignant, are classified according to the purported cell of origin or resemblance, and the organization of this chapter will follow the latest World Health Organization (WHO) scheme in that regard.

FATTY BENIGN SOFT TISSUE TUMORS

LIPOMA

Lipoma is the most common soft tissue tumor in adults. However, because it is, soft tissue sarcomas are sometimes assumed to be lipomas, unnecessarily delaying the diagnosis. Hence, recognition of the distinction between benign lipomas and soft tissue sarcomas is very important.

Pathogenesis and Pathophysiology

- Etiology is unknown.
- More common in obese patients
- Peak age: 40 to 60 (rare in children)
- Multiple lipomas in 5%

Histopathology
- Lobules of mature adipocytes
- Occasionally other areas of tissue formation
    - Bone = osteolipoma
    - Cartilage = chondrolipoma
    - Myxoid change = myxolipoma

Genetics
- Chromosomal aberrations in up to 75%
- Three patterns
    - 12q13-15 aberrations
    - 6p21-23 aberrations
    - Loss of material from 13q

Classification

- Histologic variant subtypes have no prognostic significance.
- Infiltrative

Intermuscular Versus Intramuscular
- Intermuscular: easily shelled out between muscles
- Intramuscular: two types within muscle
  - Well demarcated
  - Infiltrative: infiltrates and encases atrophic muscle fibers

Lipoma Arborescens
- Subsynovial located lipoma
- One type of intra-articular lipoma

Diagnosis

Clinical Features
- Most common: painless mass with characteristic doughy feel
- Most superficial lipomas are small (<5 cm).
- Most deep lipomas are large (>5 cm).
- Lipoma arborescens presents as articular swelling.

Radiologic Features
- Superficial lipomas: difficult to see on radiographs or magnetic resonance imaging (MRI)
- Deep lipomas (Fig. 11-1)
  - Fatty intramuscular shadow
  - Homogeneous fatty signal on all MRI sequences
  - No gadolinium enhancement
  - Occasional entrapped muscle fibers or fibrous strands
- Lipoma arborescens
  - Fatty infiltration throughout affected synovium with fat-distended villi

Diagnostic Work-up
- Most superficial lipomas are distinguished by their doughy characteristics on physical examination and do not warrant radiographic evaluation.
- Larger or deep masses warrant plain radiographic and MRI evaluation, which is usually diagnostic.
- Biopsy is rarely indicated.
- Also see Chapter 2, Evaluation of Soft Tissue Tumors.

Treatment

Surgical and Nonoperative Options
- Superficial lipomas
  - Observation favored
  - Excision only if symptomatic
- Deep lipomas
  - Observation if radiology identifies clearly as benign lesion (not atypical lipoma or liposarcoma)
  - Excision for most

Surgical Goals and Approaches
- Marginal excision (complete excision through pseudo-capsule)
- Avoid transaction of nerves running within deep lipomas (piecemeal excision preferred).

Results and Outcome
- Rarely recur following marginal excision

LIPOMATOSIS

Lipomatosis is a diffuse systemic or regional overgrowth of mature adipose tissue that differs from normal fat only in

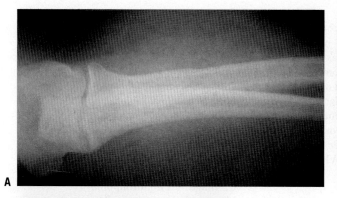
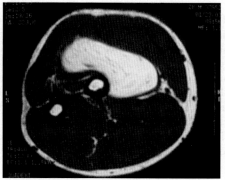
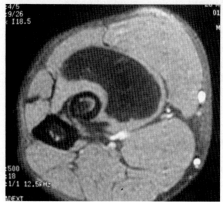

Figure 11-1 Inramuscular lipoma of the proximal forearm. (**A**) The fatty soft tissue shadow is shown within the muscle of the proximal forearm by plain radiograph. Axial T1-weighted (**B**) and T2-weighted (**C**) MR imaging studies show homogenous fatty signal characteristics identical to that of the subcutaneous fat.

its distribution. Lipomatosis should be distinguished from lipomas, as the former conditions may be correctable by addressing the underlying condition and tend to recur after attempted excision.

Pathogenesis and Pathophysiology

- Etiology is poorly understood.
- Possibly due to point mutations in mitochondrial genes
- See Table 11-1 for epidemiology.
- Histopathology: mature fat in poorly circumscribed lobules or sheets infiltrating surrounding tissues

Classification

- Classified by distribution for idiopathic types (diffuse, pelvic, symmetric) or by etiology (steroid, HIV lipodystrophy)

Diagnosis

- Notable accumulations of fat in affected areas may resemble neoplasms (see Table 11-1).
- Radiologic studies document extent of fatty deposition.
- Neither radiological evaluation nor biopsy is usually necessary to diagnosis the lipomatoses.
- See Chapter 2.

Treatment and Outcome

- Palliative surgery is rarely indicated unless life-threatening fat accumulation (such as that causing laryngeal compression in Madelung's disease).

- Correction of steroid lipomatosis follows lowering of steroid levels.

LIPOMATOSIS OF NERVE (LIPOFIBROMATOUS HAMARTOMA)

Lipofibromatosis, also referred to variously as lipofibromatous hamartoma, fibrolipomatosis, and intraneural lipoma, among other names, is a fatty and fibrous infiltrative process affecting the epineurium and leading to enlargement of the affected nerve. The median and ulnar nerves are most commonly affected.

Pathogenesis and Pathophysiology

- Etiology is unknown.
- Peak age: 10 to 40
- Frequently evident at birth or early childhood
- Female > male if macrodactyly present; male > female if none
- Gross histopathology: yellow fibrofatty infiltration of nerve (Fig. 11-2)
- Microscopic histopathology: epineurial and perineural fibrofatty infiltration isolating individual nerve bundles

Diagnosis

Clinical Features
- Gradually enlarging mass with variable neurologic deficits
- Median nerve or branches > ulnar nerve
- Foot, brachial plexus less common sites
- Macrodactyly in one third

TABLE 11-1 EPIDEMIOLOGY AND CLINICAL FEATURES OF LIPOMATOSIS SUBTYPES

Subtype	Epidemiology	Distribution	Potential Complications or Associated Symptoms
Diffuse	Typically <2 yr	Trunk, large part of extremity, head and neck, pelvis, or intestinal Macrodactyly or digital gigantism	
Pelvic	Black males all ages, 9 yr and up	Perivesicular, perirectal	Bowel or bladder symptoms (frequency, constipation), perineal/abdominal/low back pain
Symmetric (Madelung's disease)	Middle-aged men of Mediterranean descent	Upper body, especially neck	Cranial or peripheral neuropathy Airway obstruction Superior vena cava syndrome Associated with alcoholism, hyperuricemia, hyperlipidemia
Steroid	Steroid treatment Primary adrenal cortical axis overstimulation	Facial, sternal, or buffalo hump	Secondary manifestations of hypercortisolism
HIV lipodystrophy	HIV patients on treatment	Visceral, breast, cervical fat Fat wasting in face and limbs	Associated with hyperlipidemia, diabetes

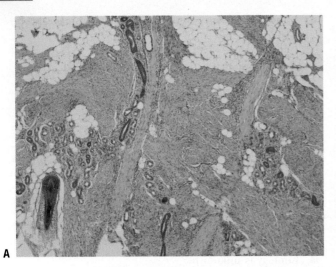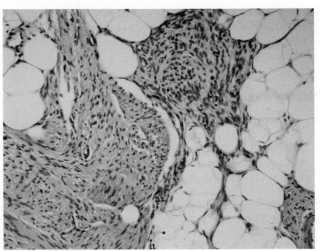

Figure 11-2 **A** Fibrous hamartoma of infancy. Organoid pattern composed of intersecting fascicles of spindle cells separated by collagen, mature fat, and islands of immature mesenchymal cells with myxoid matrix. **B** Close-up view of characteristic island of immature mesenchyma in fibrous hamartoma of infancy.

Radiologic Features
- MRI findings pathognomonic
  - Fusiform neural enlargement following branching pattern of nerve
  - Hypointense serpentine nerve bundles on both T1- and T2-weighted images
  - Variable intramuscular fatty deposition

Diagnostic Work-up
- Because MRI is diagnostic, biopsy is usually not needed.

Treatment

- Goal of surgical intervention is to decompress nerve if symptomatic.
- Avoid attempted excision, which may damage nerve.

LIPOBLASTOMA

Lipoblastoma is a tumor resembling fetal adipose tissue that occurs predominately in infants and may be localized (lipoblastoma) or diffuse (lipoblastomatosis). Since lipomas generally do not occur in this age group, lipoblastoma should be considered highly in the differential diagnosis of any tumor with fatty imaging characteristics in a child.

Pathogenesis and Pathophysiology

- Etiology is unknown.
- Peak age: birth to age 3; less common in older children
- Males > females

Histopathology
- Variable mixture of mature adipocytes and immature fat cells (lipoblasts)

- Variable myxoid background with plexiform vascular pattern suggestive of myxoid liposarcoma
- Pronounced lobular pattern and lack of atypia distinguishes lipoblastoma from liposarcoma

Genetics
- 8q11-13 rearrangement in most cases
- Fusion gene products: HAS2/PLAG1, COL1A2/PLAG1

Classification

- Solitary (lipoblastoma) versus diffuse (lipoblastomatosis)

Diagnosis

- See Chapter 2 for diagnostic work-up.

Clinical Features
- Sites: extremities predominate
- Typically small (2 to 5 cm), superficial mass
- Lipoblastomatosis often involves muscle as well.

Radiologic Features
- Fatty signal characteristics
  - Bright on T1-weighted MRI, dark on fat-suppressed sequences, identical to surrounding fat
- Indistinguishable from lipoma, well-differentiated liposarcoma (atypical lipoma) by radiology

Treatment and Outcome

- Lipoblastoma: marginal *en bloc* excision
- Lipoblastomatosis: wide surgical excision
- Recurrence rare in lipoblastoma; up to 22% in lipoblastomatosis

TABLE 11-2 HISTOLOGICAL LIPOMA VARIANTS

Tumor	Peak Ages/ Gender	Distribution	Clinical Features	Histology
Angiolipoma	Late teens to early 20s Rare >50 yr	Forearm > trunk > upper arm Superficial	Small Frequently multiple Painful mass	Mature adipocytes Branching capillary-sized vessels (see Fig. 11-3)
Chondroid lipoma	Adults Female:male 4:1	Proximal extremities or limb girdles > trunk Deep or involving fascia	Painless mass Half with enlargement	Nests and cords of lipoblasts embedded in myxoid or hyaline cartilage matrix
Spindle cell lipoma	Adults 45 to 65 yr Male:female 9:1	Posterior neck and shoulder > upper arm Superficial	Small Rarely multiple	Adipocytes, spindle cells, and collagen bundles Variable inflammatory cells (especially mast cells)
Pleomorphic lipoma	Adults >45 yr Male:female 9:1	Posterior neck and shoulder > upper arm Superficial	Small Rarely multiple	Spindle cells and giant cells with nuclei arranged in "floret-like" pattern
Hibernoma	Young adults 20 to 40 yr (60%)	Thigh > trunk > upper extremity > head and neck Subcutaneous > deep (9:1)	Painless mass Enhances with MRI contrast	Polygonal brown fat cells Lipoblast-like multivacuolated cells (see Fig. 11-4)

HISTOLOGIC LIPOMA VARIANTS

The histologic variants of lipoma are summarized in Table 11-2, and examples are shown in Figures 11-3 and 11-4.

FIBROBLASTIC BENIGN SOFT TISSUE TUMORS

NODULAR FASCIITIS

Nodular fasciitis is a tumor predominately of the upper extremity and neck region that is distinguished by its rapid growth and its tissue culture–like histology pattern.

Pathogenesis and Pathophysiology

- Etiology: unknown, but history of trauma common

Epidemiology
- Peak age: young adults, but may involve any age

Histopathology (Fig. 11-5)
- Plump, regular myofibroblasts
- Frequent mitoses but not atypical mitoses
- Tissue culture–like, "torn" or "feathery" appearance at low power

- Prominent small vessels may resemble granulation tissue.
- Nodular infiltrative pattern of organization
- Extravasated red blood cells, chronic inflammatory cells, and even giant cells may be seen.
- SMA and MSA positive
- Desmin, cytokeratin, and S100 negative

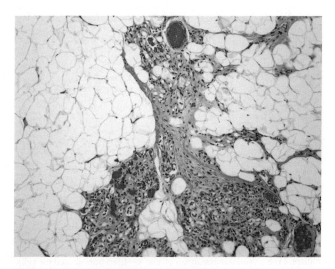

Figure 11-3   Angiolipoma composed of mature adipose tissue intermixed with numerous vascular channels. The vascularity is often more prominent in subcapsular areas.

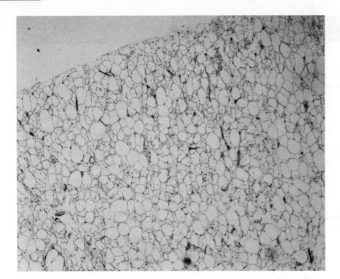

Figure 11-4 Hibernoma: rare fatty tumor composed of mature adipose tissue and a large number of multivacuolated brown fat cells with abundant granular cytoplasm and a centrally located nucleus.

Genetics
- Some clonality suggesting neoplastic nature demonstrated, but may represent artifact of culture conditions

Diagnosis
- See Chapter 2 for diagnostic work-up.

Clinical Features
- Subcutaneous >> intramuscular
- Upper extremity, trunk, head and neck most common

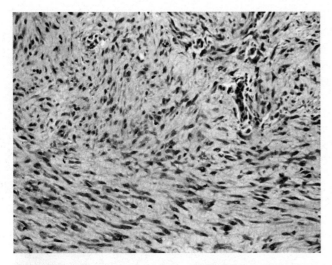

Figure 11-5 Nodular fasciitis: cellular proliferation of stellate cells with vague storiform pattern and extravasated red blood cells. Inflammatory cells and mitoses are also commonly seen, but there is no cytologic atypia.

- Rapid growth is characteristic.
- Clinical history usually <1 to 2 months
- Pain and local tenderness common
- Small size, usually <2 cm

Radiologic Features
- Nonspecific soft tissue mass (Fig. 11-6)

Treatment and Outcome
- Marginal excision
- Rare recurrence should warrant reconsideration of diagnosis.

PROLIFERATIVE FASCIITIS AND MYOSITIS

These two processes are similar to nodular fasciitis in their rapid growth, predilection for the upper extremity, and plump myofibroblastic cells, but they are distinguished by the large ganglion-like cells that are also present. Proliferative fasciitis (PF) involves the fascia, while proliferative myositis (PM) involves the muscle.

Pathogenesis and Pathophysiology
- Etiology is unknown, although a history of trauma may be elicited.
- Peak age: middle-aged or older adults, older than nodular fasciitis
- Much less common than nodular fasciitis

Histopathology
- Two cellular types: plump myofibroblasts and ganglion-like cells
- Plump myofibroblasts resemble those of nodular fasciitis.
- Ganglion-like cells: large with one to three rounded nuclei, prominent nucleoli, and abundant cytoplasm
- Numerous mitoses but not atypical mitoses
- Infiltrative growth pattern (along fascial planes for PF and between muscle groups in PM)
- Checkerboard pattern of infiltration between muscle fibers for PM
- SMA and MSA positive
- Desmin, cytokeratin, and S100 negative

Genetics
- Similar to nodular fasciitis

Diagnosis
- See Chapter 2 for diagnostic work-up.

Clinical Features
- PF: upper extremity (especially forearm) > lower extremity > trunk
- PM: trunk > shoulder girdle > upper arm > thigh
- Rapid growth is characteristic.

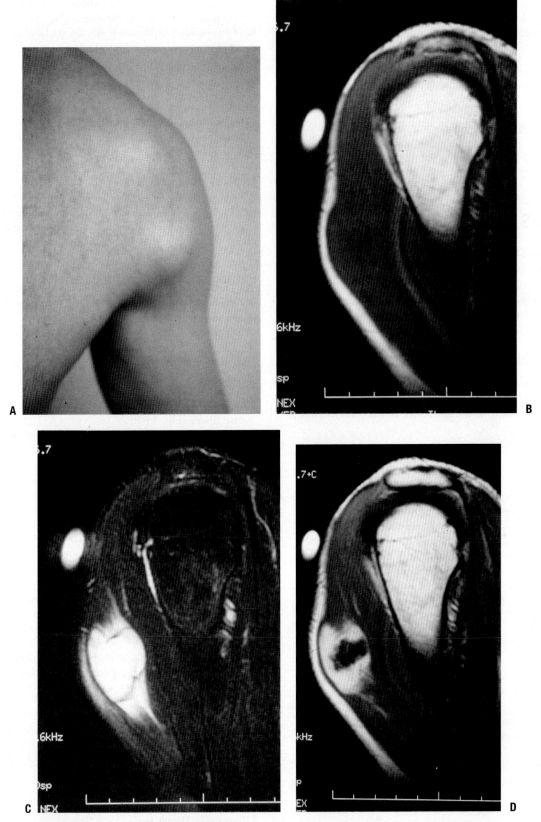

Figure 11-6 Nodular fasciitis of the shoulder. (**A**) The patient presented with a 3-week history of a rapidly enlarging, painful soft tissue mass over the anterior deltoid. Sagittal MR studies show nonspecific findings of a heterogeneous intramuscular mass hypointense to muscle on T1-weighted sequences (**B**), hyperintense on T2-weighted images (**C**), and enhancing on post-gadolinium sequences (**D**).

- Clinical history usually <1 or 2 months
- Pain and local tenderness more common with PF
- Small size, usually <5 cm

Radiologic Features
- Nonspecific soft tissue mass

Treatment and Outcome

- Marginal excision
- Recurrence is rare.

MYOSITIS OSSIFICANS

Myositis ossificans is a benign reparative process characterized by bone formation within the soft tissues in response to trauma. On the one hand, it may simulate malignancy, but conversely, sarcomas that give a similar appearance may be mistaken for this benign, self-limited condition.

Pathogenesis and Pathophysiology

- Trauma history elicited in up to 75% of patients; repetitive trauma in others
- Peak age: young, physically active adults (rare in infants or elderly)
- Males > females

Histopathology
- Zonal proliferation with central fibroblasts and peripheral osteoblast-rimmed bone trabeculae
- Progression from initially fibrous tissue to peripheral woven bone and then eventually lamellar bone
- Peripheral ossification usually evident by 3 weeks
- Mitoses frequent but no atypical mitoses

Diagnosis

- See Chapter 2 for diagnostic work-up.

Clinical Features
- Initial 1 to 2 weeks after injury: swollen, tender
- From 2 to 6 weeks after injury: tenderness and pain resolve, and painless, very firm mass forms
- Chronically, the mass becomes less prominent over time.
- Any location in body susceptible to trauma
- Most common locations: thigh, shoulder, buttock, elbow

Radiologic Features
- Initial 1 to 2 weeks after injury: x-ray, computed tomography (CT), MRI shows soft tissue shadow, heterogeneous MRI signal with edema

- From 2 to 6 weeks after injury: x-ray, CT best show peripheral rim of calcifications (Fig. 11-7)
- Chronically, MRI eventually shows low-signal rim with fatty marrow signal centrally.

Treatment and Outcome

- Observation is best, but marginal excision is appropriate if sufficiently symptomatic.
- May recur if excised incompletely early in course

ELASTOFIBROMA

Elastofibroma (elastofibroma dorsi) is a unique process that occurs almost exclusively in a subscapular location in adults and is characterized by histologic evidence of elastic fibers.

Pathogenesis and Pathophysiology

- Etiology is unknown, although repetitive trauma has been implicated.
- Peak age in seventh and eighth decades (nearly always after age 50)
- Females > males

Histopathology
- Low-cellularity collagenous tissue with intermixed elastic fibers (Fig. 11-8)
- Immunohistochemistry positive for elastin

Genetics
- Familial occurrence reported in Okinawa

Diagnosis

Clinical Features
- Slowly growing mass, typically painless and nontender
- May cause popping scapula or local discomfort
- Classic location
  - Nearly exclusively subscapular, applied to chest wall at the lower portion of the scapula
  - Deep to latissimus dorsi and rhomboid major
  - Often attached to periosteum of ribs
  - Rare musculoskeletal sites: upper arm, hip
  - May be bilateral (especially subclinical) in up to one third

Radiologic Features
- Fibrous and fatty elements create layered picture.
- MRI may be highly suggestive (Fig. 11-9).
  - Fatty areas: bright areas on T1-weighted images, intermediate on T2-weighted images
  - Fibrous areas: similar to muscle

Diagnostic Work-up
- Biopsy is generally recommended to confirm diagnosis, although the combination of classic location and radiologic appearance is highly suggestive.
- Also see Chapter 2.

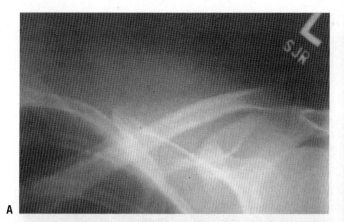

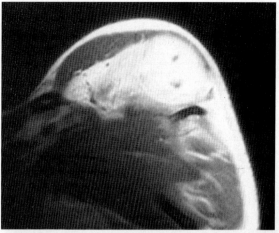

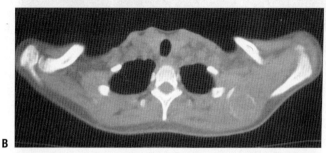

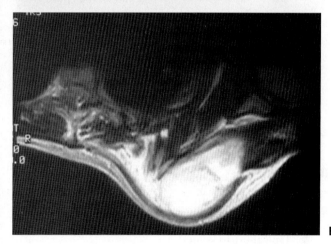

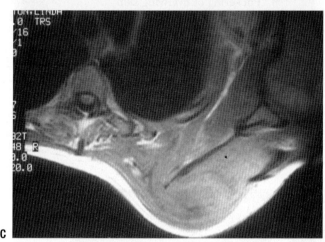

Figure 11-7   (**A**) Initial plain radiographs within the first 2 to 3 weeks may not show the characteristic peripheral rim of calcification associated with myositis ossificans. (**B**) Subsequently, the peripheral rim is best demonstrated on computed tomography. (**C**) MR studies show a heterogeneous mass that is sometimes confused with a soft tissue sarcoma.

Treatment and Outcome

- Marginal excision indicated for symptomatic patients but may be observed if asymptomatic and histologically proven
- Rarely recurs after complete excision

SUPERFICIAL FIBROMATOSES

The superficial fibromatoses include palmar fibromatosis (Dupuytren's disease or contracture) and plantar fibromatosis (Ledderhose disease), both fibroblastic proliferations with infiltrative growth that are usually easily recogniz-

able clinically and have a high rate of local recurrence if excised.

Pathogenesis and Pathophysiology

- Etiology is multifactorial.
  - Familial component
  - Trauma
  - Associated diseases: epilepsy, diabetes, alcohol-induced liver disease
- Peak age: adults with increasing frequency in advanced ages (rare before age 30)
- Males >> females (3 to 4:1)
- Ethnicity: highest incidence in northern Europe and in

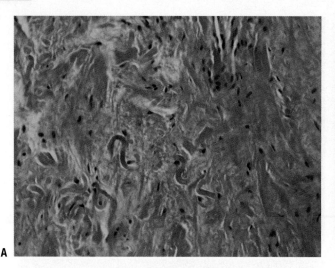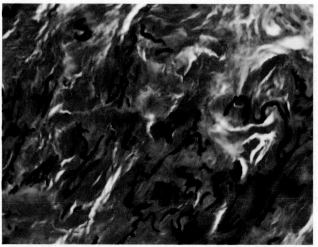

Figure 11-8 (A) Elastofibroma composed of intertwining, swollen collagen and elastic fibers with fibroblasts. (B) Elastic fibers highlighted by EVG stain in elastofibroma.

those of northern European descent; rare in non-Caucasians
- Pathophysiology is shown in Figure 11-10.

Diagnosis

Clinical Features
- Palmar fibromatosis
  - Volar surface, 50% bilateral
  - Typical progression
    - Begins with firm painless nodule
    - Progresses to multiple nodules connected by

tight cords (distinguished from pre-existing normal fascial bands)
    - Puckering of overlying skin
    - End-stage flexion contractures favoring ring and little fingers
- Plantar fibromatosis
  - Plantar aponeurosis
  - Typical course
    - Begins with firm nodule adherent to skin
    - Often painful with shoe wear
    - Progressive enlargement may result.
    - Rarely leads to contracture

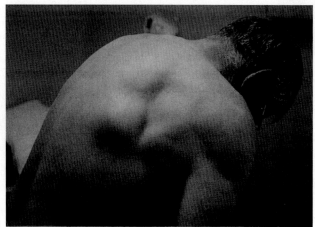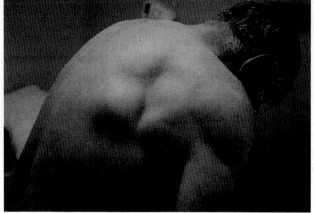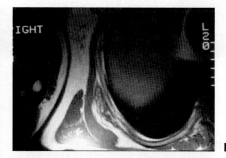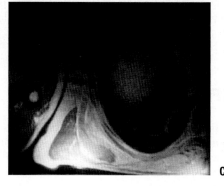

Figure 11-9 (A) The characteristic location for an elastofibroma is at the inferior medial border of the scapula in a subscapular position. MR images show a heterogeneous subscapular soft tissue mass on T1-weighted (B) and proton density (C) axial images.

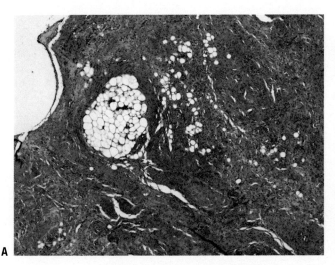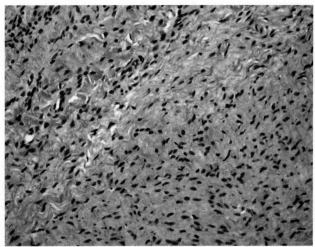

Figure 11-10 (A) Plantar fibromatosis: dense fibrous proliferation infiltrating adipose tissue. (B) Plantar fibromatosis: early lesions consist of cellular proliferations of bland-looking spindle cells and collagen deposition similar to desmoid tumors. Older lesions tend to be less cellular and contain more collagen.

Radiologic Features
- Palmar fibromatosis
  - Cords and hypocellular nodules dark on T1- and T2-weighted images
  - Hypercellular nodules intermediate on T1- and T2-weighted images
- Plantar fibromatosis
  - Isointense to slightly hyperintense always on T1-weighted images and nearly always on T2-weighted images
  - Usually hyperintense on short tau inversion recovery (STIR) sequence
  - Enhancement common

Diagnostic Work-up
- Dupuytren's contracture and many cases of plantar fibromatosis are easily recognized clinically and do not require either further imaging or biopsy.
- If plantar masses are not characteristic, MRI imaging may establish the diagnosis, but biopsy is sometimes needed.

Treatment and Outcome
- Palmar fibromatosis
  - Flexion contracture is most common indication for operative treatment.
  - Details of operative treatment are beyond the scope of this text.
- Plantar fibromatosis
  - Usually managed nonoperatively unless recalcitrant to adaptive shoe wear and inserts
  - If operative treatment is elected, complete fasciectomy achieves lowest recurrence rates.
  - High recurrence rate for plantar fibromatosis ranging from 50% with complete fasciectomy to 100% with local excision

DESMOID-TYPE FIBROMATOSES

Extra-abdominal desmoid tumors are the subset of interest in orthopaedics. They consist of a neoplastic fibroblastic proliferation that may result in pain, infiltrative growth resulting in recurrence, and absence of metastatic potential.

Pathogenesis and Pathophysiology

Etiology
- Familial component
  - Component of Gardner syndrome (autosomal dominant transmission, variant of familial adenomatous polyposis; Box 11-1)
- Endocrine factors
  - Frequent exacerbation/appearance postpartum
  - Estrogen receptors in desmoid tumors
  - Response to endocrine agents
- Trauma may be contributory factor.

Epidemiology
- Pediatric patients: extra-abdominal > abdominal
- Puberty to 40: abdominal > extra-abdominal, female > male
- Older than 40: abdominal = extra-abdominal

BOX 11-1 COMPONENTS OF GARDNER SYNDROME

Gastrointestinal polyps with 100% risk of malignancy
Multiple osteomas
Epidermoid cysts
Desmoid tumors
Other benign skin and soft tissue tumors

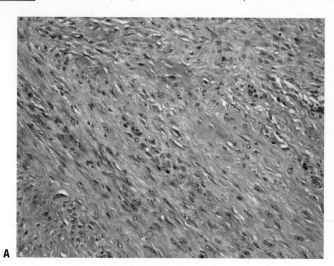 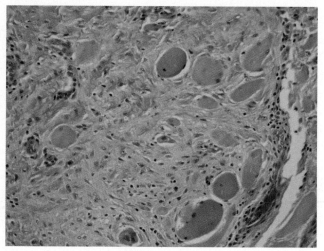

Figure 11-11   (**A**) Extra-abdominal fibromatosis showing a proliferation of bland-looking spindle cells separated by collagen. (**B**) Infiltration of surrounding soft tissues in fibromatosis. Note the presence of entrapped skeletal muscle cells.

Pathophysiology

Histopathology (Fig. 11-11)
- Low-cellularity spindle cells in collagenous stroma
- Extremely infiltrative process arranged in sweeping bundles

Genetics
- Two mutations with common endpoint of increased beta-catenin expression
  - Inactivation of APC tumor suppressor gene on 5q may be initiating event, especially those with familial occurrence.
  - Activating beta-catenin mutations render beta-catenin resistant to inhibitory effect of APC.
- Trisomies for chromosomes 8 or 20 in 30% of cells

Diagnosis
- See Chapter 2 for diagnostic work-up.

Clinical Features
- Deep (as distinguished from superficial fibromatoses)
- Painful or painless, poorly circumscribed, very hard mass
- Occasionally multifocal
- Occasional joint stiffness or neurological symptoms

Radiologic Features
- MRI nonspecific (Fig. 11-12)
  - Isointense to muscle on T1-weighted images
  - Intense contrast enhancement
  - Hyperintense on STIR and T2-weighted images

Treatment
- Surgical indication
  - Wide resection preferred if adequate margin attainable with acceptable function

- Surgical contraindications
  - Vital structures involved or unresectable disease
  - Consider alternative treatments in this situation:
    - Radiotherapy
    - Pharmacologic treatment
      - Hormonal agents
      - Nonsteroidal anti-inflammatory agents
      - Interferons
      - Cytotoxic chemotherapy
- Radiotherapy consultation is recommended for positive surgical margins, although efficacy not well established.

Results and Outcome
- Surgical resection
  - Wide margins: 85% to 90% local control
  - Marginal margins: 50%
  - Intralesional margin: <50%
- Radiotherapy
  - Typically recommended for positive margins, but proof of efficacy not clearly established
- Pharmacologic treatment
  - 40% to 50% response rate

SOLITARY FIBROUS TUMOR AND HEMANGIOPERICYTOMA

According to the latest WHO classification, extrapleural solitary fibrous tumors (SFT) and hemangiopericytoma (HP) share enough clinical, histological, and immunohistochemical features to be classified together and may actually represent a spectrum of the same entity. They typically behave in a benign fashion, but up to 30% are malignant.

Pathogenesis and Pathophysiology
- Etiology is unknown.
- Peak age 20 to 70 years (median 50)

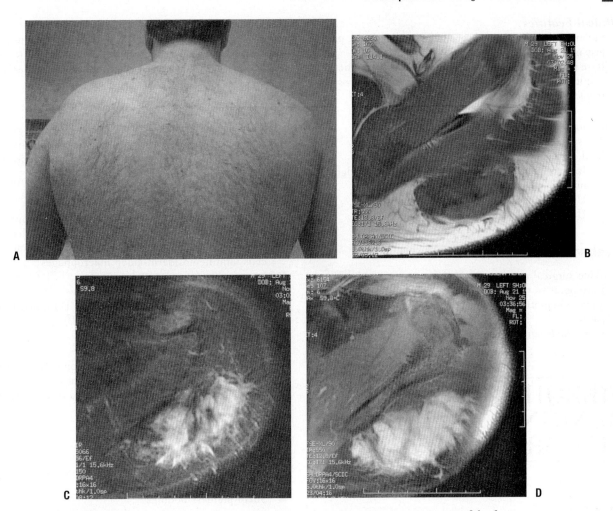

Figure 11-12 (**A**) Desmoid tumor typically presents as a slow-growing, sometimes painful soft tissue mass. MR imaging shows nonspecific hypointense signal on T1-weighted sequences (**B**) and hyperintense signal on T2-weighted sequences (**C**). (**D**) Gadolinium enhancement is intense.

Histopathology
- SFT
  - Intermixed hypercellular and hypocellular areas separated by bands of hyalinized collagen
  - Round to spindle cells with indistinct cytoplasm
  - Immunohistochemistry
    - Vimentin, CD34, and CD99 positive
    - Variable focal positivity for others
- HP
  - Similar to SFT with addition of prominent variably branching thin-walled vessels with staghorn configuration (Fig. 11-13)
  - Immunohistochemistry
    - Vimentin, CD34, and CD99 positive
    - Cytokeratin, actin, and desmin negative

Genetics
- Inconsistent chromosomal aberrations

Diagnosis

- See Chapter 2 for diagnostic work-up.

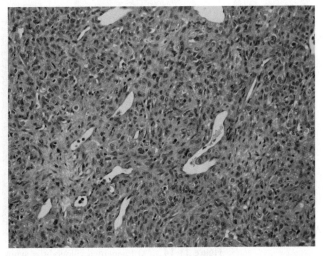

Figure 11-13 Hemangiopericytoma: cellular neoplasm composed of spindle and round cells with large vascular spaces with a "staghorn" configuration.

Clinical Features

■ Superficial or deep, slowly growing, small or large, painless mass in any location

■ Rare paraneoplastic syndrome due to IGF-1 production results in hypoglycemia or acromegaly; oncogenic osteomalacia is very rare with these tumors.

Radiologic Features

■ Nonspecific radiologic features

■ MRI nonspecific

  ■ Isointense to slightly hyperintense on T1-weighted images

  ■ Hyperintense on T2-weighted images

  ■ Heterogeneous, enhancing

Treatment and Outcome

■ Wide surgical resection

■ Postoperative management with adjuvant radiotherapy and/or chemotherapy may play a role in some malignant cases.

■ 85% 5-year survival rate including malignant forms

FIBROHISTIOCYTIC BENIGN SOFT TISSUE TUMORS

GIANT CELL TUMOR OF TENDON SHEATH

Also referred to as localized tenosynovial giant cell tumor or nodular tenosynovitis, these common tumors represent the most common neoplasms of the hand. In some classifications, such as that of the current WHO, this terminology also includes what in the past has been referred to as the localized form of pigmented villonodular synovitis (PVNS).

Pathogenesis and Pathophysiology

■ Current evidence favors a neoplastic etiology over the traditional belief that this was a reactive process.

■ Peak age: 30 to 50 years (but any age may be involved)

■ Female > male

Histopathology (Fig. 11-14B)

■ Grossly well circumscribed with yellow and brown areas

■ Composed of mixture of background mononuclear cells, variable numbers of giant cells, lipid-laden xanthoma cells, and hemosiderin-laden macrophages

■ Immunohistochemistry

  ■ Mononuclear cells: CD68 positive

  ■ Giant cells: positive for CD68, CD45, and tartrate resistant acid phosphatase (TRAP)

Genetics

■ Cytogenetic aberrations of chromosome 1p in particular, frequently with translocation, are common.

■ No trisomies of chromosomes 5 or 7, as seen with PVNS

Diagnosis

Clinical Features

■ Predominately in the hand (85%) near tendon sheath or joint > wrist, foot/ankle, knee

■ Small painless nodules

Radiologic Features

■ Approximately 20% erode adjacent bone.

■ Nonspecific MRI features (Fig. 11-15)

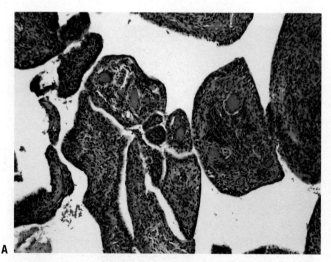
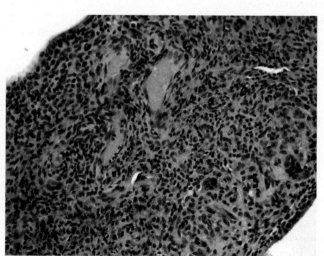

A   B

Figure 11-14   (A) Pigmented villonodular synovitis showing characteristic intra-articular villous pattern. Abundant hemosiderin pigment seen within macrophages in fibrovascular core. (B) Pigmented villonodular synovitis: solid areas composed of oval to spindle-shaped, histiocytoid, mononuclear cells and multinucleated giant cells.

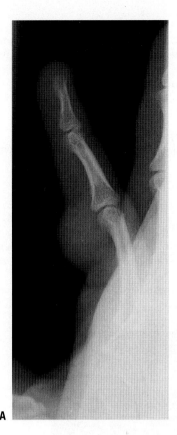
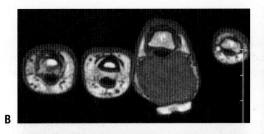
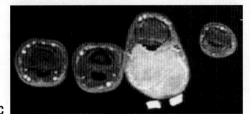
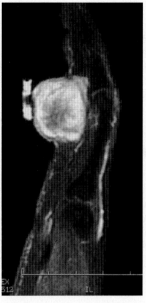

Figure 11-15   Giant cell tumor of tendon sheath shows a soft tissue shadow on plain lateral radiograph (**A**), hypointense signal on axial T1-weighted MRI (**B**), hyperintense signal on axial T2-weighted MRI (**C**), and gadolinium enhancement on post-contrast fat-suppressed T1-weighed sagittal MRI (**D**).

■ T1-weighted images: hypointense to slightly hyperintense to muscle
■ T2-weighted images: hypointense to hyperintense to muscle
■ Heterogeneous due to hypointense areas
■ Diffuse contrast enhancement

Diagnostic Work-up
■ Usually plain radiographs and MRI are sufficient for these small masses.
■ Also see Chapter 2.

Treatment and Outcome

■ Marginal excision
■ Up to 30% recurrence rate, easily controlled by re-excision

DIFFUSE-TYPE GIANT CELL TUMOR (PIGMENTED VILLONODULAR SYNOVITIS)

Pigmented villonodular synovitis (PVNS) is a destructive proliferative synovial process predominately seen affecting the knee. It was formerly subdivided into localized and dif-fuse forms; the former is now classified as localized giant cell tumor.

Pathogenesis and Pathophysiology

■ Current evidence favors a neoplastic etiology over the traditional belief that this was a reactive process.
■ Peak age: <40 years (but any age may be involved)
■ Female > male

Histopathology
■ Intra-articular forms: villous pattern with yellow and brown areas (Fig. 11-14A)
■ Extra-articular forms: grossly well circumscribed with yellow and brown areas (Fig. 11-14B)
■ Expansile sheets of infiltrative cells with intermixed cellular regions and discohesive areas creating blood-filled pseudoalveolar spaces
■ Composed of mixture of background mononuclear cells, variable numbers of giant cells, lipid-laden xanthoma cells, and hemosiderin-laden macrophages
   ■ Giant cells less common than in giant cell tumor of tendon sheath, sparse or absent in up to 20%
   ■ Bimodal mononuclear cells: small histiocyte-like cells and larger dendritic cells
■ Immunohistochemistry
   ■ Mononuclear cells: CD68 positive
   ■ Larger dendritic cells: desmin positive
   ■ Giant cells: CD68, CD45, and TRAP positive

Genetics

■ Chromosome 1p translocations common and similar to giant cell tumor of tendon sheath
■ Trisomies of chromosomes 5 and 7 seen only in PVNS, not in giant cell tumor of tendon sheath

Classification

■ Intra-articular and extra-articular forms

Diagnosis

Clinical Features

■ Usually large and associated with pain, local tenderness, and decreased joint motion
■ Recurrent hemarthroses common

Radiologic Features (Fig. 11-16)

■ Juxta-articular erosions evident in intra-articular form in advanced cases

■ MRI

■ Characteristic hemosiderin attenuation of signal resulting in at least foci of hypointense signal within all sequences
■ Fatty areas due to lipid accumulation
■ Joint effusion

Diagnostic Work-up

■ Usually plain radiographs and MRI are sufficient for these processes.
■ Also see Chapter 2.

Treatment

■ Intra-articular form: arthroscopic or open complete synovectomy; radiosynovectomy or external-beam radiotherapy used in recalcitrant cases
■ Extra-articular form: marginal excision

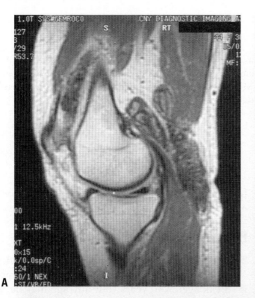
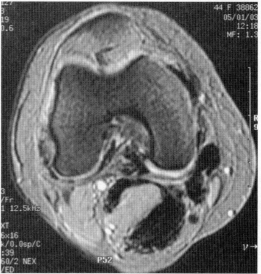
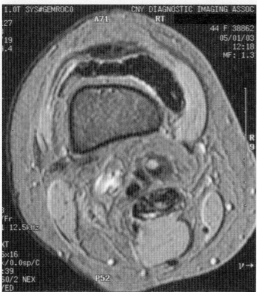

Figure 11-16 Pigmented villonodular synovitis shows characteristic signal attenuation from the hemosiderin deposition within the synovium on all MRI sequences. In this case, low-signal areas can be seen within the suprapatellar pouch and popliteal region on these sagittal T1-weighted (**A**), axial proton density (**B**), and axial T2-weighted (**C**) MR images.

■ Up to 50% recurrence rate in both forms
■ Rare cases of lung involvement (n = 2)

NEURAL BENIGN TUMORS

NEUROFIBROMA AND NEUROFIBROMATOSIS

Neurofibromas are benign peripheral nerve sheath tumors that may occur as solitary lesions or as a component of neurofibromatosis. Neurofibromas are more characteristically intertwined with the peripheral nerve and difficult to separate.

Pathogenesis and Pathophysiology

■ Etiology is unknown.
■ Peak age: young adults 20 to 30 years

Histopathology (*Fig. 11-17*)

■ Mixture of Schwann cells, perineurial-like cells, and fibroblasts
■ Hypocellular, widely spaced cells with thin, elongated nuclei
■ S100 positive

Genetics

■ NF-1 gene mutation in neurofibromatosis (NF)
■ Solitary neurofibromas not as clearly established

Classification (Table 11-3)

■ Localized cutaneous neurofibroma (Fig. 11-18)
  ■ Most common type
  ■ 10% occur in NF-1
■ Diffuse cutaneous neurofibroma
  ■ Plaque-like thickenings of dermis and subcutaneous tissue
■ Localized intraneural neurofibroma (Fig. 11-19)
  ■ Second most common type
  ■ Fusiform segmental enlargement of nerve (Fig. 11-20)

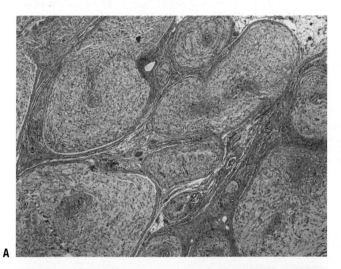

A

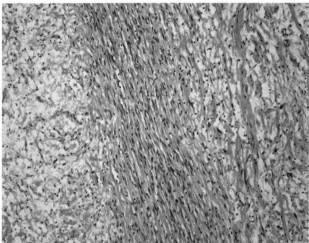

B

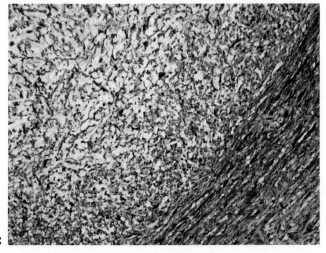

C

Figure 11-17   (A) Cross-section of a plexiform neurofibroma showing its distinctive arrangement in large fascicles. (B) Characteristic neurofibroma with wavy spindle cells in a loose stroma. Toward the center, cells are more tightly apposed, resembling peripheral nerve fibers. (C) Diffuse and strong immunostaining of neurofibroma with S-100 protein stain.

TABLE 11-3 SUBTYPES OF NEUROFIBROMA

Subtype	Depth	Site	Size	Pain?	% in NF-1	Malignant Transformation?
Diffuse cutaneous neurofibroma	Skin and subcutaneous	Any	1 to 2 cm	No	10%	No
Localized cutaneous neurofibroma	Skin and subcutaneous	Head and neck	Several centimeters	No	10%	Rare
Localized intraneural neurofibroma	Superficial or deep	In NF-1, predilection for cervical spine	1 cm to many centimeters	Neural pain if deep	Minority	Infrequent
Plexiform neurofibroma	Usually deep	Predilection for larger nerves	Large	Neural pain	Almost exclusively	Highest
Massive soft tissue neurofibroma	Skin and deeper tissues	Shoulder, pelvis, lower extremity	Large	Variable	100%	Rare

- Plexiform neurofibroma (Fig. 11-21)
  - Uncommon tumor usually affecting large nerve
  - "Bag of worms" appearance in plexus regions (Fig. 11-22)
  - Firm, ropy cylinder in nonbranching nerves
  - Highly suggestive of diagnosis of NF-1
- Massive soft tissue neurofibroma (Fig. 11-24)
  - Least common form always seen in NF-1
  - Formerly called "elephantiasis neuromatosa"
  - Localized gigantism or massive regional tissue enlargement

Diagnosis

- See Chapter 2 for diagnostic work-up.

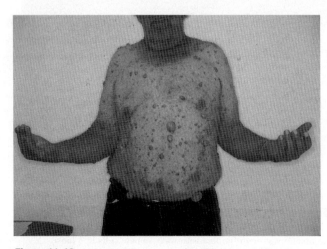

Figure 11-18 Localized cutaneous neurofibromas, as shown in this patient with type I neurofibromatosis, are the most common type of neurofibroma.

Clinical Features

- Solitary painless or painful masses or in the setting of NF-1 (von Recklinghausen's disease)
- Intraneural neurofibromas may cause pain or paresthesias along distribution of affected nerve.
  - Tinel's sign may be positive.
  - More medial–lateral movement than proximal–distal on palpation

Radiologic Features

- MRI features may be highly suggestive of benign peripheral nerve sheath tumors.
  - Target sign more frequent with neurofibromas than schwannomas (Fig. 11-25)
  - Dark on T1-weighted images, bright on T2-weighted images
- Dumbbell tumors (partially intraspinal and partially extraspinal) may cause foraminal enlargement.

Treatment

- Localized cutaneous neurofibroma and diffuse cutaneous neurofibroma
  - Excision usually curative
  - No neurological deficit expected
- Localized intraneural neurofibroma and plexiform neurofibroma
  - Avoid resection due to need to resect functional nerve fibers.
  - Indications for excision: suspicion for malignant degeneration
    - Rapid increase in size
    - Pain
- Massive soft tissue neurofibroma
  - May be amenable only to debulking

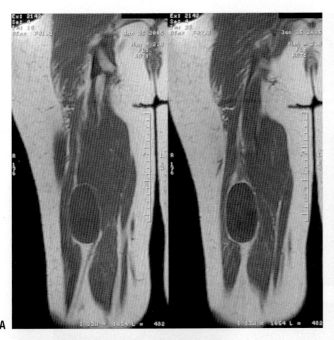

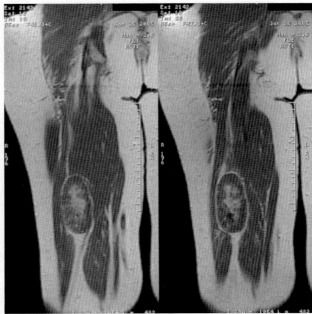

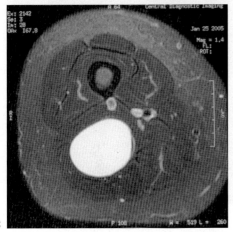

Figure 11-19   Localized intraneural neurofibroma is usually recognizable as a benign peripheral nerve sheath tumor, but it may be difficult to distinguish from a schwannoma. This case shows a discrete enhancing mass in continuity with deep nerve fibers on coronal T1-weighted (**A**), post-gadolinium T1-weighted (**B**), and axial T2-weighted (**C**) images. Although these features could be seen with either neurofibroma or schwannoma, this tumor was found to be a neurofibroma histologically.

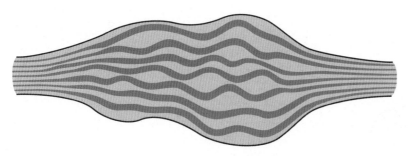

Figure 11-20   Schematic shows appearance of an intraneural neurofibroma, where normal nerve fibers entering and exiting the tumor are intimately intertwined with those of the neurofibroma.

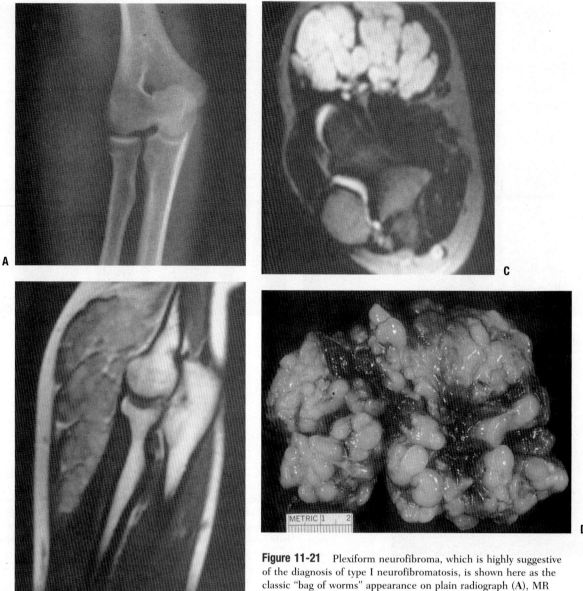

Figure 11-21   Plexiform neurofibroma, which is highly suggestive of the diagnosis of type I neurofibromatosis, is shown here as the classic "bag of worms" appearance on plain radiograph (**A**), MR images (**B,C**), and gross resected specimen (**D**).

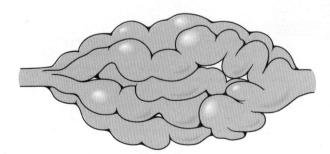

Figure 11-22   Schematic shows typical "bag of worms" appearance of a plexiform neurofibroma.

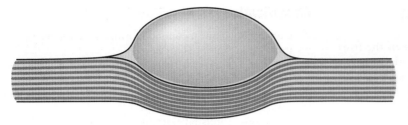

Figure 11-23 Schematic shows typical eccentric position of a neurilemoma, where normal nerve fibers are displaced peripherally by the mass.

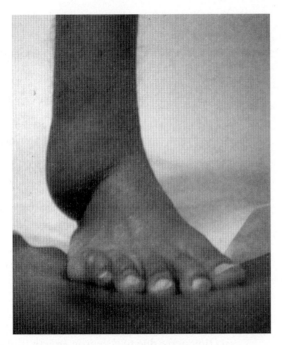

Figure 11-24 Massive soft tissue neurofibroma is manifest in this leg as a bag-like collection.

Figure 11-25 (**A**) The target sign of peripheral nerve sheath tumors on an axial MR image for a neurofibroma, which more commonly shows this sign than does schwannoma. Coronal T1-weighted (**B**) and T2-weighted (**C**) images.

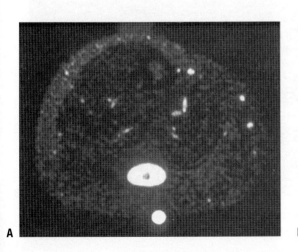

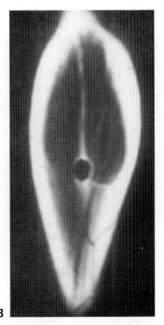

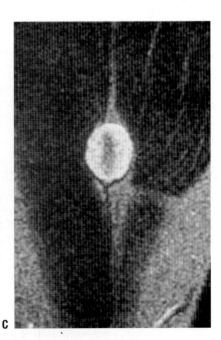

A   B   C

SCHWANNOMA (NEURILEMOMA)

Schwannoma is, along with neurofibroma, one of the two most common benign peripheral nerve sheath tumors. While there are four histological variants, this section will concentrate on the conventional schwannoma.

Pathogenesis and Pathophysiology

- Etiology is unknown.
- Peak ages: third to sixth decades
- A schwannoma is a neoplasm composed of Schwann cells, and its immunohistochemical and ultrastructural profile reflects that.

Histopathology (Fig. 11-26)
- Biphasic Antoni A and B areas
  - Antoni A pattern
    - Collagenous background
    - Compact, elongated spindle cells aligned in bundles
    - Verocay bodies: palisaded arrangement of peripheral aligned nuclei surround central eosinophilic cell processes
  - Antoni B pattern
    - Mucopolysaccharide myxoid background
    - Less organized cells with plump nuclei and delicate cobweb-like interconnecting processes
- Cystic degeneration and hemorrhage frequent (formerly termed "ancient schwannoma")
- Immunohistochemistry: S100 positive

Genetics
- Not associated with NF-1 but may be associated with NF-2

Classification

- Conventional: most common form; characterized by Antoni A and Antoni B areas
- Cellular: higher cellularity, mostly Antoni A areas, absent Verocay bodies
- Plexiform: rare variant with intraneural pattern but not usually associated with NF-1
- Melanotic: unusual variant with melanin-producing cells

Diagnosis

- See Chapter 2 for diagnostic work-up.

Clinical Features
- Head and neck, flexor surfaces of extremities (Fig. 11-27)
- Slowly growing masses <10 cm
- May elicit neural symptoms of pain or paresthesias
- Physical examination may show positive Tinel sign, limited proximal–distal mobility.
- Spinal schwannomas usually affect sensory nerves.

Radiologic Features (Fig. 11-28)
- Well-demarcated soft tissue masses on plain x-ray
- MRI heterogeneity related to cystic degeneration
  - Hypointense on T1-weighted images, hyperintense on T2-weighted images
  - Enhancing
- Target sign on MRI less common than neurofibroma
- Foraminal enlargement with dumbbell schwannomas and giant sacral schwannomas

Treatment and Outcome

- Marginal complete excision usually possible without resecting nerve due to eccentric growth (unlike intraneural and plexiform neurofibromas; Fig. 11-23)
- Recurrence unusual except in sacral schwannomas

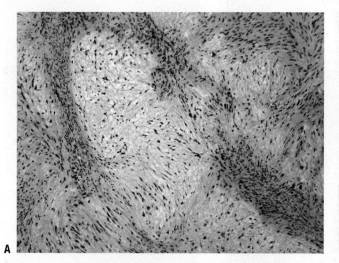
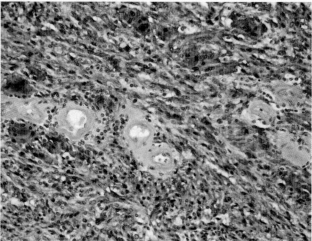

Figure 11-26 (A) Schwannoma with characteristic areas of high cellularity (Antoni A) and low cellularity (Antoni B). Note the palisading of spindle cells known as Verocay bodies. (B) Strong immunoreactivity of schwannoma cells with S-100 protein stain.

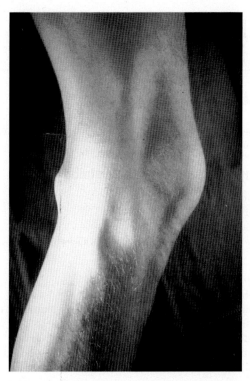

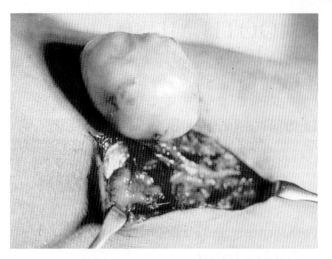

Figure 11-29   The schwannoma is usually easily separable from the associated nerve, unlike the intraneural neurofibroma.

Figure 11-27   Schwannomas of the extremity typically occur on the flexor surface near a joint, such as the knee in this patient.

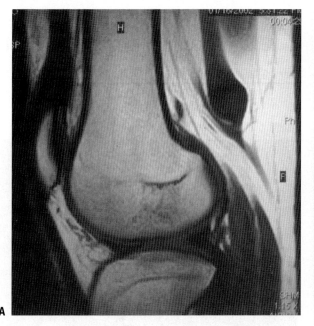

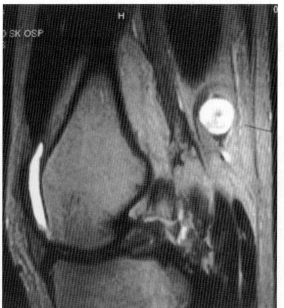

A   B

Figure 11-28   Schwannomas are hypointense to muscle on T1-weighted MR image (**A**) and hyperintense on T2-weighted image (**B**). Note how the nerve fibers splay around the round to oval mass.

SMOOTH MUSCLE BENIGN SOFT TISSUE TUMORS

LEIOMYOMA OF DEEP SOFT TISSUE

Leiomyoma of the soft tissue is a tumor comprising normal-appearing smooth muscle cells, but it is extremely rare in the extra-abdominal soft tissues.

Pathogenesis and Pathophysiology

- ▪ Etiology is unknown.
- ▪ Extremely rare
- ▪ Cells resemble smooth muscle cells with eosinophilic cytoplasm and blunt-ended, cigar-shaped nuclei arranged in intersecting bundles (Fig. 11-30).
- ▪ Immunohistochemistry
  - ▪ Positive for actin, desmin, and h-caldesmon
  - ▪ S100 negative

Diagnosis

- ▪ Clinical features: superficial or deep soft tissue masses
- ▪ Radiologic features: frequently calcified, but otherwise non specific
- ▪ See Chapter 2 for diagnostic work-up.

Treatment and Outcome

- ▪ Marginal excision
- ▪ Local recurrence rate ~3%

SKELETAL MUSCLE BENIGN TUMORS

RHABDOMYOMA

Analogous to leiomyomas, rhabdomyomas are extremely rare tumors of the soft tissue.

Pathogenesis and Pathophysiology

- ▪ Etiology is unknown.
- ▪ Very rare
- ▪ Peak ages:
  - ▪ Adult form: median 60 years (33 to 80 years)
  - ▪ Fetal form: median 4 years

Histopathology (Fig. 11-31)

- ▪ Lobules of closely packed cells
- ▪ Spider cells (large, polygonal cells with abundant eosinophilic cytoplasm)
- ▪ Cytoplasmic inclusion bodies, cross-striations
- ▪ Immunohistochemistry: MSA, desmin, and myoglobulin positive

Classification

- ▪ This section refers only to extracardiac rhabdomyomas at the exclusion of cardiac rhabdomyomas.
- ▪ The extracardiac rhabdomyomas are subdivided into adult and fetal types.

Diagnosis

- ▪ Clinical features: head and neck (90%), soft tissue mass
- ▪ Radiologic features are nonspecific.
- ▪ See Chapter 2 for diagnostic work-up.

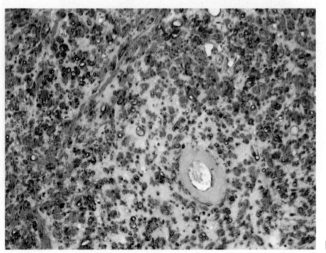

A   B

Figure 11-30   (A) Leiomyoma. Fusiform cells with eosinophilic cytoplasm arranged showing a vague fascicular pattern closely resembling normal smooth muscle. (B) Strong and diffuse reactivity for smooth muscle actin stain in leiomyoma.

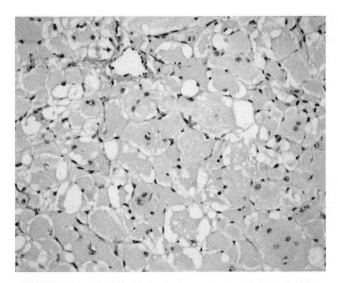

Figure 11-31   Rhabdomyoma. Solid growth of closely packed, large polygonal cells with abundant eosinophilic or granular cytoplasm and eccentrically located nuclei.

Treatment and Outcome

■ Marginal excision
■ Up to 42% local recurrence

VASCULAR BENIGN SOFT TISSUE TUMORS

HEMANGIOMAS

Hemangiomas, which are most commonly seen in the skin, are seen in the orthopaedic context predominately as intra-muscular angiomas or less commonly as synovial hemangiomas.

Pathogenesis and Pathophysiology

■ Although theories of neoplasm, reactive processes, and malformations have been put forth, these are currently thought to most likely be simply malformations.

Epidemiology

■ Intramuscular angiomas are among the most common of soft tissue tumors, particularly in adolescents and young adults, while the other variants are uncommon to rare.
■ Intramuscular angiomas have a female predominance.

Histopathology (Fig. 11-32)

■ Various combinations of variably thick-walled vascular channels with hemosiderin deposition
■ Variable amounts of fatty tissue within intramuscular angiomas

Classification (Table 11-4)

■ Synovial hemangioma
■ Intramuscular angioma
■ Venous hemangioma
■ Arteriovenous hemangiomas

Diagnosis

Clinical Features

■ Intramuscular angioma causes classic activity-related fluctuation in size and pain even over the course of a single day.
  ■ Spongiform, compressible mass
  ■ Slowly enlarging
■ Arteriovenous malformations result in shunting.

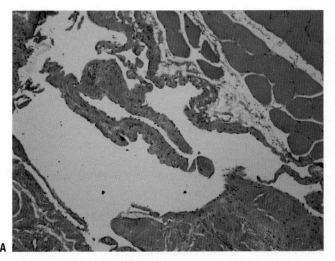
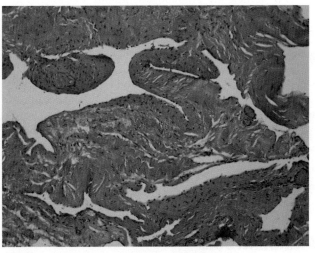

A   B

Figure 11-32   (A) Intramuscular hemangioma. Large vascular channels lined by flat endothelial cells surrounded by skeletal muscle. (B) Hemangioma. Cavernous vascular spaces lined by flat endothelial cells and focally containing red blood cells.

TABLE 11-4 FEATURES OF HEMANGIOMA SUBTYPES

Hemangioma Subtype	Peak Age	Occurrence	Most Common Location	Clinical Symptoms
Synovial hemangioma	Children and adolescents	Rare	Knee	Joint swelling and pain, mechanical symptoms
Intramuscular angioma	Adolescents and young adults	Common	Deep, thigh	Activity-related pain and swelling
Venous hemangioma	Adults	Uncommon	Superficial or deep, extremities	Soft tissue mass
Arteriovenous hemangioma	Children and young adults	Uncommon	Superficial or deep, head and neck > extremities	Shunting manifestations

- Physical examination reveals audible bruit, palpable thrill.
- Clinical manifestations of shunting: limb hypertrophy, heart failure, consumption coagulopathy (Kasabach-Merritt syndrome)

Radiologic Features (Fig. 11-33)
- Plain radiographs may reveal phleboliths.
- MRI findings typically diagnostic
  - Characteristic serpentine pattern of blood vessels
  - Intermediate on T1-weighted images, bright on T2-weighted images; heterogeneous
  - Intermixed fatty signal on established lesions

Diagnostic Work-up
- Clinical examination combined with plain radiographs and MRI is usually diagnostic and obviates the need for biopsy except in unusual circumstances.
- Also see Chapter 2.

Treatment and Outcome

- Only sufficiently symptomatic lesions warrant treatment consideration; the remainder should be observed or treated with nonsteroidal anti-inflammatory medications and compressive devices.
- Surgical excision
  - Small synovial and intramuscular hemangiomas amenable to marginal *en bloc* excision
  - Especially if single expendable muscle involved
- Embolization and sclerotherapy
  - Larger lesions for which surgical excision is not feasible but sufficiently symptomatic to warrant treatment
  - Contraindicated if neurologic symptoms or compression
- Recurrence rate 30% to 50% following excision unless entire involved muscle excised

ANGIOMATOSIS

Angiomatosis represents involvement of a large segment of the body by hemangioma(s). This may manifest as extensive muscle involvement or involvement of multiple tissue levels, including skin, subcutaneous tissue, muscle, and bone.

Pathogenesis and Pathophysiology

- Etiology is unknown.
- Peak age: adolescents and young adults
- Histopathology is same as for hemangioma.

Diagnosis

- See Chapter 2 for diagnostic work-up.

Clinical Features
- Common sites: lower extremity > chest wall > upper extremity
- Skin involvement may be evident by varicosities.
- Same symptoms as described for hemangioma

Radiologic Features
- Same as for hemangiomas but more extensive (Fig. 11-34)

Treatment and Outcome

- Often too extensive for adequate excision
- High rate of local recurrence following attempted excision

LYMPHANGIOMA

Lymphangioma, also referred to as cystic hygroma, is similar to hemangioma except in its absence of blood components.

Pathogenesis and Pathophysiology

- Etiology is unknown.
- Peak age: birth to childhood
- Histopathology: variably sized, thin-walled lymphatic vessels (Fig. 11-35)
- Genetics: associated with Turner syndrome

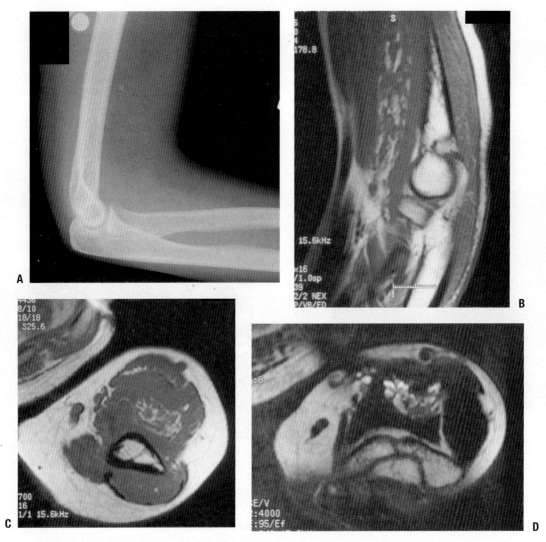

Figure 11-33 This intramuscular hemangioma of the proximal forearm shows classic radiographic features. Phleboliths can be seen on the plain radiograph (**A**), and the sagittal (**B**) and axial (**C**) T1-weighted MR images and axial T2-weighted (**D**) MR image show serpiginous vascular structures intermixed with fat signal.

Classification

■ Cystic versus cavernous subtypes

Diagnosis

■ See Chapter 2 for diagnostic work-up.

Clinical Features
■ Cystic: neck, axilla, groin
■ Cavernous: upper trunk, extremities

Radiologic Features
■ Cystic signal characteristics with nonenhancing, fluid-filled, well-defined structures on MRI
■ Cystic structures on ultrasound

Treatment and Outcome

■ Marginal excision
■ High rate of local recurrence

PERIVASCULAR BENIGN SOFT TISSUE TUMORS

GLOMUS TUMORS

Glomus tumors are tumors of the smooth muscle cells that make up the normal glomus body and are characterized best by their clinical presentation as small painful nodules predominately found in a subungual location.

Pathogenesis and Pathophysiology

■ Etiology unknown
■ Peak age: young adults predominate
■ Subungual lesions more common in women

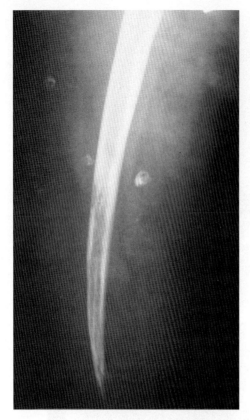

Figure 11-34 Angiomatosis involves multiple tissue levels within a large segment of or an entire limb. This patient had undergone amputation for complications of angiomatosis of the lower extremity. Note the phleboliths within the soft tissues and involvement of the bone as well.

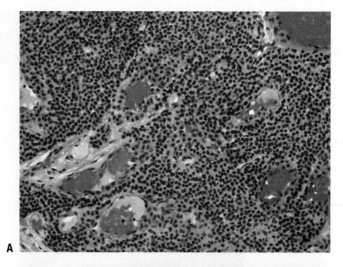

A

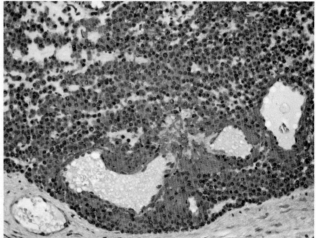

B

Figure 11-36 (A) Glomus tumor. Nests of small, uniform, round cells with centrally located nucleus and amphophilic or slightly eosinophilic cytoplasm surrounded by capillary blood vessels. (B) Glomus tumor showing strong immunoreactivity with smooth muscle actin stain.

Histopathology (Fig. 11-36)
- Three components in varying amounts
  - Glomus cells
    - Small, uniformly round cells
    - Centrally placed round nuclei
    - Prominent cell membranes define cytoplasm.
  - Vascular structures
  - Smooth muscle cells

Genetics
- Familial cases: autosomal dominant pattern of inheritance
- Subungual glomus tumors associated with NF-I

Classification

- Typical glomus tumors have three histologic variants:
  - Solid glomus tumor: glomus cells predominate
  - Glomangioma: vascular structures predominate

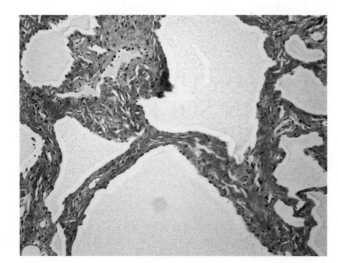

Figure 11-35 Lymphangioma. Thin-walled vascular channels lined by flat endothelial cells and filled by proteinaceous material.

- Glomangiomyoma: smooth muscle cells predominate
- Glomangiomatosis: extremely rare clinical variant similar to angiomatosis but characterized by glomus histology
- Symplastic glomus tumors: rare histologic variant with atypia but benign behavior
- Malignant glomus tumors: 1% of glomus tumors

Diagnosis

- See Chapter 2 for diagnostic work-up.

Clinical Features
- Subungual region (hand, wrist, foot) predominates.
- Superficial in vast majority
- Small reddish-blue nodules
- Associated with chronic pain in severe paroxysms
- Exposure to cold or minor pressure often exacerbates pain.

Radiologic Features
- Ultrasound may detect tumors as small as 3 mm.
- MRI: bright on T2-weighted images, dark on T1-weighted images; enhancing

Treatment and Outcome

- Complete excision is the only treatment.
- Local recurrence in 5% to 50%

CHONDRO-OSSEOUS BENIGN SOFT TISSUE TUMORS

SOFT TISSUE CHONDROMA

Soft tissue chondroma, otherwise known as chondroma of the soft parts, is an extraosseous, extrasynovial mature hyaline cartilage tumor.

Pathogenesis and Pathophysiology

- Etiology is unknown.
- Peak age: middle-aged (may involve any age)
- Histopathology: mature hyaline cartilage lobules, S100 positive (Fig. 11-37)
- Genetics: 12q13-15 structural rearrangements involving HMGA2 gene locus

Classification

- Chondroblastic chondroma: chondrocytic cells in lacunae predominate

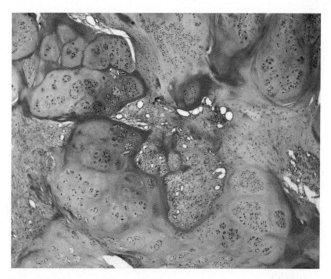

Figure 11-37 Soft tissue chondroma composed of well-defined lobules of mature cartilage embedded in a fibrous stroma.

- Fibrochondroma: prominent fibrosis
- Osteochondroma of soft tissue: prominent ossification centrally
- Myxochondroma: prominent myxoid change

Diagnosis

- See Chapter 2 for diagnostic work-up.

Clinical Features
- Fingers (two thirds), hands, toes, feet predominate.
- Painless small lumps rarely >3 cm

Radiologic Features
- Plain films show variable mineralization.
- MRI shows hyaline cartilage signal (lobulated, dark on T1-weighted images, bright on T2-weighted images).

Treatment and Outcome

- Marginal excision
- Recurrence unusual

TUMORS OF UNCERTAIN DIFFERENTIATION

INTRAMUSCULAR MYXOMA

Intramuscular myxoma is a benign, low-cellularity myxoid tumor characterized clinically by its somewhat distinctive radiographic appearance in showing very hypointense signal compared to muscle on T1-weighted MRI. It may occur as a solitary soft tissue mass or may be accompanied by fibrous dysplasia lesions, as in Mazabraud syndrome.

Pathogenesis and Pathophysiology

■ Etiology is unknown.
■ Peak age: 40 to 70 years

Histopathology (Fig. 11-38)
■ Uniformly bland cellularity with small bland spindle cells
■ Bland extracellular myxoid background
■ Infiltrating borders

Genetics
■ Point mutations in GNAS1 gene common both in Mazabraud syndrome and isolated myxomas

Classification

■ Cellular myxoma: histologic variant with increased cellularity and vascularity

Diagnosis

Clinical Features
■ Deep, painless soft tissue mass
■ Thigh, shoulder, buttocks, upper arm
■ Usually 5 to 10 cm
■ Mazabraud syndrome: myxomas and fibrous dysplasia (monostotic, polyostotic, or Albright syndrome)

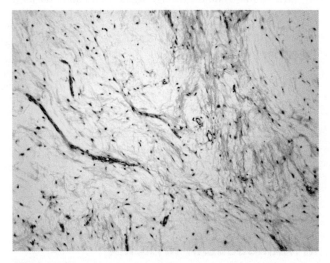

Figure 11-38 Intramuscular myxoma. Hypocellular neoplasm composed of very bland-looking spindle cells in an abundant myxoid background.

Radiologic Features (Fig. 11-39)
■ Homogenous, hypointense to muscle on T1-weighted images, hyperintense on T2-weighted images
■ Variable patterns of enhancement (peripheral and/or central) dependent on cellularity
■ Peritumoral edema and fat cap

Diagnostic Work-up
■ This process may be highly suspected based on MRI, so biopsy may be unnecessary.
■ Also see Chapter 2.

Treatment and Outcome

■ Marginal excision
■ Recurrence unlikely

JUXTA-ARTICULAR MYXOMA

The juxta-articular myxoma arises close to large joints and frequently has associated cystic changes.

Pathogenesis and Pathophysiology

■ Etiology is unknown.
■ Peak age: range 9 to 83 years

Histopathology
■ Similar to cellular myxoma variant of intramuscular myxoma
  ■ Bland spindle cells
  ■ Myxoid background
■ Cystic-like ganglion spaces

Genetics
■ Lacks the GNAS1 mutations seen in intramuscular myxomas

Diagnosis

■ See Chapter 2 for diagnostic work-up.

Clinical Features
■ Frequently painful or tender soft tissue mass
■ Present for weeks to years
■ May be associated with meniscal tear
■ May be incidental finding during knee or hip arthroplasty

Radiologic Features
■ Similar to intramuscular myxoma
■ Distinguished by juxta-articular location

Treatment and Outcome

■ Marginal excision
■ Local recurrence in up to one third

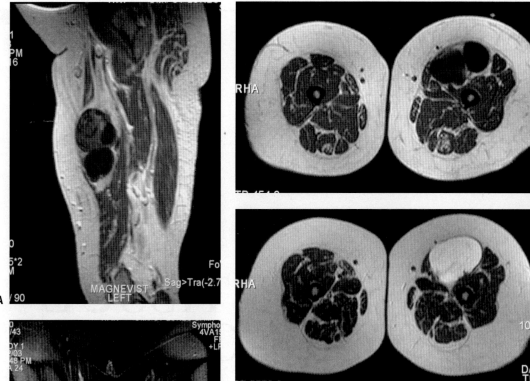

Figure 11-39 This intramuscular myxoma within the quadriceps shows characteristically hypointense signal on T1-weighted sagittal (**A**) and axial (**C**) MRI sequences and hyperintense signal on T2-weighted coronal (**B**) and axial (**D**) sequences.

SUGGESTED READING

Aflatoon K, Aboulafia AJ, McCarthy EF Jr, et al. Pediatric soft tissue tumors. *J Am Acad Orthop Surg* 2003;11(5):332–343.

Ballo MT, Zagars GK, Pollack A, et al. Desmoid tumor: prognostic factors and outcome after surgery, radiation therapy, or combined surgery and radiation therapy. *J Clin Oncol* 1999;17(1):158–167.

Bos GD, Esther RJ, Woll TS. Foot tumors: diagnosis and treatment. *J Am Acad Orthop Surg* 2002;10(4):259–270.

Butler MG, Fuchigami KD, Chako A. MRI of posterior knee masses. *Skeletal Radiol* 1996;25(4):309–317.

Carr MM, Mahoney JL, Bowen CV. Extremity arteriovenous malformations: review of a series. *Can J Surg* 1994;37(4):293–299.

Damron TA, Beauchamp CP, Rougraff BT, et al. Soft tissue lumps and bumps. *AAOS Instr Course Lect* 2004;53:625–637.

Forthman CL, Blazar PE. Nerve tumors of the hand and upper extremity. *Hand Clin* 2004;20(3):233–242.

Goy BW, Lee SP, Eilber F, et al. The role of adjuvant radiotherapy in the treatment of resectable desmoid tumors. *Int J Radiat Oncol Biol Phys* 1997;39(3):659–665.

Kim DH, Murovic JA, Tiel RL, et al. A series of 397 peripheral neural sheath tumors: 30-year experience at Louisiana State University Health Sciences Center. *J Neurosurg* 2005;102(2):246–255.

Kransdorf MJ, Murphey MD, Smith SE. Imaging of soft tissue neoplasms in the adult: benign tumors. *Semin Musculoskelet Radiol* 1999;3(1):21–38.

Laor T. MR imaging of soft tissue tumors and tumor-like lesions. *Pediatr Radiol* 2004;34(1):24–37.

Merchant NB, Lewis JJ, Woodruff JM, et al. Extremity and trunk desmoid tumors: a multifactorial analysis of outcome. *Cancer* 1999; 86(10):2045–2052.

Murphey MD, Carroll JF, Flemming DJ, et al. From the archives of the AFIP: benign musculoskeletal lipomatous lesions. *Radiographics* 2004;24(5):1433–1466.

Pakos EE, Tsekeris PG, Goussia AC. Desmoid tumours of the extremities and trunk: a review of the literature. *Int Orthop* 2005;29(4): 210–213.

Rogalski R, Hensinger R, Loder R. Vascular abnormalities of the extremities: clinical findings and management. *J Pediatr Orthop* 1993; 13(1):9–14.

Tang P, Hornicek FJ, Gebhardt MC, et al. Surgical treatment of hemangiomas of soft tissue. *Clin Orthop Relat Res* 2002;(399): 205–210.

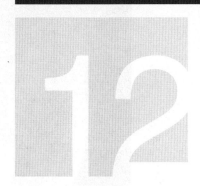

SOFT TISSUE SARCOMAS

CAROL D. MORRIS

Soft tissue sarcomas are malignant neoplasms that arise in nonepithelial extraskeletal tissue (e.g., fat, muscle, fibrous structures, etc.) of mesenchymal origin. They account for less than 1% of all cancers, with approximately 8,000 to 9,000 diagnosed annually in the United States. Benign soft tissue tumors outnumber malignant ones by a factor of at least 100. More than 50 histologic subtypes of soft tissue sarcoma are recognized (Table 12-1).

Soft tissue sarcomas can occur anywhere in the body, though the majority occur in the extremities (50% to 75%). Ten percent occur on the trunk. As with other malignancies, soft tissue sarcoma tends to occur in older individuals, with a median age of 65, although there are subtype-related variations in peak age. For example, embryonal rhabdomyosarcoma occurs almost exclusively in children (<10 years old), synovial sarcoma occurs in young adults (20 to 40 years old), and pleomorphic sarcoma and liposarcoma occur in older adults (>60 years old). Approximately 10% of patients have clinically detectable metastases at presentation, usually in the lung.

The management of soft tissue sarcoma requires a multidisciplinary approach that includes surgery, radiation therapy, and chemotherapy. Treatment plans are best coordinated and administered when possible by specialty centers with expertise in treating the disease. The overall 5-year survival for patients with soft tissue sarcoma is largely dependent on the stage of disease. This, in turn, is determined by a combination of factors that include the grade, size, and location of the tumor. Using the four-tiered staging system of the American Joint Committee on Cancer (AJCC), 5-year survival rates are approximately 90% for stage I, 70% for stage II, 50% for stage III, and 10% to 20% for stage IV.

This chapter will review the rationale and outcomes for the management of soft tissue sarcoma with current treatment paradigms. In addition, the clinical and histopathologic presentation of the more common soft tissue sarcomas likely to be encountered in practice and on examinations will be discussed.

PATHOGENESIS

The etiology of soft tissue sarcoma is largely unknown. While numerous genetic aberrations continue to be identified, the clinical significance of these is still being elucidated. The more consistent genetic findings are outlined in connection with individual tumor types.

Etiology
- Largely unknown
- Chemical carcinogens
  - Increased incidence reported after exposure to dioxins (herbicides)
  - Controversial
- Radiation
  - Termed "post-radiation" or "radiation-induced" sarcoma
  - More common in women, reflecting the distribution of conditions for which radiation is widely used: breast cancer, genitourinary cancers
  - Risk increases with dose, with most patients having received at least 50 Gy.

TABLE 12-1 WHO CLASSIFICATION OF MALIGNANT SOFT TISSUE TUMORS

Adipocytic tumors	Atypical lipomatous tumor/well-differentiated liposarcoma Dedifferentiated liposarcoma Myxoid liposarcoma Round cell liposarcoma Pleomorphic liposarcoma Mixed-type liposarcoma Liposarcoma, not otherwise specified
Fibroblastic/myofibroblastic	Solitary fibrous tumor and hemangiopericytoma Inflammatory myofibroblastic tumor Low-grade myofibroblastic sarcoma Myxoinflammatory fibroblastic sarcoma Infantile fibrosarcoma Adult fibrosarcoma Myxofibrosarcoma Low-grade fibromyxoid sarcoma Hyalinizing spindle cell tumor Sclerosing epithelioid fibrosarcoma

Fibrohistiocytic tumors	Undifferentiated pleomorphic sarcoma
	  Pleomorphic malignant fibrous histiocytoma (MFH)
	  Giant cell MFH
	  Inflammatory MFH
	  Not otherwise specified

Smooth muscle tumors	Leiomyosarcoma
Skeletal muscle tumors	Embryonal rhabdomyosarcoma (including spindle cell, botryoid, anaplastic) Alveolar rhabdomyosarcoma (including solid, anaplastic) Pleomorphic rhabdomyosarcoma
Vascular tumors	Retiform hemangioendothelioma Papillary intralymphatic angioendothelioma Composite hemangioendothelioma Kaposi sarcoma Epithelioid hemangioendothelioma Angiosarcoma of soft tissue
Chondro-osseous tumors	Mesenchymal chondrosarcoma Extraskeletal osteosarcoma
Tumors of peripheral nerves	Malignant peripheral nerve sheath tumor (MSNST)
Tumors of uncertain differentiation	Synovial sarcoma Epithelioid sarcoma Alveolar soft part sarcoma Clear cell sarcoma of soft tissue Extraskeletal myxoid chondrosarcoma ("chordoid" type) Primitive neuroectodermal tumor/ extraskeletal Ewing tumor Desmoplastic small round cell tumor Extrarenal rhabdoid tumor Malignant mesenchymoma Neoplasms with perivascular epithelioid cell differentiation (PEComa) Clear cell myomelanocytic tumor Intimal sarcoma

- Median time between exposure and tumor development is ~10 years.
- More common in patients with germline mutations
- Viral and immunological factors
  - Increased incidence of sarcomas in immunocompromised individuals
    - Immunodeficiency syndromes
    - Therapeutic immunosuppression associated with organ transplantation
    - Stewart-Treves syndrome: an acquired "regional" immunodeficiency of the edematous upper extremity in breast cancer patients following radical mastectomy associated with lymphangiosarcoma
  - Oncogenic viruses
    - Human herpes virus 8 associated with Kaposi sarcoma
    - Epstein-Barr virus associated with leiomyosarcomas
- Genetic predisposition
  - Neurofibromatosis-1 associated with malignant peripheral nerve sheath tumors (MPNST)
  - Li-Fraumeni syndrome: germline mutation in *p53* suppressor gene
  - Hereditary retinoblastoma: germline mutation of *RB1* locus

Epidemiology

- Approximately 8,700 new cases diagnosed annually in the United States
- Annual incidence is 1.5 per 100,000 individuals
  - 8 per 100,000 in individuals greater than 80 years old
- Slight male predominance
- No proven racial variation

Classification

Soft tissue sarcomas are a highly heterogeneous group of tumors that are most commonly classified on a histological basis according to the tissue they most resemble. The most widely recognized classification system is that of the World Health Organization (WHO), which was first published in 1969 and most recently updated in 2002 (see Table 12-1).

Staging

- Staging systems incorporate histological and clinical information for prognostic value.
- The staging system used throughout this chapter is the AJCC staging system (Table 12-2).
  - 75% of soft tissue sarcomas are high grade.
  - One third of soft tissue sarcomas are superficial and two thirds are deep.

DIAGNOSIS

- The diagnosis of soft tissue sarcoma is made with a combination of a good history and physical examination, appropriate radiology imaging, and biopsy.
- The pertinent components of the history and physical examination as well as the clinical and radiologic features are detailed in Chapter 2.

Clinical Findings

- Summary of clinical features and examination findings:
  - Most soft tissue sarcomas are painless.
  - Masses that are suspicious for sarcoma:
    - >5 cm regardless of location
    - Deep to fascia
    - Firm or fixed
    - Enlarging
  - Clinical features of tumors with advanced size
    - Distal edema
    - Nerve compression
    - Bladder symptoms (pelvic sarcomas)
  - Metastatic disease
    - 10% of patients present with metastatic disease.
    - Lung is the most common metastatic site.
    - Bone (6%) and lymph node (3%) metastases are less common.

TABLE 12-2 AMERICAN JOINT COMMITTEE ON CANCER (AJCC) STAGING SYSTEM FOR SOFT TISSUE SARCOMA

Stage	Size	Depth*	Grade	Metastases
I	Any	Any	Low	No
II	<5 cm, any depth *or* >5 cm, superficial		High	No
III	>5 cm	Deep	High	No
IV	Any	Any	Any	Yes

*Depth is termed superficial (above the deep fascia) or deep (deep to the deep fascia). Retroperitoneal tumors are considered deep.
From American Joint Committee on Cancer (AJCC) Staging System for Soft Tissue Sarcoma, 6th ed.

Radiologic Findings

- Necessary imaging
  - Chest x-ray
  - Computed tomography (CT) of chest: preferred for detection of metastases
  - Magnetic resonance imaging (MRI) of primary site
    - CT with contrast substituted in patients with contraindication for MRI
    - CT often preferred for intra-abdominal tumors
  - Role of positron emission tomography (PET) scan unclear

Other Diagnostic Tests

- Histologic analysis of tissue is required for staging and should be performed prior to initiating any treatment, with rare exceptions.
- A good biopsy is the first step in a successful limb salvage operation.
- Diagnostic tissue can be obtained by the following methods:
  - Needle
    - Fine-needle aspiration (FNA)
    - Core
  - Open incision
  - Open excisional
- The advantages and disadvantages of each type of biopsy are discussed in Chapter 3, Biopsy of Musculoskeletal Tumors.

Diagnostic Tools

- Numerous investigative tools are available to the pathologist to assist in the diagnosis of specific sarcoma subtypes (Tables 12-3 and 12-4).

TREATMENT

Soft tissue sarcoma is treated with an interdisciplinary approach that incorporates surgery, radiation, and chemotherapy. The details, rationale, and outcomes for each of these modalities are reviewed in Chapter 4, Treatment Principles. The following is a summary.

Surgery

- Complete surgical excision is the main cornerstone of treatment.
- Often curative for localized disease
- Limb salvage is the preferred method.
- Amputation is ultimately required in 5% to 10% of patients.

Radiation

- Methods of delivery
  - External beam (pre-, post-, and intraoperation)
  - Brachytherapy

TABLE 12-3 COMMON IMMUNOHISTOCHEMISTRY STAINS AND TISSUE DISTRIBUTION

Tissue	Representative Sarcomas	Antigen Stains
Mesenchymal tissue	All soft tissue sarcomas	Vimentin
Skeletal muscle	Rhabdomyosarcoma	Actin Desmin Myosin Myogenin MyoD
Smooth muscle	Leiomyosarcoma	Smooth muscle antigen (SMA) Desmin
Epithelium	Synovial sarcoma Epithelioid sarcoma	Epithelial membrane antigen (EMA) Cytokeratin
Neural, uncertain differentiation	Malignant peripheral nerve sheath tumor Clear cell sarcoma Extraskeletal myxoid chondrosarcoma (variable)	S-100
Endothelium	Angiosarcoma (all) Epithelioid Hemangioendothelioma (CD31, CD34) Hemangiopericytoma (CD34)	CD34 CD31 Factor VIII (von Willebrand's factor)

TABLE 12-4 CHROMOSOMAL TRANSLOCATIONS IN SOFT TISSUE SARCOMA

Tumor Type	Translocation	Involved Genes
Ewing/primitive neuroectodermal tumor	11;22	*FLI1, EWS*
Clear cell sarcoma	12;22	*ATF1, EWS*
Extraskeletal myxoid chondrosarcoma	9;22	*CHN, EWS*
Synovial sarcoma	X;18	*SSX1 or SSX2, SYT*
Myxoid liposarcoma	12;16	*CHOP, TLS*
Alveolar rhabdomyosarcoma	2;13	*PAX3, FKHR*
Alveolar soft part sarcoma	X;17	*TFE3, ASPL*
Dermatofibrosarcoma protuberans (DFSP)	17;22	*COL1A1, PDGFB1*

■ Typical dose ~6,000 cGy
■ Primarily indicated for:
    ■ High-grade tumors (unless margins are very wide)
    ■ Intermediate-grade tumors with close margins
    ■ Large tumors
    ■ Recurrent disease
■ Improves local control by 20% to 35%

Chemotherapy

■ Indicated for patients at the highest risk of developing metastatic disease or patients with metastatic disease
■ Best administered in the setting of a clinical trial
■ Doxorubicin-based therapy is associated with a minimal improvement in overall survival (<10%).
■ Ifosfamide-based therapy is associated with moderately improved survival at intermediate follow-up; long-term results are unknown.

Results and Outcome

The outcome of patients with soft tissue sarcoma is multifactorial but largely dependent on the stage of disease. The overall survival for all patients with soft tissue sarcoma is approximately 70%. Using the four-tiered staging system of the AJCC, 5-year survival rates are approximately 90% for stage I, 70% for stage II, 50% for stage III, and 10% to 20% for stage IV.

■ Negative prognostic factors
    ■ Metastatic disease
    ■ High histologic grade
    ■ Size >10 cm
    ■ Bone and neurovascular invasion
    ■ Advanced age
    ■ Retroperitoneal and visceral location
    ■ Positive microscopic surgical margins
    ■ Presentation with locally recurrent disease

ADIPOCYTIC TUMORS

Well-Differentiated Liposarcoma

■ Synonym: atypical lipomatous tumor

Pathogenesis
■ No potential for metastasis unless it undergoes dedifferentiation (<2% in the extremity, ~20% in retroperitoneum)
■ Locally aggressive nature can cause symptoms and even death when complete excision is not possible, as in the retroperitoneum and mediastinum.
■ Genetics: ring chromosome 12 with amplification of the *MDM2* gene

Epidemiology
■ Frequency: accounts for 40% to 45% of all liposarcomas
■ Age: incidence peaks during sixth decade of life
■ Site: most commonly occurs in the thigh

Classification
■ Subtypes: lipoma-like, sclerosing, inflammatory, and spindle cell

Diagnosis
■ Histology: mature adipocytic tissue with slight atypia and scattered to rare lipoblasts (Fig. 12-1)

Myxoid Liposarcoma

■ Synonyms: round cell liposarcoma, myxoid/round cell liposarcoma

Pathogenesis
■ Tendency for extrapulmonary metastases (soft tissue and bone, especially the spine)
■ Multifocal presentation not uncommon
■ Genetics: >90% of cases associated with t(12:16)(q13;p11) leading to the *TLS/CHOP* fusion protein; t(12;22) has been described less frequently

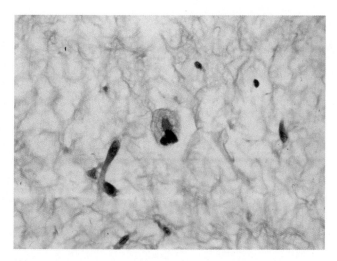

Figure 12-1 Well differentiated liposarcoma; relatively mature adipocytic tissue with varying cell size admixed with hyperchromatic and multinucleated stromal cells.

Epidemiology
- Frequency: accounts for about one third of all liposarcomas
- Age: incidence peaks during the fourth and fifth decades of life
- Site: most commonly arises in the deep tissues of the thigh

Classification
- Grade is often equated to the size of the round cell component, usually expressed as a percentage (>5% round cells = high grade).

Diagnosis
- Myxoid component is characterized histologically by mixture of lipoblasts and uniform nonlipogenic mesenchymal cells in prominent myxoid stroma associated with a fine capillary network (Fig. 12-2).

- Round cell component is characterized histologically by more cellular regions of round cells (see Fig. 12-2).

FIBROBLASTIC/MYOFIBROBLASTIC TUMORS

Hemangiopericytoma
- Historically evolving term used to refer to neoplasms with a thin-walled branching vascular pattern; its current status as a discrete entity is controversial, as the pattern appears within numerous other types of tumors
- Synonym: extrapleural solitary fibrous tumor

Pathogenesis
- Genetics: breakpoints in chromosomes 12 and 19 reported but sporadic
- May cause hypoglycemia due to secretion of insulin-like growth factor

Epidemiology
- Age: occurs in middle-aged adults, most often in the pelvic retroperitoneum

Diagnosis
- Characterized histologically by monomorphic, evenly distributed cellularity arranged around thin-walled vessels with a staghorn pattern (Fig. 12-3)
- Immunohistochemistry: positive for CD34

Adult Fibrosarcoma
Pathogenesis
- Genetics: inconsistent aberrations

Epidemiology
- Frequency: accounts for 1% to 3% of all soft tissue sarcomas
- Age: occurs in middle-aged and older adults
- Site: most commonly affects the trunk, head, and neck

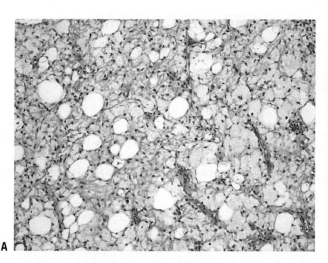
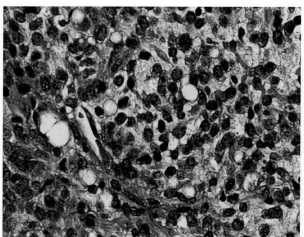

Figure 12-2 (A) Myxoid liposarcoma. Mixture of lipoblasts and uniform nonlipogenic mesenchymal cells in prominent myxoid stroma associated with a fine capillary network. (B) High-grade myxoid liposarcoma with a predominant round cell component.

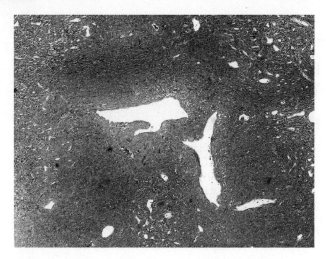

Figure 12-3 Hemangiopericytoma. Monomorphic evenly distributed cellularity arranged around thin-walled vessels with a staghorn pattern.

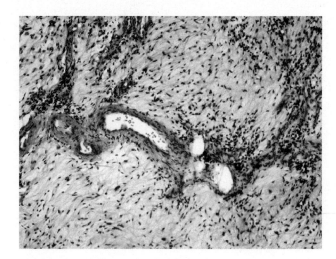

Figure 12-5 Low-grade myxofibrosarcoma. Nodular growth pattern of spindle cells in a myxoid stroma composed of hyaluronic acid with characteristic elongated, curvilinear blood vessels surrounded by a condensation of tumor cells.

Classification
■ Termed "infantile fibrosarcoma" when it occurs in children

Diagnosis
■ Fibroblasts with variable collagen production arranged in long intersecting fascicles classically with a herringbone architecture (Fig. 12-4)

Myxofibrosarcoma

■ Synonym: myxoid malignant fibrous histiocytoma

Pathogenesis
■ Local recurrence is notoriously high at >50%, independent of grade.

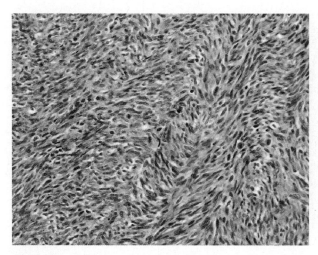

Figure 12-4 Adult fibrosarcoma. Fibroblasts with variable collagen production arranged in long intersecting fascicles with a classic herringbone architecture.

■ Low-grade tumors may acquire a higher grade in recurrence, thereby increasing their metastatic potential.
■ Genetics: inconsistent aberrations

Epidemiology
■ One of the more common soft tissue sarcomas of adulthood
■ Frequency: incidence peaks in sixth to eighth decades of life
■ Site: two thirds occur in the subcutaneous tissue, usually in the limbs

Diagnosis
■ Characterized histologically by nodular growth pattern of spindle cells in a myxoid stroma composed of hyaluronic acid with characteristic elongated, curvilinear blood vessels surrounded by a condensation of tumor cells (Fig. 12-5)

FIBROHISTIOCYTIC TUMORS

Undifferentiated High-Grade Pleomorphic Sarcoma, Not Otherwise Specified

■ Formerly termed pleomorphic malignant fibrous histiocytoma (MFH)
■ Definition: Once considered the most common soft tissue sarcoma of adulthood, MFH has been declassified as a distinct diagnostic entity; it is now thought to represent a variety of poorly differentiated or dedifferentiated neoplasms and has been renamed "undifferentiated pleomorphic sarcoma."

Pathogenesis
■ Genetics: extensive heterogeneity

Etiology
■ 2% to 3% arise in a previously radiated field (radiation-induced sarcoma).

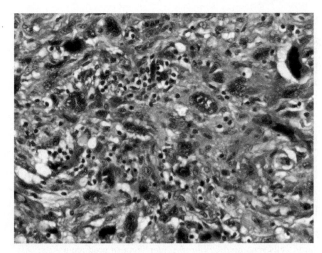

Figure 12-6   Undifferentiated pleomorphic sarcoma. Marked cellularity and nuclear pleomorphism with bizarre tumor giant cells admixed with spindle and histiocyte-type cells.

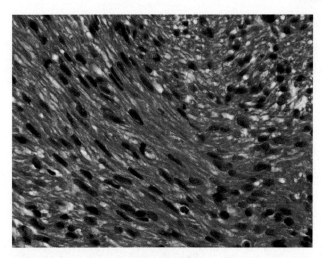

Figure 12-7   Leiomyosarcoma. Spindle cells with blunt-ended nuclei interspersed with myxoid changes.

Epidemiology
- Frequency and age: The pleomorphic sarcomas are the most common soft tissue sarcomas in patients >40 years of age, with an increasing incidence with increasing age, peaking during the sixth and seventh decades of life.
- Site: most commonly arise in the deep tissues of the lower limbs

Diagnosis
- Considered a diagnosis of exclusion
- Characterized histologically by marked cellularity and nuclear pleomorphism with a storiform pattern and often bizarre tumor giant cells admixed with spindle cells and histiocyte-type cells (Fig. 12-6)

SMOOTH MUSCLE TUMORS

Leiomyosarcoma

Pathogenesis
- Genetics: heterogeneous, though losses on chromosomes 3, 8, and 13 are common; the latter is associated with an *RB1* mutation

Epidemiology
- Frequency: accounts for 10% to 15% of limb sarcomas
- Age: may occur in any age, though more common in middle-aged adults
- Site: commonly arise primarily in the pelvis from the uterus and large blood vessels (inferior vena cava)

Diagnosis
- Characterized histologically by elongated cigar-shaped spindle cells with blunt-ended nuclei interspersed with myxoid changes (Fig. 12-7)
- Immunohistochemistry: positive for smooth muscle antigen (SMA) and desmin

SKELETAL MUSCLE TUMORS

Embryonal Rhabdomyosarcoma

- Synonyms: myosarcoma, rhabdomyosarcoma, rhabdosarcoma

Pathogenesis
- Genetics: losses on chromosome 11

Epidemiology
- Frequency: most common soft tissue sarcoma in children and adolescents, with 4.6 cases per million persons <15 years of age
- Site: Most arise in the head and neck, followed by the genitourinary tract; limb and trunk involvement is less common (<10%).
  - Spindle cell variant most commonly arises in the scrotum.
  - Botryoid variant arises beneath mucosal epithelial surfaces (e.g., bladder, biliary tract, pharynx).
- Age: ~45% occur in children <5 years of age.

Classification
- Embryonal is the most common subtype of rhabdomyosarcoma and encompasses the spindle cell, botryoid, and anaplastic variants.

Diagnosis
- Immunohistochemistry: desmin and actin positivity variable; MyoD1 and myogenin highly specific
- Histologically characterized by a constellation of rhabdomyoblasts in various stages of differentiation, with the more primitive cells possessing oval nuclei and more differentiated cells demonstrating elongated nuclei ("tadpole" cells) with eosinophilic cytoplasm (Fig. 12-8)

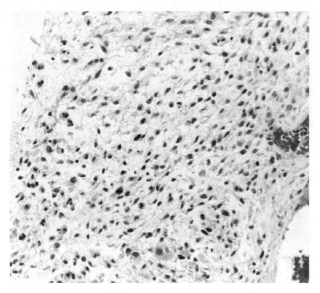

Figure 12-8 Embryonal rhabdomyosarcoma. A constellation of rhabdomyoblasts in various stages of differentiation. The more primitive cells possess oval nuclei, while more differentiated cells demonstrate elongated nuclei ("tadpole" cells) with eosinophilic cytoplasm.

Alveolar Rhabdomyosarcoma

■ Synonyms: rhabdomyoblastoma, rhabdomyopoetic sarcoma, monomorphous round cell rhabdomyosarcoma

Pathogenesis
■ Genetics: t(2;13)(q35;q14) leading to the *PAX3/FKHR* fusion protein; t(1;13) in rare cases

Epidemiology
■ Frequency: less common than embryonal rhabdomyosarcoma
■ Age: occurs most commonly in adolescents and young adults
■ Site: most commonly arises in the extremities, followed by paraspinal, perineal, and paranasal locations

Diagnosis
■ Histologically resembles lymphoma and other small blue round cell tumors but characterized by alveolar pattern similar to that in the lung, with cellular areas separated by fibrovascular septa (Fig. 12-9)
■ Immunohistochemistry: positive for desmin, actin, myogenin, and MyoD

VASCULAR TUMORS

Epithelioid Hemangioendothelioma

■ Synonyms: angioglomoid tumor, myxoid angioblastomatosis

Pathogenesis
■ Genetics: t(1;3) has been reported, though consistency is unknown.

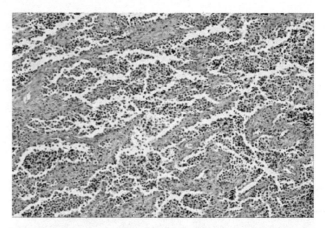

Figure 12-9 Alveolar rhabdomyosarcoma. Nest of small blue round cells separated by fibrovascular septa to produce a morphologic pattern similar to alveoli in lung.

Epidemiology
■ Age: affects all ages
■ Site: usually arises in the extremity, often originating from a small vein
■ Often presents with a multifocal distribution in an entire limb bud involving both soft tissue and bone

Diagnosis
■ Clinical presentation: unlike other soft tissue sarcomas, typically presents as a painful mass
■ Characterized histologically by short strands of eosinophilic epithelioid endothelial cells embedded in a blue to pink acidic matrix (Fig. 12-10)
■ Immunohistochemistry: positive for CD31, CD34, and FLI1

Angiosarcoma

■ Synonyms: lymphangiosarcoma, malignant hemangioendothelioma, hemangiosarcoma, hemangioblastoma

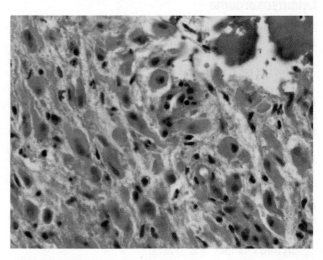

Figure 12-10 Epithelioid hemangioendothelioma. Short strands of bland eosinophilic endothelial cells in a deep pink hyaline matrix.

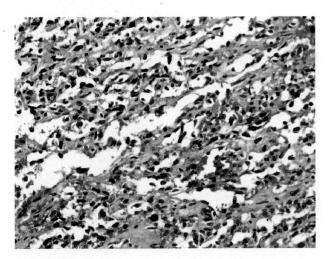

Figure 12-11 Angiosarcoma. Spindle and epithelial cells arranged morphologically in loose, irregular vascular channels. Areas of hemorrhage are common.

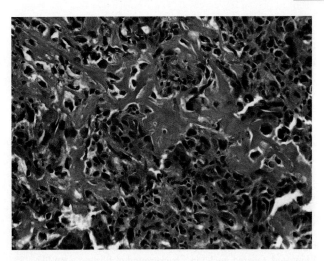

Figure 12-12 Extraskeletal osteogenic sarcoma. Neoplastic bone in a lacy, sheet-like pattern interspersed with atypical, mitotically active tumor cells.

Pathogenesis
 Genetics: inconsistent chromosomal aberrations

Etiology
- One third of tumors are associated with a pre-existing condition such as chronic lymphedema, neurofibromatosis-1, vascular implants, Klippel-Trenaunay syndrome, Maffucci syndrome, and previous radiation.

Epidemiology
- Age: Incidence peaks in the seventh decade of life, though may occur at any age.
- Site: Most occur in the subcutaneous tissue; the majority of deep angiosarcomas occur in the thigh.

Diagnosis
- Histologically characterized by nodular hemorrhagic masses composed of epithelioid and spindle cells attempting to form interconnecting rudimentary vascular channels (Fig. 12-11)
- Immunohistochemistry: positive for von Willebrand factor, CD31, and CD34

CHONDRO-OSSEOUS TUMORS

Extraskeletal Osteogenic Sarcoma

- Synonym: soft tissue osteosarcoma

Pathogenesis
- ~10% associated with previous radiation (radiation-induced sarcoma)
- Genetics: inconsistent aberrations

Epidemiology
- Frequency: accounts for <2% of all soft tissue sarcomas and 2% to 4% of all osteogenic sarcomas

- Age: Incidence peaks during fifth to seventh decades of life.
- Site: most commonly arises in the deep soft tissue of the lower extremity

Diagnosis
- Histologically characterized by same features as skeletal osteosarcoma; lace-like osteoid produced by pleomorphic cells (Fig. 12-12)
- Immunohistochemistry: variable positivity for many antigens, most specifically osteocalcin
- Prognosis is worse than in skeletal osteogenic sarcoma (likely due to lack of chemotherapy response).

TUMORS OF PERIPHERAL NERVES

Malignant Peripheral Nerve Sheath Tumor (MPNST)

- Synonym: neurofibrosarcoma (generally abandoned)

Pathogenesis
- Genetics: alterations at the NF-1 locus on chromosome 17; *p53* mutations

Epidemiology
- 50% of cases occur in the setting of neurofibromatosis-1.
- Two thirds arise from neurofibromas.
- More common in large nerves
  - Sciatic nerve most commonly affected

Diagnosis
- Histologically characterized by elongated, tapered nuclei in a fibrosarcoma-type background (Fig. 12-13)
- Herringbone pattern suggestive of fibrosarcoma arising within a major nerve is highly suggestive of MPNST.

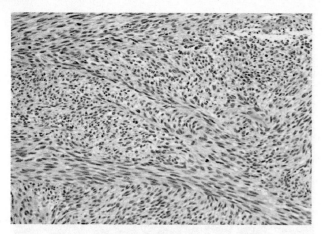

Figure 12-13 Malignant peripheral nerve sheath tumor. Elongated, tapered nuclei in a background of fibrosarcoma-like spindle cells.

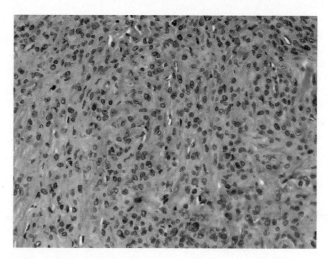

Figure 12-14 Epithelioid sarcoma. Nodular mixture of eosinophilic epithelial cells and spindle cells.

- Immunohistochemistry: positive for S-100
- Triton tumor: MPNST with rhabdomyosarcomatous differentiation; associated with a poor prognosis (5-year survival ~12%)

TUMORS OF UNCERTAIN DIFFERENTIATION

Epithelioid Sarcoma

Pathogenesis
- Genetics: inconsistent aberrations

Epidemiology
- Age: occurs in young adults in the second to fourth decades of life
- Site: commonly arises on the flexor surfaces of fingers, hands, wrist, and forearm

Diagnosis
- Clinically, often associated with superficial ulceration
- Histologically challenging: may be misdiagnosed as a benign granulomatous process (Fig. 12-14)
- Immunohistochemistry: positive for cytokeratins and epithelial membrane antigen (EMA)

Alveolar Soft Part Sarcoma

Pathogenesis
- Genetics: t(X;17)(p11;q25) resulting in the ASPL/TFE2 fusion protein
- Associated with very high metastatic potential; brain and lung metastases are common

Epidemiology
- Frequency: very rare, accounting for <1% of all soft tissue sarcomas

- Age: Incidence peaks during the second to fourth decades of life.
- Site: most commonly arises in deep tissues of the thigh
  - In children, most commonly arises in the head and neck

Diagnosis
- Histologically characterized by nests of tumor cells separated by sinusoidal vascular partitions, resulting in a pseudoalveolar architecture (Fig. 12-15)

Clear Cell Sarcoma

- Synonym: malignant melanoma of soft parts

Pathogenesis
- Genetics: t(12;22)(q13;q12) resulting in the EWS/ATF1 fusion protein
- Associated with high metastatic potential, especially to lymph nodes

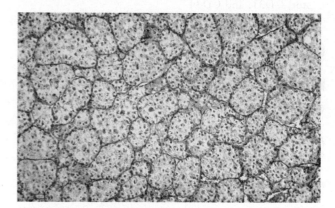

Figure 12-15 Alveolar soft part sarcoma. Nests of tumor cells separated by sinusoidal vascular partitions resulting in a pseudoalveolar architecture.

Epidemiology

- Age: Incidence peaks during the third and fourth decades of life.
- Site: >90% arise in the extremities, with almost half of those cases involving the foot and ankle.
    - Often attached to tendons and aponeuroses

Diagnosis

- Histologically characterized by large cells with clear cytoplasm
- Immunohistochemistry: positive for melanoma antigens and S100

Extraskeletal Myxoid Chondrosarcoma

Pathogenesis

- Genetics: t(9:22) (q22;q12) resulting in the EWS/NR4A3 fusion protein is seen in ~50% of cases.
- Despite the name, there is no evidence of cartilaginous differentiation.
- Late disease recurrence is common.

Epidemiology

- Frequency: accounts for <3% of soft tissue sarcomas
- Age: Incidence peaks during sixth decade of life.
- Site: most commonly arises in the deep tissues of the proximal limb girdles (thigh > arm)

Diagnosis

- Histologically characterized by uniform round and oval cells in a blue chondromyxoid hypovascular stroma (Fig. 12-16)
- No characteristic immunohistochemistry findings, although variable S100, cytokeratin, EMA

Synovial Sarcoma

- Synonyms: malignant synovioma, tendosynovial sarcoma, synovial cell sarcoma (but all of these terms have been abandoned)

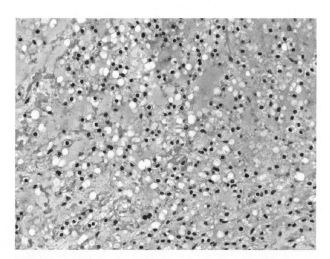

Figure 12-16   Extraskeletal myxoid chondrosarcoma. Uniform round and oval cells in a blue chondromyxoid hypovascular stroma.

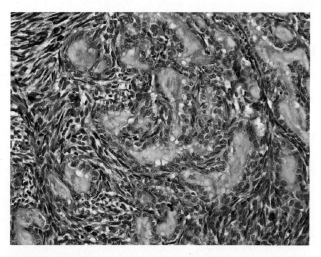

Figure 12-17   Biphasic synovial sarcoma. Mixture of both spindle cells and epithelial cells. The epithelial cells display ovoid nuclei and form mucin-containing glands.

Pathogenesis

- Can be deceptively slow-growing; not unusual to present as mass present for years without change
- Genetics: t(x;18)(p11;q11) results in the SYT/SSX1, SYT/SSX2, or SYT/SSX4 fusion protein.
- Monophasic synovial sarcoma with the SSX2 gene variant is associated with a better prognosis.

Epidemiology

- Frequency: accounts for 5% to 10% of all soft tissue sarcomas
- Age: may occur at any age but peaks during second to fourth decades of life
- Site: 80% arise in the extremity.
    - ~5% arise intra-articular.

Diagnosis

- Histologically characterized by both mesenchymal background cells with nests of epithelial cells (biphasic) (Fig. 12-17) or simply mesenchymal or epithelial tissue (monophasic), the latter similar in appearance to the herringbone pattern of fibrosarcoma
- Immunohistochemistry: for tumors with an epithelial component, positive for cytokeratins and EMA

SUGGESTED READING

Adjuvant chemotherapy for localised resectable soft-tissue sarcoma of adults: meta-analysis of individual data. Sarcoma Meta-analysis Collaboration. *Lancet* 1997;350(9092):1647–1654.

AJCC Cancer Staging Handbook, 6th ed. New York: Springer, 2002.

Alektiar KM, Leung D, Zelefsky MJ, et al. Adjuvant brachytherapy for primary high-grade soft tissue sarcoma of the extremity. *Ann Surg Oncol* 2002;9(1):48–56.

Borden EC, Baker LH, Bell RS, et al. Soft tissue sarcomas of adults: state of the translational science. *Clin Cancer Res* 2003;9(6):1941–1956.

Eilber FC, Brennan MF, Eilber FR, et al. Validation of the postoperative nomogram for 12-year sarcoma-specific mortality. *Cancer* 2004;101(10):2270–2275.

Fong Y, Coit DG, Woodruff JM, Brennan MF. Lymph node metastasis from soft tissue sarcoma in adults. Analysis of data from a prospective database of 1772 sarcoma patients. *Ann Surg* 1993;217(1): 72–77.

McCarter MD, Jaques DP, Brennan MF. Randomized clinical trials in soft tissue sarcoma. *Surg Oncol Clin North Am* 2002;11(1): 11–22.

O'Sullivan B, Davis AM, Turcotte R, et al. Preoperative versus postoperative radiotherapy in soft-tissue sarcoma of the limbs: a randomised trial. *Lancet* 2002;359(9325):2235–2241.

Pathology and Genetics of Tumours Soft Tissue and Bone. Lyon: International Agency for Research on Cancer, 2002.

Pisters PW, Leung DH, Woodruff J, et al. Analysis of prognostic factors in 1,041 patients with localized soft tissue sarcomas of the extremities. *J Clin Oncol* 1996;14(5):1679–1689.

Pollack A, Zagars GK, Goswitz MS, et al. Preoperative vs. postoperative radiotherapy in the treatment of soft tissue sarcomas: a matter of presentation. *Int J Radiat Oncol Biol Phys* 1998;42(3): 563–572.

Weiss SW. *Enzinger and Weiss' Soft Tissue Tumors,* 4th ed. St. Louis: Mosby, 2001.

Weitz J, Antonescu CR, Brennan MF. Localized extremity soft tissue sarcoma: improved knowledge with unchanged survival over time. *J Clin Oncol* 2003;21(14):2719–2725.

Williard WC, Hajdu SI, Casper ES, et al. Comparison of amputation with limb-sparing operations for adult soft tissue sarcoma of the extremity. *Ann Surg* 1992;215(3):269–275.

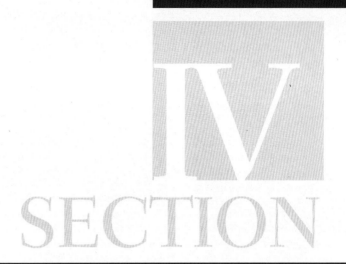

SECTION

IV

BASIC SCIENCE

13

CELLULAR AND MOLECULAR BIOLOGY

MATTHEW J. ALLEN

THE CELL CYCLE

The transformation from a fertilized egg to a complex multi-cellular organism, be it a mouse or a human, depends on the complex and exquisitely regulated control pathways that govern the proliferation and subsequent differentiation of cells. The critical nature of the pathways that control cellular proliferation and growth is perhaps best illustrated by the fact that most cancers are the result of either inherited or induced defects in these control systems.

The cell cycle provides a mechanistic framework for explaining the temporal pattern of cellular activity that is required for one cell to divide (i.e., produce two identical daughter cells). The cell cycle is divided into four active phases and one inactive (quiescent) phase that may be more accurately considered outside of the cell cycle (Fig. 13-1, Table 13-1), since it is not involved in the production of a daughter cell. Although cells from different tissues may show vastly different proliferation rates, the length of the cell cycle is fairly constant, approximately 24 hours; the difference in proliferation rate is the result of differences in the length of time that cells remain in the quiescent phase.

Checkpoints in the Cell Cycle

Given the critical nature of accuracy in cellular proliferation, it should not be surprising to find that the cell cycle contains a number of "checks and balances" through which the integrity of DNA replication, spindle formation, and chromosome separation can be ensured. The feedback pathways by which these checks are made are known as **checkpoints.**

G1 Checkpoint
- Passage is necessary before DNA synthesis can be initiated.
- Failure to progress leads to accumulation of cells in G1.

G2/M Checkpoint
- Passage is necessary for the tetraploid cell to split into daughter cells via the process of mitosis.
- Failure to progress leads to accumulation of cells in G2.
- Radiation therapy and chemotherapy can cause blockade of the G2/M checkpoint.

Cyclins and Cyclin-Dependent Kinases (Cdk)
- Central effectors of cell cycle control at the molecular level
- Disturbances in cyclin–Cdk interactions have been implicated in loss of cell cycle control in neoplastic conditions:
  - p53, a tumor suppressor gene, modulates the activation of cyclin D.

309

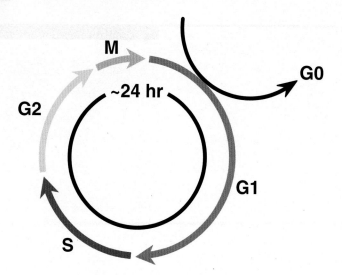

Figure 13-1   The cell cycle. Under culture conditions, growing cells divide approximately every 24 hours. Cycle times in vivo are more variable since fully differentiated cells may exit the cell cycle and remain in G0 for protracted periods.

Phase	Duration (approx.)
G1	10 hr
S	7.5 hr
G2	3.5 hr
M	1 hr

■ Mutations in p53 are present in a very large proportion of cancers.

Techniques for Studying the Cell Cycle

Labeling with Bromodeoxyuridine (BrdU)

Basis of the Technique

■ Synthetic analog of thymidine that is incorporated into newly formed DNA
■ Incorporation provides information on both magnitude and timing of DNA synthesis within a cell population.

Detection of BrdU Incorporation

■ Autoradiography
 ■ Location of radiolabeled BrdU is visualized by exposing the cells or tissues to x-ray film.
■ Immunohistochemistry

■ Detection within cells or histological specimens using antibodies.
■ Enzyme-linked immunoabsorbent assay (ELISA)
 ■ Detection and quantification using antibodies for in-vitro specimens

Flow Cytometry

■ A DNA-binding dye (such as propidium iodide) is used to label the DNA.
■ Cells flow past a laser light source; scattering of beam provides measures of both cell number and size.
■ By combining information on cell size, number, and intensity of propidium iodide, it is possible to quantify the proportion of cells in the G1, S, and G2/M phases (Fig. 13-2).
 ■ Flow cytometry is also a useful technique for documenting programmed cell death (see later).
 ■ Flow cytometry can also be used to quantify BrdU incorporation (see earlier).

TABLE 13-1   PHASES OF THE CELL CYCLE

Stage	Descriptive Name	Function	Ploidy
G0	Quiescent phase	Metabolic activity but no cell division	Diploid (2n)
G1	Growth phase	Synthesis of RNA and proteins	Diploid (2n)
S	Synthetic phase	Duplication of cellular DNA	Tetraploid (4n)
G2	Second growth phase	Synthesis of RNA and proteins	Tetraploid (4n)
M	Mitotic stage	Formation of mitotic spindle and separation of two copies of cellular DNA	Diploid (2n)

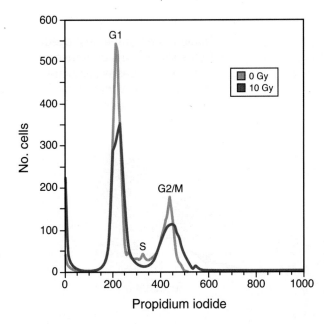

Figure 13-2   Analysis of the cell cycle using flow cytometry. Cells that have been stained with propidium iodide can be classified into three populations—G1, S, and G2/M—based on the amount of DNA that they contain. Treatment with X-irradiation (10 Gy in this example) decreases the G1 fraction and promotes the build-up of cells in G2/M. Note also the appearance of a large spike to the left of the G1 peak; this spike (known as sub-G1) represents cells with reduced DNA content, likely the result of either apoptosis or necrosis (see later).

CELL DEATH

Apoptosis Versus Necrosis

Two forms of cell death are recognized in vitro and in vivo: *apoptosis*, or programmed cell death, and *necrosis*. While the net effect of each mechanism is death of the cell, the fundamental morphological and molecular features of apoptosis and necrosis are vastly different.

Apoptosis
■ Death from the inside out

Definition
■ Organized cascade of intracellular processes
■ Ultimately leads to digestion of the cellular DNA and fragmentation of the cell into apoptotic bodies

Importance
■ Critical role in the regulation of tissue structure and function
■ Important during growth and differentiation
■ Stimuli that promote or inhibit apoptosis have the capacity to deregulate normal growth and differentiation, leading to an increased risk of neoplasia.

Necrosis
■ Cell dies from the outside in.

Definition
■ Most often the result of direct injury to the plasma membrane
■ Once the membrane is damaged, the stability of the cell's internal milieu is lost and cellular components may be released directly into the extracellular space.

Inflammatory Component
■ Release of cytosolic and organellar components into surrounding tissues has an important secondary effect.
■ Typically induces a local inflammatory response in vivo
■ This effect is not seen in vitro, since a cell culture environment cannot replicate the innate immune response that is seen in vivo.

Morphologic Features of Apoptosis

■ Nuclear condensation, blebbing, and fragmentation
  ■ Recognized best by labeling nuclei with fluorescent dyes (e.g., Hoechst 33258; Fig. 13-3)
■ Depending on the type of tissue, apoptotic cells may be removed by phagocytes.
  ■ Inflammatory changes are not a feature of apoptosis.

Key Steps in Apoptosis (Fig. 13-4)

■ Initiation
  ■ Although the plasma membrane remains intact dur-

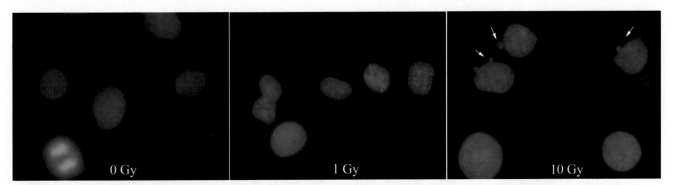

Figure 13-3   Morphological signs of apotosis. Radiation causes a dose-dependent increase in the incidence of cells with nuclear blebbing (*arrows*). Hoechst stain, 100× original magnification.

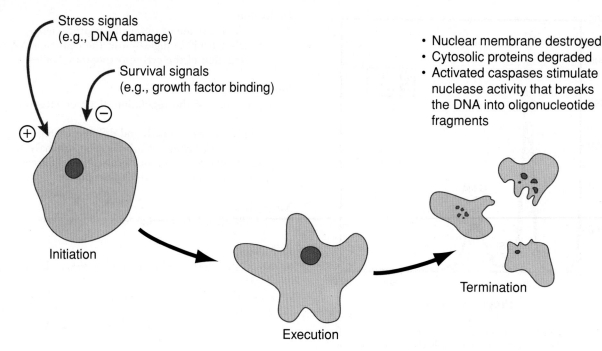

Stress signals
(e.g., DNA damage)

Survival signals
(e.g., growth factor binding)

• Nuclear membrane destroyed
• Cytosolic proteins degraded
• Activated caspases stimulate
  nuclease activity that breaks
  the DNA into oligonucleotide
  fragments

Initiation

Execution

Termination

Figure 13-4   Key steps in apoptosis. The healthy cell needs to be stimulated by growth factors to survive. Loss of these factors, or the addition of stress signals, can push the cell toward programmed cell death.

ing the early stages of apoptosis, there is redistribution of a glycolipid, phosphatidyl serine (PS), from the inner layer to the outer layer. As a result, PS becomes "visible" on the outside of the cell.

■ Execution/activation
  ■ As a result of changes in mitochondrial membrane permeability, cytochrome c migrates from the inside of the mitochondria into the cytosol.
  ■ Caspase activation then ensues, leading to further changes in the permeability of intracellular organelles such as the mitochondria.

■ Termination
  ■ The nuclear membrane is destroyed.
  ■ DNA damage is mediated via caspase-activated DNase (CAD).
  ■ CAD activity is usually controlled by an inhibitor, iCAD, but this is cleaved via the effector caspases (Fig. 13-5).
  ■ Cytosolic proteins are cleaved and organelles break up.

Molecular Pathways of Apoptosis

Apoptogenic Signals (Stimulators of Apoptosis Caspase Activity)

■ DNA damage from irradiation (UV or x-ray) or chemotherapy
  ■ DNA damage activates p53 pathways, leading to the transcription of p21.
  ■ p21 blocks the ability of cyclin D/Cdk to phosphorylate the retinoblastoma (Rb) gene product; this blocks the movement of cells through the G1/S transition.

  ■ p53 activation also stimulates apoptosis via a direct effect on Bax (see later).
■ Loss of key trophic factors (e.g. serum withdrawal in cultured cells)
  ■ Growth factors are critical "survival signals" for cells; their loss will tip the balance towards programmed cell death.
■ Fas ligand
  ■ Signals via the Fas (or Apo2) receptor (CD 95)
  ■ Receptor activation enables FADD (Fas-associated death domain) binding, which in turn activates caspase-8.
■ Tumor necrosis factor-α
  ■ Signals via TNF receptor-1 (TNFR1)
  ■ Binding can have both pro- and anti-apoptotic effects:
    ■ Pro-apoptotic effects are mediated via FADD binding to the death domain on the activated receptor (see above).
    ■ Alternatively, the death domain can bind a protein known as RIP (receptor interacting protein); in this case, binding leads to activation of the nuclear factor kappa B (NF-κB) or the Jun kinase pathway, both of which inhibit apoptosis.
■ "Cellular stress," including free radicals

Caspases

■ Cysteine-dependent *a*spartate-specific *p*roteases, or CASPases, are the central component of the normal cell's machinery for programmed cell death.
■ Not all of the caspase family members are involved in apoptosis; caspase 1, for example, is a key regulator of IL-1 activity. However, caspases 3, 6, 7, 8, and 9 are

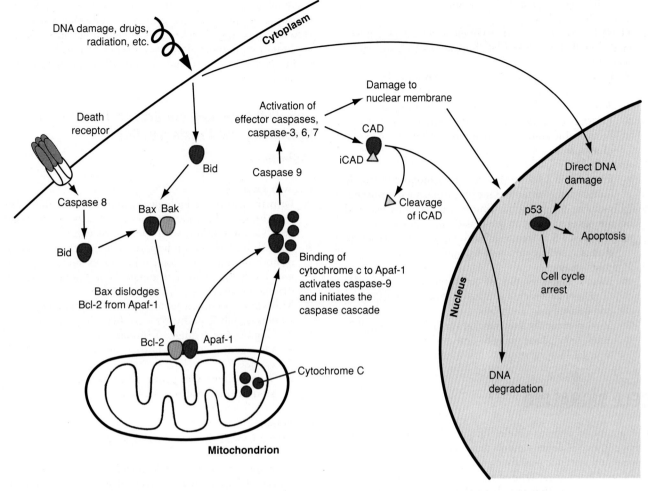

Figure 13-5   Apoptosis pathways. Activation of Bid (via death receptors or direct DNA damage) and Bax/BAK leads to release of Apaf-1 from the mitochondrial membrane. Apaf-1 is then free to bind to cytochrome c that is released from the interior of the mitochondrion. The interaction of Apaf-1 and cytochrome c activates the caspase cascade, ultimately leading to membrane damage, DNA degradation, and the dissolution of cellular proteins and organelles.

situated at pivotal control points in apoptotic signaling pathways.
- Based on their structure and function, caspases can be considered either activators or effectors:
  - Activators such as caspases 8 and 9 amplify the initial signal and activate downstream effector caspases.
  - Effectors such as caspases 3, 6 and 7 mediate direct effects on cellular processes and structures.

Bcl-2 Family Members
- Intracellular control of apoptosis is determined by the balance between pro- and anti-apoptotic signaling molecules in the Bcl-2 family.
- Anti-apoptotic molecules include Bcl-2 and Bcl-XL.
  - Bcl-2 tethered to the outer mitochondrial membrane binds to an adapter protein known as Apaf-1.
  - Binding of Bcl-2 anchors the Apaf-1, preventing its release into the cytoplasm.
  - Overexpression of Bcl-2 is associated with malignan-

cies, particularly in B-cell leukemias (hence the name).
  - In this instance, neoplasia is the result of decreased cell death from apoptosis (i.e., enhanced survival) rather than increased cell proliferation.
- Binding of pro-apoptotic molecules such as Bax, Bak, or Bid dislodges Apaf-1, which is now free to enter the cytoplasm (see Fig. 13-5).
  - Changes in the permeability of the mitochondrial membrane allow cytochrome c to diffuse out into the cytoplasm.
  - Apaf-1 and cytochrome c then bind, leading to the activation of caspase 9.

Techniques for Detecting Apoptosis

- Microscopy: with or without special stains (e.g., Hoechst stains will stain the DNA and facilitate the identification of nuclear blebbing; see Fig. 13-3)
- Gel electrophoresis: Fragmentation of DNA results in

~200 bp oligonucleotide fragments that can be resolved by gel electrophoresis.

- TUNEL (terminal deoxynucleotidyl transferase-mediated dUTP nick end-labeling) stains on histological sections
  - Immunohistochemical staining technique in which the 3′ ends of fragmented DNA are labeled and then detected using an antibody-based technique.
  - TUNEL staining is not specific to apoptosis but can be useful if combined with morphological evidence of apoptosis.
- Annexin V
  - Phosphatidyl serine (PS) is a phospholipid normally found on the inner surface of the plasma membrane.
- In response to apoptotic stimuli, PS becomes exposed on the outer surface of the plasma membrane.
  - Exposed PS is free to bind to annexin V, a reaction that is readily confirmed by flow cytometry.
- Caspase assays
  - Direct measurement of activated caspase family members provides a robust method for confirming and quantifying apoptosis.
  - Most commonly used markers are caspases 3 and 7.
  - Activated caspases may be detected by Western blotting, ELISA, or immunohistochemistry.

CELL SIGNALING

The ability of cells to divide, differentiate, function, and survive in vivo is dependent on and regulated by a vast array of local and systemic signals, including growth factors, cytokines, and hormones. One of the most remarkable characteristics of cells is that they have the capacity to integrate this multitude of signals, be they stimulatory or inhibitory, into a coherent response in the form of alterations in cellular activity. The stimulus → response pathway can be broken down into three stages.

- Perception of the signal at either the cell surface or within the cell
  - This is usually made possible by the possession of specific receptors that can interact with the stimulus.
- Intracellular signaling pathways
  - These convey signals from the activated receptor, through the cytoplasm to the nucleus.
  - Several key signaling pathways have been implicated, including intracellular Ca++, phosphoinositols, cyclic AMP, and intracellular kinases (e.g., tyrosine kinase).
- Effector pathways
  - Proto-oncogenes such as c-fos and c-jun appear to be important targets; these proto-oncogenes encode transcription factors that interact with the DNA molecule, facilitating the expression of genes that control DNA replication, cellular differentiation, and synthetic activity.

Advances in genomics and proteomics have revolutionized our ability to identify and characterize many of these intracellular signaling pathways and their effects on the cell.

A complete discussion of this field is clearly well beyond the scope of this book. The goal of the following discussion is to use some specific examples of signaling pathways that are important in musculoskeletal tissues as a means of conveying general themes that are broadly applicable across many tissue types.

Cell–Cell Signaling via Growth Factors, Cytokines, and Prostaglandins

Definitions

Growth Factors

- Growth factors are biologically active factors that control the growth, differentiation, and survival of target cells via interactions with specific receptors.
- Growth factors play an important role in the regulation of both normal physiological processes such as growth and development and pathological conditions caused by disease or injury.
- Mutations in growth factors, their receptors, or downstream signaling pathways have been implicated in the development of a range of human cancers.
  - Oncogenes: genes whose overexpression leads to cancer
  - Tumor suppressor genes: genes whose underexpression (or inactivation) is associated with cancer

Cytokines

- Cytokines can be considered a specialized subset of growth factors.
- Cytokines are small, usually locally acting secreted proteins that are classically described as being the products of immune cells.
- However, it is now recognized that cytokines are synthesized by (and act on) a wide range of cell types throughout the body.
- Although cytokines usually function locally either on the cells that secrete them (*autocrine* pathway) or on adjacent cells (*paracrine* pathway), they can occasionally act on distant tissues via an endocrine mechanism.

A complete review of all known growth factors and cytokines is clearly outside the scope of this chapter. What follows is intended as a general overview of those factors with greatest relevance to the musculoskeletal system, with the aim of this discussion being to describe the key biological actions of these molecules as well as to highlight the signaling pathways by which these factors control the activity of target cells.

Growth Factors of Relevance to the Musculoskeletal System

Insulin-like Growth Factors (IGF-I and IGF-II)

- Sources
  - Most IGF-I is synthesized in the liver in response to growth hormone.
  - Mineralized matrix contains abundant reserves of IGF that are released by bone resorption.
- Functions

- Potent regulators of both osteoblast and chondrocyte function
- IGFs promote osteoblast survival and stimulate the proliferation and differentiation of chondrocytes.

Platelet-Derived Growth Factor (PDGF)
- Sources
  - Found in high concentrations in platelets and endothelial cells
  - Consists of homo- or heterodimers of two isoforms, A and B (i.e., PDGF-AA, PDGF-AB, or PDGF-BB), although biological effects appear to be similar for all variants
- Functions
  - Primary physiological role appears to be to stimulate wound repair.
  - Stimulates cell proliferation and differentiation in a wide variety of cell types, including chondrocytes and osteoblasts

Fibroblast Growth Factor (FGF)
- Sources
  - Two distinct forms exist, acidic FGF (aFGF) and basic FGF (bFGF).
  - FGFs are expressed in a variety of tissues, including the central nervous system, vasculature, musculoskeletal system, and the developing mammary gland.
  - Upregulation of FGF expression has been associated with malignant transformation in solid tumors (breast, prostate cancer) and hematological malignancies (including acute myeloid leukemia).
- Functions
  - FGFs play a critical role in embryonic development, homeostasis, and tissue regeneration.
  - FGFs also stimulate endothelial cell proliferation, increasing vascularization at sites of injury and healing.
  - Both forms are also mitogenic for both fibroblasts and osteoblasts, although bFGF is the more potent of the two forms.

Transforming Growth Factor-Beta (TGF-β)
- Sources
  - Three isoforms of TGF-β are found in humans.
  - Synthesized in a latent form by osteoblasts and platelets
  - Latent TGF-β is activated by extracellular proteases.
  - Activation by osteoclast-derived proteases may provide a mechanism for coupling bone resorption with subsequent bone formation.
  - Bone matrix is the most abundant source of TGF-β1 and TGF-β2.
- Functions
  - Multifunctional growth factor has been implicated in the control of cellular growth and differentiation in healthy and neoplastic tissues.
  - Signaling involves the Smad pathway (Fig. 13-6).

Bone Morphogenetic Proteins (BMPs)
- Sources
  - Originally identified through the groundbreaking work of Marshall Urist and colleagues, who identified the osteoinductive capacity of demineralized bone powder
- Functions
  - BMPs are members of the TGF-β superfamily, sharing both structural features and signaling pathways (see Fig. 13-6).
  - BMPs have been shown to play critical roles in the regulation of bone and cartilage formation.
    - BMP-6 is an important paracrine regulator of growth plate function (see Chapter 14, Growth and Development of the Skeleton).
    - BMP-2 and BMP-7 (also known as osteogenic protein-1 [OP-1]) stimulate new bone formation and show tremendous promise in applications such as spine fusion, fracture repair, and cartilage repair/regeneration.

Interleukin-1 (IL-1)
- Major sources include monocytes and macrophages.
- Functions
  - Stimulates matrix metalloproteinase (MMP) activity and the production of other pro-inflammatory cytokines, including IL-6 (see below)
  - Implicated in both osteoarthritis and rheumatoid arthritis
    - Stimulates the proliferation of synovial fibroblasts and T cells
    - A soluble IL-1 receptor antagonist (anakinra) is currently approved for the treatment of rheumatoid arthritis. The drug has a short half-life in vivo, however, and a better approach may be to deliver the molecule via gene therapy.

Interleukin-6 (IL-6)
- Sources
  - Originally identified as a key factor in B-cell immunology
  - It is now recognized that IL-6 is a pleiotropic growth factor that is expressed by multiple cell types, including macrophages, fibroblasts, endothelial cells, glial cells, keratinocytes, and synovial cells.
  - IL-6 binds to a surface receptor and activates gp130.
- Functions: pro-inflammatory cytokine that plays a key role in the pathophysiology of postmenopausal osteoporosis and other conditions of pathological bone loss, including aseptic implant loosening, osteomyelitis, and tumor osteolysis

Tumor Necrosis Factor-Alpha (TNF-α)
- Sources: synthesized by many cell types, perhaps most importantly synovial macrophages, fibroblasts, bone marrow monocyte-macrophages, and osteoblasts
- Functions
  - Pro-inflammatory cytokine that stimulates bone resorption and cartilage destruction in vitro and in vivo
  - Implicated in the pathogenesis of rheumatoid arthritis
    - Stimulates the release of pro-inflammatory IL-6 from synovial macrophages, fibroblasts, and chondrocytes

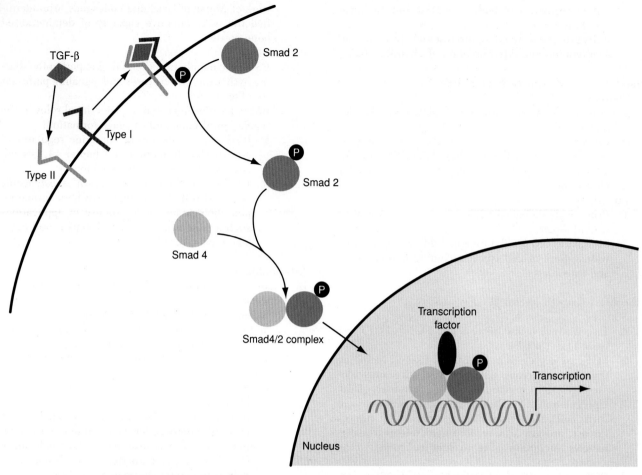

Figure 13-6   Smad pathways involved in BMP and TGF-β signaling. Binding of TGF-β leads to phosphorylation of the receptor, which in turn phosphorylates Smad 2. Phosphorylated Smad 2 binds to Smad 4 and the complex crosses into the nucleus, where it binds transcription factors and activates gene expression.

■ Soluble TNF-α antagonists (etanercept, infliximab) are available for the treatment of rheumatoid arthritis.

Prostaglandins
■ Sources: products of the cyclooxygenase (COX) pathway of arachidonic acid metabolism
■ Functions
  ■ Potent mediators of inflammation in a range of diseases
  ■ Prostaglandins of the E series appear to be particularly important within the musculoskeletal system.
    ■ Locally applied prostaglandin E2 (PGE2) stimulates bone resorption.
    ■ Systemic administration of PGE2 is anabolic for the skeleton; this effect is the result of enhanced osteoblast recruitment and/or differentiation.
  ■ Selective inhibitors of the inducible COX enzyme (COX-2) are highly effective in the management of joint inflammation and bone loss in patients with arthritis.

Cell–Cell Signaling via Adhesion Junctions

Direct cell-to-cell signaling is facilitated by the presence of specialized connections between adjacent cells. In musculoskeletal tissues, the most common junctions are gap junctions and adherens junctions.

Gap Junctions
■ Function: to provide selective passage of small-molecular-weight molecules, Ca + + ions, and signaling molecules such as cyclic AMP.
■ Cell types: Gap junctions have been identified in osteoblasts, osteocytes, and fibroblasts.
■ Components
  ■ Connexins are the major transmembrane components of gap junctions.
  ■ Connexin 43 is the predominant connexin in osteoblasts.
    ■ Plays key roles in osteoblast differentiation, apoptosis, and response to mechanical strain

Adherens Junctions
■ Function

- Act as dimers
- Cytoplasmic end of the cadherin binds via α- and β-catenins to the actin cytoskeleton.
- Extracellular domain binds via a Ca + +-dependent mechanism to cadherins in adjacent cells.
- Loss of adherens function impairs osteoblast differentiation, indicating a critical role in this process.
- Cell types and components
  - Cadherins are transmembrane proteins (>40 variants).
    - E-cadherin found on epithelial cells
    - N-cadherin on muscle, neural tissues

Cell–Matrix Interactions

As specialized connective tissues, both bone and cartilage are functional composite materials consisting of cells embedded within an extracellular matrix (ECM). In both cases, the matrix is composed of proteoglycans mixed with collagen fibers. Interactions between cells and the surrounding matrix appear to play a critical role in the following.

Physiological Response to Mechanical Loading in Bone, Cartilage, Ligament, and Tendon
- Mechanical forces
  - Potent regulators of the extracellular matrix in musculoskeletal tissues
  - Regulate the synthesis of extracellular matrix proteins by osteoblasts, chondrocytes, and fibroblasts
  - Capacity to modulate cell survival via effects on apoptosis
    - In osteocytes, mechanical stretch activates extracellular signal regulated kinases (ERKs) via effects on integrins and the cytoskeleton.
  - Primary sensor of the mechanical force: matrix itself

Coupling of Bone Formation and Resorption
- Osteoblast–matrix interaction
  - Degradation products of type I collagen modulate the activity of osteoblasts.
  - Osteoblasts control local bone resorption by regulating the differentiation of osteoclasts via the RANKL-OPG axis (see later).
- Osteoclast–matrix interaction
  - Osteoclast interactions with the matrix (via the sealed zone) are mediated via integrin binding.
  - Removal of bone by osteoclastic activity may also lead to changes in the mechanical properties of bone; these changes then serve to signal for increased new bone formation.

Role of the Cytoskeleton

Cytoskeletal Elements
- Microtubules: polymeric complexes of tubulin that play a crucial role in organizing the mitotic spindle
- Actin filaments: polymers of actin that are essential for cell movement and, in combination with myosin, for contractility in myocytes

- Intermediate filaments: vimentin and vimentin-related proteins are most significant in connective tissues. They are:
  - Critical to the cell's ability to resist mechanical stress
  - Particularly abundant in cells that need to stretch (epithelial cells, myocytes, fibroblasts)

Cytoskeletal–Matrix Interactions
- Interactions between the cytoskeleton and the ECM are modulated via interactions between matrix proteins and membrane-tethered integrins.
- Integrins
  - Transmembrane heterodimers consisting of one α and one β subunit
  - Interact with RGD (arginine-glycine-aspartate) sequences that are present in a variety of extracellular matrix components, including collagen, fibronectin, and laminin
  - Alterations in integrin expression can modulate cell–ECM interactions.
    - Particularly important in the context of tumor cell metastasis, in which it is known that expression of certain integrins (e.g., αVβ3) is associated with an increased risk of skeletal metastasis

CELLULAR FUNCTION

Cellular Ontogeny and Morphology

Osteoblasts
- Source
  - Derived from the mesenchymal cell lineage
- Morphology and molecular markers
  - Variable morphology, with active cells being cuboidal and more quiescent (lining) cells having a flattened appearance (Fig. 13-7)

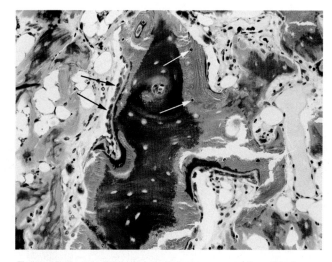

Figure 13-7 Osteoblast morphology. Active osteoblasts (*black arrows*) are seen as cuboidal cells that overlie the osteoid seam. Osteocytes (*white arrows*) are flattened cells embedded in lacunae within the bone. Modified Masson-Goldner trichrome stain, 200× original magnification.

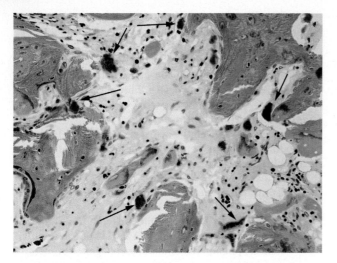

Figure 13-8 Large, multinucleated osteoclasts (*arrows*) attached to and resorbing bone. Modified Masson-Goldner trichrome stain, 200× original magnification.

■ No specific molecular markers, although osteocalcin, osteonectin, and alkaline phosphatase are often used for this purpose
■ Function
　■ Primary function: form mineralized bone matrix
　　■ Bone matrix (40% of the dry weight of bone) is first formed as nonmineralized osteoid containing:
　　　■ Type I collagen (90% of the protein in bone)
　　　■ Noncollagenous proteins such as proteoglycan, osteocalcin, osteopontin, osteonectin, bone sialoprotein, and thrombospondin
　　■ Bone mineral (60% of the dry weight of bone) is mainly hydroxyapatite, $Ca_{10}(PO_4)_6(OH)_2$.
　■ Osteoblasts also control bone turnover via the RANKL-OPG axis (see later).

Osteocytes
■ Source
　■ Terminally differentiated form of the osteoblast
　■ Formed as osteoblasts become encased in mineralized bone
■ Function
　■ Osteocytes lie within lacunae but connect with each other via long cellular extensions that run through channels (canaliculae) in the bone.

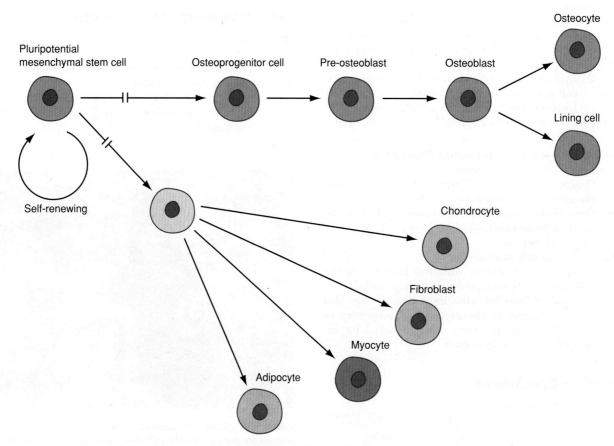

Figure 13-9 Differentiation pathways for mesenchymal cells. The potential for proliferation decreases as cells move from left to right (i.e., with advancing differentiation).

TABLE 13-2 KEY FACTORS IN REGULATION OF OSTEOCLAST DIFFERENTIATION VIA THE RANKL-OPG AXIS

	Name	Location	Function	Effect on Osteoclast Differentiation
RANK	Receptor activator of nuclear factor kappa-B (NF-κB)	Surface receptor on osteoclast precursor cells	Binding with RANKL activates upregulation of genes under transcriptional control of NF-κB	Upregulation
RANKL	Receptor activator of nuclear factor kappa-B ligand	Osteoblasts and stromal cells	Binds to cognate receptor RANK	Upregulation
OPG	Osteoprotegerin	Soluble molecule	Decoy receptor for RANKL; prevents binding of RANKL to RANK	Downregulation

- ■ Forms an extended network of interconnected cells, rather like a neuronal net
- ■ Osteocyte communication plays a critical role in the response of the skeleton to mechanical loading (or unloading).

Osteoclasts
- ■ Source
  - ■ Derived from the hematopoietic cell lineage

- ■ Multinucleated cells formed by the fusion of mononuclear precursor cells
- ■ Morphology and molecular markers
  - ■ Multinucleated cells (Fig. 13-8)
  - ■ Osteoclast markers: tartrate-resistant acid phosphatase (TRAP) 5b, the vitronectin receptor (CD 51), and the calcitonin receptor
- ■ Function
  - ■ Primary function: resorb mineralized bone

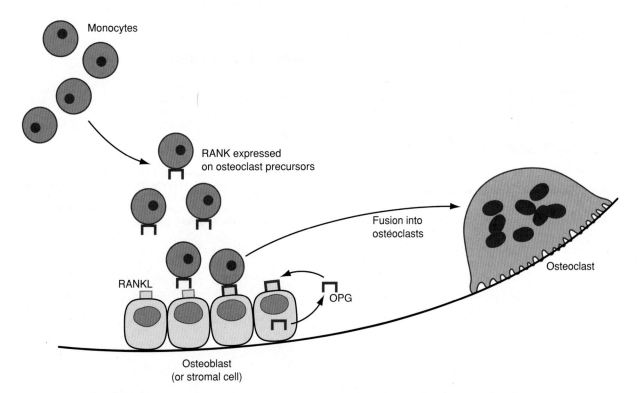

Figure 13-10 The RANKL-OPG axis. Monocytes that are stimulated with M-CSF (via the c-fms receptor) become osteoclast precursors. These cells bind RANKL on the surface of local osteoblasts and/or stromal cells. Binding of RANKL to its receptor, RANK, leads to NF-κB activation, gene transcription, and the formation of functional multinucleated osteoclasts. Osteoprotegerin (OPG), the decoy receptor for RANKL, antagonizes RANKL binding to RANK, thereby blocking osteoclast formation.

- Cells attach to bone matrix via a complex of membrane invaginations, the so-called ruffled border.
    - Ruffled border has large surface area for secretion and absorption.
    - Sealed space contained within the ruffled border is acidified by the osteoclast's proton pump.
        - Low pH favors the activity of secreted matrix metalloproteinases (MMPs) and lysosomal proteases such as cathepsin K.

Chondrocytes

- Source: derived from mesenchymal cell precursors
- Function: differentiation into one of two fates:
    - Growth plate chondrocytes (see Chapter 14)
    - Articular chondrocytes (see Chapter 15)
- Morphology and molecular markers
    - Molecular markers
        - Articular chondrocytes: type II collagen
        - Proliferative growth plate chondrocytes: type I collagen
        - Hypertrophic growth plate chondrocytes: type X collagen
    - Chondrocytes are embedded within a water-rich matrix that contains both collagenous and noncollagenous proteins.

Fibroblasts

- Source: derived from mesenchymal cell precursors
- Function: Within the musculoskeletal system, fibroblasts are found in the bone marrow, synovial membrane, ligament, and tendon.
- Morphology and molecular markers
    - Spindle-shaped morphology
    - Characterized by the expression of type I and type III collagen, as well as fibronectin
        - Tendon and ligament fibroblasts are highly differentiated and express type I and type IX collagen, along with biglycan and decorin.

Regulation of Musculoskeletal Cell Differentiation

Common Precursor Pluripotential Cell Source (Fig. 13-9)

- Osteoblasts, osteocytes, chondrocytes, fibroblasts, myocytes, and adipocytes are all ultimately derived from a common precursor.
- Exception: Osteoclasts are derived from hematopoietic cell line.
- Commitment to one lineage rather than any other appears to depend on the expression of tissue-specific transcription factors:
    - Osteoblasts: Cbfa-1 and osterix
    - Chondrocytes: Sox proteins

Regulation of Osteoclast Differentiation: RANKL-OPG Axis

- Osteoclasts are derived from a circulating hematopoietic precursor.
- Stimulation of monocytes precursors involves M-CSF, which binds to a specific surface receptor (c-fms).
- Activated monocytes (now considered to be committed osteoclast precursor cells) fuse together to form the osteoclast.
- The differentiation of osteoclast precursors into mature, functional osteoclasts is controlled by several regulatory pathways, of which the RANKL-OPG axis is best understood (Table 13-2; Fig. 13-10).
- Therapies that target the RANKL-OPG signaling pathway show promise in the treatment of osteoporosis and tumor osteolysis:
    - Options include monoclonal antibodies to RANKL or delivery of OPG as either recombinant protein or as a gene therapy product.

SUGGESTED READING

Buckwalter JA, Glimcher MJ, Cooper RR, et al. Bone biology. I: Structure, blood supply, cells, matrix, and mineralization. *AAOS Instr Course Lect* 1996;45:371–386.

Buckwalter JA, Glimcher MJ, Cooper RR, et al. Bone biology. II: Formation, form, modeling, remodeling, and regulation of cell function. *AAOS Instr Course Lect* 1996;45:387–399.

Katagiri T, Takahashi N. Regulatory mechanisms of osteoblast and osteoclast differentiation. *Oral Dis* 2002;8:147–159.

Rosier RN, Reynolds PR, O'Keefe, RJ. Molecular and cell biology in orthopaedics. In: Buckwalter JA, Einhorn TA, Simon SR, eds. *Orthopaedic Basic Science*, 2nd ed. Rosemont, IL: American Academy of Orthopaedic Surgeons, 2000:20–76.

14

GROWTH AND DEVELOPMENT OF THE MUSCULOSKELETAL SYSTEM

DONALD E. SWEET[†]
THOMAS V. SMALLMAN

The process of growth and development involves an ordered sequence of steps that begins in the embryo. Growth follows a logical order of sequential appearance, maturation, and removal of progressively more differentiated structures and tissues. The morphology of this sequence will be demonstrated in this chapter. The genetic mechanisms underlying this process are not fully known; reference will be made, where appropriate, to areas of ongoing investigation.

[†]Dr. Sweet passed away suddenly on August 18, 2004. The Chairman of the Department of Orthopaedic Pathology, Armed Forces Institute of Pathology, Washington, DC, and an educator *par excellence*, he was in the process of preparing this chapter with me (T.V.S.), and the chapter is dedicated to his memory. Humble, brilliant, and a contributor in many ways to the world of orthopaedics for 35 years, he will be missed.

EMRYOGENESIS

Skeletal Development

The skeleton arises from the mesoderm, the middle cell layer of the three-layer embryo (Table 14-1).

Limb Bud Development

Limb Bud Elements
- Central core gives rise to bones and joints.
- Around central core: looser tissue from which muscles, tendons, ligaments, and vessels will develop
- Ectodermal covering with a central condensation of mesoderm (Fig. 14-1)

TABLE 14-1 ORIGIN OF SKELETAL ELEMENTS ACCORDING TO MESODERMAL SITE

Skeletal Element	Origin
Craniofacial bones	Develop directly from a mesodermal membranous background derived from the neural crest and brachial arches
Base of the skull	Derived from cartilage models differentiating directly from mesoderm
Axial skeleton	Somites, paired condensations of mesoderm, appear adjacent to the midline at 19 to 21 days, with 42 to 44 pairs appearing by 30 days; somites include a dermatomal element, destined to become dermis, and a sclerotomal element, precursor to the axial skeleton.
Appendicular skeleton	Arises from limb buds that develop from the unsegmented mesoderm (somatopleure) of the lateral body wall and thus are unrelated to somite development

Outgrowth

■ Governed by relationship between the thickened distal ectoderm (apical ectodermal ridge [AER]) and the underlying mesoderm

■ Extremely rapid reproduction of large numbers of cells in the central core as well as in the ectoderm results in a rapid elongation of the limb bud.

■ Several growth factors regulate activities at the AER and adjacent zones:

  ■ Fibroblast growth factors (FGFs; especially FGF4 and FGF8) control cell differentiation in the immediately adjacent limb bud along its longitudinal axis.

  ■ Zone of polarizing activity (ZPA) at posterior distal part of the limb bud controls anterior posterior patterning through the protein sonic hedgehog (Shh).

Innervation

■ Nerves extend outward from the central nervous system and attach themselves to developing muscles.

■ Innervation of bone and periosteum is by sympathetic and sensory fibers that contribute to regulation of vascular control and perception of nociceptive stimuli.

■ Nerves accompany vessels into bone both into the marrow space and into the Haversian and Volkmann canal systems.

Differentiation

■ Unfolds from proximal to distal in a sequential manner (hip, then femur, then knee, then calf, and so forth; see Fig. 14-1)

■ Cartilage formation from the mesenchymal condensations begins during the sixth week.

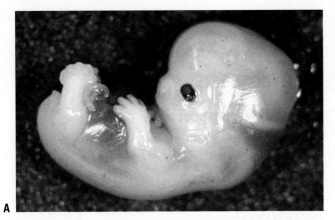
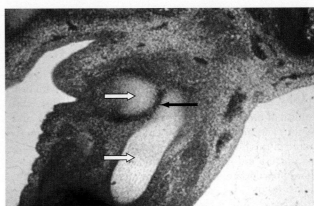

Figure 14-1 (A) Seven-week embryo with well-developed limb buds. Lower limb development lags behind upper limb throughout life. Rapidly developing cells are susceptible to insult. (B) Limb bud cross-section showing central condensation of immature cartilage cells (appearing as dark dots at this power) forming two early cartilage models with immature matrix production (*white arrows*), as well as the dark zone between the two cartilage models that will become a joint (*black arrow*). (Courtesy of the Armed Forces Institute of Pathology, Washington, DC.)

FUNDAMENTAL CONCEPTS IN SKELETAL GENESIS

- To understand the further development of the limb bud, one must consider several fundamental aspects of bone development.
- Bone is not created *de novo* but rather as an appliqué on or within a pre-existing mesenchymal framework. In skeletal embryogenesis, then, bone forms:
  - On a collagen framework called *woven bone* in the craniofacial bones and clavicle, or
  - On a *calcified cartilage* framework in the remainder of the skeleton.
  - Once bone has formed, bone modeling or remodeling involves bone deposition on *previously made bone*.

Bone is made by osteoblasts and is deleted by osteoclasts. Once formed, the skeleton attempts to maintain homeostasis in the long run by balancing formation and deletion. A surgeon, Julius Wolff, proposed in 1891 that mechanical stress determined the architecture of bone in that bone is made in areas where there is mechanical stress and is deleted where there is little stress. Homeostasis in the skeleton involves a balance among mechanical, metabolic, and circulatory influences acting on the effector cells, osteoblasts and osteoclasts. The discipline of cell biology is now demonstrating that the final pathways directing these cells in these fields of influence involve polypeptide signaling substances, hormones, and their receptor systems.

Normal Bone Formation

In the embryo and throughout life there are three types of normal bone formation.

Membranous (Woven) Bone Formation

In membranous bone formation (Figs. 14-2 and 14-3), bone is formed directly by osteoblasts, the life cycle of which includes:

- Osteoblast origin: subset of pluripotent stromal stem cell line
- Preosteoblast (flat, spindle cell): inducible osteoprogenitor cells (IOPCs) proliferate and make bone morphogenic protein (BMP) and osteopontin
  - Molecular regulator of osteoblast differentiation is transcription factor Cbfa1; bone morphogenic proteins 2 and 7 (BMP2, BMP7) regulate Cbfa1 gene expression (Box 14-1).
- Proliferating osteoblast (cell is plumper, increasing rough endoplasmic reticulum)
- Differentiating osteoblast
- Mature osteoblast (cell is cuboidal, looks like a plasma cell) expresses alkaline phosphatase
- Osteoblast, matrix mineralizing: most osteoblasts undergo apoptosis, some become osteocytes, some remain on the endosteal surface as bone lining cells
  - Osteocalcin is expressed by the osteoblast in this stage.
- Osteocyte, resident in bone

- One in ten osteoblasts does not participate in the extreme activity creating the osteoid seam but becomes a resident osteocyte, responsible for maintaining the bone that has been produced around it.
- Cells communicate through dendritic processes and gap junctions, forming a functional syncytium with the bone lining cells.
- Life span of an individual osteocyte may be months (fetal bone) to years (adult bone).
- Bone surface lining cell (BSLC)
  - Can either be resting or in an activated state making bone
  - Resting cells provide cytokine signal to activate bone remodeling.
  - May adopt fat cell morphology in the aging

All bone in the body is made by osteoblasts (see Fig. 14-3) and is either skeletal or extraskeletal; dysregulation of these precursor cells may manifest clinically in diseases such as fibrodyplasia ossificans progressiva, a genetic disease characterized by the ossification of skeletal muscle and other connective tissues, or in the periarticular heterotopic ossification that can complicate skeletal trauma.

Enchondral (Endochondral) Bone Formation

In endochondral bone formation, bone is formed on a calcified cartilage template.

- Calcified cartilage acts as a nidus on which bone is deposited by osteoblasts derived from perivascular stem cells arising from vessels in the adjacent marrow.
- Figure 14-4 is a high-power cut showing a primary trabecula in a growth plate; primary trabeculae anchor the growth plate to the rest of the bone and act as an initial lattice for transmission of mechanical force.
- This region undergoes rapid remodeling in the fetus and young and remains the site of most remodeling of bone throughout life.
- Primary trabeculae thus remodel rapidly, with removal by osteoclasts of bone and calcified cartilage and replacement by bone, thus forming a secondary trabecula.

Lamellar Bone Formation

In lamellar bone formation, bone is formed on pre-existing bone (Fig. 14-5) in a process that takes days to months to complete.

- Lamellar bone consists of layers of collagen, each layer arranged at a different angle from its neighbor, like plywood; this gives mechanical strength to the composite structure. It can be applied to pre-existing woven bone or to lamellar bone.
  - In woven bone the lamellar bone is applied in sheets as an inlay apposed to the inner surface of the randomly oriented trabecula; the effect is to strengthen the construct.
  - In lamellar bone the application of new bone is part of the modeling or remodeling process.
- Woven bone formation is rapid, and the bone that results is a mechanically weak, open mesh that must be reinforced by a lamellar bone fill-in before significant weight transmission.

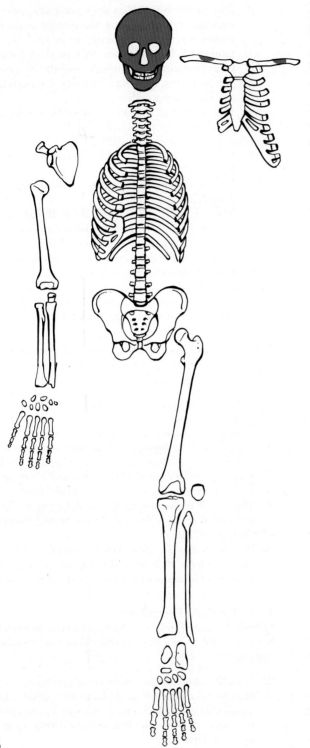

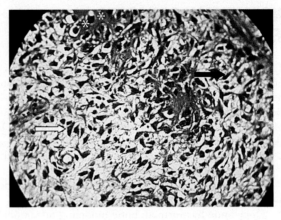

Figure 14-2 Woven bone formation. **(A)** Facial bones and central clavicle start from a collagenous framework. **(B)** Spectrum of cells making woven bone. Spindle-shaped mesenchymal cells (*black arrow*) change into plumper pre-osteoblasts. Pre-osteoblasts (*white arrow*) are larger cells not yet elaborating collagen. Osteoblast deposits collagen subunits into extracellular space, where they aggregate into the triple helix of collagen (dark-staining extracellular material; *asterisks*). (Courtesy of the Armed Forces Institute of Pathology, Washington, DC.)

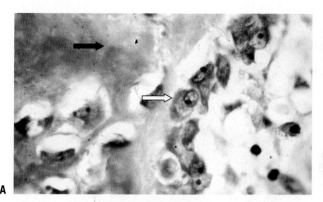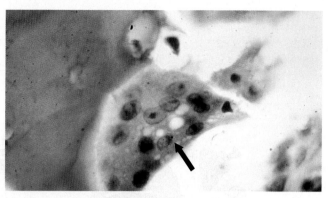

A   B

Figure 14-3   Woven bone formation. (**A**) High-power view of osteoblasts depositing osteoid, forming woven bone. *White arrow* points to an osteoblast that looks like a plasma cell. Cytoplasm is packed with rough endoplasmic reticulum for collagen production, packaged as subunits in the juxta-articular Golgi apparatus for excretion. Osteoid (collagen) is the deposited amorphous dark-staining extracellular material (*black arrow*) that then undergoes a complex biochemical preparation for mineralization for 10 days after deposition. (**B**) An osteoclast, a motile multinucleated giant cell packed with mitochondria for energy production, is shown actively deleting bone (*arrow*), creating a Howship's lacuna under the ruffled border of its attachment site through dissolution of hydroxyapatite in a highly acidic local environment, and through enzymatic destruction of the collagen, marking the surface path of osteoclast. (Courtesy of the Armed Forces Institute of Pathology, Washington, DC.)

Bone Modeling

Definition
■ Process whereby bone, formed initially in the embryo, is shaped into the adult form as growth occurs
■ Responsible for the large changes in bone structure during growth

Defining Characteristics
■ Changes in bone structure occur on existing bone structure.
■ Bone structure alterations occur by independent action of osteoblasts and osteoclasts.
■ Bone resorption and formation may occur on different surfaces.

Bone Remodeling

Definition
■ Process whereby current bone structure is maintained
■ Cannot cause large changes in bone structure at a given site

BOX 14-1 FACTORS EXPRESSED BY THE VARIOUS STAGES OF PROLIFERATING AND DIFFERENTIATING OSTEOBLASTS AND THEIR PRECURSORS

BMP 2	Osteopontin
BMP 7	Bone sialoprotein
Type I collagen	Alkaline phosphatase

Defining Characteristics
■ Changes in bone structure occur on or within existing bone structure (same as for modeling).
■ Osteoblasts and osteoclasts do not act independently but are coupled through cytokine activity and mechanical forces (different than for modeling). Table 14-2 outlines the essential features of osteoblasts and osteoclasts.
■ Coupled bone deletion and formation at the same site:
  ■ Intracortical remodeling is affected by the bone remodeling unit (BRU)—teams of osteoclasts excavating a hole in the cortex (10 longitudinal surges of clastic activity over 2 months) followed by osteoblasts filling in the hole (months)
  ■ Cancellous bone remodeling occurs at many sites in the honeycomb trabecular array, with activation of bone surface lining cells, recruitment of marrow osteoclasts, creation of a Howship's lacuna (see Fig. 14-3), and activation of stem cells to become osteoblasts, which fill the defect.

Long Bone Growth

By the ninth week in the embryo the skeleton is preformed, the craniofacial bones as woven bone and the rest as a multiplicity of cartilage models (Fig. 14-6). Subsequent growth of the models progresses in stages.

Stages of Long Bone Development
■ Before development of ossification centers:
  ■ Cartilage models undergo considerable growth in size:
    ■ By appositional induction at their surface ("perichondrium") and
    ■ By internal cartilage cell proliferation and maturation

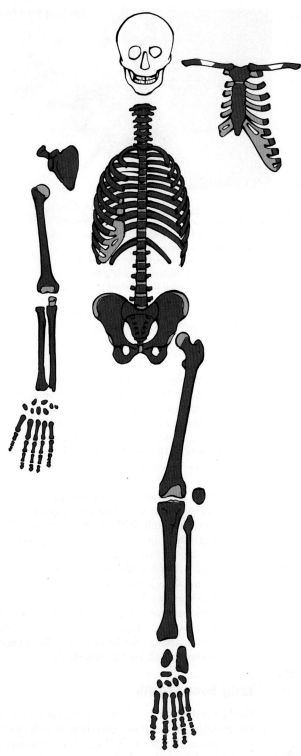

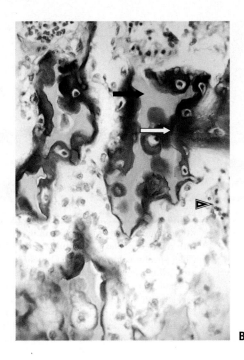

B

A

Figure 14-4 (**A**) Enchondral bone formation. Much of the skeleton arises from cartilage model bones; these grow in length at growth plates. (**B**) Enchondral bone formation: primary trabeculae formation. "Primary trabeculae" form a latticework (like a honeycomb) of intersecting bone structures, each formed by a process in which the calcified cartilage core (dark blue–staining material, *black arrow*), a remnant of the growth plate cartilage, acts as a nidus on which woven bone (dark pink–staining material; *white arrow*) is deposited. In the surrounding marrow space, a fibrovascular stroma (*arrowhead*) supplies stem cells and blood supply to support the enchondral bone process. (Courtesy of the Armed Forces Institute of Pathology, Washington, DC.)

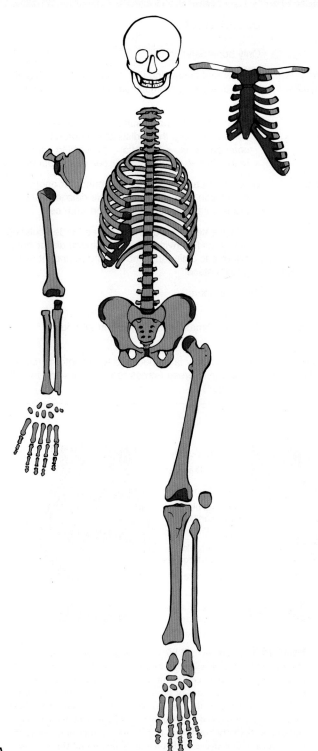

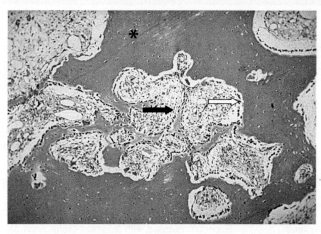

A

B

Figure 14-5   Bone modeled bone (lamellar). (**A**) Once created, bone throughout the entire skeleton is altered through modeling and remodeling. (**B**) Photomicrograph shows dense cortical bone (solid pink–staining material; *asterisk*), which has been tunneled through aggressive osteoclast action after a stress fracture. Bone is being formed rapidly to refill the spaces, as generation after generation of osteoblasts line up and deposit lamellar bone on the margins of the space. Mature, adult cortical bone is a solid structure (*asterisk*) and consists of osteons that have formed over time through repeated stress-directed cutting cone activity. The marrow space is a fibrovascular stroma (*black arrow*) that supports the lamellar bone formation (*white arrow*). The process effectively fills in holes created by osteoclast activity in an overuse situation. (Courtesy of the Armed Forces Institute of Pathology, Washington, DC.)

TABLE 14-2 ESSENTIAL FEATURES OF OSTEOBLASTS AND OSTEOCLASTS

	Osteoblast (OB)	Osteoclast (OC)
Function	Only bone-forming cell	Only bone-deleting cell
Cell cycle	Stem cell → pre-OB → proliferating OB → mature OB → mineralizing OB → apoptotic OB/osteocyte/bone lining cell	Marrow and circulating OC precursors → fusion of OC precursors → multinucleated OC → apoptotic OC
Cell function	Expression of type I collagen, ALP, osteonectin, osteopontin, bone sialoprotein, biglycan, decorin, matrix Gla-protein, and bone acidic glycoprotein	Attachment to the bone surface → polarization of the cell surface into three distinct membrane compartments → formation of a sealing zone → resorption → detachment → cell death (apoptosis)
Cytoplasm	Cytoplasm packed with rough endoplasmic reticulum, stains blue with hematoxylin	Cytoplasm packed with mitochondria, for energy production associated with bone deletion. Clear areas contain material for export from cell.
Nucleus	Eccentric nucleus with adjacent Golgi apparatus	Multinucleated giant cell with ruffled border isolating highly acidic environment for mineral dissolution, enzymatic collagen removal, and abundant acid phosphatase
Survival	As blast, up to 10 days As resident osteocyte, months to years	24 to 48 hours
Efficiency	Up to 100 osteoblasts required to fill bone deleted by one osteoclast; requires 3 months	Digests 3 times its cell volume in 24 hours
	Clast 100 times more efficient than blast in terms of volume and creates its cavity in 1 day, while refill takes months	Clast efficiency is responsible for symptoms related to acute overuse (stress reactions leading to stress fractures)

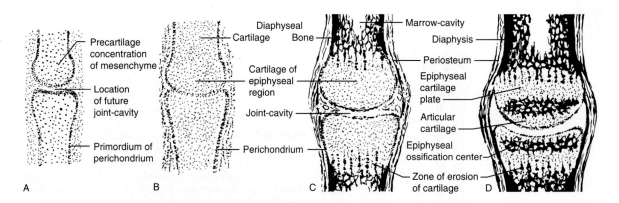

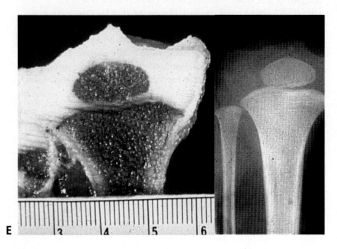

Figure 14-6 Cartilage cell life cycle. Sequential cartilage maturation from early cartilage model formation to emerging primary and secondary centers of ossification. (**A**) Mesenchymal condensation early at sites of bone model, adjacent perichondrium, and interzone (future site of joint). (**B**) Differentiation and cellular function have produced cartilage matrix of the bone model and collagen at the perichondrium. (**C**) Primary center of ossification has formed with a sleeve of diaphyseal bone around the marrow cavity, a trabecular array of woven bone, growth plates, epiphyseal cartilage, and early joint space. (**D**) Fetal joint now has fully formed with secondary center of ossification, articular cartilage, joint capsule, and other elements as already listed. (**E**) Emergence of ossification centers allows radiographic visualization. Gross specimen correlates with radiograph, demonstrating secondary center of ossification in the tibia but none in the fibula. (A–D, Courtesy of *Proceedings of Annual Canadian Orthopaedic Association Basic Science Course*, DE Sweet, lecture notes, Skeletal Radiologic/Pathologic Correlation, 1987–2003. E, Courtesy of the Armed Forces Institute of Pathology, Washington, DC.)

■ After development of ossification centers:
  ■ Emergence of sequential primary and then secondary ossification centers subdivides long bone cartilage models (see Fig. 14-6).
    ■ Epiphysis (secondary ossification center)
    ■ Epiphyseal growth plates (physeal growth center/physis)
    ■ Metaphysis
    ■ Diaphysis
  ■ Emergence of secondary ossification centers allows radiographic identification, providing a basis for evaluating chronological versus biologic bone age.

Primary Center of Ossification

The cartilage model in long bones begins as a central condensation of mesenchymal cells, which then produce cartilage matrix from the center of the bone, spreading outward toward the ends. This step, differentiation of cells to become chondrocytes, is regulated by a DNA transcription factor, Sox9, which controls the expression of genes coding for collagen (col), proteoglycan (PG), or non-collagenous proteins. Sox9, in conjunction with L-Sox5 and Sox6, binds to specific enhancer regions in the promoters of these target genes to activate gene transcription. Individual cartilage cells undergo sequential stages of development, which lead to development of the primary center of ossification.

Stages of Individual Cartilage Cell Development (Chondrification)

1. Differentiation from uncommitted stromal cell
2. Rest

3. Reproduction
4. Maturation/matrix production
5. Hypertrophy
6. Matrix mineralization: first identifies primary center of ossification on x-ray
7. Senescence and death (apoptosis)

Stages of Development in Primary Center of Ossification

1. Initiation of chondrification

   ■ Begins near the center
   ■ Cartilage cells there reach the final stages of mineralization and terminal differentiation first (Fig. 14-7).

2. Woven bone formation

   ■ Change in cartilage maturation induces the formation of a sleeve of coarsely woven bone at the level of maximum cartilage cell hypertrophy (see Fig. 14-7).
   ■ Stimulus for this induction is unknown.
   ■ Perichondrium changes to periosteum.

3. Vascular invasion

   ■ Death of cartilage cells may provide the signal for vascular invasion; it is likely that cytokines direct the process.
   ■ Invading vascular granulation tissue brings in endothelial cells and precursor cells that differentiate into blasts and clasts.

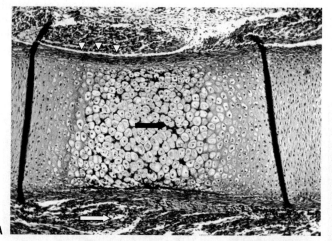
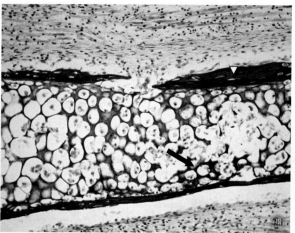

A   B

Figure 14-7 Primary center of ossification. (**A**) Central portion of cartilage model where cartilage cell death (absence of cells centrally) has left behind dark-staining calcified cartilage (*black arrow*), which will act as a nidus for apposition of woven bone in the formation of primary trabeculae; this defines enchondral bone formation. On either end, the cartilage cells undergo growth through their cell cycle, showing growth plate morphology. *White arrow* indicates surrounding mesenchymal anlage forming early skeletal muscle. (**B**) Later, vascular invasion occurs through a gap in the woven bone that has formed from the inner layer of the periosteum. The cortex at this time is a coarsely woven sleeve of bone, incomplete where the vessel enters. Cartilage cells are dead; the calcified cartilage (*black arrow*) is removed by osteoclasts emerging as precursors from the vessels; no bone is deposited yet on the cartilage cores. *Arrowheads* indicate primitive cortex, arising from the cambium layer of the periosteum, which is woven bone in the embryo, lamellar bone in the child. (Courtesy of the Armed Forces Institute of Pathology, Washington, DC.)

4. Removal of chondrocytes and calcified cartilage

■ Monocytes and specialized giant cells (chondroclasts, analogous to osteoclasts) remove most of the dead and dying chondrocytes and calcified cartilage (see Fig. 14-7).

5. Primary trabecula formation

■ Osteoblasts differentiate out of the cellular blastema and reinforce the remaining calcified cartilage remnants (Fig. 14-8).
■ Primary trabecula
   ■ Definition: the combination of calcified cartilage core with apposed woven bone
   ■ Array of interconnected primary trabeculae consists of plates of bone that act to transmit force from the cortex to the epiphysis and articular surface

6. Secondary trabecula formation

■ Secondary trabecula (Fig. 14-9)
   ■ Lacks calcified cartilage cores
   ■ Makes up the metaphyseal trabecular array in long bones and the core of cuboidal bones
   ■ Undergoes repeated remodeling throughout life
■ Remodeling of these occurs with removal of those that are not needed mechanically, and reinforcement of those that become the selected transmitters of mechanical force.

7. Growth plate formation

■ Growth plates (see Fig. 14-8) become clearly visible on either end with identifiable zones of function correlating with the stages of development of cartilage cells; the entire bone model (diaphysis, metaphyses, growth plates) is contained within a periosteal sleeve

that merges with the perichondrium on either end. This confluence of periosteum and perichondrium is termed the perichondrial ossification groove of Ranvier, containing the circumferential bony ring of Lacroix.

■ Bony ring of Lacroix
   ■ This is a woven sleeve of bone maintaining its position at the level of the hypertrophic cartilage cells (see Fig. 14-8). It acts as a rigid cup supporting the cartilaginous epiphysis.
■ Ossification groove of Ranvier
   ■ An outer fibrous perichondrial layer formed by fibroblasts and collagen, continuous below with the periosteum
   ■ An inner layer of undifferentiated loosely packed cells that become chondrocytes, providing lateral growth adjacent to the germinal and proliferating layers
   ■ Below this, the inner layer differentiates into osteoblasts that form the ring of Lacroix.

THE GROWTH PLATE

Growth in length is accomplished in the composite structure of the growth plate, where reserve cartilage cells in the physeal growth center give rise to multiple successive generations of proliferating clones of cartilage cells. The growth plate can be divided into zones, as in Figure 14-9. There are a variety of descriptions of the cell layers, with confusion arising because some refer to *morphology* and others to *cell function*. The cartilage cells follow the cycle that applies to cartilage at most sites in the body: rest, proliferation, hypertrophy, and programmed cell death or apoptosis. Matrix synthesis occurs throughout with variation of content according to cell layer. As the chondrocyte

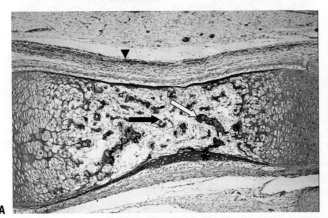 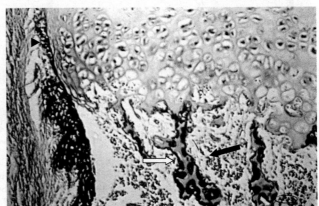

Figure 14-8 Primary center of ossification. (**A**) The initial cortex (*asterisk*) is a sleeve of woven bone that ends on either end of the cartilage model at the hypertrophic zone of the growth plate. This is the site of the circumferential ring of Lacroix. Most of the calcified cartilage is gone centrally and replaced by a fibrovascular stroma (*black arrow*); there are a few primary trabeculae centrally (*white arrow*). The *arrowhead* indicates the several layers of periosteum. (**B**) Growth plate with woven bone reinforcement of primary trabeculae. The *arrowhead* indicates the termination of cortex at the hypertrophic zone. (Courtesy of the Armed Forces Institute of Pathology, Washington, DC.)

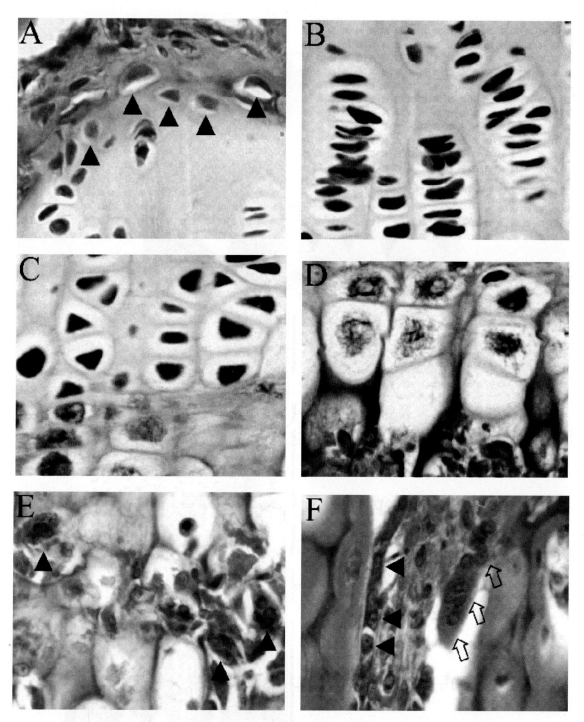

Figure 14-9 Growth plate morphology. **(A) Resting zone:** One cell per lacuna, large amount of PG; high ratio of extracellular matrix to cells. *Arrowheads* identify resting zone stem cells. 40× magnification, H&E. **(B) Proliferative zone:** Flattened disc morphology with occasional mitotic profile, may have many cells within a single large lacuna, highest rate of PG synthesis and turnover. 40× magnification, H&E. **(C) Upper hypertrophic (transition) zone:** Characterized by loss of capacity to divide and increase in size, cartilage cells termed prehypertrophic, calcium storage begins, PG synthesis continues. 40× magnification, H&E. **(D) Lower hypertrophic zone:** Matrix calcification, breakdown of nuclear envelope, and apoptosis of cells. 40× magnification, H&E. **(E) Chondro-osseous junction:** Vascular invasion and multinucleate osteo-/chondroclastic matrix removal. *Arrowheads* show chondroclasts at transverse septa of evacuated lacunae. 40× magnification, H&E. **(F) Primary spongiosa:** Endochondral bone formation over cartilaginous trabeculae by osteoblastic osteoid (pink) deposition over cartilage scaffold (blue-purple) and continuation of remodeling via osteo-/chondroclastic matrix resorption, removing cartilage scaffold core. Osteoblasts identified by *black arrowheads*, osteo-/chondroclasts by *arrows*. 40× magnification, H&E.

(continued)

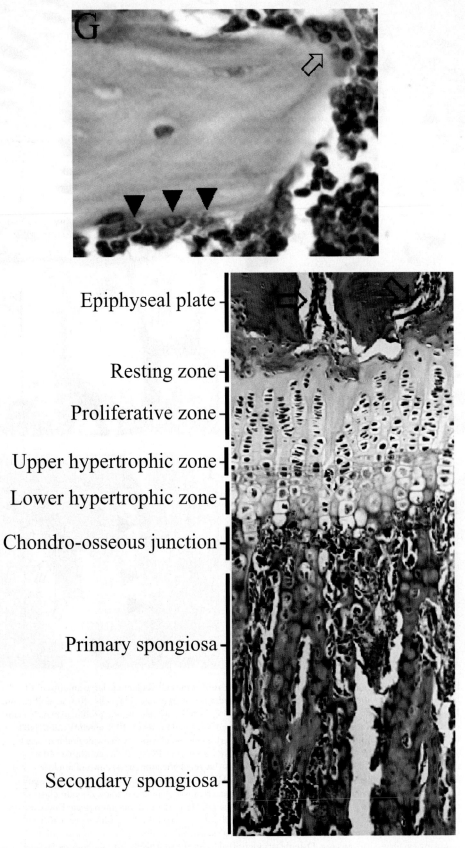

Epiphyseal plate

Resting zone

Proliferative zone

Upper hypertrophic zone

Lower hypertrophic zone

Chondro-osseous junction

Primary spongiosa

Secondary spongiosa

Figure 14-9 *(continued)*   (**G**) **Secondary spongiosa:** Remodeling of secondary, osseous trabeculae by osteoblastic bone deposition over osteoid scaffold and continuation of osteoclastic matrix resorption. Osteoblasts identified by *black arrowheads*, osteoclasts by *arrow*. 40× magnification, H&E. **Bottom:** Micrograph of 10-week-old male rat proximal tibial growth plate and metaphyseal primary and secondary spongiosa. *Arrows* identify epiphyseal vascular structures. 10× magnification, H&E.

is the only cell present in the growth plate, it is responsible for all activities:

- Synthesis, maintenance, and breakdown of the collagen and extracellular matrix
- Elaboration of the cytokines that participate in the direction of these processes

Regulation of this process is far from understood. The extracellular matrix acts as a reservoir in which there is interaction among cells, the surrounding structure, integrins, circulating systemic hormones, and local polypeptide signaling substances. The vessels also seem to be intimately involved. Actual growth is a function of increased cell mass (proliferation plus hypertrophy) and matrix elaboration. All of this occurs in place, with the cells finally undergoing senescence and programmed cell dropout (apoptosis) as calcification of the surrounding cartilage occurs. This combined activity essentially lifts or pushes the overlying epiphysis away from the underlying metaphysis. The dynamics of chondrocyte differentiation are such that a cell moves through resting, proliferating, and hypertrophic stages, ending with calcification over 24 hours, with apoptosis involving 18% of this time (see Fig. 14-9, Table 14-3).

Circulatory Support for the Growth Plate (Fig. 14-10)

- Epiphyseal vessels supply the secondary center of ossification and the resting, proliferative, and hypertrophic zones.
  - Resting zone
    - Vessels perforate but do not supply cells.
    - Chondrocytes at this level have a low pO_2 and their metabolism is anaerobic.
  - Proliferative zone
    - Vessels ramify at this level, providing a high-pO_2 environment for the aerobic activities of cellular proliferation and matrix production.
  - Hypertrophic zone
    - Progressive drop-off of oxygen tension as the now-hypertrophying cells pass through altered cell function, terminal differentiation, and apoptosis.
    - Adjacent cartilage becomes more and more calcified.
    - Metabolism becomes more and more anaerobic up to cell death.
- Metaphyseal vessels supply the periphery of the zone of vascular invasion; end loops from the nutrient artery system supply the center.
  - Vascular invasion
    - Space is created by deletion of most of the calcified cartilage by clasts emanating from the invading vessels.
    - The remaining calcified cartilage cores act as templates for the application of woven bone by perivascular cells that become osteoblasts; this is the primary trabecular array.
    - Anatomy of terminal vessels
      - Arteriole loops back on itself beneath the last

intact transverse septum of calcified cartilage.
      - Capillary ends in a venous sinusoid where flow is turgid and pO_2 is very low, supporting bone formation.
  - Adjacent marrow becomes more and more vascular to support the active process of primary trabecular bone formation and subsequent internal remodeling.

Hormones and the Growth Plate

Growth is intensely anabolic with the production of cells, which then produce structure formed from proteins, proteoglycans, and non-protein substances. Disorders of growth thus represent problems in cell multiplication and differentiation, or in formation of the elements of structure. Growth plate function is a linked series of steps affecting the chondrocyte, stem cells, vascular endothelial cells, osteoblasts, and osteoclasts, influenced by a combination of systemic (endocrine) and local (paracrine or autocrine) factors (Table 14-4). Each step in the growth cascade has specific factors that influence and direct it; effects are different between the developing embryonic and postnatal growth plate.

Physeal Closure

Physeal closure occurs at the end of adolescence, in a hormonally and cytokine-driven osteoclastic surge (Fig. 14-11).

- Mechanism of growth plate closure
  - Hormones driving growth diminish in activity.
  - Reduced proliferation of cartilage and reduced hypertrophic chondrocyte size and column density produce a radiographic narrowing of the growth plate.
  - Cartilage becomes progressively more mineralized as the remaining cells go through a slower sequence, again seen on radiographs.
  - Clast activity works only on calcified cartilage, so that the final step is a surge of clast activity (see Fig. 14-11).
  - Estrogen is a key factor leading to growth plate closure.
    - Genetic disorders in estrogen handling, either in the gene encoding aromatase enzyme that converts androgen to estrogen, or in gene encoding estrogen receptor-[α]; in both the physes fail to close, leading to increased height.
    - Mechanism of estrogen-driven growth plate closure is unknown.

Secondary Center of Ossification: The Epiphysis

Growth and development in the epiphysis is physiologically similar to, but slower than, physeal growth. It primarily emanates from the subarticular (subchondral) cartilage rather than the growth plate (physis). The timing of appearance of the secondary centers of ossification (Fig. 14-12) is

TABLE 14-3 GROWTH PLATE STRUCTURE AND FUNCTION

Growth Plate Zone Anatomy	Cellular Function and Synthesis	Metabolism and pO$_2$	Intracellular & Ionic Calcium	Chondrocyte Diseases
Resting Zone (RZ) • Small rounded cells often found in clusters • Variable cellularity and thickness according to species being examined. Smaller animals commonly used in research have thinner, more cellular RZ; larger animals, such as humans, have thicker, less cellular RZ.	• Mechanical support/perichondrium • Involved in the regulation of the chondrocyte proliferation/maturation pathway by responding to Indian hedgehog (Ihh) through the Patched receptor by increasing expression of parathyroid-related protein (PTHrP)	• Branches of epiphyseal artery pass through RZ to top of proliferative columns (true only in large animals). • Low pO$_2$	• Lowest intracellular and ionized Ca	**Sox9 associated:** campomelic dysplasia
Proliferative Zone (PZ) • Flattened cells with eccentric nuclei formed in longitudinal columns aligned parallel to the long axis of bone • The cellular lacunae and interterritorial matrix are easily visible. • Generally the overall numbers of cells in each column vary according to age.	• Proliferative cells contribute to growth in part by proliferating rapidly in columns and producing a matrix composed of collagens (collagen II, IX, XI) and proteoglycans (aggrecan, decorin, and biglycan). • Proliferative cells possess the receptor for PTHrP, which inhibits apoptosis and allows for continued proliferation. • Growth hormone induces the expression of insulin-like growth factor (IGF-I), which increases proliferation and is important for normal postnatal skeletal growth.	• Rich blood supply through epiphyseal vessels • Highest pO$_2$ • Aerobic glycolysis with raised mitochondrial ATP	• Intracellular Ca equal to RZ • Ionized Ca higher	**PG associated:** autosomal recessive chondrodysplasias as diastrophic dysplasia **Collagen associated:** gene mutations of collagen II, IX, or XI lead to spondyloepiphyseal dysplasia (SED), multiple epiphyseal dysplasia (MED), hypochondriasis, all causing short stature **PZ control associated:** Laron syndrome, a hereditary dwarfism with truncal obesity and low serum IGF-I levels. Achondroplasia (ACP), a dwarfing condition in which proliferation is markedly reduced through an activating mutation in the FGF-3 receptor (FGFR-3), which modulates the PTHrP-Ihh proliferation/maturation feedback loop by inducing cellular maturation by causing cells to exit the cell cycle.

Zone				
Upper Hypertrophic Transition Zone (HTZ) • Cells transition from flat to more rounded shapes. • Nuclei are larger and located centrally.	• As PTHrP concentrations decrease, chondrocytes begin to mature, increasing their expression of Ihh, vascular endothelial growth factor (VEGF), and alkaline phosphatase (ALP). • Part of the maturation process in chondrocytes is the increase in cell size, or cellular hypertrophy. • Limited cellular division can be observed in this zone. • Collagen II expression decreases and collagen X expression increases (X unique to this zone). • Fibronectin and collagenase are produced. • Mineralization of matrix begins.	• No direct vascular supply • Diminishing pO_2 • Glycogen is consumed: Highest content of glycolytic enzymes	• Upper levels have highest levels of total cellular Ca and stored Ca. • As glycogen is totally used, Ca is released by mitochondria. • Elevated intracellular Ca activates proteases, lipases, and nucleases, leading to apoptosis.	**ALP associated:** Hypophosphatasia is a congenital absence of ALP that produces a form of rickets with the following: • Decreased mineralization of matrix • Widening of growth plate • Defective mineralization of bone with retarded extravesicular crystal propagation
Lower Hypertrophic Transition Zone (HTZ) • Cells increase in size substantially, becoming round and ovoid. • Nuclei are located centrally and the chromatin becomes condensed. • Organelles and glycogen become prominent.	• Cells produce collagen X and a mineralized matrix that will function as an anlage for new bone. • Cells undergo apoptosis but remain viable until they reach the chondro-osseous junction. • TGF-beta in vesicles in an inactive form then is activated by MMP-13.	• Anaerobic • Very low pO_2 • Glycogen depleted	• Annexin II, V, and VI exist in the lipid bilayer and are necessary for Ca uptake.	
Primary Spongiosa • Composed of osteoblasts, endothelial cells, and chondroclasts • Metaphyseal vascular arcades supply the GP cellular nutrition by diffusion. • Capillaries form loops during vascular ingrowth into the empty lacunae of the terminal hypertrophic cell. • Formation of primary trabeculae; apposition of woven bone to cartilage core template by osteoblasts	• Hypertrophic chondrocytes produce factors that attract endothelial cells, osteoblasts, and chondroclasts (VEGF, FGF-2, and the ligand for the receptor activator of nuclear kappa-beta [RANK-ligand]). • Primary modeling: Osteoblasts produce woven bone composed of collagen I and mineral apatite. • Chondroclasts are specialized multinucleate cells that produce MMP-9, which resorbs the mineralized cartilage matrix.	• Highly vascular tissue due to plexus of capillaries forming at the chondro-osseous junction • High pO_2		

(continued)

TABLE 14-3 (continued)

Growth Plate Zone Anatomy	Cellular Function and Synthesis	Metabolism and pO$_2$	Intracellular & Ionic Calcium	Chondrocyte Diseases
Secondary Spongiosa • Trabeculae become thicker and are composed of lamellar bone, in which osteocytes are located between the lamellae and osteoblasts are located on the outer surface. • Abundant numbers of osteoclasts remodel bone.	• The shape of the ends of long bones is altered through the process of modeling involving independent action of osteoclasts and osteoblasts. • Surface remodeling of primary trabeculae • Osteoclast removal of bone • Osteoblast fill-in and add-on	• Good blood supply through metaphyseal vessels and end vessels from nutrient artery • High pO$_2$		**Remodeling associated:** Osteopetrosis, a disorder of osteoclast function characterized by abnormal remodeling; there is absent or reduced osteoclast activity in the metaphysis so that the calcified cartilage bars at the end of the HTZ persist. Calcified cartilage has more mineral than bone; the marrow space becomes packed with this material, producing radiographic density (marble bones) and bone fragility; no space is left for marrow elements.

ECM, extracellular matrix.

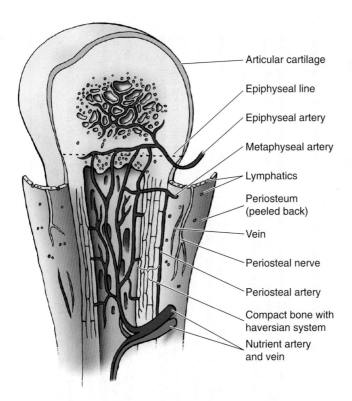

Articular cartilage

Epiphyseal line

Epiphyseal artery

Metaphyseal artery

Lymphatics

Periosteum
(peeled back)

Vein

Periosteal nerve

Periosteal artery

Compact bone with
haversian system

Nutrient artery
and vein

Figure 14-10　Blood supply to a typical growth plate. (From Moore KL, Dalley AF. *Clinically Oriented Anatomy*, 4th ed. Baltimore: Lippincott Williams & Wilkins, 1999.)

unique for each bone. The morphology is identical to that of the primary center as detailed earlier in the section "Stages of Development in Primary Center of Ossification."

Initially, the cartilage around the secondary center of ossification grows circumferentially with normal physeal morphology until impaction on the epiphyseal side of the growth plate occurs. Then growth in that part of the epiphysis ceases, and a bony plate is laid down on the epiphyseal side of the physis. From that moment on, growth in the epiphysis is from subarticular cartilage (Fig. 14-13).

Cancellous Bone

Cancellous bone is initially generated at the epiphyseal and subarticular growth plates as primary metaphyseal and epiphyseal trabeculae, respectively (see Fig. 14-13). It is subsequently modeled and remodeled into a lattice of interconnected bony plates compartmentalizing the marrow space.

Location Within Bones
- Small round and square bones (e.g., talus, calcaneus)
  - Represents the central core of these bones
- Long tubular bones
  - Confined to the epiphysis and metaphysis only
  - Minimal cancellous bone is present in the diaphysis along the inner "endosteal" surface of the cortex.

Functions
- Mechanical
  - To support the subarticular bony plate

- To transmit mechanical force from the articular surface to the cortex
- Acid–base homeostasis
  - Enormous surface area of the body's trabecular and canalicular array provides the ionic resources for mineral and acid–base homeostasis.
  - Estimated surface area: 1,500 to 5000 m^2
- Reservoir for hematopoiesis
  - Initial extent: both axial and appendicular skeleton in the fetus and child
  - With skeletal maturation and cessation of growth, hematopoiesis recedes from limbs and remains within the axial skeleton.

Determination of Quality and Quantity
- Architectural orientation is largely determined by the changing patterns of force on each bone.
- Quantity of cancellous bone depends on the total force applied.

Marrow Space Reactions
- The presence of disease or the requirements of remodeling can induce a regional marrow transformation from fatty marrow to fibrovascular tissue that may lead to emergence of spindle cells, osteoblasts, and osteoclasts.

Cortical Bone and Periosteum

Cortex

Formation of Cortical Bone in the Embryo
- The cortex first appears as a sleeve of woven bone during the development of primary center of ossification (see Figs. 14-7 to 14-8).
  - Change in cartilage maturation induces the formation of a central sleeve of coarsely woven bone that ends at the level of maximum cartilage cell hypertrophy near the periphery of the center of ossification.
  - Stimulus for this induction is unknown but presumably is cytokine-driven.
  - Perichondrium merges with the growth plate at the level of the reserve cells, contributing cells at the lateral margin in a groove-like structure termed the ossification groove of Ranvier (see Fig. 14-8).
  - Inferior to this, the perichondrium changes to periosteum, making bone instead of cartilage. The bone at this level is termed the circumferential bony ring of Lacroix around the hypertrophic zone (see Figs. 14-8A and 14-8B).
  - Periosteum consists of an outer fibrous layer and an inner cambium layer that produces an initial cortex of woven bone extending from one growth plate to the other, ending at the level of the hypertrophic zone.
    - Starting as a solid fibrous structure, as the periosteum migrates outward; its inner layer undergoes fibroclasia, with most of the collagen being removed through clastic activity.
    - Some of the collagen remains and acts as an osteoconductor for the deposition of osteoid,

TABLE 14-4 HORMONE/VITAMIN EFFECTS ON THE GROWTH PLATE

HORMONE/FACTOR	SOURCE	BIOLOGIC EFFECT	ZONE AFFECTED
Growth hormone	Pituitary	After birth, growth hormone promotes cellular proliferation acting directly, and indirectly through mediators, on the somatomedins, produced in liver and in CCs; direct effect creates target CCs in which IGF-I induces replication of CCs.	Throughout growth plate
Somatomedins: Insulin-like growth factor (IGF) I and II	Liver, plus local from CCs	IGF receptors are present throughout GP CCs; receptors for IGF-I have highest concentration in PZ; response to IGF-I lessens with increasing maturity and HT of the CCs; IFG-II is essential for normal fetal growth; IGF-I most active during postnatal life.	Throughout growth plate
Thyroid hormone: T_3 (3,5,3-triiodothyronine)$_3$ T_4 (thyroxine)	Thyroid gland	T_4 and T_3 together with IGF/IGF-II allow normal growth and maturation of CCs; excess T_4 produces protein catabolism; deficient T_4 produces growth retardation, cretinism, and abnormal degradation of mucopolysaccharides.	Proliferative zone and upper hypertrophic transition zone
Parathyroid hormone (PTH)	Parathyroid	Direct mitogenic effect on CCs; stimulates prostaglandin synthesis through increase in intracellular Ca and stimulation of protein kinase; is synergistic with other growth factors	Proliferative zone and upper hypertrophic transition zone
Glucocorticoids (GC)	Adrenal cortex	Familial GC deficiency is associated with tall stature; GC excess is associated with osteopenia and growth retardation; direct effect is reduction in CC proliferation and extracellular matrix synthesis; impaired growth is also an indirect effect by interfering with other growth-modulating pathways.	Proliferative zone
Calcitonin	Parafollicular cells of thyroid	Accelerates GP calcification and CC maturation	Lower hypertrophic and transition zone
Estrogen (Eg)	Ovary	Growth spurt is probably caused by elevated growth hormone plus low Eg levels. GP fusion is probably caused by higher level of Eg.	Probably proliferative zone
Androgen (Ag)	Testicles	Ag stimulates longitudinal growth, independent of Eg action, by direct local effect on CCs; until skeletal maturity, Ags stimulate mineralization, increased glycogen, and lipids in CCs, prostaglandin synthesis; suprapysiologic doses of Ag depress growth and accelerate GP closure.	Hypertrophic transition zone, primary spongiosa
Vitamin A	Diet	Normal levels maintain CC metabolism; deficient vitamin A impairs CC maturation, suppresses growth, and alters bone shape; excess vitamin A produces fragile bones; mechanism is increased lysosomal body membrane fragility.	Hypertrophic transition zone
Vitamin C	Diet	Cofactor in enzymatic synthesis of collagen; stimulates mineralization in cultures of CCs; mechanism is stimulation of matrix vesicle formation, and of synthesis of ALP, collagen II, and collagen X	Proliferative zone and hypertrophic transition zone
Vitamin D	Diet; secondary from the sun; locally produced by CCs and osteoblasts	Allows mineralization of newly synthesized osteoid; 1,25-hydroxyvitamin D3 and 24,25-dihydroxyvitamin D3 control autocrine regulators of matrix events: activity of enzymes in matrix vesicles, of matrix proteins during growth, calcification, and activation of growth factors; increases activity of alkaline phosphatase and MMPs	All growth plate zones except hypertrophic transition zone; highest levels in proliferative zone
Prostaglandins	Ubiquitous	Family of hormone-like substances derived from arachidonic acid; mechanism of action is variable depending on the prostaglandin; the precise role of prostaglandin in the GP is unknown.	All growth plate zones

CC, cartilage cells; HT, hypertrophy.

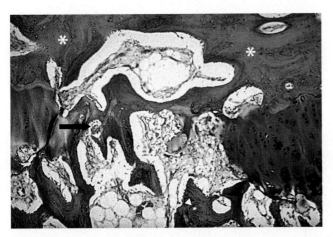

Figure 14-11 Growth plate closure occurs by a wave of osteoclast activity, driven by a complex interplay of systemic hormones and local factors. The slide shows the central region of a growth plate with the epiphyseal bone plate above (*white asterisks*) and growth plate (*black asterisk*) below, with a gap in the middle. The gap has been created by repetitive osteoclast activity. An osteoclast (*arrow*) is deleting calcified cartilage on the left side of the gap. Secondary trabeculae (*arrowhead*) are seen below the gap. (Courtesy of the Armed Forces Institute of Pathology, Washington, DC.)

which then mineralizes; this produces a radiating or streaming appearance of the new woven bone.
- Nature of the woven bone in the embryo
  - Explosive process with radiating streamers of woven bone laid down in bursts of activity (also called osteophytic or streamer bone)

- High cell-to-bone ratio; irregular and random collagen deposition; appearance of an open mesh (Fig. 14-14)
  - Newly formed woven bone is like chicken wire and is mechanically weak.
- Woven bone of this immature nature is seen throughout life in any situation requiring the formation of bone very rapidly (fracture, periosteal response to acute bacterial infection or aggressive tumor).

Primary Osteon Formation
- Once the woven bone structure is in place, Wolff's law demands a strengthening process: this occurs through a filling-in of the interstices of the woven bone by a lamellar bone fill-in, producing a composite structure that is flexible and strong.
- Process of primary osteon formation
  - Osteoblasts line up on the margins of the woven bone trabeculae and slowly deposit bone in successive layers of inlay lamellar configuration into the open spaces between the trabeculae; this passive filling-in produces "primary" or passive osteons.
  - Completes the process of formation of a mechanically solid cortex in the fetus (Fig. 14-15)

Bone Structure from Fetus to Child
- In the embryo and the young child, the cortex is a composite structure:
  - Solid central array of primary osteons, formed by passive lamellar bone fill-in of the fibrovascular

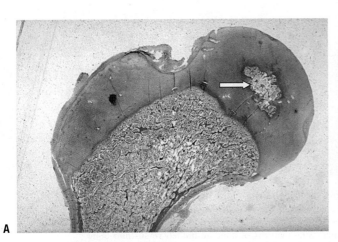
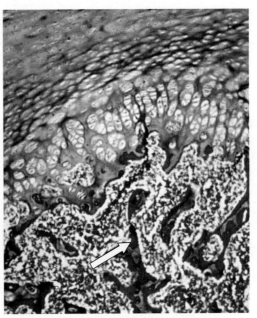

Figure 14-12 (A) Secondary center of ossification (*arrow*) with central growth plate morphology. (B) At higher power the growth plate morphology is seen above. The cancellous bone is formed initially as primary trabeculae (*arrow*) with woven bone deposited on the calcified cartilage core. Primary trabeculae are also seen in Figure 14-8. (Courtesy of the Armed Forces Institute of Pathology, Washington, DC.)

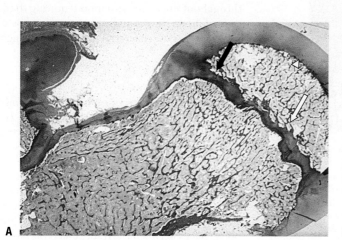
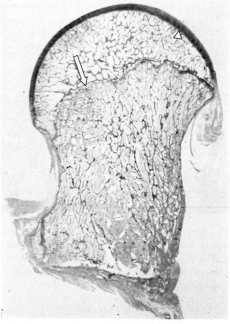

Figure 14-13   Epiphyseal development of the proximal femur. (A) Initial circumferential growth ceases as epiphyseal growth impacts physis (*black arrow*). (B) Bony plate (*white arrow*) develops under mechanical forces on the epiphyseal side of the physis. Remaining growth occurs only from subarticular cartilage (*arrowhead*). In both A and B, the medullary space of the epiphysis and metaphysis consists of an array of cancellous bone, a latticework of interconnected secondary trabeculae. These secondary trabeculae (lamellar bone only, no calcified cartilage core) replace the primary trabeculae that first form on the metaphyseal end of the growth plate. (Courtesy of the Armed Forces Institute of Pathology, Washington, DC.)

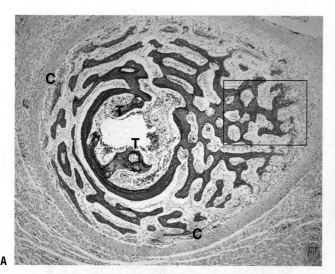
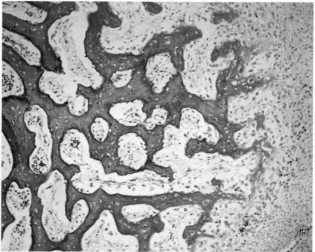

Figure 14-14   (A) Cross-section of fetal cortex through primary center of ossification. The cambium layer (C) of the periosteum has deposited coarse woven bone. Note primary trabeculae (T), fibrovascular marrow space centrally. (B) Higher-power view of boxed area in A emphasizes open mesh appearance of this woven bone. Note increasing maturity of bone on the left versus new bone formation from osteoblasts on the right (cambium layer of periosteum). This is also the appearance of fracture callus at 2 to 3 weeks, at the onset of mineralization prior to lamellar bone fill-in. This is the prototype image of woven bone: random orientation of trabeculae, high cell-to-bone ratio, fibrovascular marrow space. (Courtesy of the Armed Forces Institute of Pathology, Washington, DC.)

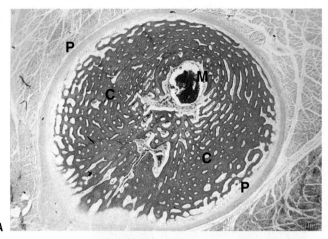
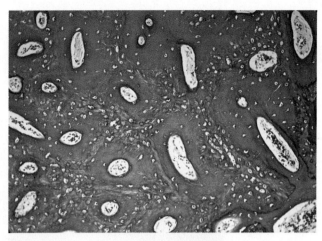

Figure 14-15   (A) Fetal cortex solid appearance after lamellar fill-in. (B) Higher power shows high cell-to-bone ratio of woven bone ghost, with much denser lamellar bone fill-in forming primary osteons. This mimics the appearance of fracture callus at 5 to 6 weeks. M, marrow space; P, periosteum; C, cortex (passive osteons). (Courtesy of the Armed Forces Institute of Pathology, Washington, DC.)

space between the newly deposited, first-formed trabeculae of woven bone

- Outer primary structural element of the cortex
  - Peripheral successive rings of bone deposited by osteoblasts arising from the cambium layer of the periosteum
  - This is woven bone in the embryo and becomes lamellar as growth slows.
- On either end of a fetal long bone are epiphysis and metaphysis with growth plate (see Figs. 14-8, 14-12, and 14-13), and primary and secondary trabecular arrays forming the cancellous network filling the medullary space. The primary trabeculae (primary spongiosa), forming first, are replaced promptly by mechanically more solid bone because of the high rate of turnover of this area.
- The processes of modeling and remodeling continue to unfold, changing the shape and size of the growing bone, respectively, and making the composite structure mechanically efficient.

Modeling of Cortex
- Modeling is the mechanism by which bone alters its shape during growth.
- Involves unequal removal and addition of bone on opposing surfaces (Figs. 14-16 and 14-17)
- Bone removal and replacement occurs in bursts of activity.
  - Teams of clasts completely remove portions of cortex in the cutback zone.
  - Simultaneously, the inner surface of the adjacent bone (either cortex or trabecula) becomes the site of active bone formation.
- Funnelization: Unbalanced removal and replacement allows the metaphysis to "funnel" down to diaphyseal diameter (see Fig. 14-17); removal is highly efficient

and occurs in bursts, while replacement takes months (see Table 14-2).
- Cortex, once it funnels to diaphyseal diameter, remains in a state of imbalance throughout life.
  - Cortical diameter enlarges over time through subperiosteal apposition of rings of lamellar bone.
  - Once growth ceases, the cortex gradually thins as clastic removal on the medullary side of the cortex outstrips the periosteal addition of bone.

Remodeling and Apposition
Growth, development, remodeling, and maintenance of bone and joints depend on a normal balanced relationship among metabolic, mechanical, and circulatory factors. Balance of these factors explains any shift in density in bone through clast and/or blast activation. Each side of this triangle is ultimately driven by a combination of local and systemic environmental and humoral influences (cytokines) acting on blasts and clasts.

Remodeling of Bone—Cortical
- Osteonization: The mechanical stress-driven formation of a resorption cavity and its refill with concentric lamellar bone; this is the process by which cortical bone increases enormously its mechanical properties, providing a durable skeleton for a lifetime (Figs. 14-18 to 14-20). Once formed, the osteon's lifetime is, in part, a function of the activity of the individual. Turnover is rapid in the fetus and growing child, and the osteon may be remodeled in a matter of months.
- Cutting cone activation (see Fig. 14-18): This process, which osteonization relies upon, begins in the infant femur at 1 year of age and the rest of the skeleton over the next several years and continues throughout life. In 1964 Lent Johnson provided this description of the formation of a cutting cone:

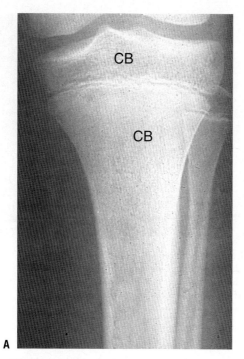
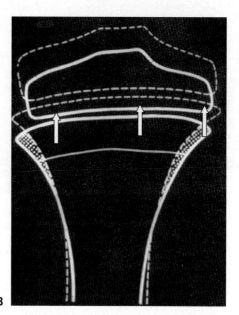

Figure 14-16 Modeling. **(A)** Cancellous bone (CB) fills the medullary space of the epiphyses and metaphyses of long bones, transmitting force from the cortex to the articular surfaces. To maintain the shape of the bone end as growth occurs, modeling must occur. Modeling is a complex process with coordinated addition and deletion of bone to achieve an adult configuration. **(B)** Diagram shows where bone must be deleted and added as growth unfolds. At a given time the proximal tibia has the appearance diagrammed by the solid line. Growth plate action, through increased cell mass and volume and the secretion of matrix, pushes the epiphysis away from the metaphysis. The epiphysis grows in width and in height. The metaphysis widens superiorly and undergoes cutback inferiorly, narrowing its width to that of the diaphysis. The diaphysis undergoes lamellar bone apposition to increase its width, while there is endosteal deletion of bone to maintain cortical width. All deletion is performed by osteoclasts; addition of bone is by osteoblasts. The subsequent bone has the contour outline by the dashed line. (Courtesy of the Armed Forces Institute of Pathology, Washington, DC.)

The cavity is formed by a broad, shallow, cone-shaped osteoclastic wave front, the cutting cone, containing an average of 6 osteoclasts in the plane of section. This is followed by a zone of scattered clasts planing down the edges of Howship's lacunae and producing a slight further increase in diameter. The cutting cone is . . . followed by a mesenchymal cell proliferation so that the spindle-shaped cavity is at all times filled with connective tissue and blood vessels. Finally, there is a very long, slowly closing cone of osteoblastic lamellar refill. Osteoclasts are limited to the cutting cone and the planing zone. Osteoblasts are present all along the face of the closing cone.

■ Osteon: The osteon represents a complex cable, laid down in response to mechanical signals, glued to its neighbors. The composite structure of each bone represents a biomechanical structure of force transmission that is flexible, strong, and capable of ongoing self-maintenance and repair by virtue of its contained living elements.

■ Wolff's law is described by Robert Salter as "remodeling of bone, occurring in response to physical stresses—or to the lack of them—in that bone is deposited in sites subjected to stress and is resorbed from sites where there is little stress." The precise mechanism explaining Wolff's law is not yet determined.

Remodeling of Bone—Cancellous (Fig. 14-21)

■ The cancellous network is a honeycomb-like lattice of lamellar bone in which remodeling occurs on the trabecular surface.

■ Remodeling occurs in the following series of linked steps, termed **coupling**:

■ Quiescence: Bone surface lining cells at rest act as a barrier covering a thin layer of unmineralized osteoid.

■ Activation: Bone surface lining cells' surface receptors for PTH, vitamin D, and IL-6 initiate the remodeling process in response to:

■ Hormone signals: changes in acid–base and calcium–phosphate homeostasis activate receptors for PTH and vitamin D

■ Mechanical signals: mediated via IL-6 signaling

■ Bone surface lining cells initiate a response to a hormonal or stress-induced signal:

■ Secretion of enzymes collagenase and stromelysin for the removal of the osteoid covering the bone surface

■ Secretion of cytokine IL-6, which acts on the marrow to initiate the formation and activation of osteoclasts

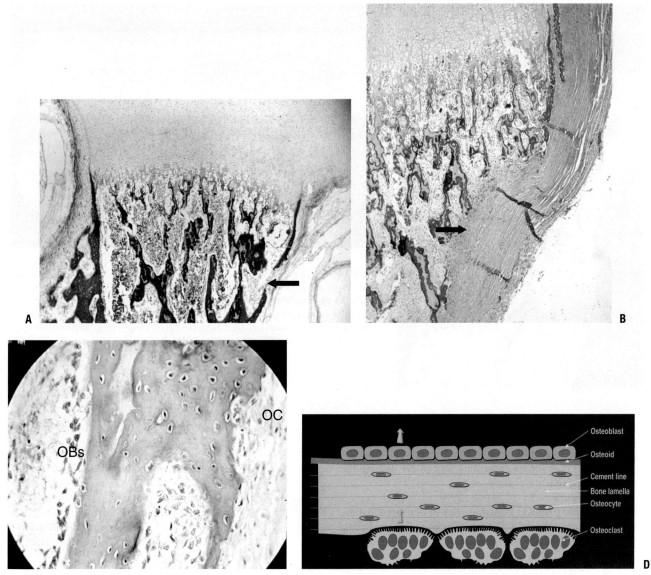

Figure 14-17 Modeling. (**A**) Proximal long bone whole mount specimen. *Arrows* show site of active metaphyseal cutback; osteoclast activity has temporarily deleted a portion of the cortex (*arrow*). (**B**) Another specimen shows a higher-power view of zone of complete cortical deletion adjacent to primary trabeculae (*arrow*). (**C**) Cortex at higher power in a different specimen shows bone modeling with osteoclasts on one surface and blasts on the opposing surface. (**D**) Diagram of modeling, with osteoblasts on one side of the cortex and a site of cortical deletion with a Howship's lacuna and osteoclast on the other side. (**A–C**, Courtesy of the Armed Forces Institute of Pathology, Washington, DC.)

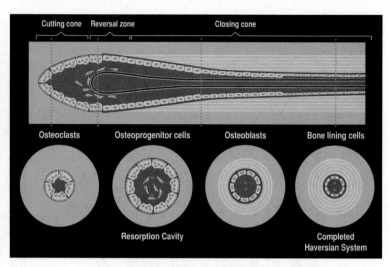

Figure 14-18 Cortex: bone remodeling unit (cutting cone). (**A**) Photomicrograph shows cortical bone (CB) being deleted by a team of osteoclasts. The trailing vessels (V) are seen with activation of perivascular cells to osteoblast lineage; osteoblasts lay down a cement line and then sequential layers of lamellae. (**B**) Diagrammatic representation. (A, Courtesy of the Armed Forces Institute of Pathology, Washington DC; B, courtesy of Dr. P. Roughley.)

- ■ Downregulation of osteoprotegerin, the decoy receptor for receptor activator of NF-Kβ-ligand (RANKL)
- ■ Resorption
  - ■ With RANKL available, newly activated osteoclasts link to RANKL and the bone surface lining cells through the receptor activator of NF-kappa beta (RANK).
  - ■ This coupling made, the bone surface lining cells drop off and the osteoclast settles onto the newly exposed raw bone surface.

  - ■ Osteoclast seals the site and elaborates acid for solubilizing the mineral and the enzyme cathepsin K, which eliminates the osteoid.
  - ■ Bone deletion liberates local stores of cytokines, including BMP and TGF-beta.
  - ■ BMPs initiate osteoblast differentiation in the adjacent marrow; these cells then migrate in and fill the hole.
  - ■ TGF-beta stimulates the osteoblasts to make osteoid and fill the hole.
- ■ Reversal: process by which osteoclasts stop remov-

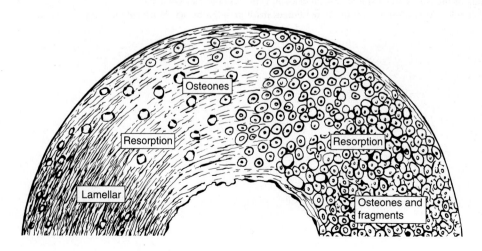

Figure 14-19 Cortical remodeling (osteonization). Over the course of a person's lifetime, cortex begins as a mechanically linked array of "primary" or passive osteons, created by lamellar bone fill-in of the spaces between the initial woven bone trabeculae of the fetal cortex. Mechanical activity induces the activation of cutting cones that create "secondary" or active osteons whose orientation and structure is directed by Wolff's law. On the left the cortex is primarily passive osteons in the fetus; the subsequent bone structure changes with the activity of a lifetime to fully osteonized bone with innumerable interstitial fragments, as on the right.

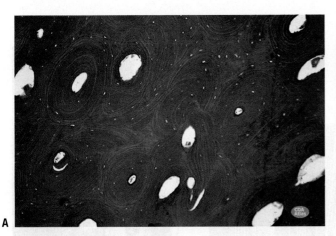
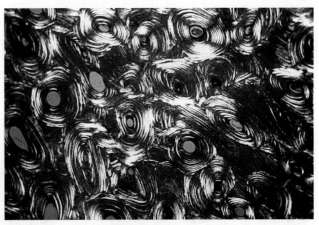

Figure 14-20 (A) Adult cortical bone. Note mature haversian systems (secondary osteons). (B) Polarized light view of adult cortex showing secondary osteons and osteonal fragments. (Courtesy of the Armed Forces Institute of Pathology, Washington, DC.)

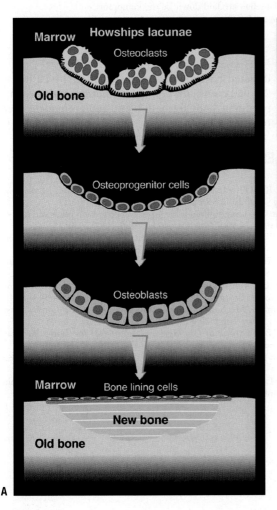

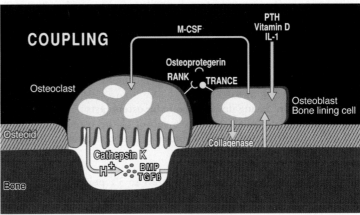

Figure 14-21 (A) Trabecular remodeling. Activation of bone surface lining cells recruits marrow osteoclasts, which dig a cavity (Howship's lacuna), subsequently filled in by locally recruited osteoblasts. (B) The process of activation, resorption, and formation explained diagrammatically. (Courtesy of Dr. Peter Roughley.)

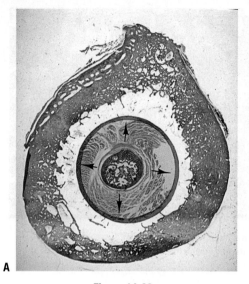
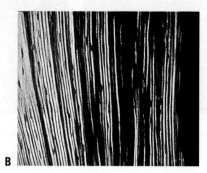
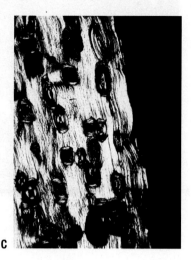

Figure 14-22 (A) Fetal femur plus thigh muscle compared to cross-section of adult femur (woman in late 60s). Mechanism for cortical drift is periosteal addition of lamellar rings with concomitant endosteal osteoclastic removal. The process is not balanced so that as one ages, the cortex becomes thinner as the bone contour expands. Note early cancellization (porosity) of adult femur. (B) Polarized image of outer concentric lamellar, not yet osteonized. These lamellae are laid down by the cambium layer of the periosteum. (C) Polarized image of similar lamellae undergoing osteonization. (Courtesy of the Armed Forces Institute of Pathology, Washington, DC.)

ing bone and osteoblasts fill the defect. Initiation of this step involves the deposition of a cement line by the first wave of osteoblasts.
- Formation: laying down of bone by osteoblasts
- Once the cycle is complete, a subset of the osteoblasts become bone surface lining cells and the surface again becomes quiescent.
- Rates of remodeling
  - Remodeling of cortical bone: 2% to 3% per year
  - Remodeling of trabecular skeleton: 25% per year

Periosteal Apposition of Lamellar Bone
- Changes over lifetime
  - Initially coarse and more cellular in the fetus
  - Lamellae become finer and finer as the individual ages.
  - The slow, more orderly pattern of periosteal bone formation in late childhood, adolescence, and adulthood results in successive layers of lamellar bone encompassing the cortical circumference (circumferential lamellar bone), like the rings of a tree.
  - Subsequent generation of "secondary" (stress-

directed haversian systems; see Figs. 14-19 to 14-21) will eventually convert the normal periosteal appositional bone formation into adult remodeled cortex (Fig. 14-22).

SUGGESTED READING

Ballock RT, O'Keefe RJ. The biology of the growth plate. *J Bone Joint Surg [Am]* 2003;85:715–726.

Brighton CT. Longitudinal bone growth: The growth plate and its dysfunctions. *AAOS Instr Course Lectures* 1987;36:3–25.

Forriol F, Shapiro F. Bone development: Interaction of molecular components and biophysical forces. *Clin Orthop* 2005:14–33.

Iannotti JP. Growth plate physiology and pathology. *Orthop Clin North Am* 1990;21:1–17.

Johnson LC. Morphologic analysis in pathology. In: Frost H, ed. *Bone Dynamics*. Boston: Little, Brown and Company; 1964:543–654.

Katunuma N. Mechanism and regulation of bone resorption by osteoclasts. *Curr Top Cell Regul* 1997;35:179–192.

Salter RB. *Textbook of Disorders and Injuries of the Musculoskeletal System*, 1st ed. Baltimore: Williams & Wilkins, 1970.

Teitelbaum SL. Bone resorption by osteoclasts. *Science* 2000;289:1504–1508.

van der Eerden BC, Karperien M, Wit JM. Systemic and local regulation of the growth plate. *Endocr Rev* 2003;24:782–801.

15

GENETIC BASIS OF MUSCULOSKELETAL DISORDERS

SATHAPPAN S. SATHAPPAN
KIRILL ILALOV
PAUL E. DI CESARE

The *orthopaedic genome* consists of all genes involved in the development and functioning of the musculoskeletal system. The Human Genome Project (1990–2003) has facilitated an in-depth understanding of the orthopaedic genome as well as the molecular biology of musculoskeletal conditions. Current and future molecular interventional modalities are expected to represent a paradigm shift in the management of orthopaedic disorders.

PATHOGENESIS

Etiology

- Human DNA consists of 46 chromosomes (22 pairs of autosomes and 1 pair of sex chromosomes), comprising approximately 30,000 genes.
- Each gene represents a chain of nucleotides (Fig. 15-1) characterized by:
  - Promoter and other regulatory elements that control gene expression
  - A coding region, consisting of introns and exons, that defines the unique order of amino acids and hence determines protein form and function
  - Gene expression: the transfer of genetic information (DNA) to messenger RNA by the process of transcription, followed by the translation of mRNA into a specific protein (Table 15-1 gives definitions of terms used in this chapter)
- Genetic abnormalities
  - Can involve individual chromosomal aberrations, such as deletions (as in Turner syndrome), additions (as in Down syndrome), translocations (where portions of two chromosomes are exchanged, as seen in the 11:22 translocation associated with Ewing sarcoma), and nucleotide repeat expansions (as in trinucleotide disorders)
  - Can affect autosomes and sex chromosomes
  - Inheritance may be autosomal dominant or recessive.
  - X-linked mode of inheritance typically is recessive (e.g., Duchenne's muscular dystrophy, hemophilia) but rarely may be dominant (e.g., X-linked hypophosphatemic rickets).
  - Many diseases exhibit more than one pattern, depending on the mutation.
  - Can be inherited or spontaneous (new mutations)
  - Can follow a simple or complex pattern of inheritance
    - Single-gene disorders follow Mendelian genetics.
    - Polygenic disorders result from interaction of multiple genes (e.g., congenital hip dislocation

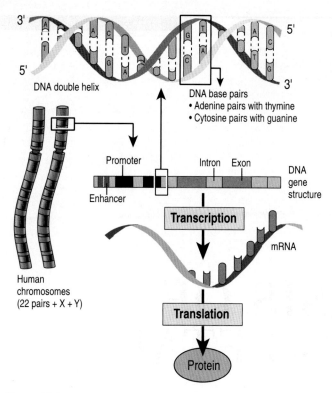

Human chromosomes (22 pairs + X + Y)

DNA double helix

DNA base pairs
• Adenine pairs with thymine
• Cytosine pairs with guanine

Promoter

Enhancer

Intron Exon

DNA gene structure

Transcription

mRNA

Translation

Protein

Figure 15-1 Outline of the human genome.

or neural tube defects, such as myelomeningo-cele).

- Mosaicism refers to an expression of two cell lines in one individual (e.g., X chromosome inactivation in female).

- May have variable penetrance (percentage of individuals with the mutation expressing the phenotype) and expressivity (degree to which the individuals with the mutation express the phenotype)
- The underlying basis for various musculoskeletal disorders has been attributed to disorders in genotype.
- The disease manifestations of abnormalities in the orthopaedic genome (Fig. 15-2) can be broadly classified as:
  - Skeletal dysplasias
  - Connective tissue disorders
  - Neuromuscular disorders
  - Trinucleotide disorders
  - Other genetic disorders

Epidemiology

The incidence of many musculoskeletal conditions is increasing due to longer life expectancies. Estimating incidence rates for inheritable musculoskeletal diseases is difficult, since new detection methods, changing classification schemes, and more complete understanding of the disease mechanisms constantly shape our perception of these disorders.

DIAGNOSIS (Algorithm 15-1)

Physical Examination

- Age at presentation
  - Most genetic diseases present early.
  - Autoimmune disorders with genetic contribution may present in adulthood only.
- Presence of characteristic facial features (e.g., Down syndrome and achondroplasia)
- Stature: lesser- or greater-than-normal arm span-to–height ratio
- Skin lesions (e.g., café-au-lait spots)
- Neurologic assessment: weakness in myotomes can be either neural or muscle related
- Limb configuration and range of motion of joints (e.g., joint contractures)

Laboratory Tests

- Hematology (e.g., erythrocyte sedimentation rate elevated in rheumatoid arthritis)
- Biochemistry (e.g., creatine phosphokinase [CPK] in Duchenne's muscular dystrophy)
- Molecular diagnostic tests
  - Gene product analysis using immunoblotting techniques
  - DNA mutation analysis with polymerase chain reaction (PCR)
  - Chromosomal studies
    - Indications include multiple orthopaedic abnormalities, two or more siblings with the same condition, multiple miscarriages in the mother, multiple organ system abnormalities, mental retardation.

TREATMENT

- Varies with specific disease
- Supportive
  - Orthotics to address joint and spinal deformities (e.g., ankle–foot orthosis [AFO] in Charcot-Marie-Tooth disease associated with peroneal muscle weakness)
  - Physical therapy to condition and maintain tone of functioning musculature (e.g., in spinal muscular atrophy)
- Medical treatment
  - Medications to suppress or curb disease activity (e.g., anti-inflammatory agents and steroids in autoimmune disorders)
- Surgical procedures
  - Fusion procedures
    - Spinal instability and scoliosis (e.g., for severe atlantoaxial instability in Down syndrome)
  - Realignment osteotomies
    - Sofield osteotomies in osteogenesis imperfecta
  - Lengthening procedures have been considered for short stature in selective cases of skeletal dysplasia.

TABLE 15-1 DEFINITIONS OF TERMS ASSOCIATED WITH GENETIC DISORDERS

Term	Definition
Alleles	Alternate forms of a gene found at the same locus
Anticipation	Phenomenon that refers to a progressive increase in the number of nucleotide triplets down the successive familial generation with worsening in disease presentation
Arthrogryposis	Congenital nonprogressive limitation of joint movement attributable to soft tissue contractures that involve at least two joints
Autoimmune disorders	A group of clinical conditions that have a predilection for accumulation of selective antibodies, the detection of which facilitates clinical diagnosis and categorization
Autosomal dominant	Condition that occurs when a mutation of only one of the alleles is enough to cause the disease, as in achondroplasia, Marfan syndrome, and neurofibromatosis
Autosomal recessive	Condition that requires mutations be present in both alleles of a gene, as in spinal muscular atrophy
Cartilage oligomeric matrix protein	A member of the thrombospondin family of proteins; expressed in high levels in the chondrocyte matrix
Charcot-Marie-Tooth disease	Type 1 or 2 hereditary sensory and motor neuropathy; an autosomal-dominant disease that presents with motor and sensory demyelinating neuropathy
Coding region (of a gene)	Consists of introns and exons; defines the unique order of amino acids and thus determines protein production
Dwarfism	Pathological decrease in stature; can be divided as proportionate (midget) versus disproportionate (short limb or trunk); the short-limb type can be defined by location of maximal shortening as rhizomelic (proximal portion of limb), mesomelic (middle portion of limb), or acromelic (distal portion)
Dysplasia	Intrinsic skeletal developmental abnormality
Ehlers-Danlos syndrome	A group of the most common inheritable connective tissue disorders, consisting of six major subtypes; all have features of skin and joint hypermobility.
Fibroblast growth factors	A group of polypeptide growth factors involved in chondrocyte development and wound healing
Gene	A chain of nucleotides that contain a promoter and a coding region
Hereditary sensory and motor neuropathy	A group of disorders characterized by a slow neural conduction, with muscle biopsy revealing uniformly small-diameter fibers and nerve biopsy revealing demyelination
Mendelian disorders	Disorders involving a single gene
Mosaicism	Expression of two cell lines in the same individual
Muscular dystrophies	A group of inherited, noninflammatory disorders that cause progressive muscular weakness
Neuromuscular disorders	A group of conditions that may have genetic anomalies leading to abnormalities in signal transmission in one of three regions: neural junction, neuromuscular junction, or muscle
Orthopaedic genome	The genes involved in the genesis and functioning of the musculoskeletal system
Osteogenesis imperfecta	A disorder associated with mutation in type I collagen, primarily characterized by bone fragility and long bone deformities
Pleiotropic	A single genotype producing multiple phenotypic effects
Promoter region	The region of the DNA that regulates gene expression
Rheumatoid arthritis	An autoimmune disorder characterized by symmetrical inflammatory arthropathy with varied extra-articular manifestation
Scleroderma	A chronic disease of unknown etiology, characterized by skin fibrosis
Seronegative spondyloarthropathies	A group of conditions that are negative for rheumatoid factor and are associated with inflammatory arthritis and various typical extra-articular manifestations

(continued)

TABLE 15-1 (continued)

Term	Definition
Skeletal dysplasias	A spectrum of disorders that are caused by abnormalities in bone and cartilage metabolism and phenotypically identified by short stature
Spinal muscular atrophy	An autosomal-recessive disease characterized by loss of anterior horn cells in the spinal cord and presenting with progressive weakness
Transcription	A process of transferring genetic information found in DNA to mRNA
Transduction	The insertion of genetic material into a host cell by use of a viral vector, most commonly an adenovirus
Translation	The process of converting RNA to protein
Trinucleotide disorders	A group of conditions associated with an increased number of nucleotide triplets in DNA

- Gene therapy
  - Gene therapy is a potential therapeutic option when a single functional gene product is absent and treatment is affected by transfer of a wild-type gene; possible orthopaedic examples are Duchenne's muscular dystrophy, osteogenesis imperfecta, familial osteoarthritis.
  - Gene transfer into cell lines requires the aid of vectors, which can either be viral (recombinant viruses) or nonviral.
  - Key issues concerning gene therapy use in orthopaedics
    - Orthopaedic genetic diseases have an early onset, which necessitates administration of gene therapy at a very early age.
    - In heterozygous individuals with selective genetic conditions, half of the genes are abnormal and can behave as mutations producing inhibitory protein products that interfere with normal gene products. A successful gene therapy outcome therefore requires eliminating this endogenous mutant allele.
    - Longevity of gene expression
    - Economics of gene therapy
  - Current status of orthopaedic applications for gene therapy
    - Genetic diseases
      - Osteogenesis imperfecta
        - Trials ongoing with implantation of precursors of normal bone (stem cells) into osteogenesis imperfecta mice models
      - Duchenne muscular dystrophy
        - In animal models, dystrophin gene delivery success has been hampered by immunogenicity and rejection issues.
    - Nongenetic diseases
      - Arthritis was the first orthopaedic condition to be targeted by gene therapy.
        - Involves delivery of antiarthritic genes into synovial linings of diseased joints (rheumatoid arthritis, osteoarthritis)
        - Phase I trials in human have suggested

efficacy in transfer of genes (interleukin-1 receptor antagonists) in patients with rheumatoid arthritis.
  - Current challenge is to sustain longevity of gene expression.
- Osteoporosis
  - Osteoporotic mice models injected with vector carrying transgenes to block interleukin-1, an osteoclastic cytokine, showed decreased bone loss and in some cases bone mass was restored to normal.
- Tissue repair
  - Gene expression is required for a limited time period until healing is complete.
  - Bone healing can be enhanced in animal models using an adenovirus that carries the BMP-2 gene.
  - In experimental models, cartilage defects have been treated using "gene plugs"—bone marrow aspirates combined with a vector carrying a localized "healing" transgene that allows the stem cells to differentiate into chondrocytes and thus repair the cartilage defect.

SKELETAL DYSPLASIAS

DEFINITION

Skeletal dysplasias, which are mostly heritable disorders, are caused by abnormalities in bone and cartilage development and phenotypically characterized by a variably short stature.

EPIDEMIOLOGY

The incidence of skeletal dysplasias is 1:3,000 to 5,000 births depending on disease subtype and geographic area.

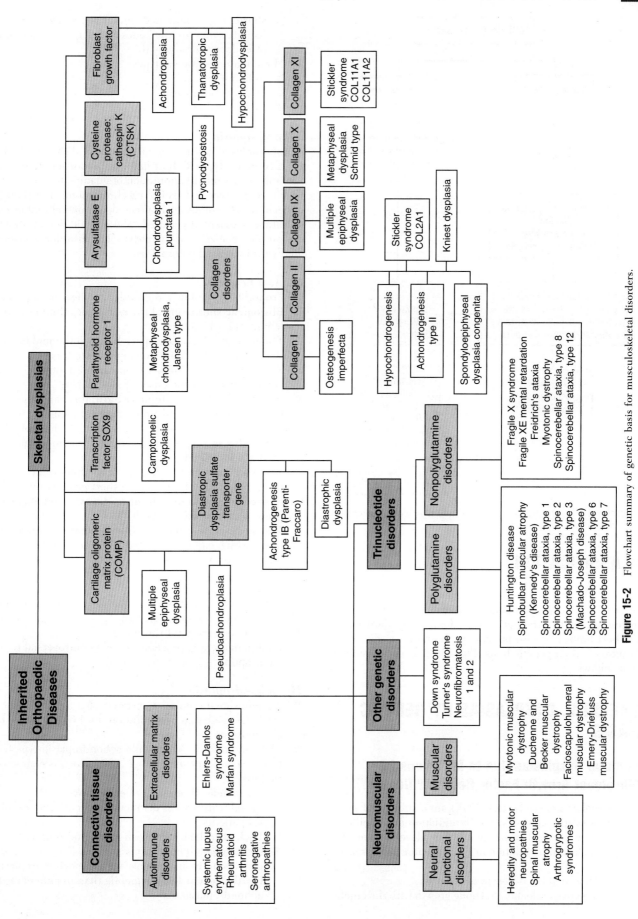

Figure 15-2   Flowchart summary of genetic basis for musculoskeletal disorders.

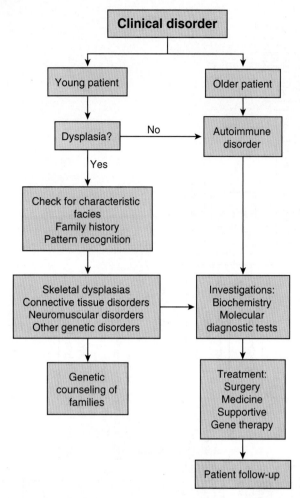

Algorithm 15-1   Diagnostic work-up of musculoskeletal disorders.

CLASSIFICATION

The clinical classification of dysplasias is based on whether the dwarfism is proportionate or disproportionate, and, if disproportionate, whether it is predominantly short-trunk or short-limb. It is also possible to define these disorders in terms of their genetic basis (Fig. 15-3), as in the section that follows.

SKELETAL DYSPLASIAS BY GENETIC BASIS

Skeletal Dysplasias Due to Mutations in Fibroblast Growth Factor Receptor Genes

- Fibroblast growth factors (FGF) are a subtype of polypeptides that control cell differentiation and proliferation and are critical in chondrocyte development and wound healing. Mutation in FGF receptor 3 genes leads to:
  - Abnormal chondrocyte maturation
  - Impeded endochondral bone growth with rhizomelic ·

shortening (femur and humerus are the most affected as they are the bones with the largest amount of endochondral growth)
- Three main disease subtypes
  - Achondroplasia
  - Hypochondroplasia
  - Thanatrophic dysplasia

Achondroplasia

Achondroplasia, an autosomal-dominant disorder, is the most common type of short-limb, disproportionate dwarfism and occurs due to a mutation of guanine to adenine in FGF receptor type 3 (FGFR3) on chromosome 4. Although endochondral ossification is affected, intramembranous ossification is essentially spared. The genetic defect affects the proliferative zone of the physis. The disorder is associated with increased paternal age.

Clinical Features
- Frontal bossing, low nasal bridge, midface hypoplasia
- Rhizomelic shortening of the extremities (humerus and femur) (Fig. 15-4)
- Trident hand: increased space between the middle and ring finger and inability to approximate them
- Thoracolumbar or lumbar kyphosis in infancy that usually resolves with the onset of ambulation
- Infants are often hypotonic at birth: this can be due to foramen magnum and upper cervical stenosis, which can present with apnea and lead to hydrocephalus. When this is suspected, magnetic resonance imaging (MRI) is indicated.
- Radiographs in older children and adults often reveal increased lumbar lordosis with short pedicles and a decreased interpedicular distance, know as "champagne glass" pelvis (width > depth).
- The most serious clinical problem is lumbar spinal stenosis, which can be evaluated with computed tomography (CT) or MRI.

Treatment
- Fusion for significant cervical instability and decompression for spinal stenosis
- Osteotomies for genu varum
- Limb-lengthening procedures are a controversial treatment option.

Hypochondroplasia
- An autosomal-dominant disorder that results from a cytosine-to-adenine substitution in FGFR3 gene on chromosome 4
- The condition, in which mild achondroplasia-type features become apparent at age 2 to 3 years, is characterized by:
  - Rhizomelic shortening of extremities
  - Facial features less distinctive than in achondroplasia patients
  - Lack of trident hand seen in achondroplasia
  - Neurologic complications such as lumbar stenosis can occur in individuals with hypochondroplasia, but they occur less frequently than in patients with achondroplasia.

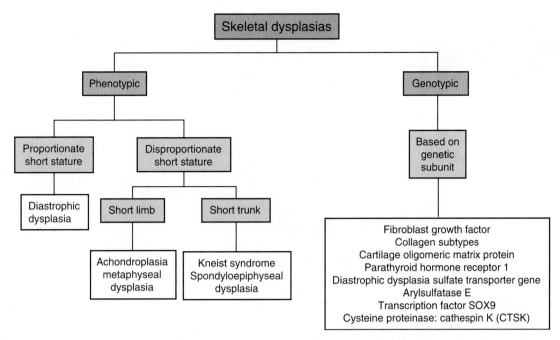

Figure 15-3   Classification of skeletal dysplasias.

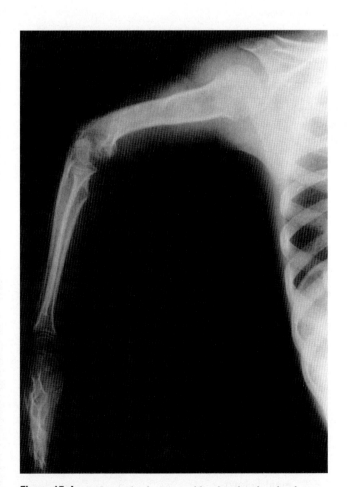

Figure 15-4   Radiograph of 10-year-old girl with achondroplasia. Note features of rhizomelic shortening of the upper extremity. (From Baitner AC, Maurer SG, Gruen MB, et al. The genetic basis of the osteochondrodysplasias. *J Pediatr Orthop* 2000;20:594–605.)

Thanatophoric Dysplasia
- Lethal bone dysplasia
  - New mutations in FGFR3 gene result in new cysteine residues, which trigger the formation of abnormal disulfide bonds between the mutant FGFR receptors.
  - FGFR receptor complexes then inhibit endochondral ossification.

Clinical Features
- Rhizomelic dwarf with large head and normal trunk
- Generalized platyspondyly (flattening of the vertebral bodies)
- Extreme rib shortening

Skeletal Dysplasias due to Mutations in Collagen Genes

Mutations in Type I Collagen: Osteogenesis Imperfecta

Etiology
- Type I collagen (Fig. 15-5) is a major structural protein in bone, skin, and tendons.
  - A heterotrimer of two identical α-1 chains and one α-2 chain folded into a triple helix configuration
  - The α-1 and α-2 chains consist of amino acid repeats (Gly-X-Y).
- COL1A1 gene, coding for the α-1 chain, is on chromosome 17, whereas the α-2 subunit is coded by the COL1A2 gene on chromosome 7.
- COL1A1/A2 gene mutations disrupt the synthesis of type I collagen.

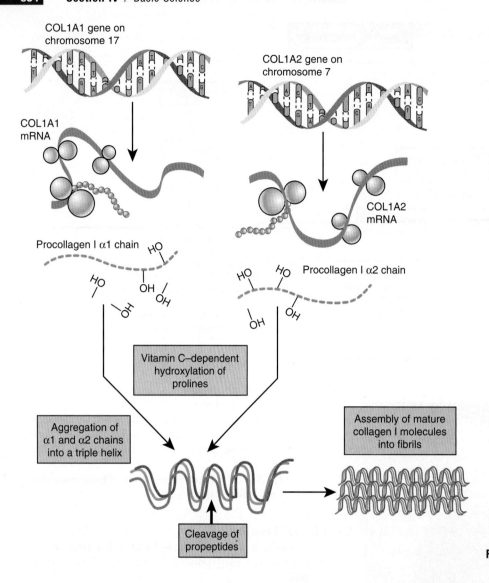

COL1A1 gene on
chromosome 17

COL1A2 gene on
chromosome 7

COL1A1
mRNA

COL1A2
mRNA

Procollagen I α1 chain

Procollagen I α2 chain

Vitamin C–dependent
hydroxylation of
prolines

Aggregation of
α1 and α2 chains
into a triple helix

Assembly of mature
collagen I molecules
into fibrils

Cleavage of
propeptides

Figure 15-5   Type I collagen synthesis.

- Affect all bone and connective tissue containing type I collagen as their major structural protein
- Classical findings: bone fragility, long bone deformities (Fig. 15-6)
- May also have blue sclerae, dentinogenesis imperfecta, and scoliosis

Clinical Features and Classification
- Most patients are categorized among the four distinct types using the Sillence classification; the rest are classified recently under V, VI, VII types (Table 15-2).
- May be autosomal dominant or autosomal recessive. New mutations are rare.

Radiographic Features
- Osteoporosis
- Multiple fractures
- Bowing of long bones (often described as "gracile")
- Deficient ossification of the skull

Diagnosis and Work-up
- Prenatal ultrasound and DNA analysis (chorionic villi sampling)
- Collagen synthesis analysis of dermal fibroblasts (from skin biopsy)
- Osteogenesis imperfecta should be considered in the differential diagnosis of child abuse.

Treatment
- Medical treatment options aim to improve bone mass.
  - Bisphosphonates (pamidronate most common)
  - Bone marrow transplantation has been used with some success in severe cases but is not standard treatment.
  - Gene therapy (discussed in detail in section on treatment below)
- Bracing may be used for fracture prevention (not effective in management of scoliosis).
- Surgical treatment options include Sofield osteotomies

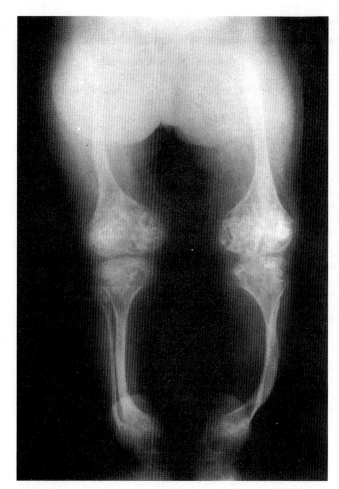

Figure 15-6   Radiograph of a young patient with osteogenesis imperfecta. (From Baitner AC, Maurer SG, Gruen MB, et al. The genetic basis of the osteochondrodysplasias. *J Pediatr Orthop* 2000; 20:594–605.)

to correct long bone deformities, decompression of basilar impression, and spine fusion for significant scoliosis.
■ Genetic linkage studies: for risk assessment and genetic counseling

Mutations in Type II Collagen

Etiology
■ Type II collagen: found in large quantities in cartilage, tectorial membrane, nucleolus pulposus, and ocular vitreous humor
■ Polypeptide chains are encoded by COL2A1 gene on chromosome 12.
■ Mutations involving the gene lead to several connective tissue disorders (Table 15-3).

Mutations in Type IX Collagen—Multiple Epiphyseal Dysplasia Type II (Ribbing's/Milder Form)

Etiology
■ Type IX collagen: essential for cartilage fibril formation and found only in cartilage

■ Encoded by three genes: COL9A1 (on chromosome 6), COL9A2 (on chromosome 1), and COL9A3 (on chromosome 20)
■ Mutations of these genes result in multiple epiphyseal dysplasia type II (Ribbing's).

Clinical Features
■ Present at 2.5 to 6 years of age with knee and hip pain, worse after exercise
■ Mildly short stature, limbs affected more than the trunk
■ Waddling gait
■ Occasional angular deformities
■ The course is progressive pain and joint deformity leading to early-onset osteoarthritis.
■ Radiologic features: small, flattened epiphyses in many joints (severe in knees)

Mutations in Type X Collagen

Etiology
■ Type X collagen: produced by the COL10A1 gene
■ Gene expression is essential in chondrocyte hypertrophic stage in the physis, which controls endochondral ossification and facilitates long bone development.
■ Gene mutations result in an inability of nascent alpha chain to be incorporated in the collagen X triple helix, which decreases the quantity of collagen X in the zone of endochondral ossification (metaphyses affected, with normal epiphyses).

Clinical Features
■ Metaphyseal chondrodysplasia, Schmid type (MCDS), is the mildest and most common of the metaphyseal chondrodysplasias.
■ Patients present in childhood with small stature and bowed legs.

Radiologic Features
■ Varus deformities of the hips and knees
■ Flared metaphyses
■ Physes widened

Mutations in Type XI Collagen
■ Type XI collagen: found primarily in physeal cartilage
■ Three encoding genes: COL11A1 (chromosome 1), COL11A2 (chromosome 6), and COL2A1 (the gene on chromosome 12 that also encodes type II collagen)
  ■ Most type XI collagen abnormalities are associated with mutations in these genes and exhibit an autosomal-dominant pattern.
  ■ COL2A1 gene mutations are the most common and result in Stickler syndrome type I (classified as type II collagen disorder; see section on type II collagen).
  ■ Mutations of the COL11A1/A2 genes are more rare but result in distinct phenotypes.
  ■ Stickler syndrome, COL11A1 or type 2
    ■ Referred to as vitreoretinal type because of characteristic myopia, glaucoma, and retinal detachment
    ■ Skeletal changes affect the joints and manifest similar to arthritis on x-rays.

TABLE 15-2 SILLENCE CLASSIFICATION FOR OSTEOGENESIS IMPERFECTA

Type	Inheritance and Incidence	Genetic defect	Clinical Features/Comments
I	Autosomal dominant, 1:30,000	• "Functional null alleles" of COL1A1 or COL1A2 genes that lead to 50% reduction in type I collagen (mild disease)	• Bone fragility and blue sclera throughout life • Susceptibility to multiple fractures with minimal trauma; though initial bone healing is normal, there is a lack of bone remodeling phase • Life expectancy: normal or slightly reduced
II	Autosomal dominant (new mutation or parental gonadal mosaicism) 1:60,000; autosomal recessive (rare)	• Various mutations in COL1A1 gene leading to the disruption of Gly-X-Y repeat in the α-1 chain • Disruption in triple helix patter	• Perinatal lethal form • Present with numerous fractures at birth • Soft skull, beaded ribs, dark sclera • Death within first year of life
III	Autosomal dominant (new mutation) or autosomal recessive, 1:70,000	• Deletions in α-1 and α-2 chains leading to abnormal collagen synthesis • In certain mutations amino acid glycine is replaced by a different amino acid during procollagen synthesis	• Present in utero or neonatal period with multiple fractures • Progressive limb deformities throughout life • Shortened life span due to respiratory infections and skull fractures
IV	Autosomal dominant, rare	• COL1A1/A2 mutation • Results in shortened pro-α1chain affecting all chain structures in triple helix	• Similar to type I, except patients have normal hearing and scleral hue • Life expectancy may be slightly reduced.

- Stickler syndrome, COL11A2 or type 3
  - Referred to as nonocular because of the absence of ocular pathology (unlike types I and II)
  - Patients exhibit marfanoid habitus, hearing loss, and facial features similar to Stickler, COL2A1, or type I.

Skeletal Dysplasias due to Mutations in the Cartilage Oligomeric Matrix Protein (COMP) Gene

A member of the thrombospondin family of proteins, cartilage oligomeric matrix protein (COMP) is expressed in high levels in the chondrocyte matrix. Two autosomal-dominant disorders have been mapped to the region of the COMP gene on chromosome 19 and are described below.

Multiple Epiphyseal Dysplasia (MED) Type I (Fairbanks's/Severe Form)
- MED has been linked to the mutations in the COMP gene (MED, Fairbank type 1) and collagen type IX genes (MED, type II; see section on collagen IX).
- Presentation and prognosis of MED type I
  - Dependent on the type of the COMP mutation
  - Selective mutation types present with a milder phenotype that is similar to COL9 mutations.
  - Short stature, genu valgum and ossification abnormalities about the knees (femoral condyle flattening, "double-layer" patella), shortened metatarsals and metacarpals
  - Severe disease entity presents with major involve-

ment of the capital femoral epiphyses and irregular acetabuli (Fig. 15-7). This can be mistaken for bilateral Perthes disease, but Perthes does not appear as symmetric.

Pseudoachondroplasia
- Infants appear normal at birth; growth retardation becomes apparent only at age 2 years or later.
- Form of short-limb dwarfism, similar to achondroplasia
  - Head and face are normal; fingers, although short, do not exhibit the trident hand of achondroplasia
  - Cervical instability, scoliosis, increased lumbar lordosis
  - Genu varum or valgum
- Radiographically, all tubular bones are short, with uneven, splayed metaphyses and irregularly developed epiphyses.

Skeletal Dysplasias due to Mutations in the Parathyroid Hormone Receptor 1 Gene

Etiology
- Parathyroid hormone receptor 1 (PTHR1) is a G-protein receptor and is highly expressed in the growth plate and involved in chondrocyte proliferation and differentiation.
- An autosomal-dominant mutation of the PTHR1 gene in 3p22 results in a severe form of metaphyseal chondrodysplasia called the Jansen's type.

Clinical Features
- Large skull
- Widely spaced and exophthalmic eyes

TABLE 15-3 DISEASES ASSOCIATED WITH MUTATION OF THE COL2A1 GENE

Disease	Inheritance	Genetic Defect	Clinical Features/Comments
Stickler syndrome, type I (hereditary arthro-ophthalmopathy)	Autosomal dominant	• Single base pair mutations (stop codons) • Result in the absence of protein synthesis and inability of the healthy allele to compensate (haploinsufficiency)	• Craniofacial abnormalities (midface hypoplasia, cleft palate) • Hearing loss • Premature joint degeneration, abnormal epiphyseal development, marfanoid hypermobility, may have scoliosis or kyphosis • Ocular abnormalities (congenital myopia, vitreoretinal degeneration, retinal detachment)
Achondrogenesis, type II (Langer-Saldino dysplasia)	Autosomal dominant (new mutation)	• Glycine-to-serine substitutions in COL2A1 • Inability to form the triple helix	• Neonatal dwarfism, micromelia, short trunk, fetal hydrops • Early death in utero or after birth
Hypochondrogenesis	Autosomal dominant	• Different glycine-to-serine substitutions	• Milder allelic variant of type II achondrogenesis • Infants: oval facies and widely spaced eyes • Neonatal death from respiratory infections
Spondyloepiphyseal dysplasia congenita	Autosomal dominant	• Single base pair mutations or entire exon deletions and duplications • Abnormal protein produced that interferes with function of trimer	• Short stature (140 cm or less) • Barrel-chested trunk, more shortened than extremities • Cleft palate, myopia
Kniest dysplasia	Autosomal dominant	• Single amino acid mutations or deletions of entire exons • Secretion of type II procollagen that lacks a c-propeptide • Results in abnormal fibril formation	• Short-trunk dwarfism • Severe kyphoscoliosis • Flattened facies, retinal detachment, deafness • Physical therapy for joint contractures and reconstructive surgery for hip osteoarthritis

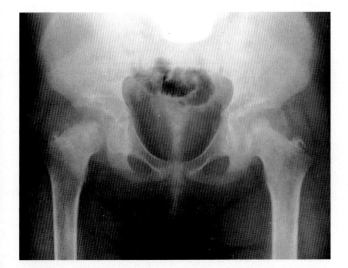

Figure 15-7 Radiograph of a 10-year-old girl with multiple epiphyseal dysplasia (Fairbanks type). (From Baitner AC, Maurer SG, Gruen MB, et al. The genetic basis of the osteochondrodysplasias. *J Pediatr Orthop* 2000;20:594–605.)

- ▣ Severe limb shortening
- ▣ Angular deformities at the diaphyseal–metaphyseal junction
- ▣ Radiographs: metaphyseal fragmentation, normal epiphysis
- ▣ Differential diagnosis: hyperparathyroidism
  - ▣ Both disease entities are characterized by hypercalcemia, hypophosphatemia, and increased renal phosphate secretion.
  - ▣ Abnormal parathyroid hormone (PTH) levels: only in hyperparathyroidism

Skeletal Dysplasias due to Mutations in the Diastrophic Dysplasia Sulfate Transporter Gene

Etiology

- ▣ The diastrophic dysplasia sulfate transporter (DTDST) gene is found on chromosome 5 and encodes a Na+-independent membrane transporter of sulfate.
  - ▣ DTDST found in human cartilage and intestines
  - ▣ Probable role in endochondral bone formation
- ▣ Mutations are associated with recessively inherited osteochondrodysplasias.

Diastrophic Dysplasia

■ Cartilage of diastrophic dysplasia (DTD) patients is associated with decreased sulfation of glycosaminoglycans, which leads to severe limb distortion ("twisted" dwarf).
  ■ A rare form of micromelic dwarfism
  ■ Spinal malalignment (cervical kyphosis and scoliosis)
  ■ Cleft palate and irregular calcifications of the pinnae of the ears ("cauliflower ears")
  ■ Rigid foot deformities (e.g., talipes equinovarus)
  ■ "Hitchhiker's thumb"

Achondrogenesis Type IB (Parenti-Fraccaro Type Achondrogenesis)

■ Autosomal-recessive DTDST mutation leading to impaired sulfation of proteoglycan
■ A lethal neonatal dwarfism associated with severe micromelia, large head, and fetal hydrops
■ Distinguished from type II achondrogenesis, which results from a mutation leading to abnormal type II collagen and has a normal cranial vault

Skeletal Dysplasias due to Mutations in the Arylsulfatase E Gene

■ Arylsulfatase E (ARSE): a steroid sulfatase, a family that includes enzymes that convert sulfated steroids to free steroids
  ■ The gene for ARSE is located on the X chromosome.
  ■ These sulfatases are active in osteoblast cell lines and play an important role in bone and cartilage formation.
■ Mutations of the ARSE gene have been implicated in at least one type of osteochondrodysplasia: chondrodysplasia punctata.
  ■ Similar to diastrophic dysplasia and type I achondroplasia (mutation in sulfate transport)
  ■ Chondrodysplasia punctata is due to an inherited deficiency of the sulfatase enzyme.
    ■ Causes a high degree of sulfation of certain components within the cartilage matrix (exact disease etiology unclear)

Chondrodysplasia Punctata 1 X-Linked Recessive Type

■ Characterized by asymmetry of extremities
■ Hypoplasia of distal phalanges
■ Patients present in infancy with failure to thrive, atypical facies (commonly nasal hypoplasia), ichthyosis (pigmented hyperkeratosis of the skin), and apparent mental retardation.
■ The name refers to the punctate epiphyseal calcifications that are prominent on the radiographs.

Skeletal Dysplasias due to Mutations in the SOX9 Gene

■ SOX9: a tissue-specific transcription factor that is highly expressed in cartilaginous tissue and is involved in testicular development

■ The gene for SOX9 is on chromosome 17.
  ■ It codes for a transcription factor that results in the production of specific regulatory proteins.
  ■ These regulatory proteins bind to the first intron on COL2A1 gene, thus regulating type II collagen expression and chondrogenesis.
  ■ Camptomelic dysplasia is caused by an autosomal-dominant SOX9 mutation.

Clinical Features of Camptomelic Dysplasia

■ Neonatal dwarfism with congenital angulation and bowing of long bones; the tubular bones are thickened
■ Other skeletal abnormalities include talipes equinovarus and hypoplastic scapulae.
■ Cleft palate, micrognathia, flat face
■ Most individuals with XY karyotype have a partial or full female phenotype since testicular development is affected.
■ Most patients do not survive past the neonatal period because of respiratory problems (tracheobronchial hypoplasia).
■ Radiologic features
  ■ Long bones are shortened and bowed.
  ■ Iliac bones, scapulae, and cervical spine are often hypoplastic.

Skeletal Dysplasias due to Mutations in the Cysteine Proteinase Cathepsin K Gene

■ The cysteine proteinase cathepsin K (CTSK) gene is located on chromosome 1q21 and produces an endoprotease, which belongs to the cysteine proteinase family.
  ■ Vital role in the degradation of bone matrix, collagen, and osteonectin
  ■ Selectively expressed in osteoclasts and thus controls bone resorption
  ■ Associated with rheumatoid arthritis
■ CTSK gene mutation may result in pyknodysostosis, a form of dwarfism characterized by osteosclerosis on radiographs and bone fragility.

CONNECTIVE TISSUE DISORDERS

Connective tissue disorders can be classified as:

■ Extracellular matrix disorders
■ Autoimmune disorders

EXTRACELLULAR MATRIX DISORDERS

Pleiotropic mutations in genes responsible for extracellular matrix production can lead to various abnormalities of bone, vascular system and viscera. ("Pleiotropic" refers to a single gene influencing several distinct and seemingly unrelated phenotypic traits.)

- Ehlers-Danlos syndrome
- Marfan syndrome
- Osteogenesis imperfecta and other collagen disorders

Ehlers-Danlos Syndrome

- Most common heritable connective tissue disorders, with six major subtypes, all characterized by skin and joint hypermobility (Table 15-4). All are autosomal-dominant disorders except for kyphoscoliosis and the dermatosparaxis subtypes, which are autosomal recessive. The classic, hypermobility, and vascular subtypes are the most common.

Marfan Syndrome

- An autosomal-dominant disorder with pleiotropic mutation of *FBN1* gene on chromosome 15q21 that affects fibrillin production
  - Fibrillin is a major protein component of microfibrils.
  - Fibrillin serves as a scaffold for deposits of newly synthesized elastin.
  - Microfibrils are seen in large quantities in the eye (zonule of Zinn: the suspensory ligament of the eye that holds the lens in place), skin, cartilage, and viscera (heart, lung, and kidney).
- Marfan syndrome has a high penetrance and variability

TABLE 15-4 SUBTYPES OF EHLERS-DANLOS SYNDROME ACCORDING TO THE VILLEFRANCHE CLASSIFICATION

Subtype	Inheritance	Genetic Defect	Clinical Features/Comments
Classic	Autosomal dominant	Type V collagen abnormality due to mutations in COL5A1 or A2 genes	• Hypermobility of skin • Joint hypermobility • Tower vertebra (high vertebral height), scoliosis (30%) • Aortic root dilation (30%) • Tissue fragility • >50% of patients may present with chronic pain.
Hypermobility	Autosomal dominant	Genetic mutation uncertain	• Both small and large joint hypermobility (multidirectional instability of shoulder, patellar subluxation, chronic ankle instability) • Soft, lax skin • Most common subtype associated with orthopaedic intervention due to its debilitating presentation
Vascular	Autosomal dominant	Genetic mutation involving COL3A1 with abnormalities in type III collagen synthesis	• Hypermobility of joints • Clubfoot • Laxity of viscera • Vascular abnormalities predisposing to rupture of large arteries • 75% of patients have aortic root dilatation; 25% of affected women are at risk of death due to uterine rupture
Kyphoscoliosis	Autosomal recessive	Procollagen-lysine, 2-oxoglutarate 5 dioxygenase-1 (PLOD) gene mutations resulting in deficient production of lysyl hydroxylase, an enzyme involved in the modification of collagen	• Hypotonia at birth • Progressive infantile scoliosis (double thoracic pattern) • Hypermobility of joints • Ocular complications: fragile sclera with globe rupture • Patients with this disease have similar phenotypic presentation to Marfan syndrome.
Arthrochalasis	Autosomal dominant	COL1A1/A2 genetic abnormality with absence of pro-α I or 2 collagen type I chains at their N-terminal end	• Hypermobility of joints • Excessive laxity of skin • Bilateral developmental dysplasia of hip with a high recurrence rate following surgical intervention
Dermatosparaxis	Autosomal recessive	Lack of production of procollagen I N-terminal peptidase	• Fragile redundant skin • Easy bruising

in clinical expression both within and between families (25% of cases arise from new mutations).

- Diagnosis of Marfan syndrome is based on the characteristic phenotypic presentation and is confirmed by genetic studies.
  - Skeletal abnormalities: dolichostenomelia (disproportionately long limbs), arachnodactyly, scoliosis (60% of patients), chest wall deformity (pectus carinatum or excavatum), tall body habitus, ligamentous laxity, abnormal joint mobility, and protrusio acetabula
  - Patients have an arm span–to–height ratio of more than 1.05.
  - Most common extraskeletal manifestations are superior dislocation of lens (ectopia lentis, often bilateral) and abnormalities in cardiovascular system (aortic root dilation/aortic regurgitation and aortic aneurysms).
- Treatment options include beta-blockers (to help reduce stress on aorta) and scoliosis treatment with bracing or surgery.

AUTOIMMUNE DISORDERS

Autoimmune disorders are a group of clinical conditions characterized by an accumulation of selective antibodies. Identification of disease subtypes is facilitated by tests for these antibodies.

- Common examples
  - Systemic lupus erythematosus
  - Rheumatoid arthritis
  - Seronegative spondyloarthropathy

Systemic Lupus Erythematosus

- Characterized by microvascular inflammation and generation of autoantibodies affecting multiple organ systems
- Prevalence of 1:2,000; greater in premenopausal women and African Americans
- Genetic basis for system lupus erythematosus: high rate of concordance in monozygotic twins (57%)
  - Associated with 10 different genetic loci—in particular, alleles of the human leukocyte antigens: HLA-DR2 and HLA-DR3
- Musculoskeletal symptoms
  - Arthralgia and myalgia
  - Early morning joint stiffness and pain
  - In systemic lupus erythematosus arthritis is migratory and polyarticular (small joints of the hands, wrist, and knee joints).
  - 10% of patients develop Jaccoud's arthropathy of the hand (bony erosion of metacarpal heads), resembling rheumatoid arthritis disease pattern (Fig. 15-8).
- Presence of any four of the following clinical findings confirms the diagnosis:
  - Arthritis
  - Malar/discoid rash

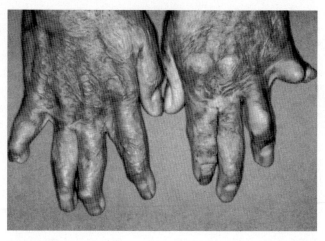

Figure 15-8   A 49-year-old woman with systemic lupus erythematosus and Jaccoud's arthropathy of the hands.

  - Photosensitivity
  - Oral ulcers
  - Serositis
  - Renal disorder
  - Neurologic disorder
  - Hematologic disorder
  - Immunologic disorder
  - Antinuclear antibody
- Treatment for systemic lupus erythematosus arthritis
  - Supportive: nonsteroidal anti-inflammatories (NSAIDs), hydroxychloroquine (antimalarial drug effective in refractory myalgias and arthralgias), corticosteroid therapy for renal and neuropsychiatric symptoms (can cause osteoporosis)
  - Joint reconstruction/replacement for severely affected joints (e.g., avascular necrosis of the hips)

Rheumatoid Arthritis

- Autoimmune disorder characterized by symmetrical inflammatory arthropathy (Fig. 15-9), positive rheumatoid factor, and a varied extra-articular manifestation (e.g., rheumatoid nodules and neuropathy)
- Recent evidence suggests that in at least 50% of patients genetic susceptibility is attributable to major histocompatibility complex class II loci (DR4β chains), with the strongest associations with rheumatoid arthritis being DRB*0401 and DRB*0404.
- Treatment principles: similar to those for systemic lupus erythematosus

Seronegative Spondyloarthropathies

- Group of conditions negative for rheumatoid factor and associated with inflammatory arthritis and various typical extra-articular manifestations
- Four main conditions in this group: ankylosing spondylitis, psoriatic arthropathy, reactive arthritis, and inflammatory bowel disease
- All have their etiology associated with HLA-B27 (class

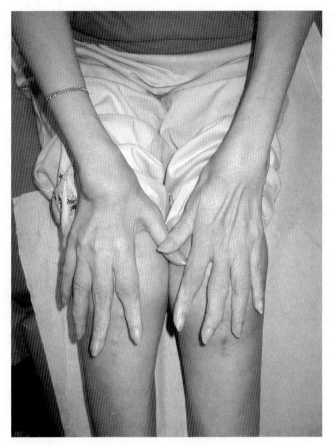

Figure 15-9   A 40-year-old woman with bilateral, symmetrical proximal polyarthropathy.

I major histocompatibility antigen), which can facilitate diagnosis (Fig. 15-10):

- About 50% to 95% of patients with ankylosing spondylitis test positive for HLA-B27.
- However, about 5% of the normal population also test positive.

NEUROMUSCULAR DISORDERS

Neuromuscular disorders are a group of conditions in which genetic defects cause abnormalities in signal transmission in one of three regions: the neural junction (synapse), neuromuscular junction, or muscle.

NEURAL JUNCTION DISORDERS

Hereditary Sensory and Motor Neuropathy

- Hereditary sensory and motor neuropathy (HSMN) is characterized by slow neural conduction identified by nerve conduction studies and also associated with abnormal electromyographic results.

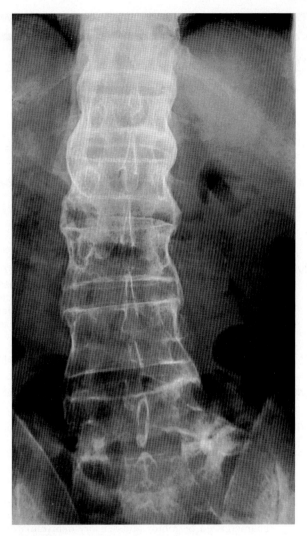

Figure 15-10   Radiograph of a 51-year-old man with a longstanding history of ankylosing spondylitis. Note "bamboo spine" characterized by bridging syndesmophytes between vertebrae.

- The histologic hallmark is demyelination on nerve biopsy.
- Muscle biopsy is characterized by uniformly small-diameter fibers.
- HSMN has been associated with 10 different genetic mutations.
  - The most common mutation involves overexpression of the peripheral myelin protein 22 gene on chromosome 17.
  - Other associated genes: myelin protein zero gene and connexin-32 gene
- Patients with HSMN present to the orthopaedist with hip dysplasia, scoliosis (10%), and cavovarus foot deformity (most common orthopaedic manifestation).
  - Approximately two thirds of patients have marked hand involvement characterized by intrinsic muscle weakness.
  - Six main types: the three main types encountered by orthopaedic surgeons are types 1, 2, and 3 (Table 15-5)

TABLE 15-5 THE SEVEN SUBTYPES OF HEREDITARY SENSORY AND MOTOR NEUROPATHIES

Type	Inheritance	Genetic Defect	Clinical Features/Comments
I	Autosomal dominant	Duplication of a portion of chromosome 17p or a point mutation that results in an abnormality in the peripheral myelin protein-22	• Neuropathy marked by demyelination • Includes disorders referred to as peroneal atrophy, Charcot-Marie-Tooth disease type IA (hypertrophic form), or Roussy-Levy syndrome
II	Autosomal dominant (majority)	Can have a variable inheritance pattern	• Normal reflexes, sensory, and motor nerve conduction times
III	Autosomal recessive	Genetic mutation of PMP (peripheral myelin protein) 22	• More severe than type I or II with clinical features of delayed ambulation, pes cavus, and "glove-and-stocking" dysesthesia; most patients confined to a wheelchair by third or fourth decade • Synonymous with Dejerine-Sottas disease
IV	Autosomal recessive	Mutation of peroxin 7 (PEX7) gene or phytanoyl-CoA hydroxylase (PAHX), which controls the production of the enzyme phytanoyl-CoA, resulting in accumulation of phytanic acid in tissues and fluids	• Synonymous with Refsum disease
V	Autosomal dominant	Undetermined genetic mutation	• Inherited spastic paraplegia with distal weakness in the limbs
VI	Autosomal recessive	Undetermined genetic mutation	• Optic atrophy in association with peroneal muscular atrophy
VII	Autosomal dominant	Undetermined genetic mutation	• Retinitis pigmentosa associated with distal muscle weakness

- Charcot-Marie-Tooth disease refers to HSMN type 1 or 2 disease, an autosomal-dominant condition characterized by motor and sensory demyelinating neuropathy
    - Can present either in the second decade of life as the hypertrophic form or, more classically, in the third or fourth decades as the axonal form
    - Distinguished by extensive foot involvement, with the phenotypic appearance of "upside-down champagne bottle" (Fig. 15-11)
    - Other features include cavovarus feet, hammertoes, peroneal weakness, and intrinsic muscle wasting.
    - May require orthotics, surgical releases, and/or muscle transfers for the foot

Spinal Muscular Atrophy

- An autosomal-recessive disease that manifests as a loss of anterior horn cells in the spinal cord; the most common diagnosis in girls presenting with progressive muscle weakness
    - Incidence: 1:200,000 births
    - Classified into three disease types based on age at presentation (Table 15-6)
- Pathology is consistent with muscle denervation, and nerve conduction is unaffected.
- Survival motor neuron (SMN) gene mutation on chromosome 5q has been detected in a significant number of patients; this gene plays a critical role in RNA metabolism and is a mediator of apoptosis.
- No cerebral dysfunction; patients have a normal intellect
- The disease presents with:
    - Progressive scoliosis

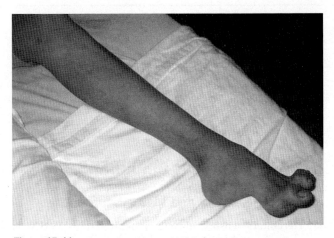

Figure 15-11 A 32-year-old man with Charcot-Marie-Tooth disease. Note typical extensive lower limb and foot involvement ("upside-down champagne bottle").

TABLE 15-6 TYPES OF SPINAL MUSCULAR ATROPHY BASED ON AGE AT PRESENTATION

Type	Name	Genetic Defect	Clinical Features/Comments
1	Acute Werdnig Hoffman disease	Defective gene(s) for all three types located on chromosome 5q, but appear to be different mutations at the same locus	• Presents at birth and in infants • Short life span
2	Chronic Werdnig Hoffman disease		• Presents between age 6 months and 2 years
3	Kugelberg-Welander disease		• Presents in children after 2 years • Typically long life span

- Symmetric paresis and weakness predominating in the proximal musculature of both lower limbs
- Hip dysplasia

Arthrogrypotic Syndromes

- Arthrogryposis refers to a congenital, nonprogressive limitation of joint movement attributable to soft tissue contractures involving two or more joints.
- 150 different genetic manifestations have been linked to the disease.
  - Decreased intrauterine movement a common etiology in all types
  - Pathophysiology due to the replacement of muscle in affected areas with fat and fibrous tissue
- A severe disease entity that may be managed by a pediatric orthopaedic surgeon is called arthrogryposis multiplex congenita or amyoplasia. Arthrogryposis multiplex congenita has the following disease features:
  - Three types: myopathic, neuropathic, and mixed
  - Loss of anterior horn cells from the spinal cord
  - Multiple rigid joints with muscle wasting
  - Normal facies and intellect

MUSCULAR DISORDERS (INHERITED MYOPATHIES)

- A group of nine inherited myopathies that cause progressive muscular weakness
- >30,000 people in the United States with inheritable myopathies
- Clinical diagnosis based on family history, physical examination, laboratory findings (CPK, aldolase), electrophysiologic studies (electromyography, nerve conduction studies), muscle biopsy, and molecular diagnostic tests
- CPK is an enzyme found in high levels in skeletal muscle and is closely associated with the myopathic disorders.
  - Levels normal in neuropathic disorders
  - Normal or mildly elevated levels in congenital myopathies and spinal muscular atrophies
  - High levels seen when there is significant myocyte destruction
    - Following this phase when the muscle has been replaced with fat and fibrous tissue, CPK levels return to normal.

Myotonic Muscular Dystrophy

- The most common muscular dystrophy, with an incidence of 1:8,000
- Marked phenotypic variability
- Inherited as an autosomal-dominant trait, it is caused by a trinucleotide expansion in the myotonic dystrophy protein kinase (DMPK) gene on chromosome 19q13.2–q13.3.
- Patients present with hypotonia in infancy, myotonia in childhood, weakness, cataracts, hypogonadism, frontal balding, mental retardation, and electrocardiographic changes.

Duchenne's and Becker Muscular Dystrophies

- Duchenne's muscular dystrophy and the milder Becker muscular dystrophy are two disorders that result from different mutations in the dystrophin gene on the X chromosome (Xp21) (Table 15-7).
- Special diagnostic tests include:
  - Muscle biopsy
    - Necrotic foci
    - Fatty infiltration of muscle
    - Dystrophin immunoblotting: lack of detection of dystrophin with an antibody in a muscle biopsy
  - DNA mutation analysis with PCR or restriction fragment length polymorphism
  - Dystrophin RNA testing (requires a blood sample only)

Facioscapulohumeral Muscular Dystrophy

- The third most common muscular dystrophy (after Duchenne's and myotonic muscular dystrophies), facioscapulohumeral muscular dystrophy (FSHMD) is an autosomal-dominant disorder associated with the gene on chromosome 4q.
- Patients present in late childhood or early adulthood with progressive muscular weakness of the face, shoulder girdle (scapular winging), and arm muscles (Fig. 15-12).
- Patients generally have normal life expectancy.

Emery-Dreifuss Muscular Dystrophy

- A rare muscular dystrophy: an X-linked disorder that affects males and is caused by a mutation in the emerin gene on chromosome Xq28 (dystrophin is normal)

TABLE 15-7 TWO FORMS OF MUSCULAR DYSTROPHY THAT ARISE FROM DYSTROPHIN MUTATION

Parameter	Duchenne's	Becker
Incidence	1:3,500	1:30,000
Inheritance	X-linked recessive	
Protein	Dystrophin (found in skeletal, smooth, and cardiac muscle and the brain)	
Mutations	Disrupt the translational reading frame or promoter region, leading to truncated/unstable dystrophin with absence of functional dystrophin	Usually associated with a less disruptive type of mutation, resulting in a smaller and/or semifunctional protein (nonsense mutation)
Creatine phosphokinase	Highly elevated (100 times normal)	Moderately to highly elevated (50 to 100× normal)
Dystrophin immunoblotting	Complete absence of dystrophin	Dystrophin decreased in amount, size, or both
Onset	Between 3 and 6 years of age	Later in childhood
Characteristics	Proximal muscle weakness (Gowers maneuver)	Proximal muscle weakness (less severe)
Skeletal manifestations	Joint contractures, scoliosis, equinovarus	Similar to Duchenne's but less severe
Other manifestations	• Cardiac involvement with sinus tachycardia and right ventricular hypertrophy with arrhythmias and congestive heart failure in 10% of patients • Progressive loss of respiratory capacity • Gastric dysmotility • Risk of malignant hyperthermia	• Cardiomyopathy can occur, but complications such as congestive heart failure and arrhythmias are infrequent. • Risk of malignant hyperthermia
Course	• Progressive weakness of axial and appendicular muscles • Walking until age 10 years • Death from respiratory problems in late 20s	• More variable, protracted course • Able to run as children, preserve ability to walk sometimes into adulthood • Fewer respiratory problems

■ Slow progression, with initial nonspecific features (e.g., muscle weakness in the first few years of life, awkward gate, tendency to toe-walk)
  ■ Differential diagnosis: Duchenne's and Becker muscular dystrophy
  ■ The early diagnosis is confirmed by electromyography and muscle biopsy.
  ■ Definitive clinical features are noted in the second decade:
    ■ Fixed equinus deformities
    ■ Elbow flexion contractures
    ■ Neck extension contractures (limit neck flexion)
    ■ Cardiac abnormalities (risk of sudden cardiac death)

TRINUCLEOTIDE DISORDERS

■ A group of conditions associated with an increased number of nucleotide triplets in the DNA

■ There is a progressive increase in trinucleotide number down the successive familial generation, with worsening in disease presentation (phenomenon called anticipation).
■ The repeat expansions are associated with a "loss-of-function" mechanism: these expansions prevent the expression of normal protein.
■ The genetic abnormality may be located on various chromosomes, and some disease entities share a characteristic increase in CAG repeat.
  ■ CAG trinucleotide codes for amino acid glutamine.
■ To date, 14 trinucleotide disorders have been documented.
■ Trinucleotide disorders may be classified as polyglutamine or nonpolyglutamine disorders.
  ■ Most polyglutamine disorders are rare and not associated with any major orthopaedic issues.
■ Friedrich's ataxia is an autosomal recessive nonpolyglutamine trinucleotide disorder characterized by spinocerebellar involvement.
  ■ Findings include a classic triad of ataxia, loss of deep tendon reflexes (areflexia), and an extensor Babinski response.

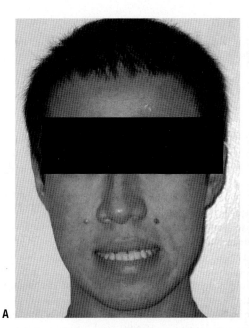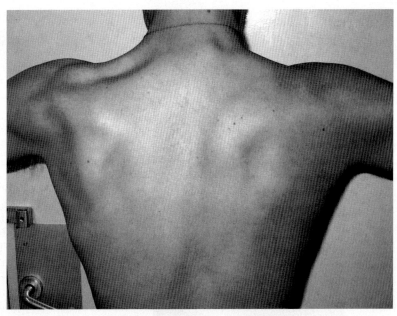

A   **B**

Figure 15-12   A 22-year-old man with facioscapulohumeral muscular dystrophy. Note loss of facial muscle contracture (patient is attempting to say "E") (**A**) and winging of scapulae (**B**).

- Patients typically present to an orthopaedic surgeon because of scoliosis (which occurs in approximately 80%) and/or cavovarus feet.
- Average age of onset is 12 years; patients often die by age 25 years due to cardiomyopathy-related heart failure.
- Molecular basis linked to the presence of expanded guanine-adenosine-adenosine trinucleotide repeats in the gene in chromosome 9 involved in the production of the mitochondrial protein frataxin, which plays an essential role in iron metabolism and oxidative stress
  - ~66 to 1,500 abnormal repeats, the number correlating to disease severity (normal patients have up to 32 abnormal repeats)
  - Presence of this genetic defect can lead to accumulation of free radicals (produced when excess iron reacts with oxygen), which then cause irreversible damage in the nervous system, the heart, and the pancreas.
  - Knowledge of the genetic basis of the disease has given physicians the opportunity to extend the lives of patients at risk for cardiac failure (secondary to accumulation of bioactive radicals) by administration of antioxidants.

OTHER GENETIC CONDITIONS

Down Syndrome (Trisomy 21)

- Duplication of long arm of chromosome 21
- Increasing incidence with increasing maternal age

- Clinical features: ligamentous laxity, mental impairment, heart disease, endocrine disorders, early aging
- Orthopaedic implications: atlantoaxial instability, scoliosis, hip instability, slipped capital femoral epiphyses, patella dislocation, metatarsus primus varus, planovalgus

Turner's Syndrome (XO)

- Single X chromosome instead of the normal XX or XY configuration
- Clinical features: short stature, sexual infantilism, web neck, renal anomalies in 66%, cardiac anomalies in 33%
- Orthopaedic issues: short stature, scoliosis, genu valgum, shortened fourth and fifth metacarpals, risk of malignant hyperthermia following administration of anesthesia

Neurofibromatosis

- Neurofibromatosis is an autosomal-dominant disorder of the bones, soft tissues, skin, and nervous system. Two distinct subtypes:
  - Neurofibromatosis-1 (NF-1 or von Recklinghausen disease)
  - Neurofibromatosis-2 (NF-2)
- NF-1, the more common peripheral subtype, is characterized by a mutation in the neurofibromin tumor-suppressor gene on chromosome 17.
  - Incidence: 1:3,000 births (highest incidence of all single gene disorders)
  - Half of cases can be new mutations.
  - Affects multiple organ systems with varying severity; this can help in making the diagnosis
    - Higher mortality rate due to malignant periph-

- Axillary or inguinal freckling
- Optic glioma
- At least two iris hamartomas (Lisch nodules)
- Distinctive bony lesion
  - Sphenoid dysplasia or thinning of the cortex of the long bones
  - Congenital pseudarthrosis or anterolateral bowing of tibia (Fig. 15-13)
  - Dystrophic scoliosis (short, sharp curve with or without thinning of ribs, enlargement of neural foramina, vertebral body scalloping)
  - First-degree relative with NF-1
- Treatment
  - Excision of enlarging or symptomatic neurofibromas
  - Treatment of scoliosis and pseudoarthrosis of the tibia
  - Resection of malignant peripheral nerve sheath tumors
- NF-2 is characterized by various central nervous system tumors. Its incidence is 1:40,000, and it has been localized to chromosome 22 (half are de novo mutations).
  - Patients present with unilateral/bilateral vestibular schwannomas (may be associated with various tumors).
  - Treatment: excision of acoustic neuromas causing tinnitus, vertigo, epilepsy

SUGGESTED READING

Baitner AC, Maurer SG, Gruen MB, et al. The genetic basis of the osteochondrodysplasias. *J Pediatr Orthop* 2000;20:594–605.

Beighton P, Giedion ZA, Gorlin R, et al. International classification of osteochondrodysplasias. *Am J Med Genet* 1992;44:223–229.

Dietz FR, Mathews KD. Update on the genetic basis of disorders with orthopaedic manifestations. *J Bone Joint Surg [Am]* 1996;78(10):1583–1598.

Evans CH, Ghivizzani SC, Robbins PD. Orthopaedic gene therapy. *Clin Orthop Relat Res* 2004;(429):316–329.

Mackenzie WG, et al. Genetic diseases and skeletal dysplasias. In: Vaccaro AR, ed. *Orthopaedic Knowledge Update, Home Study Syllabus* 2005:663–675.

Online Mendelian Inheritance in Man (OMIM) Database [Internet]. Bethesda, MD: National Center for Biotechnology Information for the National Institute of Health. Available from http://www.ncbi.nlm.nih.gov/Omim/

Sollazzo V, Bertolani G, Calzolari E, et al. A two-locus model for nonsyndromic congenital dysplasia of the hip (CDH). *Ann Hum Genet* 2000;64:51–59.

Wilkinson JA. Etiologic factors in congenital displacement of the hip and myelodysplasia. *Clin Orthop Relat Res* 1992;(281):75–83.

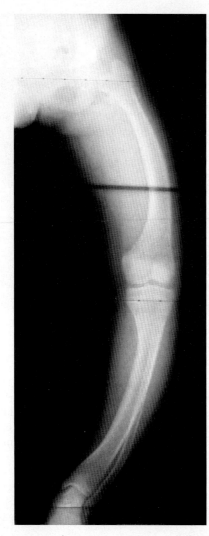

Figure 15-13 Radiograph of a 16-year-old girl with a diagnosis of neurofibromatosis. Note anterolateral bowing of tibia.

eral nerve sheath tumor (formerly neurofibrosarcoma)
- Two or more of these criteria are necessary for diagnosis:
  - At least two neurofibromas (tumors of Schwann cells) or one plexiform neurofibroma
  - At least six café-au-lait spots (irregular brown spots on skin) that measure at least 5 mm in children, at least 15 mm in adults

BIOMECHANICS

FREDERICK W. WERNER
JOSEPH A. SPADARO

SOME BASIC BIOMECHANICAL TERMS

- **Force (load):** A force is an action on a body. It has a direction and a magnitude.
- **Oblique forces:** A force being applied at some angle to a coordinate system can be represented as two perpendicular or orthogonal forces in that coordinate system.
  - Magnitude of the oblique force on the implant is the square root of the sum of the squares of the perpendicular forces (Fig. 16-1).
  - Graphically, the force on the implant is the hypotenuse of the right triangle formed by the perpendicular forces.
  - Examples: shoulder joint (Fig. 16-2) and knee joint (Fig. 16-3)
- **Dynamic forces:** Dynamic forces include the effect of the inertia of the person moving or an impact on an object against another.

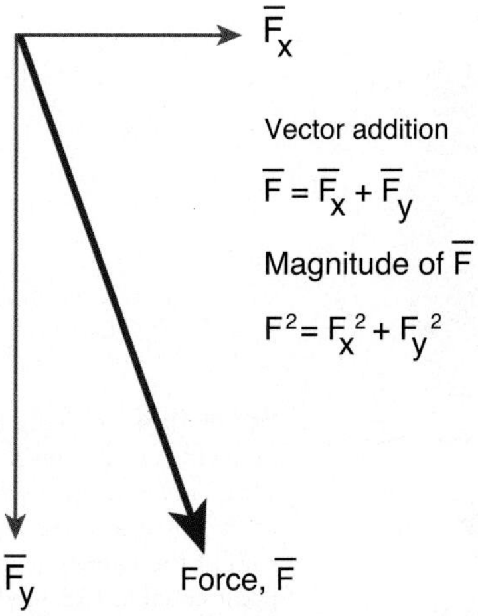

$$\overline{F}_x$$

Vector addition

$$\overline{F} = \overline{F}_x + \overline{F}_y$$

Magnitude of $\overline{F}$

$$F^2 = F_x^2 + F_y^2$$

$$\overline{F}_y \qquad \text{Force, } \overline{F}$$

Figure 16-1 Vector addition of two orthogonal forces to obtain the force, F. A force is represented by drawing either an arrow or line over the letter corresponding to that force.

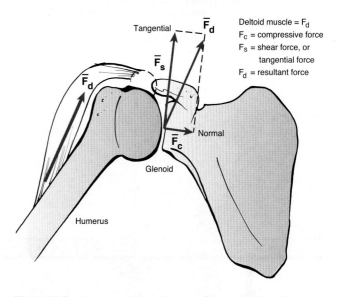

Tangential — $\overline{F}_d$

$\overline{F}_s$

$\overline{F}_d$

Normal

$\overline{F}_c$

Glenoid

Humerus

Deltoid muscle = F_d
F_c = compressive force
F_s = shear force, or tangential force
F_d = resultant force

Figure 16-2 Example of force decomposition in the shoulder joint. The deltoid force, F_d, is represented (decomposed) as a compressive force, F_c, and a shearing or tangential force, F_s. (Adapted from Buckwalter JA, Einhorn TA, Simon SR, eds. *Orthopaedic Basic Sciences*, 2nd ed. Chicago: American Academy of Orthopaedic Surgeons, 2000.)

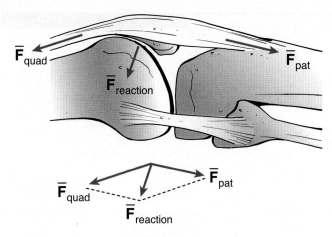

Figure 16-3 Example of calculation of forces in the knee joint. The patellofemoral joint reaction force, $F_{reaction}$, is the vector parallelogram sum of the quadriceps force, F_{quad}, and the patellar tendon force, F_{pat}.

- Example of normal walking gait: During gait, the forces on the knee joint are due to the weight of the person, the muscles causing the knee to move, the ligamentous structures that provide stability, and the inertia of the person as the heel strikes the floor and as he or she pushes off before toe off.
- **Moment:** A moment is defined as a force being applied at some distance away from some pivot point. Its magnitude is the force times the moment arm.
- **Moment calculation:** If several moments are being ap-

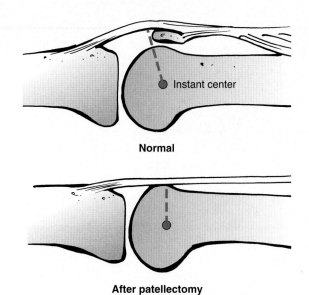

Figure 16-5 After a knee patellectomy, the moment arm for the knee extension moment is decreased. Therefore, the quadriceps force required to extend the knee has to be larger than before patellectomy. (Adapted from Nordin M, Frankel VH, eds. *Basic Biomechanics of the Musculoskeletal System*, 2nd ed. Philadelphia, Lea & Febiger, 1989.)

plied to a bone or some object in equilibrium, then the sum of those moments about a given point is equal to zero.

- Examples: using a see-saw (Fig. 16-4), the knee joint (Fig. 16-5)

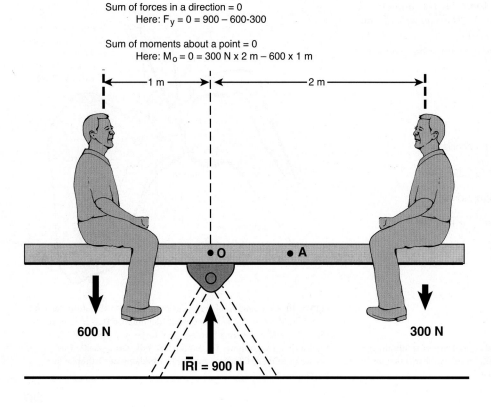

Sum of forces in a direction = 0
Here: $F_y = 0 = 900 - 600 - 300$

Sum of moments about a point = 0
Here: $M_o = 0 = 300 \text{ N} \times 2 \text{ m} - 600 \times 1 \text{ m}$

Figure 16-4 Calculation of moments about a pivot point, 0. In a static, nonmoving situation, the sum of the vertical forces equal 0, and the sum of the moments about a pivot point equal 0. (Adapted from Buckwalter JA, Einhorn TA, Simon SR, eds. *Orthopaedic Basic Sciences*, 2nd ed. Chicago: American Academy of Orthopaedic Surgeons, 2000.)

- **Torques:** A torque is typically caused by a twisting motion such as opening a jar. There is an equal but opposite torque required to resist the torque being applied to open the jar.
  - Torque = applied force × the moment arm
- **Units:** Forces are typically measured in Newtons (N). Moments and torques are measured in Newton-meters (N-m) or Newton-millimeters (N-mm).

KINEMATICS

Kinematics is the study of how things move. Motions can be viewed as displacements (translations), as rotations, or as a combination of them. A person or object might be moving at a constant velocity or with a changing velocity, in which case it is accelerating or decelerating.

- **Velocity:** The rate (speed) and direction of movement of an object, such as a car moving down the road. The magnitude of the velocity is the distance or displacement of the object per unit time.
- **Acceleration** and **deceleration:** If the speed of that object, or its direction, is changing, then the object is either accelerating or decelerating.
- **Center of rotation:** For most joints in the body, one can find a center of rotation about which the bone is rotating. For example, door hinges are the fixed center of rotation for a rotating door. In the knee joint and many others, the center of rotation is not fixed but changes through the range of knee flexion.
- **3D center of rotation:** In the knee joint as well as in other joints in the body, the motion is not necessarily planar. As the knee flexes and extends, tibial rotation and ab/adduction cause the center of rotation to move in three dimensions.

MECHANICAL PROPERTIES OF MATERIALS

- **Stress:** A force applied to an implant or bone will cause a stress in the material.
  - Stress = applied force divided by the area over which the force is being applied (typical units are N/mm²)
- **Strain:** When a force or stress is applied to some implant or bone, there will be a small deformation. To normalize that deformation, a strain is computed.
  - Strain = change in length (ΔL) divided by the original length (Lo); typical units are mm/mm
- **Force-displacement (loading) curve** (Fig. 16-6): Plot of the resultant forces due to an applied displacement to a structure such as a bone or ligament. It can also be a plot of the force applied to a structure to produce a displacement.
  - Structural properties

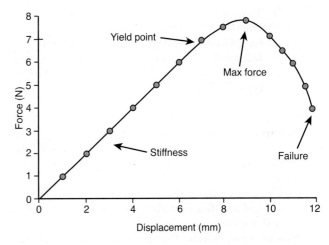

Figure 16-6 Example of a force–displacement loading curve for a linear, elastic structure.

- **Stiffness:** slope of the linear portion of the force–displacement curve
- **Yield point:** force at which the structure starts to plastically (permanently) deform
- **Maximum force:** maximum force the structure can support
- **Energy:** area under the force–displacement curve
- **Stress–strain curve** (Fig. 16-7): A stress–strain curve is computed from a force–displacement curve.
  - Material properties
    - **Elastic modulus:** slope of the linear portion of the curve
    - **Proportional limit:** force at the end of the linear part of the curve
    - **Yield point:** force at which the material starts to plastically deform
    - **Ultimate strength** (tensile strength if in tension, compressive strength if in compression): maximum stress the material can support

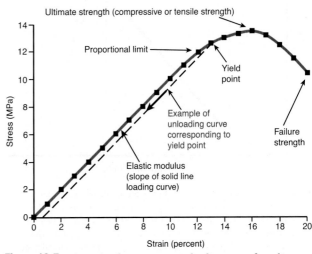

Figure 16-7 Example of a stress–strain loading curve for a linear, elastic material.

- ■ **Toughness:** area under the stress–strain curve
- ■ **Ductility:** the ultimate strain (strain at rupture) for a material undergoing inelastic deformation. Intuitively, how much a deforming material stretches or deforms before breaking. This is typically described as a percent elongation or reduction of area.
- ■ **Fatigue properties:** With repetitive loading, materials and structures can fail (fracture) at forces and moments that are far less than the maximum force due to the single application of a force. Most implants fail in fatigue.
  - ■ **Endurance limit:** the maximum stress that can be applied an infinite number of times and the material will not fail
- ■ **Nonlinear materials** (Fig. 16-8): A material that has an initial nonlinear loading curve (i.e., does not have a straight-line relationship between force and displacement or between stress and strain)
  - ■ **Toe-in region:** Region at the beginning of a typical force–displacement or stress–strain curve in which the flatness of the curve reflects considerable displacement or strain with the initial application of very little force or stress. For example, little force is required to cause initial displacement in a ligament as the fibers straighten.
- ■ **Viscoelastic material properties:** Creep and stress relaxation of materials (Fig. 16-9)
  - ■ **Viscoelasticity:** When material properties and behavior (above) are *loading rate-dependent*. True of almost all biological tissues, especially ligaments, cartilage, and polymeric biomaterials. Their properties change with the speed at which they are loaded, or with constant loading.

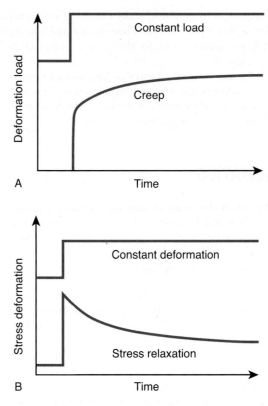

Figure 16-9 Creep and stress relaxation material behavior. (From Mow VC, Hayes WC. *Basic Orthopaedic Biomechanics.* New York: Raven Press, 1991;203.)

- ■ **Creep deformation:** Under constant load, deformation continues with time until a plateau is reached.
- ■ **Stress relaxation:** After a sudden but then constant deformation, the stress in the material beneath the deformation will gradually decrease until a plateau is reached.
- ■ **Wear of materials** (Fig. 16-10)
  - ■ **Three-body wear:** Particulate material between adjoining surfaces causes abrasion or accelerated loss of surface integrity.
    - ■ Three-body wear is encountered when bone cement or bone particles abrade the polyethylene

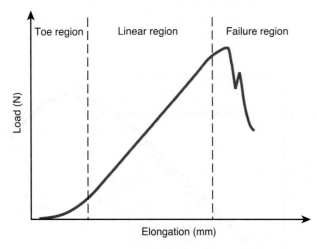

Figure 16-8 Example of a nonlinear material. Under initial loading, there is some initial laxity as the material starts to elongate. This region of the curve is known as the toe-in region, followed by a linear region where there is a linear elongation response to the applied force. (Adapted from Buckwalter JA, Einhorn TA, Simon SR, eds. *Orthopaedic Basic Sciences*, 2nd ed. Chicago: American Academy of Orthopaedic Surgeons, 2000.)

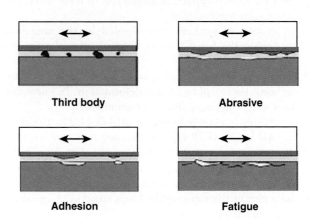

Figure 16-10 Material wear.

surface in an implanted hip prosthesis, or when ceramic particles released from certain femoral head trunion designs accelerate wear and loosening of the implant.

- **Abrasive wear:** One or both of the adjoining surfaces with an uneven texture cause loss of material from the surfaces during movement.
  - Abrasive wear accelerates the destruction of the natural articular surface when cartilage becomes thin or subchondral bone is exposed, resulting in "bone on bone." In artificial joints, irregularities (asperities) in metal components due to corrosion or adhesion rapidly abrade an adjacent polyethylene surface.
- **Adhesive wear:** Portion of one material is in contact with irregularities on opposing material, causing them to adhere to each other.
  - Adhesive wear is an important early wear mechanism. Ultra-high-molecular-weight polyethylene acetabular cups have shown such wear leading to formation of a secondary socket and distortion of mechanical function in total hip joint replacements.
- **Fatigue wear:** Material is removed from articulating surfaces after repetitive excessive stresses cause minute fracturing of the surface layer.
  - Fatigue wear generally occurs as a late failure mechanism. For example, if a polymer component in a joint prosthesis is too thin, local stresses exerted by a metal component on the polymer may be greater than with a thicker layer. After many cycles the fatigue limit of the polymer can be exceeded, leading to cracking and surface failure of the polymer.
- **Hardness:** The resistance to surface deformation by indentation or scratching
  - Scratching hardness is commonly quantified using the Mohs original scale:
    - Diamond = 10, talc = 1, aluminum = 2 to 3, steels = 5 to 8
  - Indentation hardness is quantified by using either a Brinell hardness or Rockwell hardness scale.

BEHAVIOR OF SIMPLE STRUCTURES

- Tensile, compressive, bending, and torsional loading
  - **Tension:** causes material to elongate
  - **Compression:** causes material to compress (shorten)
  - **Bending:** causes compression on one side, tension on other side of material
  - **Shear:** tends to cause distortion of one portion of the material relative to another portion, parallel to the direction of loading
  - **Torque:** causes material to twist
- **Three-point bending** (Fig. 16-11): produced by a combination of three parallel forces applied at different points on the structure

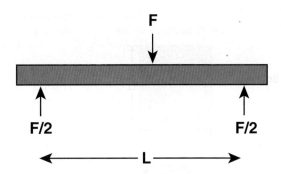

Figure 16-11   Three-point bending. An implant or bone can be exposed to three-point bending by having an intermediate force centrally located and supported by two end supports.

- **Four-point bending** (Fig. 16-12): produced by a combination of four parallel forces applied at different points on the structure
- **Bending stresses:** If a bone is exposed to bending, one side of the bone experiences tensile stresses, while the other experiences compressive stresses.
  - The magnitude of either stress is:

$$\text{Stress magnitude} = \sigma = Mc/I$$

where M is the moment, c is the distance from the center of the beam or bone where there are no stresses, and I is the moment of inertia (a descriptor of the beam or bone's cross-sectional shape to resist bending; see below).

- **Moment of inertia** (Fig. 16-13): The moment of inertia of a bone, structure, or implant is a characteristic of its cross-sectional geometry and represents the resistance to bending. For simple cross-sections, this property can be easily computed. The bending moment of inertia, for example, increases with the diameter of the bone raised to the fourth power.
- **Torsional stresses:** Torques applied to a bone or beam may cause a torsional spiral fracture. In a beam, the torsional stresses are greatest at the largest radius from the center of the beam.

$$\text{Stress magnitude} = \tau = Tc/J$$

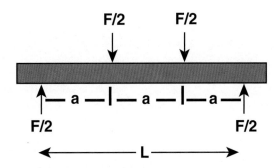

Figure 16-12   Four-point bending. An implant or bone can be exposed to four-point bending. Here the distance between the two intermediate forces is the same as the distance to the end supports.

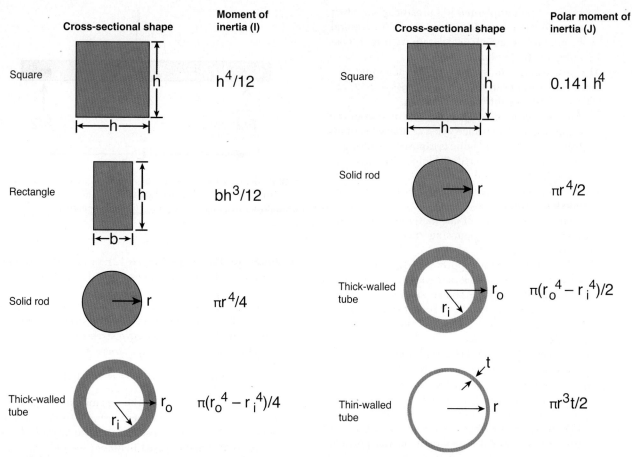

	Cross-sectional shape	Moment of inertia (I)
Square	h (h × h square)	$h^4/12$
Rectangle	h, b	$bh^3/12$
Solid rod	r	$\pi r^4/4$
Thick-walled tube	r_o, r_i	$\pi(r_o^4 - r_i^4)/4$

Figure 16-13   Cross-sectional views and the corresponding moments of inertia.

	Cross-sectional shape	Polar moment of inertia (J)
Square	h	$0.141\,h^4$
Solid rod	r	$\pi r^4/2$
Thick-walled tube	r_o, r_i	$\pi(r_o^4 - r_i^4)/2$
Thin-walled tube	t, r	$\pi r^3 t/2$

Figure 16-14   Cross-sectional views and the corresponding polar moments of inertia.

where T is the applied torque, c is the distance from the neutral axis, and J is the polar moment of inertia (see below).

■ **Polar moment of inertia** (Fig. 16-14): The polar moment of inertia of a bone, structure, or implant is a characteristic of its cross-sectional geometry. It represents the structure's resistance to twisting under torsional load. For simple cross-sections, the polar moment property can be easily computed. The polar moment of inertia of a long bone increases as the diameter raised to the fourth power. Small changes in the size can have profound changes in torsional strength.

SUGGESTED READING

Buckwalter JA, Einhorn TA, Simon SR, eds. *Orthopaedic Basic Sciences*, 2nd ed. Chicago: American Academy of Orthopaedic Surgeons, 2000.

Mow VC, Huiskes R, eds. *Basic Orthopaedic Biomechanics and Mechano-Biology*, 3rd ed. Philadelphia: Lippincott Williams & Wilkins, 2005.

Nordin M, Frankel VH, eds. *Basic Biomechanics of the Musculoskeletal System*, 2nd ed. Philadelphia: Lea & Febiger, 1989.

17

BIOMATERIALS

JOSEPH A. SPADARO
MICHAEL T. CLARKE
JULIE M. HASENWINKEL

The advances made in contemporary orthopaedic surgery are intimately related to the development of and use of implant biomaterials. These are materials used to augment, repair, or replace natural tissues or assist in healing. Currently, biological performance is as influential as the mechanical properties of its component materials in the design of an implant. It is now recognized that no implanted biomaterials are actually inert. In fact, instead of demanding inertness, most surgical specialties are embracing "bioactivity" as a means toward a fuller regeneration of the normal state. Orthopaedics is no exception. Only by the orchestration of the mechanical, chemical, and biological behaviors of these biomaterials can further improvements be made.

An understanding of the general principles is therefore crucial to implant selection and expectations on behavior.

METALS AND METALLIC ALLOYS

- Metals and their alloys of other metallic and nonmetallic elements are used as implants in orthopaedic surgery mainly for bearing and structural components that are typically affixed to bone.
- Benefits: bulk biocompatibility, strength, resistance to fatigue failure over millions of cycles
- Drawbacks: susceptibility to corrosion, potential for immune stimulation, particulate cytotoxicity and mutagenicity, possibility of fatigue failure in the long term

Implant Manufacture

- Raw material is processed in one of three ways (frequently, a combination of two or three is necessary for final implant shape; Table 17-1 gives definitions).
  - Machining: includes lathing, milling, or grinding of material
  - Casting: molten alloy is poured into a mold (subsequently broken)
  - Forging: by bending, compressing, and impacting (often at elevated temperatures)
- Final modifications of an implant frequently used are:
  - Coating (to enhance bone ingrowth or ongrowth)
    - Plasma spray of powdered hydroxyapatite or metal alloy
    - Cold deposition of hydroxyapatite
    - Sintering of beads or wire
  - Grit blasting (to enhance frictional interference with cement or bone)
  - Polishing (to enhance appearance, reduce corrosion, and reduce friction on cement)
  - Shot peening (to enhance fatigue properties of critical areas [e.g., Morse taper junctions])

Alloys in Current Use

- Although new alloys are constantly being developed, there are four broad classifications of alloy types currently in common orthopaedic use:

TABLE 17-1 SOME METALLURGICAL DEFINITIONS

Term	Definition
Cold working	The alteration of the shape or size of a metal by plastic deformation. Processes include rolling, drawing, pressing, spinning, extruding, and heading; are carried out below the recrystallization point, usually at room temperature. Hardness and tensile strength are increased with the degree of cold work, while ductility and impact values are lowered.
Hot working	The rolling, forging or extruding of a metal at a temperature above its recrystallization point without significant strain hardening
Warm working	Processing in a range usually 0.3 to 0.6 of melting point
Forging	A process of working metal to a finished shape by hammering or pressing; primarily a "hot" operation. It is applied to the production of shapes either impossible or too costly to make by other methods or needing properties not obtainable by casting. Categories of forgings include hammer, press, drop, or stamping.
Wrought	An alloy that has been significantly "worked" to break down its cast structure
Solution heat treatment	A process in which an alloy or metal is heated to a suitable temperature, is held at that temperature long enough to allow a certain constituent to enter into solid solution, and is then cooled rapidly to hold that constituent in solution. Most solution heat treatments soften or anneal.
Annealing	A heat treatment that relieves internal stress. Solution-annealed material is frequently in its most corrosion-resistant and ductile condition.
Work hardening	A term that signifies crystalline changes when a material is strained beyond its yield point
Grain boundary	As metals solidify (crystallize), many individual regions (grains) form with differing orientations of the atomic lattice. The region where grains meet (boundary) is less dense and more chemically reactive than the bulk material.
Passivation	A process of formation of an oxide layer on the surface of an alloy or metal. This can be spontaneous in the environment or enhanced chemically, for example by immersion in nitric acid. Passivation generally leads to improved corrosion resistance.

- Titanium alloys
- Cobalt chromium alloys
- Stainless steel alloys
- Tantalum-carbon

Titanium and its Alloys

- Although developed as an aerospace alloy, titanium is well known in the medical field for its biocompatibility and high strength-to-weight ratio.
- It is broadly used in the manufacture of fracture and spinal fixation devices as well as nonarticulating joint replacement components.

Orthopaedic Uses of Titanium Alloy

- Fracture and spinal fixation devices: screws, plates, intramedullary nails
- Joint replacement components
  - Cementless total hip: acetabular shells, femoral stems, ingrowth or ongrowth coatings
    - *Not* femoral heads (historically abandoned due to high wear)
  - Total knee: tibial tray, ingrowth or ongrowth coatings
    - *Not* femoral bearing surfaces (historically abandoned due to high wear)

Metallurgy

- Titanium is typically alloyed with other elements as well as being thermomechanically treated to achieve the desired properties for implantation.
- Metallic alloying increases the strength and maintains ductility by replacing titanium atoms in the crystal lattice with other metal atoms such as aluminum, vanadium, zirconium, and niobium.
- Nonmetallic interstitial elements such as oxygen, carbon, and nitrogen lie in voids between atoms of titanium.
- Strength is gained, but ductility and toughness are reduced.
- The natural crystal state for pure titanium (CPTi) is an alpha phase with a hexagonal close packed (hcp) crystal lattice.
  - An alternate beta, body centered cubic (bcc) crystal phase is present in varying extents in titanium alloys depending on the alloy and heat treatments performed.
  - Beta-phase alloys can be harder and more brittle than alpha-phase ones.
  - In the commonly used titanium–aluminum–vanadium, an alpha-beta alloy, aluminum stabilizes the alpha phase and vanadium the beta phase.

BOX 17-1 GENERAL ADVANTAGES AND DISADVANTAGES OF TITANIUM ALLOYS

Advantages	Disadvantages
Excellent biocompatibility	Poor wear properties
Relatively low elastic modulus	Notch sensitive
Spot welding to itself in taper junctions	Concern with vanadium and aluminum content in specific alloys
Low galvanic corrosion to CoCrMo alloy	

■ The newer substantially beta-phase alloys containing molybdenum impart superior strength to an alloy and have the lowest elastic modulus (80 MPa) of any of the commonly used bulk implant alloys (e.g., CoCrMo 200 MPa).

Titanium Implant Characteristics (Box 17-1 and Table 17-2)

Advantages
■ Biocompatibility: result of a highly inert, insoluble, and adherent 10-nm-thick surface passivation layer of titanium oxide (titania, TiO_2), allowing superior corrosion resistance
  ■ Inert passivation layer of TiO_2 significantly reduces galvanic corrosion to cobalt base alloys at taper junctions (e.g., femoral head/femoral stem of total hip replacement [THR]).
■ Low elastic modulus (80 to 110 Mpa)
  ■ Useful in the prevention of stress shielding around cementless implants such as femoral hip replacement stems, but is to be avoided when used with polymethylmethacrylate (PMMA) cement as it is prone to increased cement stresses from bending as well as abrasive wear against cement due to poor wear properties
■ Spot welding at titanium–titanium taper junctions (e.g., stems on tibial base-plate for total knee replacement [TKR]) minimizes micromotion and fretting.

Disadvantages
■ Poor wear properties: resulted in general abandonment of titanium alloys as wear surfaces except for custom implants (e.g., in nickel-sensitive patients where cobalt alloy or stainless steel are to be avoided)
■ For custom titanium bearing surfaces, surface hardening is performed (e.g., ion implantation or nitriding)
■ Even the nitrided surface may be subject to delamination.
■ Notch sensitivity: problem for all alloys, but particularly so for titanium
■ Sharp angles, scratches, and sintered powder or beads allow stress risers to concentrate in one area, significantly reducing the fatigue life of an implant.
■ Vanadium, and to a lesser extent aluminum, are considered undesirable elements due to cell cytotoxicity seen in vitro and theoretical concerns about biocompatibility. Newer, currently unproven alloys that omit one or both of these alloys have been developed to avoid these theoretical concerns.

Cobalt-Based Alloys

Cobalt-based alloys, most notably of the cobalt–chromium binary system, are widely used for load bearing as a result of their fatigue resistance, and for wear surfaces as a result of their exceptional hardness when properly formed. Many of the properties of the alloys arise from the following:

TABLE 17-2 DIFFERENT USES OF SOME TITANIUM ALLOYS

Material	Crystal Structure[a]	Uses	Notes
Pure titanium (ASTM F67-00)	Alpha (hcp)	Mesh and porous coatings	Not heat treatable but can be cold worked. Has oxygen (<0.5%), nitrogen (<0.05%), carbon (<0.1%), and iron (<0.5%) as impurities that significantly alter mechanical properties. The yield strength is significantly dependent on impurities, especially oxygen. Higher oxygen increases yield strength.
90% titanium, 6% aluminum, 4% vanadium (Ti-6-4, Grade 5, ASTM 136-02)	Mainly alpha (hcp) with isolated particles of beta (bcc) at grain boundaries	Intramedullary nails, spinal fixation, joint replacement structural components	Can be heat treated to strengthen. The "workhorse" alloy for many years. <0.4% impurities allowed.
80% titanium, 12% molybdenum, 6% zirconium, 2% iron (ASTM F1813-01)	Mainly beta (bcc)	Femoral stems	Newer alloy used for low modulus components

[a]Crystal structures are hexagonal close packed (hcp) and body centered cubic (bcc).

BOX 17-2 GENERAL ADVANTAGES AND DISADVANTAGES OF COBALT-BASED ALLOYS

Advantages
Good biocompatibility
Fatigue-resistant
Wear-resistant
Low galvanic corrosion to
  titanium

Disadvantages
Galvanic corrosion to
  stainless steel

Concerns regarding
  nickel content
Cobalt and chromium ion
  release
High elastic modulus
Expensive
Difficult to process

- Crystal structure of cobalt
- Strengthening effects of chromium, nickel, tungsten, and molybdenum
- Formation of hard metal carbides (e.g., chromium carbide)
- Corrosion resistance imparted by chromium, nickel, and molybdenum alloying elements

Orthopaedic Uses of Cobalt Alloys
- Fracture and spinal fixation devices: braided wire for fracture fixation
- Joint replacement components
  - Femoral heads for metal-on-plastic and metal-on-metal bearings
  - Femoral stems for cemented and cementless THR
  - Femoral component for TKR
  - Ingrowth or ongrowth coatings on implants (e.g., THR/TKR)

Metallurgy
- Cobalt alloy in cast or wrought forms is typically alloyed with varying amounts of chromium and molybdenum.
- Tungsten and nickel are used in some alloys to achieve the desirable properties of strength, fatigue resistance, and corrosion resistance.
- Mechanical properties of cast alloys can be improved by hot forging that removes pores and reduces grain size.
- In some alloys (e.g., MP35N), cold working can change

the crystal structure from a face centered cubic (fcc) lattice to an hcp one, creating a biphasic alloy that has improved resistance to plastic deformation and increased strength.
- The presence of carbon is carefully controlled as this can affect the mechanical properties, including toughness, wear resistance, and corrodibility.
  - High carbon (>0.14% w/w) alloy is used as bearing surfaces against itself.
  - Low carbon (<0.14% w/w) alloy is used as structural members as well as for coating applications in addition to bearing applications against the ultra-high-molecular-weight form of poly(ethylene) (UHMWPE).
- Cast alloy may be porous, and mechanical properties are improved by hot forging or hot isostatic pressing (HIP) that removes pores and reduces grain size.
  - HIP is a process of heat treatment in argon gas at high temperature (e.g., 1200°C) and pressure (e.g., 1000 Atmospheres), followed typically by solution annealing.

Implant Characteristics (Box 17-2 and Tables 17-3 and 17-4)

Advantages
- Biocompatibility
  - Provided by a chromium oxide passivation layer that may be enhanced prior to implantation by cleaning, polishing, and an oxidizing nitric acid bath (see Table 17-1)
  - The solubility in water, however, is greater than TiO_2 and there is susceptibility to crevice corrosion, with concern about possible loss of implant fixation in the long term when directly apposed to bone.
- Improved fatigue resistance
  - THR stem fractures with cast stems: a concern in the past
  - Better metallurgical processing of alloys and improved alloy compositions have essentially eliminated this as a problem, to the point where wrought cobalt alloys provide some of the most fatigue-resistant alloys available for implantation.
- Wear resistance

TABLE 17-3 DIFFERENT USES OF SOME COBALT ALLOYS

Material	Crystal Structure	Uses	Notes
Cast cobalt–chromium–molybdenum alloy (ASTM F75)	fcc	Femoral heads, metal-on-metal bearings, femoral component of TKR	Comes in high- or low-carbon versions. Can be heat treated (hipped, solution annealed). Low nickel content.
Wrought cobalt–chromium–molybdenum alloy (F799, F1537)	fcc	Cemented femoral stems, metal-on-metal bearings	Wrought version of cast F75. Comes in high- and low-carbon versions. Low nickel content.
Wrought cobalt–chromium–nickel–molybdenum	fcc and hcp	Femoral stems	Extremely strong; fatigue and corrosion resistant. High nickel content has caused limited use in vivo.

TABLE 17-4 MECHANICAL PROPERTIES OF SOME IMPLANT ALLOYS

Alloy		Yield Strength (Mpa)	Ultimate Tensile Strength (MPa)	Fatigue Strength (MPa)	Elastic Modulus (Mpa)
Titanium Alloys					
Alpha-phase commercially pure titanium CpTi (ASTM F67 by ATI Allvac)	Grade 1 (0.18% oxygen)	172	241	—	110
	Grade 4 (0.4% oxygen)	480	550	380	110
Alpha-beta–phase titanium–aluminum–vanadium (ASTM F136 by ATI Allvac)		793	862	600	110
Beta-phase titanium–molybdenum–zirconium–iron alloy (ASTM F1813 by ATI Allvac)		965	1000	—	80
Cobalt Alloys					
Cast cobalt–chromium–molybdenum alloy (ASTM F75)	As cast	450–520	655–890	207–310	210
	HIPped	841	1277	725–950	253
Wrought cobalt–chromium–nickel alloy (ASTM F562 by Carpenter-MP35N)	Annealed	414	931	—	232
	55% cold-worked	1413	1827	—	232
	53% cold-worked and aged	1999	2068	793 max	232
Wrought cobalt–chromium–molybdenum alloy (ASTM F799/F1537 by Carpenter-BioDur CCM plus)	Annealed	882	1351	—	—
	Hot-worked	930	1365	900 max	210
Stainless Steels					
Nitrogen-strengthened stainless steel (ASTM F1586 by Sandvik-Bioline Hign N)	Annealed	430	740	—	—
	Cold-worked	1100	1350	—	—
AISI 316L stainless steel (ASTM F138 by Sandvik-Bioline 316LVM)	Annealed	190	490	270	200
	Cold-worked	800	1100	300	200
Nickel-free stainless steel (ASTM F2229 by Carpenter-Biodur 108)	Annealed bar and wire	607	931	381	
	40% cold-worked bar and wire	1551	1731		
	80% cold-worked (wire only)	1862	2206		
	Forged material water quenched for hip implants	1036	1253	513	
Tantalum					
Pure Ta (ASTM 560-04)	Solid material		345		186
Ta-C	75% porous components		63		3

The numbers shown are frequently greater than the ASTM minimum specifications.

- Partly a function of the strain hardening effect that occurs in vivo
- Cobalt alloy can also be machined and polished to give a low surface roughness (<0.01 micron Ra) when articulating with itself or UHMWPE.
- Low galvanic corrosion potential of a CoCrMo head on a titanium alloy femoral stem

Disadvantages
- High galvanic potential and corrosion risk of a CoCrMo head on a stainless steel stem, with the possible excep- tions of the newer nitrogen-strengthened or nickel-free stainless steels
- Presence of nickel is sometimes a problem:
  - In the common alloy grades (ASTM F75, F1537), it is specified at <1% but is unfortunately difficult to totally remove.
  - Nickel-sensitive patients may respond, and there are batch-to-batch differences, making comparisons dif- ficult.
  - Some non-wear surface alloys (e.g., femoral stems of THR) actually specify high nickel content (e.g.,

ASTM F90, F562, F563), as it improves fatigue strength as well as corrosion resistance.

- Cytotoxicity and carcinogenicity theoretical risks: Cobalt and chromium ions have been shown to be cytotoxic and carcinogenic in cell culture and in some animal models.
- Low levels are released into the body during the life of the implant.
- Cobalt is more soluble and the implant becomes relatively cobalt-depleted.
- Serum, tissue, and whole blood and urine levels of cobalt and chromium are greatly increased with metal-on-metal (CoCrMo) bearings.
- No long-term ill effects on humans have yet been reported.
- Stress shielding
  - High elastic modulus (250 MPa) is a concern for stress shielding.
  - In THR, there is a link between thigh pain and well-fixed porous coated implants.
  - There is a general trend toward use of lower-modulus titanium alloys for this reason.
- High cost: Cobalt as a raw element is expensive and thus the manufacture of implants from this alloy is very costly.
- Difficult processing of cobalt alloys
  - Casting needs to be carefully controlled to avoid poor-quality material with voids or large grain size.
  - Machining is performed at relatively slow speed and is time-consuming.

Stainless Steel

Although carbon steel was used as an orthopaedic implant material in the 19th century, stainless steel was first used in the 1920s and has undergone several evolutions since.

Orthopaedic Uses of Stainless Steel
- Fracture and spinal fixation devices
- Cables, screws, wires, plates, intramedullary nails
- Joint replacement components
  - Femoral heads for stainless steel THR
  - Cemented femoral stems

Metallurgy
- Stainless steel is a term used to classify a heterogeneous group of alloys that use the iron–chromium binary system in addition to other alloying and interstitial elements.
- Several distinct subgroups based on their crystal structure:
  - Only austenitic stainless steels are widely used as implant materials due to their corrosion resistance, non-magnetic nature, and relative ease of manufacture.
    - Austenitic stainless steel is a single-phase, fcc alloy typically forged by hot or warm methods and then cold worked to attain strength.
  - Other grades of stainless steel are used for surgical tools.

- Chromium is necessary for corrosion resistance and forms a complex chromium oxide passivation layer similar to cobalt–chromium alloys.
  - Chromium, however, favors the formation of a weaker ferritic bcc structure.
- Nickel is added to stabilize the austenitic phase in addition to improving corrosion resistance by nickel oxide formation complexing with chromium oxide.
- Other alloying elements used for corrosion resistance and ease of processing include molybdenum, silicon, and manganese.
- Carbon content is kept low to prevent sensitization from chromium carbides at grain boundaries that are prone to corrosion (see Table 17-1).
  - High-carbon stainless steel has resulted in premature implant failure.

Implant Characteristics (Box 17-3)

Advantages
- Low cost: Ubiquitous nature of iron ensures that the manufacture of stainless steel is cheaper than that of titanium and cobalt alloys.
- Biocompatibility: considered good, but inferior to that of cobalt or titanium alloys

Disadvantages
- Susceptibility of standard grades to crevice and stress corrosion has been noted in vivo, resulting in component failure.
- Permanent implant components are thus not made from the standard-grade AISI 316L, which is used primarily for temporary fracture fixation devices.
- The austenitic nature of stainless steel unfortunately makes it a poor wear material against itself, but acceptable to UHMWPE.
- Martensitic stainless steel (tetragonal crystal structure) is an excellent wear material, but is magnetic and has low corrosion resistance and is not therefore used except for some surgical tools.

Advances and Improvements (Table 17-5)
- Newer grades of wrought, nitrogen-strengthened stainless steels, however, can be made to approach the fatigue and corrosion resistance of the cobalt alloys and

---

BOX 17-3 GENERAL ADVANTAGES AND DISADVANTAGES OF STAINLESS STEEL

Advantages	Galvanic corrosion to
Cheap raw elements	CoCr and titanium
Good biocompatibility	Nickel sensitivity
	Poor wear properties
Disadvantages	
Some grades not suitable for long-term implantation due to fatigue failure	

TABLE 17-5 DIFFERENT USES OF SOME STAINLESS STEELS

Material	Crystal Structure	Uses	Notes
Fe-Cr-Ni-Mo-Mn (316L)	Austenite	Fracture fixation devices	Cold-worked to attain strength
Fe-Cr-Ni-Mo-Mn-N (nitrogen-strengthened) (ASTM F1586)	Austenite	Cemented femoral stems, steel wire	High-strength, corrosion-resistant alloy
Fe-Cr-Mn-N (nitrogen-strengthened nickel-free alloy)	Austenite	Fracture fixation devices	Newer alloy with limited components currently

have found use as the femoral heads and stems in cemented THR applications (e.g., Exeter by Stryker and Charnley by DePuy).

- Until recently, all stainless steel contained nickel.
- As a result of heightened concern about nickel sensitivity, nickel-free stainless steels have become available for implant use but are not yet widely used.
- Nickel has been substituted by manganese and nitrogen as austenite formers.

Tantalum

Tantalum is a dense metal that is a relative newcomer to large-scale implantation in orthopaedic surgery. Until recently, its use had been generally limited to research as a radiodense marker in bone in the form of balls for radiostereometric analysis (RSA) of implant migration. More recently, 80% porous, three-dimensional networks of tantalum over a backbone of vitreous carbon have been extensively used. The material properties have allowed its use as a fixation material to bone by both ingrowth and cementation with PMMA.

Orthopaedic Uses of Tantalum
- Joint replacement components
- Tibial and patellar components for TKR, some compression molded into UHMWPE
- Acetabular shells and augments for THR

Metallurgy
- Formed by cathode vapor deposition (CVD) of crystalline tantalum from gaseous tantalum pentachloride
- Resultant structure: 99% tantalum and 1% carbon with pore sizes of about 550 microns and an elastic modulus of 3MPa

Implant Characteristics

Advantages
- Low elastic modulus and prevention of stress shielding
- High porosity for bone ingrowth
- High coefficient of friction for initial stability
- Inert nature
- Relatively easy to trim blocks to fit

Disadvantages
- Significant cost
- Poor tensile strength
- Limitation to areas subject mainly to compression
- Current lack of clinical evidence for long-term benefit

POLYMERS

Polymers represent the largest class of biomaterials and are used for a variety of orthopaedic applications, including bearing surfaces and fixation materials for total joint prostheses. These materials, made of long-chain molecules with distinct repeat units known as "mers" or monomers, are derived from both natural sources and synthetic organic chemistry. The properties of polymers are a function of both the chemical and physical structure of the material. The physical structure of polymeric materials can be characterized in terms of molecular weight, which is directly proportional to the length of the polymer chains or the number of repeat units; the arrangement of monomer units into various chain structures; and the degree of crystallinity or order of the molecules within the material. These factors have a tremendous impact on the thermal and mechanical properties of polymeric materials, which in turn dictate their utility for biomaterials applications. This section will describe these basic principles of polymer science and discuss the primary applications of polymeric biomaterials in orthopaedic medicine.

Polymer Synthesis

Polymer synthesis can be accomplished by several different types of reactions, as outlined for polymers of orthopaedic interest in Table 17-6. Addition polymerization, often called free radical polymerization, is characterized by a three-step process:

TABLE 17-6 TYPES OF POLYMERIZATION REACTIONS AND THEIR CHARACTERISTICS

Type	Characteristics	Examples of Polymers
Addition	Chain reaction Initiated by reactive species	Poly(ethylene) Poly(methyl methacrylate)
Condensation	Stepwise growth process Results in condensation of small molecules (e.g., H_2O, HCl)	Poly(urethane) Nylon Poly(ethylene terephthalate)
Ring opening	Initiated by opening of a cyclic monomer	Poly(lactic acid) Poly(glycolic acid)

- Initiation
  - Free radicals are created by heat, light, or chemical reaction.
  - Radicals react with unsaturated double bond in monomer to start polymer chain.
- Propagation
  - Phase of rapid chain growth
  - Monomer units are added to the growing polymer chain
- Termination
  - Combination: two growing chains react to form one polymer molecule
  - Disproportionation: two polymer molecules result from transfer of a hydrogen atom

Physical Properties

Molecular Weight
- A unique feature of polymers is that they consist of many individual chains or molecules, many having different lengths or number of repeat units.
- Because of this distribution of molecular weights, polymers are typically characterized by their average molecular weight (Mw).
- Linear polymers used as biomaterials generally have Mw ranging from 50,000 to 300,000 g/mol.
- A notable exception to this is UHMWPE, which is used as a bearing surface in total joint prostheses.
- The Mw of UHMWPE can exceed 1 million.

Chain Structure
- Polymers can be broadly classified as:
  - Homopolymers: only one type of monomer repeat unit
  - Copolymers: two or more types of repeat units
- In addition to the structure of individual polymer chains, the molecular architecture of these chains in a polymeric material is important.
  - Polymer chains can be linear, branched, or crosslinked (Fig. 17-1).
  - UHMWPE can be cross-linked by gamma irradiation, which significantly improves its wear resistance

when used in articulating bearing surfaces of total joint replacements.

Tacticity
- Polymer molecules are composed of a backbone, usually made of carbon atoms, with various repeating side groups or pendant chains. The conformational arrangement of these side groups about the backbone is known as *tacticity*.
- Isotactic polymers have all of their side groups on one side of the chain backbone, and syndiotactic polymers have side groups that alternate.
- These conformations may crystallize, but atactic forms, which have a random arrangement of side groups, do not and hence remain amorphous.

Crystallinity
- Polymers can either be amorphous, having no long-range order, or semicrystalline.

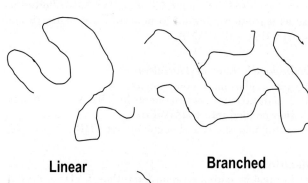

Linear   **Branched**

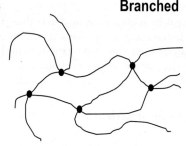

Crosslinked

Figure 17-1   Polymer chain arrangements.

- Even in highly crystalline polymers, lattice defects create small amorphous regions, making complete crystallinity virtually impossible.
- The ability of a polymer to form highly ordered crystalline domains is a function of its chemical structure (i.e., the presence and size of side groups) and chain regularity.
- In general, crystalline domains or crystallites enhance mechanical properties, thermal behavior, and fatigue strength.

Mechanical Properties

- The mechanical properties of polymers are often crucial for various orthopaedic applications and can be characterized in a number of ways:
  - Maximum stress before failure
  - Elongation to failure, modulus (E)
  - Fatigue failure stress (under cyclic loading)
  - Susceptibility to wear (abrasion, adhesion, fatigue types)
  - Creep (progressive deformation under constant load)
- These properties are described in general in Chapter 16, Biomechanics.

Thermal Properties

- Polymeric biomaterials can be described as thermoplastic, meaning that temperature can have a significant effect on their physical properties.
- All polymers exhibit a glass transition temperature (Tg), and crystalline polymers also exhibit a melting temperature (Tm).

Glass Transition Temperature (Tg)
- Temperature at which there is enough thermal energy for long-range segmental chain motions to occur
- Below Tg, amorphous polymers are hard and glassy.
- Above Tg, amorphous polymers become soft and rubbery.
- At Tg, the modulus of an amorphous polymer drops by roughly three orders of magnitude.

Melting Temperature (Tm)
- Tm is the temperature at which crystallites in the material melt and lose their ordered structure.
- Above Tm, semicrystalline polymers return to the amorphous state.
- Tm > Tg

Orthopaedic Applications of Polymers

- Polymeric bearing surfaces of the past (abandoned due to poor performance)
  - PMMA
  - Poly(tetrafluoroethylene) (PTFE)
- Current polymeric bearing surfaces

- UHMWPE
  - Introduced as bearing surface in the early 1960s
  - Highly crystalline polymer
  - Higher molecular weight, impact strength, toughness and improved wear characteristics versus the high-density and low-density forms of poly(ethylene).
  - Currently the material of choice for articulating surfaces
    - Acetabular cup of hip replacements
    - Tibial insert of knee replacements

Issues Related to UHMWPE

- Wear debris
  - Production of billions of sub-micron-sized wear particles per year
  - Causes chronic inflammation, osteolysis, implant loosening
- Methods to improve wear resistance
  - Treatment with gamma irradiation
    - Causes chain scission (breaking of bonds in polymer backbone)
    - Allows for cross-linking and increased toughness
  - Gamma irradiation in oxygen-free environment
    - Reduces post-irradiation oxidation
    - Prevents subsurface oxidation damage to polymer
- Creep
  - Deformation when subjected to a constant applied load over time
  - Contributes to loss of congruence, increased stress concentration and wear

Bone Cement

PMMA is another polymer that has enjoyed widespread use in orthopaedic medicine since the late 1960s as a fixation material for total joint prostheses. It serves as a grout, or space-filling material, at the implant site and helps to transfer mechanical loads from the metallic prosthesis to the surrounding bone. Acrylic bone cements are unique with respect to many other polymeric biomaterials because they are polymerized *in situ*, or inside the body.

Commercial bone cements are supplied as two-component, powder–liquid systems consisting of PMMA powder with the initiator benzoyl peroxide, and liquid methyl methacrylate (MMA) monomer with the activator N,N-dimethyl-p-toluidine. The powder and liquid are mixed together in the operating room to initiate polymerization of the MMA monomer via a free radical reaction. As the polymerization reaction proceeds, the viscosity of the cement increases, and the material is delivered to the site of implantation in a doughy or viscous state. The prosthesis is then inserted and properly positioned, the cement is pressurized, and finally the cement cures or sets completely.

Although alternate materials have been investigated, PMMA-based cements remain the primary choice for fixation of total joint prostheses.

Drawbacks

- Exothermic polymerization reaction
    - Releases 130 cal/g of MMA monomer
    - Temperature rise during *in situ* polymerization has potential to cause thermal necrosis of surrounding bone at implant site.
    - Thermal damage usually limited due to:
        - Relatively thin cement mantle (2 to 3 mm)
        - Heat transfer through the metallic implant stem
- Porosity within cement mantle
    - Pores act as stress concentrators.
    - Pores provide initiation sites for cracks.
        - Can lead to fracture of the cement
        - May cause loosening of the implant and need for revision
- Porosity can be reduced by improved mixing and delivery techniques (e.g., vacuum mixing)

Resorbable Polymers

Resorbable or biodegradable polymers are desirable for clinical applications where a device is required for only a short period. Examples include applications in wound closure, fracture fixation, and drug delivery. The polymers poly(lactic acid) and poly(glycolic acid), along with their copolymers, have been used clinically as suture materials since the 1970s and have been extensively studied for a variety of other applications due to their successful clinical history and approval by the U.S. Food and Drug Administration. However, orthopaedic applications of biodegradable polymers have remained limited due to lingering concerns over their mechanical performance and tissue reactions during degradation.

Clinical Applications

- Primary fixation (sutures, pins, screws, anchors, intramedullary rods)
- Drug delivery

Primary Biodegradable Polymers

- Poly(lactic acid) (PLA)
- Poly(glycolic acid) (PGA)
- Poly(lactic-co-glycolic acid) (PLGA) copolymers
- Poly(caprolactone) (PCL)
- Poly(dioxanone) (PDS)

Concerns for Biodegradable Applications

- Degradation rate (mass loss vs. time)
- Change in strength over degradation time
- Biocompatibility of degradation products (associated in some cases with sterile discharge or inflammatory changes)

CERAMICS

Although the use of ceramic materials in modern orthopaedic surgery began well after the introduction of metals and alloys, recent advances in ceramic engineering have allowed the development of many new ceramic materials and composites with improved mechanical properties and a variety of bone integration capabilities.

Ceramics are particularly attractive as implant materials because of their general chemical and temporal stability and adjustable surface and bulk properties, and because bone mineral itself (two thirds of the mass of bone tissue) is in fact a ceramic.

The purpose of this section is to outline the main features, composition, and applications of ceramic materials in clinical use or under research and development.

General Characteristics of Ceramic Materials

- Composition
    - Polycrystalline, metal oxides, silicates, phosphates, sulfides, carbons, etc.
    - Most are ionically bonded; carbons are covalently bonded.
- Physical
    - Refractory (stable to high temperature)
    - Resistant to oxidation
    - Low electrical and thermal conductivity
- Mechanical
    - Brittle, hard, low tensile strength, high compressive strength, non-ductile, undergo little or no distortion (creep) with continuous loading
    - Susceptible to micro-crack and notch formation leading to brittle failure on repetitive loading
    - Compressive strength inversely proportional to porosity
- Biological
    - Most are relatively inert, noninflammatory; some are resorbable or bioactive.

Bioceramics Used in Orthopaedics (Tables 17-7 and 17-8)

- Most commonly used:
    - Dense alumina for femoral heads (Fig. 17-2)
    - Porous calcium phosphates for grafts, defect fillers, implant coatings, bone cements (grouts), and scaffolds (Fig. 17-3)
- Advantages
    - Excellent bone ingrowth (porous) and ongrowth (coatings) ("osteoconduction")
    - Excellent attachment to bone surfaces without fibrous layer ("osseointegration")
    - Can be made bioactive or incorporate growth factors, antibiotics, etc.
    - Generally nontoxic, nonallergenic, relatively noninflammatory, noncarcinogenic
    - Can be formulated to be partially or totally resorbed over time
- Disadvantages
    - Brittle, unless reinforced by substrate or additive
    - Porous types are mechanically weak
    - Manufacture is generally demanding

Functional Types and Definitions

Resorbable (Absorbable) Ceramics

- Ceramics that dissolve or are electrolytically degraded extracellularly (with or without phagocytosis)

TABLE 17-7 PROPERTIES OF BIOCERAMIC MATERIALS APPLICABLE TO ORTHOPAEDICS

Group	Subtype	Chemical Base	Functional Type	E (Gpa^a)	σ_{max} (Mpa^a)	Comments
Metal oxides	Alumina	Al_2O_3	Dense, bioinert	380	580	Most common dense ceramic; low wear
	Zirconia (part. stabilized)	ZrO_2 (+ Y_2O_3)	Dense, bioinert	200	1000	Low wear and friction
Calcium phosphates	β-tricalcium phosphate (β-TCP)	β-$Ca_3(PO_4)_2$	Porous, resorbable	4–120	20–500	*Porosity 95% –5%: β-whitlockite
	Hydroxyapatite (HA) (synthetic, polycrystalline)	$Ca_{10}(PO_4)_6(OH)_2$	Variable porosity, bioactive, osteoconductive	4–120*	20–500*	*Porosity 95% –5%; many uses; properties vary greatly with porosity and preparation method
	Metal oxide calcium phosphates	ZnO_2, Fe_2O_3 or Al_2O_3 + CaO + P_2O_5	Porous, resorbable			Experimental, bone filler and/or drug delivery systems
Corals	Biocoral Porities Goniopora	$CaCO_3$	Porous, resorbable 190- to 230-μm pores 130- to 600-μm pores	~8	~30	50% porous, anisotropic; low strength
	Converted coral (replamineform, coralline HA)	HA	Porous, controlled resorbable			Low strength; slower resorption than $CaCO_3$
Carbons	Pyrolytic carbon	C (graphite-like structure)	Dense, bioinert	28	~520	Used as composite or coating
Glass ceramics	Polycrystalline silicon oxide–based glass (Bioglass)	SiO_2 – CaO - Na_2O_3-P_2O_5	Dense, bioactive, nonresorbable		200	Proposed as fillers, coatings; very small grain size
	Polycrystalline silicon oxide–based glass (Ceravital)	SiO_2 – CaO - Na_2O_3-P_2O_5 – MgO – K_2O	Dense, bioactive, nonresorbable	100–200		Proposed as fillers, coatings; very small grain size
Other Ca systems	Plaster of Paris	$(CaSO_4)_2$ * H_2O	Dense, rapidly resorbable		30	Little foreign body reaction; resorbs rapidly; low strength
Allograft bone (adult)	Cortical	Natural HA/collagen composite	Semiporous, osteoconductive, slowly resorbable	18	200	Anisotropic; tensile strength <150 Mpa
	Trabecular	Natural HA/collagen composite	Macroporous, osteoconductive	0.06–0.09	6–10	Varies greatly with location, age

^{a}Typical values.
E, modulus of elasticity (in compression unless otherwise noted); σ_{max}, the maximum or failure stress ("strength") in compression.

TABLE 17-8 ORTHOPAEDIC APPLICATIONS OF BIOCERAMICS

Uses	Material	Form	Examples	Comments
Articulations in joint replacement prostheses	Al_2O_3 (Alumina)	Dense, polished; femoral head and acetabular socket liners	Trident (Stryker), Ceramic-on-ceramic (Wright Medical)	Recently FDA cleared for total hip systems
	ZrO_2 ($+Y_2O_3$) (Zirconia)	Dense, polished; femoral head and acetabular socket liners	Oxinium (Smith and Nephew)	Recently FDA cleared for total hip systems
Bone void fillers, grafts, and composites; osteoconductive	Coralline (HA)	Macroporous blocks or granules	Pro Osteon, Pro-Osteon-R (Interpore)	Very slowly resorbed; FDA approved
	Coralline (HA + $CaCO_3$)	Macroporous blocks or granules	Endobon (Merck), Bio-Oss (Osteohealth)	Approved for craniofacial use; Bio-Oss contains bovine collagen
	HA derived from trabecular bovine bone			
	$(CaSO_4)_2 * H_2O$	Plaster of Paris, resorbable	Osteoset (Wright Medical)	For low-stress locations only; FDA cleared
	HA + β-TCP + collagen mix	Granules	Collagraft, NueColl (Zimmer)	Approved for mix with autogenous marrow and defects <30 cm³
	β-TCP	Macroporous, resorbable blocks or granules	Vitoss (Orthovita)	Completely resorbable; for low-loading sites; FDA cleared
	CO_3-β-TCP + bovine collagen	Macroporous, resorbable granules or cement	Healos (Orquest)	Investigational
	Bone allograft	Solid or granulized		Not considered a medical device by FDA
Cements, grouts, fracture fixation supplementation	Various calcium phosphates	Injectable slurry, self-curing, osteoconductive	SRS (Norian); a-BSM (ETEX Corp); BoneSource (Stryker)	Use for hardware enhancement and defects
	Polycrystalline silicon oxide–based glass ceramic	Injectable slurry, self-curing, osteoconductive	Bioglass (USBiomaterials), Cortoss (Orthovita)	Cortoss not yet approved in United States; several analogs approved only for craniofacial use
Implant coatings	Hydroxyapatite: Plasma spray and other coating processes	Coating on titanium or Co-Cr prostheses	In current use by several manufacturers of implants	Marketed
	Polycrystalline silicon oxide–based glass ceramic	Coated on titanium		Investigational
Scaffolds for cells or drug delivery	Various calcium phosphate/HA group materials with bioactive or osteoinductive agents	Micro- and macroporous solids and granules	HA or β-TCP + BMP; HA coatings + BMP; HA + $AgSO_4$	Investigational

FDA, U.S. Food and Drug Administration

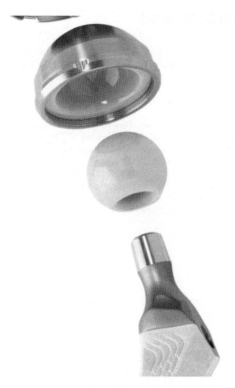

Figure 17-2 A portion of a contemporary ceramic-on-ceramic total hip replacement prosthesis. The ball and socket are made of dense polycrystalline alumina. The socket is encased in a metallic cup, which is placed into the acetabular portion of the implant. (Courtesy of Steven Brown, Stryker Orthopedics, Inc.)

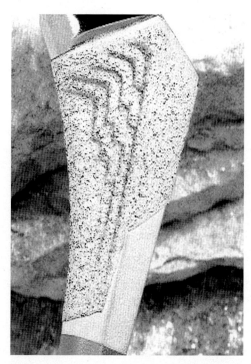

Figure 17-3 A portion of the femoral stem of a metallic hip implant with a macroporous hydroxyapatite coating designed to encourage fixation of the proximal portion of the stem. (Courtesy of Steven Brown, Stryker Orthopedics, Inc.)

- Smaller insoluble particles liberated by disintegration (e.g., β-tricalcium phosphate)
- Resorption rate must allow ingrowth and replacement by bone.
  - A very rapid resorption rate does not allow time for bone ingrowth.
  - Time frame: days to years, depending on composition, fabrication, and location
  - Rate of resorption is proportional to porosity.

Bioactive Ceramics
- Ceramics created to stimulate osteogenesis, active osteoconduction, bone remodeling, bacteriostasis, etc.
- Osteogenesis and bone remodeling: achieved by addition of bone morphogenic proteins, growth factors, or bone marrow
- Active osteoconduction: achieved when there is immediate physical contact and chemical bonding with bone
  - Bioactive glass ceramics foster this by surface dissolution and the formation of a PO_4- and Ca^{2+}- rich layer upon exposure to the physiological environment.
- Composites make use of the macroporosity of the ceramics as scaffolds for drug delivery.
  - Bacteriostasis: achieved by addition of antibiotics
  - Carriers (e.g., synthetic polymers, collagen): allow for retention and controlled release of chemotherapeutic agents

Bioinert Ceramics
- Maintain their chemical and physical properties with time
- Demonstrate fewest inflammatory or other tissue reactions
- Passive osteoconduction: exhibited if the material fosters immediate physical bone contact without chemical bonding
- Scant or nonexistent fibrous intermediate layer (at the light microscope level)
- Interdigitation with bone in pores may provide strong physical bonding.
- Bioinert hydroxyapatite ceramics (HA) undergo a small amount of surface dissolution and can lose about 15 μm during the first few months after implantation. HA coatings may disappear entirely.

Porous Ceramics
- Interconnected pores of 50 μm in diameter or more allow bone and capillary ingrowth.
  - Pores of 100 to 400 μm give best bone ingrowth.
  - Larger pore structures are called macroporous (>1 mm).
  - High specific surface area increases chemical interaction and resorption rate.
- Coralline ceramics are made from natural coral structures with large interconnected pores.
- Mechanical strength is poor and inversely proportional to pore size and the "area fraction" of pores.
  - Chemical modification of surfaces or combining with polymers improves performance.

■ Sintering (heating) improves strength and decreases resorption rate.

Dense Ceramics

■ Intergranular pores only of the order of a few microns or less
■ Volume can be almost 100% dense (3 to 4 gm/cm^2).
■ Usually nonresorbable
■ Can be highly polished for making bearing surfaces
   ■ Low friction and very low particulate release
■ Bioactive and inert ceramics have generally been classified as medical devices by the U.S. Food and Drug Administration.

SUGGESTED READING

Bauer TW, Smith ST. Bioactive materials in orthopaedic surgery: Overview and regulatory considerations. *Clin Orthop Rel Res* 2002;395:11–22.

Buckwalter JA, Einhorn TA, Simon SR, eds. *Orthopaedic Basic Science*, 2nd ed. American Academy of Orthopedic Surgeons, 2000.

Ducheyne P, Lemons JE, eds. Bioceramics: Material characteristics versus in vivo behavior. *Ann NY Acad Sci* 1988;523:1–297.

Park JB, Bronzino JD. *Biomaterials; Principles and Applications.* Boca Raton, FL: CRC Press, 2003.

Rattner BD, Hoffman AS, Schoen FJ, et al., eds. *Biomaterials Science*, 2nd ed. San Diego Academic Press, 1996.

Sperling LH. *Introduction to Physical Polymer Science*, 4th ed. New York: John Wiley & Sons, 2001.

PRINCIPLES OF ORTHOPAEDIC PHARMACOLOGY

CAROL D. MORRIS

Numerous orthopaedic conditions are amenable to pharmacologic intervention. This chapter will summarize the basic science principles behind the most commonly used drugs in orthopaedic practice.

ANTIBACTERIALS

Detailed knowledge of the most likely organism(s) causing a specific infection matched with the spectrum of the antibacterial is essential to maximize the therapeutic effect while minimizing resistance. Therefore, in general, antibacterials are most effective when they are directed against a single pathogen for a short period of time and potentially harmful when directed against multiple pathogens for a long period of time.

Classification by Mechanism of Drug Action

- Inhibition of cell wall synthesis: penicillins, cephalosporins, imipenem, vancomycin
  - Penicillins (amoxicillin, piperacillin) are inactivated by β-lactamase and are thus ineffective against *Staphylococcus aureus*.
  - Semisynthetic penicillins (nafcillin, oxacillin, dicloxacillin) are active against β-lactamase–producing *S. aureus*.
  - Cephalosporins: cephalothin, cephalexin, cefazolin, cephamandole, ceftriaxone

- Semisynthetic penicillins and cephalosporins are more effective than vancomycin against infections caused by methicillin-sensitive strains of *S. aureus*.
- Inhibition of protein synthesis: doxycycline, azithromycin, erythromycin, clindamycin, gentamicin
  - Clindamycin is active against anaerobes and most gram-positive cocci except enterococci, but it selects for *Clostridium difficile*.
  - Aminoglycosides are used against gram-negative bacilli; they are associated with renal and auditory toxicity.
- Interference with DNA metabolism: quinolones, metronidazole
  - Quinolones are primarily active against gram-negative bacteria.
  - Metronidazole is effective against all anaerobes and many parasites by exploiting their inability to metabolize oxygen free radicals.
- Antimetabolites: trimethoprim, sulfonamides
  - Mimic essential nutrients to block replication
  - Combination of trimethoprim and the sulfonamide sulfamethoxazole blocks folic acid synthesis with a wide spectrum of activity.

Clinical Applications

- Surgical prophylaxis
  - In general, antibacterial prophylaxis is indicated in

procedures with a high inherent infection rate or when the prevalence of infection is low but such an infection would have catastrophic results.

- For most elective orthopaedic procedures, the potentially offending pathogens are actually relatively limited: *S. aureus*, *Staphylococcus epidermidis*, aerobic streptococci, and anaerobes.
- For maximum benefit, the antimicrobial should be administered within 1 hour preceding the incision.
- Open fractures
  - Antimicrobials should be given as soon as possible.
  - Risk of infection in open fractures depends on the severity of soft tissue injury.
  - *S. aureus* and gram-negative bacilli are the most common pathogens causing infections after open fractures.
  - Certain environmental exposures require specific coverage:
    - Farm-related exposures: penicillin for *Clostridium perfringens*
    - Soil: clindamycin or metronidazole for anaerobic microorganisms
    - Fresh water: third-generation cephalosporin or quinolone for *Pseudomonas* species
- Osteomyelitis
  - β-lactam agents, aminoglycosides, and doxycycline are able to achieve serum-level concentrations in acutely infected bone.
  - Clindamycin is able to treat organisms such as *S. aureus* that have the ability to evade antimicrobials following macrophage ingestion.

ANTICOAGULANTS

Approximately 2 million deep venous thromboses (DVT) are diagnosed each year in the United States; of these, 200,000 to 600,000 (10% to 30%) propagate to pulmonary emboli (PE). Many pharmacologic agents used for DVT prophylaxis and treatment intervene at steps along the clotting cascade with the goal of preventing fibrin formation, the end product of the cascade (Fig. 18-1).

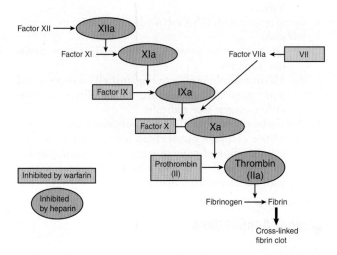

Figure 18-1   The coagulation cascade.

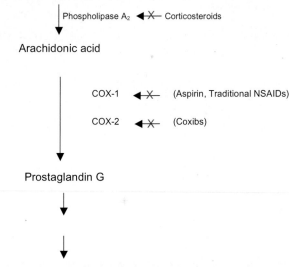

Figure 18-2   Effectors of inflammation on the arachidonic acid metabolic pathway.

- Aspirin
  - Irreversibly binds cyclooxygenase (COX-1 and COX-2), thereby blocking arachidonic acid from forming prostaglandins (Fig. 18-2)
  - In platelets, aspirin suppresses thromboxane A_2 production; thromboxane A_2 triggers platelet aggregation via phospholipase C.
  - Clinically, aspirin has little if any role in prophylaxis of venous thromboembolism.
- Warfarin
  - Warfarin is a vitamin K antagonist of vitamin K oxidoreductase (VKOR), the enzyme responsible for the activation of vitamin K.
  - Coagulation factors II, VII, IX, and X require vitamin K for activation.
  - In the absence of active vitamin K, inactive clotting factors accumulate, leading ultimately to decreased fibrin formation.
  - The anticoagulant effect is measured by the prothrombin time (PT) and the international normalized ratio (INR) target of 2 to 3.
- Heparin
  - Heparin binds antithrombin (AT), exposing AT's active site and increasing the affinity of AT for active clotting factors.
  - Clinically, heparin has unpredictable pharmacokinetics.
  - Heparin-induced thrombocytopenia (HIT) is a condition in which patients become thrombocytopenic and prothrombotic simultaneously.
  - Fixed low-dose subcutaneous heparin (i.e., 5,000 U) has limited efficacy for venous thromboembolism.

- Effects of heparin can be reversed with intravenous protamine.
- Low-molecular-weight heparins (LMWHs)
  - Exert effect by the same mechanism that heparin does
  - Pharmacokinetic profile is very predictable and therefore monitoring is largely unnecessary except in renal insufficiency and weight extremes.
  - Appears to be as efficacious as warfarin in orthopaedic patients
  - Dalteparin, enoxaparin, tinzaparin, and nadroparin are approved by the U.S. Food and Drug Administration (FDA).
  - No antidote exists, but protamine can neutralize up to 60% of effect.
- Factor Xa inhibitor (Fondaparinux)
  - Chemically unrelated to heparin and LMWH, but has similar mechanism
  - No known antidote

ANTI-INFLAMMATORY AGENTS

Most musculoskeletal conditions are characterized by some inflammatory component. Pharmacological agents to manage the symptoms of inflammatory conditions are the most frequently prescribed medicines in the United States.

Nonsteroidal Anti-inflammatory Drugs (NSAIDs; Table 18-1)

Prostaglandins and thromboxanes are examples of prostanoids, effector molecules that regulate pain and inflammation. These prostanoids are produced by the metabolism of arachidonic acid by the enzyme cyclooxygenase (COX (Fig. 18-2)). Two isoforms of the enzyme have been described: COX-1, a constitutively expressed regulator of many physiologic functions, and COX-2, an inducible form activated during pro-inflammatory conditions.

- Traditional NSAIDs
  - Possess great variability in their potency and duration of action secondary to varying COX-1 or -2 specificity
  - Clinically, the efficacy of NSAIDs for numerous acute and chronic conditions is well established.
  - Gastrointestinal side effects, namely gastroduodenal ulcers, remain a significant problem.
- COX-2 inhibitors (coxibs)
  - Have the potential advantage of preferentially suppressing COX-2, which is upregulated during inflammation, without disturbing the normal homeostatic functions of COX-1
  - Efficacy of coxibs is comparable to that of traditional NSAIDs.
  - Gastrointestinal effects are lower with coxibs use compared to traditional NSAIDs.
  - Unlike traditional NSAIDs, COX-2 inhibitors do not have a significant effect on the endogenous production of thromboxane A_2, potentially triggering a sig-

TABLE 18-1 COMMONLY USED NONSTEROIDAL ANTI-INFLAMMATORY DRUGS

	Generic Name	Trade Name
Salicylates		
	Aspirin	—
	Diflunisal	Dolobid
	Salsalate	Disalcid
Traditional NSAIDs		
Arylalkanoic acids	Diclofenac	Voltaren
	Indomethacin	Indocin
	Sulindac	Clinoril
2-Arylpropionic acids (profens)		
	Flurbiprofen	Ansaid
	Ibuprofen	Motrin
	Ketoprofen	Orudis
	Ketorolac	Toradol
	Naproxen	Naprosyn
	Oxaprozin	Daypro
N-Arylanthranilic acids (fenamic acids)	Meclofenamate	Meclomen
Oxicams	Piroxicam	Feldene
	Meloxicam	Mobic
Acetic acids	Etodolac	Lodine
	Tolmetin	Tolectin
COX-2 inhibitors (coxibs)	Celecoxib	Celebrex

nificant increase in the risk for thrombotic cardiovascular events. These findings led to the withdrawal of valdecoxib and rofecoxib from the U.S. market and issuance of a "black box" warning for celecoxib.

- Salicylates
  - The mechanism of action of salicylates is summarized by the description of aspirin in the section on anticoagulation.

CORTICOSTEROIDS

Corticosteroids are naturally occurring 21-carbon steroid hormones produced by the adrenal glands. They encompass both glucocorticoids (regulators of inflammation and metabolism) and mineralocorticoids (mediators of electrolytes).

- Corticosteroids influence all types of inflammatory events by a complex signaling pathway that has been fairly well elucidated:
  - The mediating receptor belongs to the family of cytosolic steroid–hormone receptors. Once bound, the steroid–receptor complex migrates to the nucleus,

TABLE 18-2 COMMONLY USED INJECTABLE CORTICOSTEROIDS

Solubility	Generic Name	Example Trade Name
Most soluble	Betamethasone sodium phosphate	Celestone
Soluble	Dexamethasone sodium phosphate	Decadron
	Prednisolone sodium phosphate	Hydeltrasol
Slightly soluble	Prednisolone tebutate	Hydeltra-T.B.A.
	Triamcinolone diacetate	Aristospan Forte
	Methylprednisolone acetate	Depo-Medrol
Relatively insoluble	Dexamethasone acetate	Decadron-LA
	Hydrocortisone acetate	Hydrocortisone
	Hydrocortisone	
	Prednisolone acetate	Predalone
	Triamcinolone acetonide	Kenalog
	Triamcinolone hexacetonide	Aristospan
Combination	Betamethasone sodium phosphate-betamethasone acetate	Celestone Soluspan

where it binds the promotor region of target genes called glucocorticoid-responsive elements (GRE).

- Active GREs solicit other proteins to structurally modify the chromatin, thereby leading to altered transcription of target genes. An example is the gene that codes for annexin I (also called lipocortin-1).
  - Annexin I is an anti-inflammatory protein that binds to cell membranes and physically interacts with phospholipase A_2, blocking its action on arachidonic acid and the subsequent production of inflammatory mediating prostaglandins (see Fig. 18-2).
- Commonly used synthetic corticosteroids are listed in Table 18-2. Firm guidelines regarding choice and dose for intra-articular, intrabursal, and intra-tendon sheath injection are lacking.
  - Most conditions are treated with a combination of short-acting (water-soluble) and long-acting (water-insoluble) preparations.
  - A minimum of 4 weeks between intra-articular injections is usually recommended.
  - Associated adverse effects include corticosteroid arthropathy, ligament and tendon ruptures, infection, adrenal suppression, skin atrophy, and hyperpigmentation.

INHIBITORS OF BONE RESORPTION

Metabolic bone diseases are disorders of abnormal skeletal homeostasis that lead to impairment of normal bone formation, mineralization, and remodeling. Examples of such conditions include osteoporosis, Paget's disease, rickets, and osteomalacia. A number of antiresorptive agents are available to treat the orthopaedic manifestations of these diseases.

- Bisphosphonates

- Synthetic analogs of inorganic pyrophosphate in which the P-O-P bond has been replaced with a non-hydrolyzable P-C-P bond.
- Bone is preferentially targeted because the diphosphate configuration provides a three-dimensional structure for binding divalent ions such as Ca^{2+}.
- The drug binds the mineral phase of bone exposed during bone resorption and is ingested by the endocytic activity of the osteoclast.
- The mechanism of action by which the bisphosphonate inactivates the osteoclast is divided into two pharmacologic groups: nitrogen-containing and non–nitrogen-containing.
  - Non–nitrogen-containing bisphosphonates: metabolized to nonhydrolyzable analogs of ATP; osteoclastic intracellular accumulation of these cytotoxic ATP analogs is thought to induce apoptosis.
  - Nitrogen-containing bisphosphonates: exert their effectiveness via the mevalonate pathway, which is responsible for the production of the cholesterol precursors farnesyl diphosphate and geranylgeranyl diphosphate (GGPP). Farnesyl diphosphate and GGPP are necessary for the production of proteins that are synthesized by a process called protein prenylation. One such protein, guanosine triphosphatase, plays a regulatory role in osteoclast morphology, including membrane ruffling and protein trafficking.
- FDA-approved bisphosphonates: etidronate, tiludronate, alendronate, pamidronate, risedronate, ibandronate, and zoledronic acid (Table 18-3)
- Calcitonin
  - Single-chain 32-amino-acid polypeptide hormone synthesized by the parafollicular cells of the thyroid gland.
  - Inhibits bone resorption by inducing changes in the osteoclasts' cytoskeleton by disrupting actin rings,

TABLE 18-3 FDA-APPROVED BISPHOSPHONATES

Generic Name	Proprietary Name	Route of Administration	R1	R2
Non–nitrogen-containing				
Etidronate	Didronel	Oral	—OH	—CH$_3$
Tiludronate	Skelid	Oral	—H	—S—⟨benzene ring⟩—C1
Nitrogen-containing				
Alendronate	Fosamax	Oral	—OH	—(CH$_2$)$_3$—NH$_2$
Pamidronate	Aredia	Intravenous	—OH	—(CH$_2$)$_2$—NH$_2$
Risedronate	Actonel, Opinate	Oral	—OH	—CH$_2$—⟨pyridine ring with N⟩
Ibandronate	Bondronat	Intravenous	—OH	—(CH$_2$)$_2$—N(CH$_3$)—(CH$_2$)$_4$CH$_3$
	Boniva	Oral		
Zoledronic acid	Zometa	Intravenous	—OH	—CH$_2$—⟨imidazole ring with N, N⟩

the structures responsible for the formation of bone resorption pits, or Howship's lacunae.

■ Salmon calcitonin (calcitonin extracted from salmon) is more potent than human calcitonin, though the two forms differ by just one amino acid.

■ Immunogenicity can develop with long-term salmon calcitonin use.

■ Both injectable and intranasal preparations are FDA approved for the treatment of symptoms associated with Paget's disease and osteoporosis.

■ Parathyroid hormone (PTH)

　■ Affects both osteoblastic bone formation and osteoclastic bone resorption in a coupled fashion

　■ Duration and dosing control the net metabolic effect: daily PTH injections increase bone mass, but continuous infusions lead to bone resorption.

　■ Biological activity of PTH is found within amino acids 1 to 34 at the N-terminal and is mediated by second messenger cAMP following binding to G protein–coupled receptors on osteoblasts.

　■ Bound PTH stimulates osteoblasts to produce RANKL and IL-6, both of which lead to osteoclast proliferation and maturation.

　■ Clinically indicated for patients with osteoporosis that has failed to respond to other therapies.

　■ Contraindicated in patients at increased risk for osteogenic sarcoma (e.g., skeletally immature, Paget's disease, previous irradiation).

STIMULATORS OF BONE REPAIR

Bone is unique in its ability to repair itself with actual skeletal tissue as opposed to scar tissue. This repair process very closely imitates embryonic bone development. Interest in the enhancement of fracture repair has lead to an increased understanding of the various growth factors involved in bone regeneration, most notably the bone morphogenetic proteins (BMPs).

■ BMPs

　■ Growth factors capable of inducing undifferentiated mesenchymal cells into osteoblasts leading to new bone formation.

　■ 16 isoforms have been sequenced: BMP-1 to BMP-16.

　■ All BMPs (with the exception of BMP-1) belong to the transforming growth factor-β (TGF-β) superfamily; the TGF-β family of proteins is intricately involved in the regulation of cellular growth and differentiation.

　■ BMPs act by binding serine/threonine kinase receptors, leading to activation of the SMAD transcription factor that in turn activates or suppresses a target gene.

　■ Currently two recombinant BMPs are FDA approved: rh-BMP-7 (also called OP1) and rh-BMP-2.

CHONDROPROTECTIVE SUPPLEMENTS

To remain healthy, all cartilage needs proteoglycans to attract and maintain water molecules. Proteoglycans are composed of glycosaminoglycans (keratan sulfate, dermatan sulfate, chondroitin sulfate) bound to a central core protein. In degenerative joint conditions, the relative proteoglycan production by chondrocytes is decreased. Theoretically, replacing proteoglycans might retard the degenerative process, and to that end a number of molecules have been investigated for this purpose. The published results from clinical trials have failed to show convincing efficacy, possibly due to limited bioavailability of the active moieties.

■ Glucosamine
- ▣ Glucosamine ($C_6H_{14}NO_5$) is a naturally occurring amino sugar derived from chitin (extracted from shells of crabs, lobsters, and shrimp).
- ▣ Glucosamine serves as a precursor for glycoproteins, including glycosaminoglycans. Specifically, it composes half of the disaccharide units found in keratan sulfate and hyaluronic acid.
- ▣ In an animal model, exogenous glucosamine has been shown to rebuild cartilage by enhancing cartilage proteoglycan synthesis.
- ▣ An anti-inflammatory contribution has also been described.
- ▣ Not FDA approved for the treatment of osteoarthritis, but rather is labeled as a dietary supplement
- ▣ Clinically, glucosamine seems to improve pain and function scores in patients with osteoarthritis, though the data are quite variable. Its role as a disease-modifying agent has yet to be substantiated.

■ Chondroitin sulfate
- ▣ Chondroitin sulfate is the major component of aggrecan, the large aggregating type of proteoglycan.
- ▣ Derived from shark or beef cartilage or bovine trachea
- ▣ Often supplied in combination with glucosamine
- ▣ Addition of chondroitin sulfate to cultured human chondrocytes demonstrates increased proteoglycan production and decreased collagen breakdown.
- ▣ Mechanism of action remains controversial, as the bioavailability of oral chondroitin sulfate has not been adequately demonstrated.
- ▣ Clinically, most studies support its efficacy in relieving the symptoms associated with osteoarthritis.

■ Hyaluronic acid (HA)
- ▣ HA is a stabilizing polysaccharide secreted by type B synovial cells. It is composed of repeating disaccharide units of acetylglucosamine and glucuronic acid and is capable of binding many aggrecan molecules.
- ▣ Normal concentration of HA in a healthy knee is 2 to 4 mg/mL. Arthritic knees produce about half of the normal concentration of HA, with decreased molecular size.
- ▣ Exact mechanism of action of HA is unknown. Anti-inflammatory, direct analgesic, and physical alterations of synovial fluid have all been described.
- ▣ Currently two preparations are FDA approved: Hyalgan and Synvisc.
- ▣ Extracted from rooster combs

ACKNOWLEDGMENT

Thank you to David Lehmann, PharmD, MD, for reviewing and editing this chapter.

SUGGESTED READING

Cole B, Schumacher H. Injectable corticosteroids in modern practice. *J Am Acad Orthop Surg* 2005;13:37–46.

Geerts W, Pineo G, Heit J, et al. Prevention of venous thromboembolism: The Seventh ACCP Conference on Antithrombotic and Thrombolytic Therapy. *Chest* 2004;126;338S–400S.

Jordan K, Arden N, Doherty M, et al. EULAE Recommendations 2003: an evidenced-based approach to the management of knee osteoarthritis: Report of a Task Force of the Standing Committee for International Clinical Studies Including Therapeutic Trials (ESCISIT). *Ann Rheum Dis* 2003;62:1145–1155.

Lieberman J, Daluiski A, Einhorn T. The role of growth factors in the repair of bone: Biology and clinical applications. *J Bone Joint Surg [Am]* 2002;84:1032–1044.

Morris C, Einhorn T. Bisphosphonates in orthopaedic surgery. *J Bone Joint Surg [Am]* 2005;87:1609–1618.

Perry CR. *Bone and Joint Infections.* St. Louis: Mosby, 1996.

Rodan G, Martin T. Therapeutic approaches to bone diseases. *Science* 2000;289:1508–1514.

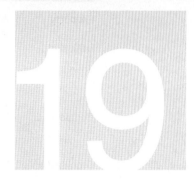

BONE FORM, FUNCTION, INJURY, REGENERATION, AND REPAIR

ALEXIA HERNANDEZ-SORIA
MATHIAS BOSTROM

Bone form consists of its cellular morphology, matrix composition, and circulation. Bone function, regeneration, and repair integrate cellular and macroscopic remodeling, biomechanics, material properties, metabolism, and age-related changes. Injury to bone can occur by way of osteonecrosis and fracture. These topics are addressed individually in this chapter.

BONE CELLULAR MORPHOLOGY

Microscopic Bone

Microscopically, bone exists in either a woven or a lamellar form (Table 19-1).

Bone Structure

Structurally, bone is categorized as trabecular or cortical bone (Table 19-2). Porosity and architectural characteristics differentiate the two types of bone. These differences

account for their respective material properties. Each structural bone type may exist as either or both types of microscopic bone, depending upon age, location, and setting (normal vs. pathologic bone).

- Trabecular bone
  - Woven
  - Lamellar
- Cortical bone
  - Compact bone: layers of lamellar bone without osteons; small animals
  - Plexiform bone: layers of lamellar and woven bone; large animals experiencing rapid growth
  - Haversian bone: vascular channels surrounded by lamellar bone (osteons); most complex type of cortical bone

Haversian Bone

- Osteon/bone structural unit (BSU): the major structural unit of cortical bone; contains a central neurovascular canal surrounded by concentric lamellae

TABLE 19-1 PROPERTIES OF MICROSCOPIC BONE

Property	Woven Bone	Lamellar Bone
Definition	Primitive; "immature" bone	Remodeled woven bone; "mature" bone
Found in	Embryo, infant, metaphyseal region, tumors, osteogenesis imperfecta, pagetic bone	Cortical bone, trabecular bone throughout the mature skeleton (most bone after the age of 4)
Composition	Dense collagen fibers, varied mineral content	Formed by intramembranous or endochondral ossification; contains collagen fibers
Organization	Randomly arranged collagen fibers	Highly ordered; stress-oriented collagen fibers
Response to stress	*Isotropic*: independent of direction of applied forces	*Anisotropic*: mechanical behavior differs according to direction of forces; bone's greatest strength is parallel to longitudinal axis

TABLE 19-2 BONE STRUCTURE

Property	Trabecular	Cortical
Description	Spongy and cancellous bone	Dense or compact bone; <30% porosity
Location	Metaphysis or epiphysis (long bone); cuboid bone (vertebrae)	Diaphysis (long bone); outer layer, "envelope," of cuboid bone (vertebrae)
Architecture	Individual trabeculae organized into 3-D lattice of rods and rods, rods and plates, or plates and plates Rods = thin trabeculae Plates = thick trabeculae Lattices orient in response to stress.	Plexiform bone: layers of lamellar and woven bone. Contains vascular channels and allows for rapid growth and accumulation of bone. Haversian bone: arrangement of osteons surrounded by lamellae
Mechanical stress	Predominantly subjected to compressive forces	Subjected to bending, torsional, and compression forces
Porosity	50% to 90% (large spaces between trabeculae)	~10% (dependent on density of voids in architecture)
Apparent density[a]	0.30 g/cm^3 (std 0.10 g/cm^3 ± 30%)	1.85 g/cm^3 (std 0.06 g/cm^3 ± 3%)

[a]Apparent density = mass of bone tissue/bulk volume of tissue (bulk volume = bone + bone marrow cavities); std = standard deviation

- Haversian canal: central canal of the osteon; contains cells, haversian vessels, and nerves
- Volkmann's canals: connect haversian canals of neighboring osteons
- Howship's lacunae: resorptive cavities within which reside osteoclasts
- Canaliculi: channels within and between osteons; allow communication and waste removal between developing cells of lamellae and haversian vessels

Haversian Vessels
- Most are structurally similar to capillaries. They contain a base membrane that functions as a selective-ion transport barrier important for Ca^{2+} and P^{2-} transport and response of bone to mechanical loads.
- The small vessels are similar to lymphatic vessels, which do not have a base membrane. These vessels contain only precipitated protein.

Bone Cells

Osteoblastic Lineage
- Three types of cells of osteoblastic lineage are each derived from pluripotential *mesenchymal* stem cells (Table 19-3).

Osteoclastic Lineage
- Osteoclasts differentiate from pluripotential *hematopoietic* stem cells (Table 19-4).
- Circulating monocytes develop into osteoclasts at resorption sites.

CELLULAR MECHANISMS OF REMODELING

Throughout life old bone is continually replaced by new bone. The process of remodeling and bone formation is regulated by cellular mechanisms of osteoblasts and osteoclasts.

Remodeling
- Remodeling is the process of resorption of immature (woven) and old bone followed by the formation of new lamellar bone.
- There are two forms of remodeling:
  - Endochondral remodeling: converts primary bone to secondary bone (cartilage to trabecular bone); believed to decrease density of trabecular bone

TABLE 19-4 PROPERTIES OF OSTEOCLASTS

Property	Description
Cell lineage	Hematopoietic lineage, same as macrophages. Similar to macrophages but have distinct differences in surface receptors. Osteoclasts have about two to five nuclei and receptors for calcitonin and vitronectin (integrin $\alpha v\beta 3$).
Morphology	Foamy, acidophilic cytoplasm. When active, are polar and have ruffled border. Generally located in groups on bone surface (forming Howship's lacuna) or in cortical bone (making haversian canals).
Function	Active osteoclasts solubilize mineral and organic bone matrix by creating an enclosed acidic environment ("clear zone") with H+ ions. When pH reaches ~3.5, bone resorbs. Mechanism of attachment to bone surface is not confirmed; evidence suggests communication with bone-lining cells.

TABLE 19-3 PROPERTIES OF OSTEOBLASTIC LINEAGE CELLS

Property	Osteoblasts	Osteocytes	Bone-Lining Cells
Morphology	Initially pluripotential mesenchymal cells. Round, polar, organelle-rich cells. High endoplasmic reticulum and golgi density reflects secretory function.	Most abundant cell in mature bone. Develop from osteoblasts embedded in lacunae; lose most cytoplasmic contents during maturation. Defining characteristic is extensive network of processes extending through canaliculi.	Flattened, elongated cells covering bone surfaces. Connect to osteocytes via gap junctions.
Function	Main function is to form bone. Two stages of bone formation: 1. Matrix formation 2. Mineralization	Main function is thought to be communication. Minimal synthetic activity when remodeling to maintain local environment. Location and morphology ideal for responding to mechanical stress and communicating with bone-lining cells.	Function is unconfirmed. Believed to be involved in bone formation and resorptive mechanisms. Act as an ion barrier between interstitial fluid and fluid in matrix, suggesting participation in mineral homeostatic mechanisms.

■ Haversian remodeling: repairs fatigue damage to skeleton, maintains bone mineral homeostasis, and thought to be necessary for maintaining viability of cells far from bone surfaces. Increases porosity of cortical bone, decreases width, and believed to decrease strength.

■ Both endochondral and haversian remodeling follow the same six-stage sequence of events: resting, activation, resorption, reversal (coupling), formation, and mineralization. The process is regulated by mechanical and systemic factors.

Stages of Remodeling

Resting

■ At any time, about 80% of human bone surface (periosteal and endosteal) is resting.

■ Bone surface is lined with an endosteal membrane and resting bone lining cells believed to be involved in bone mineral homeostatic mechanisms.

Activation

■ The exact factor of activation is unknown.

■ In response to regulators, osteoclasts are recruited and given access to a section of bone surface. It is believed that a capillary extends to the surface, delivering osteoclast precursors (monocytes).

■ Bone lining cells digest the endosteal membrane before retracting to allow the osteoclasts access to the mineralized bone (osteoclast regulation factors are summarized in Box 19-1).

Resorption

■ Resorption leads to formation of Howship's lacunae in cancellous bone and *cutting cones* (resorptive cavities or Haversian canals) in cortical bone.

■ The process lasts about 14 days. The osteoclast precursors are thought to coalesce at the bone's surface to form large multinucleated osteoclasts.

■ The osteoclasts attach to the surface, forming a "clear zone" under their ruffled border.

■ In a *concerted mechanism*, the bone surface is solubilized.

■ Concerted mechanism: Cathepsin B and acid phosphatase are released in "clear zone." Carbonic acid is reduced by carbonic anhydrase intracellularly. H^+ is released into the "clear zone" until pH reaches ~3.5 and environment is acidic enough to degrade mineralized bone.

■ Pyridinolines cannot be degraded by resorption and are released into extracellular fluid. Serum and urine levels can be measured for monitoring resorption.

Reversal/Coupling

■ A 28- to 35-day interval between resorption and formation of bone, which can be noted histologically by an absence of osteoclasts in Howship's lacunae and cutting cones

■ Surfaces are lined with mononuclear cells to prepare the surfaces for new bone formation. A glycoprotein layer (cement line), placed over the surface, is thought to

---

BOX 19-1 OSTEOCLAST REGULATION FACTORS

Receptor activator of NF-$_K$ β (RANK) / receptor activator of NF-$_K$ β -ligand (RANKL)
■ Osteoblasts produce protein RANKL.
■ RANKL is received by cell surface receptor, RANK, on precursor osteoclasts.
■ RANK + RANKL stimulates osteoclasts' development and bone resorption.

Osteoprotegerin (OPG)
■ Decoy RANKL receptor
■ OPG inhibits osteoclast development and increases bone mass.

Parathyroid hormone (PTH)
■ Stimulates number of osteoclasts found in bone
■ PTH is correlated with increased RANKL and decreased OPG expression.
■ PTH receptors are found on osteoblasts.
■ PTH stimulates osteoblast production of interleukin-6 (IL-6) and IL-6 stimulates osteoblast production of IGF-1.

Calcitonin
■ Directly inhibits bone resorption
■ Calcitonin receptors found on osteoclasts

Thyroid hormone
■ Hyperthyroidism increases bone resorption.

Vitamin A
■ Has been shown to stimulate resorption

Growth Factors
■ Resorption-stimulating growth factors:
  ■ EGF/TGFα, PDGF, IGF-1, and FGF
    ■ Osteoclasts have receptors for IGF-1.
■ TGFβ has been shown to inhibit osteoclast formation.

Cytokines
■ IL-1, IL-6, and tumor necrosis factor are known to be involved in mediating osteoclast differentiation and bone resorption.

---

facilitate attachment by new osteoblasts. The mechanisms by which this occurs are not known.

■ This time interval is considered the time when bone formation is "coupled" with resorption due to the perceived hormonal and cellular mechanisms of communication among the bone resorbing and forming cells.

Formation and Mineralization

■ The two aspects of bone formation occur in this stage: matrix synthesis followed by mineralization.

■ The new osteoblasts deposit a new layer of unmineralized bone matrix, the osteoid seam.

■ The osteoid seam will reach $\sim70\%$ mineralization in 5 to 10 days and complete mineralization in about 4 months (in cortical and trabecular bone).

■ Bone modeling-dependent bone loss: An adult BSU will mineralize 5% less bone than it resorbed.

Matrix Synthesis

- Osteoblasts secrete many types of collagenous and non-collagenous macromolecules, which are all proteins.
- The secretions include all critical structural elements for osteoid in both trabecular and cortical bone.
  - The unique architecture differentiating bone types is due to the particular organization of the secreted proteins.
- All proteins, and thus matrix organization, are regulated on a genetic level.
- Most matrix proteins undergo some form of *post-translational processing*, which allows matrix regulation without interfering with gene expression.
  - Collagen cross-linking
  - Glycosylation to produce proteoglycans and glycoproteins
  - Phosphorylation: produces osteopontin, bone sialoprotein
  - Vitamin K dependant γ-carboxylation: produces osteocalcin
- Many proteins have specific functions related to their surface receptors or adhesion and anti-adhesion properties.
- Osteoblasts secrete proteins according to matrix formation.
  - Fibronectin and osteonectin are secreted early in formation.
  - Osteocalcin (calcium binding protein) is secreted only after matrix is formed.

Mineralization

- Mineralization is the process by which bone crystals grow and proliferate within the *holes and pores* of the matrix collagen fibers.
- The bone crystals are composed of an analog of hydroxyapatite (HA). The HA in matrix leads to the rigidity of bone.
- Mineralization is regulated by the spaces and orientation of matrix collagen fibers (*pores and holes*) and by the noncollagenous matrix proteins.
- The noncollagenous proteins can function both as nucleators and inhibitors of crystal formation.
- There is a lag time of ~14 days between matrix formation and mineralization. The time is thought to be regulated by noncollagenous proteins and allows matrix to "mature;" strengthened by collagen cross-linking, resulting pyridinolines (pyridinoline, deoxypyridinoline, hydroxylysylpyridinoline, lysylpyridinoline).
  - Due to lag time, there is always an osteoid seam between the osteoblasts and newly mineralized bone.

Regulation of Remodeling

The bone remodeling sequence is intricately controlled by endocrine hormones as well as local paracrine and autocrine factors. The systemic and local factors that mediate

BOX 19-2 REGULATORS OF BONE FORMATION

Systemic factors
- Growth hormone/insulin-like growth factor
- Thyroid hormone
- Vitamin D
- Estrogens
- Glucocorticoids
- Parathyroid hormone

- Fibroblast growth factors
- Parathyroid hormone-related peptide
- Prostaglandins
- Platelet-derived growth factor (VEGF)

Local factors
- IGF-1
- Transforming growth factor beta
- Bone morphogenetic protein

Transcription factors
- Core binding factor (Cbfa1/Runx2)
- Osterix (transcription factor for osteoblast differentiation)

bone formation are listed in Box 19-2 (also see Chapter 10, Metabolic Bone Diseases).

Resorption Regulation

Regulating bone resorption necessarily focuses on mediating osteoclast proliferation and activity. The exact mechanisms of interaction remain under investigation. The roles of systemic and local factors in osteoclast regulation are summarized in Chapter 10.

BONE MATRIX COMPOSITION

Bone Composition

- Inorganic/mineral phase: 60% to 70%
- Organic matrix: 35% to 22%
- Water: 5% to 8%

Mineral Phase

- Mineral crystals are composed of an analog of calcium hydroxyapatite (HA): $Ca_{10}(PO_4)_6(OH)_2$
- Frequent impurities include Mg^{2+}, Sr^{2+}, Na^+, CO_3^{2-}, CO_3^-, HPO_3^{2-}, F^-, K^+
  - Apatite crystals are small and can contain many impurities, which can vary depending on diet, age, tissue location, and health status.
  - Impurities may alter physical characteristics of bone, such as solubility.
  - Newly formed woven bone has smaller crystals, which may result in it being more readily absorbed.

Bone Mineralization

- Two distinct phases of mineralization
  - *Initiation*: formation of the initial mineral deposits at multiple discrete sites
    - Requires the most energy
    - Local concentration of precipitatory ions increases.

- Formation and exposure of mineral nucleators
- Removal and modification of mineralization inhibitors
- Most mineral is an analog of HA.
- *Primary nucleation*: initial deposition of $Ca_3(PO_4)_2$ crystals into collagen
- *Growth*: proliferation/accumulation of mineral crystals on initial deposits
    - Rapid increase in size of crystals beginning as nuclei and forming solid particles
    - *Secondary nucleation*: greatest growth of crystals; grow in branching pattern off surface of other smaller crystals
    - *Heterogeneous apatite nucleator*: foreign material with surfaces on which crystals can grow
    - Aggregation of crystals to form mineralized bone matrix

Organic Matrix Composition

- Collagen: 90%
- Noncollagenous proteins: 5% to 8%

Organic Phase

- Mostly made up of type I collagen (~90%)
- Noncollagenous matrix proteins, minor collagen types, and lipids and macromolecules compose ~10%.

Collagen

- Low solubility
- Consists of three polypeptide chains (two α1 chains + α2 chain), ~ 4,000 amino acids
- Chains arranged in a triple helix, which is stabilized by H-bonding between hydroxyproline and other residues
- Collagen molecules aligned in parallel with other collagen molecules to form a *collagen fibril*
- Collagen fibrils bundle to form a *collagen fiber*.
- Pores: spaces between the sides of parallel molecules in a fibril
- Hole zones: gaps within fiber between ends of molecules
    - Noncollagenous proteins and mineral deposits can be found in hole zones and pores.

Collagen Synthesis
- Completed within the cell (post-translational processing completed intracellularly)
    - Triple helix procollagen is secreted.
- Postsecretory processing: Nonhelical tail of propeptide is enzymatically cleaved.
- Extracellular collagen molecules are stabilized by *cross-links* (bonding) between chains.
    - Cross-linking is unique to extracellular collagen.
    - Presence of cross-linked collagen in urine (pyridinolines) indicates bone resorption.

Osteocalcin

- Synthetic product of osteoblasts
- Represents 10% to 20% of bone noncollagenous protein

- Thought to play a role in attracting osteoclasts to resorption sites and in regulating bone and mineral maturation
- Synthesis is enhanced by 1,25-dihydroxy vitamin D and hindered by parathyroid hormone (PTH) and cortical steroids.

BONE REMODELING

Bone Growth

- Begins with embryogenesis and continues through skeletal maturity
- Intramembranous ossification
    - Flat bone growth
    - Osteoblasts develop directly from mesenchymal cells and form bone matrix.
- Endochondral ossification
    - Long bone growth
    - Cartilaginous bone develops into osteocytes/haversian bone and continues to remodel throughout life.

Skeletal Maturity

- Bone continues to remodel and adapt its material properties to the mechanical demands placed on it throughout life.
- *Wolff's Law* describes mechanisms by which bone responds to mechanical stress.

Remodeling

- Remodeling occurs on all bone surfaces: periosteal, endosteal, haversian, trabecular.
- Rate of cortical remodeling
    - Infant: up to 50%/year
    - Healthy adult: 2% to 5%/year
- Trabecular remodeling is 5 to 10 times higher than cortical remodeling throughout life.
- In "healthy" remodeling, bone formation and resorption are perfectly coupled so that there is no *net* change in bone mass.

BONE CIRCULATION

- There are three main circulatory systems in bone (Box 19-3).
- A unique characteristic of the three systems is that they are interconnected, allowing one to replace another when damaged.
    - Epiphyseal vessels are not interconnected until after skeletal maturity.

BIOMECHANICS AND MATERIAL PROPERTIES OF BONE

Bone as a tissue has material properties, whereas each specific bone has its own structural properties. As a structure,

BOX 19-3 CIRCULATORY SYSTEMS IN BONE

Nutrient blood supply
- Originates from a major artery of the systemic circulation
- Enters diaphysis through nutrient foramen
- The number of nutrient vessels varies per bone.
- Nutrient vessel enters medullary space and branches into ascending and descending arteries.
- Arterioles directly penetrate the endosteal surface and supply diaphyseal regions.

Metaphyseal complex
- Originates from periarticular complex (geniculate artery)
- Penetrates thin bone cortices to supply metaphyseal region
- Vessels anastomose with the medullary arteries and epiphyseal arteries after closure of the growth plate.

Periosteal capillaries
- Supply outer layers of cortical bone where there are muscular attachments

bone is unique in its ability to remodel and change in response to metabolic and mechanical stresses (see Chapter 16, Biomechanics).

Material Properties of Bone

- The material properties of bone vary between cortical and trabecular bone and depend additionally on microstructure and type of stress (Table 19-5).

BONE METABOLISM AND MINERAL HOMEOSTASIS

Maintaining mineral homeostasis is bone's primary function and is essential for bone's cellular life and in avoiding metabolic bone diseases. Problems arise when bone formation and resorption rates are no longer complementary, often resulting in loss of bone mass. The primary mechanism for maintaining mineral homeostasis involves an endocrine regulation of serum calcium concentration with vitamin D metabolites and PTH.

Bone Metabolism

- Bone metabolism is regulated by the interaction between bone cells and the endocrine system (see Chapter 10).

TABLE 19-5 MECHANICAL PROPERTIES OF BONE

Property	Cortical	Trabecular
Elastic behavior • Dependent on material orientation • Described by Young's modulus (stiffness, energy absorbed) and Poisson's ratio (strain)	Transversely isotropic. Greater bulging than metal when loaded uniaxially.	Due to varying architecture and density, trabecular bone is *anistroptic* in some locations and *isotropic* in others. Variable stiffness and strain. Generally less stiff than cortical bone, except in cranium, subchondral plates, and vertebral bodies.
Strength	Stronger in response to longitudinal and transverse compression loads than tension loads.	Strongest in compression. Weak in tension.
Viscoelastic behavior (variability of stress/strain relationship with time)	Typical viscoelastic behavior. Ultimate strain/ductility, increases with increases in strain rate below 0.1/sec (i.e., walking to running). When strain rates exceed 0.1/sec (trauma), cortical bone becomes more brittle; ultimate strain decreases.	Modest viscoelastic behavior.
Age effects	Young's modulus and strength properties deteriorate for men and women after age 20. Ultimate strain reduction leads to more brittle, weaker bones and high risk of fracture. Changes vary by bone location.	Preferential loss of vertical trabeculae with age. Results in new architecture and an increased susceptibility to vertebral and hip fractures. Double[a]/triple[b] jeopardy.

[a]Double jeopardy: weakened mechanism of fracture due to thinning and loss of trabeculae
[b]Triple jeopardy: reduced resistance to failure due to few, thinner, and longer trabeculae

- The regulatory mechanisms are closely related to the regulatory mechanisms of remodeling discussed above.

Calcium Homeostasis

- Maintaining an extracellular/intracellular Ca^{2+} gradient is essential for cellular life.
- A gradient is maintained through interactions between intestines, kidneys, and skeleton.
- 99% of a body's Ca^{2+} is in the skeleton (bone matrix, calcium salts, and within bone cells); the remaining 1% is extraskeletal within circulating fluid.
- Normal serum Ca^{2+} concentration is 9 to 10.4 mg/dL.
- All Ca^{2+} is acquired from diet; absorption/excretion rates are dependent on the Ca^{2+} gradient.
  - Regulation of the Ca^{2+} gradient is intricately associated with phosphate (Pi) metabolism.
  - Dietary deficiency of Ca^{2+} requires the endocrine system to find Ca^{2+} intracellularly.
  - Among other mechanisms, Ca^{2+} levels are restored by increased levels of bone resorption.
  - An age-related decrease in efficiency of dietary Ca^{2+} absorption necessitates variations in minimum daily Ca^{2+} requirements with regard to age, bone growth, and healing.

Vitamin D

- The primary function of vitamin D is to enhance calcium and phosphorus absorption in the small intestine and resorption in bone (mobilizing calcium and phosphorus).

Mechanism of Vitamin D Production

- Vitamin D is absorbed from food (fatty fish, cod-liver oil, and fortified cereals, bread, and milk) as vitamin D3 (cholecalciferol), or from sunlight as 7-dehydrocholesterol (converted to D3 in skin).
- Vitamin D_3 is biologically inert; it is carried to the liver by vitamin D binding proteins.
- Two vitamin D 25-hydroxylases catalyze the hydrolysis of vitamin D_3 to 25-hydroxyvitamin D_3 ($25(OH)D_3$) in hepatic microsomes.
- $25(OH)D_3$ (principal circulating form of vitamin D) binds to α-globulin and circulates throughout body.
- In the proximal tubule and glomerulus of the kidney, 1-α-hydroxylase produces the active 25-dihydroxyvitamin D_3 ($1,25(OH)_2D$). PTH, calcium, and phosphate levels control 1-α-hydroxylase function.
  - If PTH levels are high, or hypocalcemia or hypophosphatemia exists: $25(OH)D_3$ is hydroxylated to D_3 ($1,25(OH)_2D$).
  - If PTH levels are low, or hypercalcemia or hyperphosphatemia exists: $25(OH)D_3$ is hydroxylated to 21, $25(OH)$vitaminD_3 ($24,25(OH)_2D$).

Calcitonin

- In bone
  - Receptors: on osteoclasts
  - Action: associated with osteoclast shrinkage and decreased bone

- In kidney
  - Actions
    - Decreased Ca^{2+} and P reabsorption
    - Increases Na^+, K^+, Cl^-, and H_2O secretion

Estrogen

- Estrogen is an important regulator of bone formation.
- During late puberty: inhibits resorption and allows epiphyseal closure
- Regulatory effect on osteoblasts, osteoclasts, and other local regulatory factors remains controversial.
  - Estrogen may be involved in stimulating osteoclast apoptosis.
  - Estrogen deficiency may stimulate RANKL production by osteoblasts, thus increasing osteoclast activity and bone resorption.

AGE-RELATED BONE CHANGES

Bone Mass

- Bone grows the most during adolescence.
  - Early adolescence is marked by rapid longitudinal growth and modest mineral density increases.
  - When longitudinal growth slows, bone density increases in late adolescence until bone mass reaches its maximum in men and women between the ages of 25 and 40 years.
- Age-related bone loss begins between ages 30 and 50 years.
  - Associated with uncoupling of bone formation and resorption, especially from increased resorption rates
  - Steady loss of cortical and trabecular bone (see Table 19-5)
  - Ultimately trabecular mass can be reduced to 50% of its peak mass and cortical bone to 25% of peak mass.

Age-Related Bone Loss Disorders (see also Chapter 10)

- **Osteopenia:** decrease in bone density (loss of mineral and matrix)
- **Osteomalacia:** inadequately mineralized bone matrix (loss of mineralization)
- **Osteoporosis:** a skeletal disorder, independent of age or sex, characterized by compromised bone strength predisposing to an increased risk of fracture due to decrease in bone density (loss of mineral and matrix) (*Osteoporosis treatment and prevention, diagnosis and therapy: National Institutes of Health consensus statement*, 2000; 17:1)
  - Osteoporosis is a factor in 70% of all fractures in patients 45 years of age and older.

OSTEONECROSIS

The United States sees 10,000 to 20,000 new cases of osteonecrosis every year. **Osteonecrosis** is the death of a segment of bone in situ (from lack of circulation, not disease) and is caused by many factors that damage intraosseous vasculature. It is possible for sufficient compensatory circulation to supply the bone segment following vascular damage, avoiding cell death. Bone's blood supply varies by location, creating areas of high and low risk for osteonecrosis.

Pathogenesis

- "Osteonecrosis" is a correct description of the histopathologic process and does not suggest a specific etiology.
  - Other terms for this condition: avascular necrosis, aseptic necrosis, ischemic necrosis, osteochondritis
  - Osteonecrotic bone is NOT avascular; vessels are present but compromised.
- Prolonged secondary effects result in collapse and joint destruction within 3 to 5 years.
  - Osteonecrosis is the cause of roughly 10% of all hip replacements.
- If affected area is small enough and does not involve subchondral bone, collapse and degenerative changes can be avoided.
  - Early stages: hyperemia and vascular fibrous ingrowth
  - Creeping substitution: revascularization of necrotic bone
  - Cancellous bone: bone formation on top of the necrotic trabeculae
    - Increased density appearance on radiographs
    - No significant changes in the bone's mechanical properties
  - Cortical bone: cutting cones replace haversian bone
    - Initial osteoporosis during osteoclast removal of necrotic osteons
      - Fractures through weakened bone at 18 to 24 months
    - Late restoration of bone density: Osteoblasts begin bone formation when most of the haversian bone has been removed.
      - 2 additional years before the area's original strength and density are restored

Factors Believed to Affect Intraosseous Blood Supply

Mechanisms
- Mechanical disruption of vessels: fractures and dislocations (Box 19-4)

BOX 19-4 MOST COMMON TRAUMATIC INJURIES THAT LEAD TO OSTEONECROSIS[a]

Displaced fractured femoral neck	Displaced fracture of talar neck
Dislocation of femoral head	Four-fracture of humeral head
Displaced fracture of scaphoid	

[a]These injuries commonly lead to secondary effects and joint damage.

- Occlusion of arterial vessels: thrombosis, embolism, fat emboli, sickle-cell disease, and nitrogen bubbles (decompression sickness)
- Injury to (or pressure on) arterial walls and capillaries: can develop from within the vessel walls (vasculitis), or from internal or external injury
- Occlusion of venous vessels: Any factor resulting in greater vascular pressure than arterial pressure compromises local circulation.

Traumatic Injury

- Osteonecrosis is correlated with traumatic and nontraumatic causative factors (see Box 19-4).

Nontraumatic Vessel Damage
- Osteonecrosis is associated with several diseases and therapies:
  - Glucocorticoid administration
  - Ethanol abuse
  - Systemic lupus erythematosus
  - Antiphospholipid antibodies
  - Sickle-cell disease
  - Gaucher's disease
  - Decompression disease
  - Transplant
  - HIV
  - Legg-Calve-Perthes disease (children only)
  - Slipped femoral epiphysis (children only)

Classification

- There are numerous classification schema for osteonecrosis, but they are beyond the scope of this text.
- Classic staging systems include those of Ficat and Steinberg.

Staging
- The staging system for osteonecrosis of the femoral head has been most recently revised by the Association of Research into Osseous Circulation (ARCO; Table 19-6).

Diagnosis

- In pathologic osteonecrosis, the necrotic bone gradually collapses, leading to joint destruction.
- Symptoms do not tend to present until long after the disease has manifested itself in the bone; thus, diagnosis often occurs after joint degeneration.
- An early diagnosis provides the opportunity to minimize the extent of damage.

Clinical Features
- Most common location: anterolateral femoral head
  - Other common locations: humeral head, femoral condyles, proximal tibia
  - Other locations: vertebrae, small bones of hands and feet
- Bilaterality: common in hips, knees, or shoulders

TABLE 19-6 INTERNATIONAL CLASSIFICATION OF STAGES OF OSTEONECROSIS

Stage	Description
0	All diagnostic studies normal, diagnosis by histology only
1	Plain radiographs and computed tomography normal, magnetic resonance imaging and biopsy positive, extent of A, B, or C (<15%, 15% to 30%, and >30%, respectively)
2	Radiographs positive but no collapse, extent of involvement A, B, or C
3	Early flattening of dome, crescent sign, computed tomography or tomograms may be needed, extent of involvement A, B, or C, further characterization by amount of depression (mm)
4	Flattening of femoral head with joint space narrowing, possible other signs of early osteoarthritis

- Most common symptom: pain
  - Groin pain followed by thigh and buttock pain (common in femoral head disease)
  - Weight-bearing and motion-induced pain (frequent)
  - Rest pain (66%)
  - Night pain (33%)
  - Pain in multiple joints can suggest a multifocal process (rare).
- Physical findings: nonspecific
  - Pain with forced internal rotation and abduction of hip
  - Loss of motion
  - Limp in patients with lower extremity disease

Radiologic and Imaging Features

Magnetic Resonance Imaging (MRI)
- Most sensitive method of diagnosis
- Replaces bone marrow pressure measurement, venography, and bone biopsy methods in most cases
- Can identify changes early in disease:
  - T1-weighted images: focal lesions clearly defined and heterogeneous
    - Earliest MRI indication of osteonecrosis: Single low-intensity line separates normal and ischemic bone.
  - T2-weighted images: Second high-intensity line demonstrates hypervascular granulation tissue (pathognomonic *double-line sign*).

Radiographs
- Relatively insensitive to early changes: Films can remain normal long after symptoms of disease have presented.
- Recommended evaluation
  - Anteroposterior films
  - Frog-leg lateral films of hip: to evaluate the superior (anterolateral) portion of the femoral head, where subchondral abnormalities may be seen
- Plain radiographic findings of osteonecrosis
  - Earliest plain radiographic sign: mild increases in density; followed later by sclerosis and cysts
  - Pathognomonic *crescent sign* (subchondral radiolucency): indicates subchondral collapse
  - Late stage: collapse and change in shape of femoral head
  - Final stage: joint space narrowing and degeneration in acetabulum

Technetium-99m Bone Scanning
- Can be used (when there are no risk factors) when suspicious unilateral symptoms produce negative films
- Scan will produce the "doughnut sign" if bone is diseased.

Treatment

- Treatment of osteonecrosis remains controversial.
- There are four main treatment options; all seek to preserve the joint for as long as possible.

Nonoperative Treatment
- Lower extremity: bed rest, partial weight bearing with crutches, progression to weight bearing as tolerated
- Upper extremity: reasonable option when treating stage 0 to III humeral head lesions
  - Generally not proven effective

Surgical Treatment

Total Joint Arthroplasty
- Inconsistent results
- Generally less successful compared to patients with non-osteonecrosis disorders, resulting in higher rate of revision surgeries
- Best option for stage IV (even less severe stages in older sedentary patients) femoral head

Vascularized Fibular Grafting
- Reported results better than core decompression for selected patients
- Technically difficult, adds potential donor-site morbidity

Core Decompression
- Favorable for stage I, II, and III hips and stage I, II, III, and IV shoulders ·

Osteotomy
- Technically difficult; results not uniformly reproducible

FRACTURES AND FRACTURE FIXATION BIOLOGY

Fracture Healing

Fractures occur with concomitant damage to marrow, cortex, periosteum, and external soft tissues. Bone self-repairs and restores its mechanical and anatomical integrity without leaving scar tissue. As the bone healing process progresses, bone function is gradually restored.

Healing Process
The two types of fracture healing are distinguished by mechanical stability and the environment surrounding a fracture.

Direct (Primary) Fracture Healing
- Requisites
  - Rigid stabilization to eliminate motion (usually rigid internal plate fixation)
  - Bone matrix on one side of fracture must be exposed and in contact with the other fragment.
- Features
  - Bone heals without forming a callus (a biological splint).
  - Osteoid fills gaps >200 μm between fragments.
- Steps
  - Resorption: Osteoclasts resorb surrounding necrotic bone and, in cutting cones, create haversian systems through the osteoid.
  - Vascular ingrowth: New blood vessels penetrate the pathways, bringing endothelial, perivascular, mesenchymal, and osteoprogenitor cells, thus recreating mini-osteons.
  - Bone deposition: Osteoblasts lay down new bone; takes about 18 months for bone to heal completely.

Callus Formation (Secondary Healing)
- Requisite: Nonrigid fixation allows formation of fracture callus.
- Features: Fracture callus typifies secondary bone healing.
  - Callus serves as a splint, allowing motion and ensuring the bone's mechanical strength as it heals.
  - As bone is able to withstand more stress, the callus increases in strength (Wolff's law).
  - Clinical fracture union may be completed within months, but complete remodeling takes years to complete.
- Five-stage healing process of callus formation and remodeling (Box 19-5)

Vascularity of Fractures and Fracture Healing

Not surprisingly, the vascular response to fractures varies greatly by fracture site, extent/mechanism of damage, and fixation method. Generally the blood flow rate changes with time following fracture.

- Immediately following fracture, the blood flow rate decreases due to damage of blood vessels.
- Within hours after fracture, the flow rate increases.
- Approximately 2 weeks after the fracture, the flow rate peaks.
- By 12 weeks after the fracture, the flow rate reaches normal.

Biochemistry of Fracture Healing

- Fracture healing has phases analogous to both intramembranous and endochondral bone formation.

Proteoglycans
- Early callus formation (first week): Dermatan sulfate predominates (expressed by fibroblasts).
- Cartilage formation (second week): Chondroitin-4-sulfate predominates (chondrocytes).
- Premineralization preparation (third week)
  - Collagenase, gelatinase, stromolysine (proteolytic enzymes) expression increases and proteoglycan concentration decreases.
  - Alkaline phosphatase, IL-1, and IL-6 concentrations increase.

Collagenous Proteins
- Callus formation: type II collagen—predominant structural protein for cartilage
  - Peaks at 9 days, then turned off by 14 days
- Condensation: type I collagen—predominant structural protein in bone
  - Very low levels early on; levels increase progressively thereafter
- Cell proliferation: type III collagen (fibroblasts) found on periosteal surface
  - Substrate for cell proliferation and capillary growth
  - Present throughout fracture healing
- Minor regulatory collagens: types V, IX, XI

Noncollagenous Proteins
- Fibronectin, osteonectin, osteopontin, osteocalcin

Fracture Treatment/Fixation

- Fracture treatment objectives: align fracture fragments and maintain position until fragment union is achieved, while maintaining movement and function and avoiding complications and extended hospitalization for the patient
- Role for fracture fixation
  - Not biologically necessary due to the natural splint formed by the callus in response to motion
  - Immobilization devices are beneficial because they reduce pain, ensure proper fragment alignment, and allow patients earlier use of a fractured limb.

BOX 19-5 SECONDARY HEALING STAGES

1. Tissue destruction and hematoma formation
2. Inflammation and cellular proliferation
3. Callus formation (regulated by inductive proteins)
4. Consolidation
5. Remodeling

AUGMENTATION OF FRACTURE HEALING

Augmentation of fracture healing may be done initially for closed comminuted fractures or later for delayed union or nonunion. Augmentation may involve the addition of scaffolding (osteoconduction), bone morphogenic proteins and other growth factors (osteoinduction), or live bone cells (osteogenesis), alone or in combination.

Osteogenic Methods

- Osteogenic methods use naturally occurring grafts with living cells to promote bone regeneration.
- Autogenous grafts
  - Bone marrow provides only cells without scaffolding.
  - Cancellous bone graft provides cells, scaffolding, and growth factors.
- Fresh allogeneic grafts

Osteoconductive Methods

- Osteoconductive materials serve as a scaffold for the ingrowth of capillaries, perivascular tissues, and osteoprogenitor cells, allowing bone formation on their surfaces.
- Allograft bone
  - Classification: particulate and structural forms available
  - Widespread availability in developed countries
  - Small risk of disease transmission
- Calcium sulfate
  - Composition: basic component of plaster of Paris
  - Degradation within 60 days limits usefulness for load-bearing sites.
- Calcium phosphate–based ceramics
  - Composition: resorbable combinations of synthetic or coralline hydroxyapatite and tricalcium phosphate
  - Most commonly used group of ceramic bone graft substitutes
  - Relative brittleness limits load-bearing role.
- Bioactive glasses
  - Composition: silica-containing calcium phosphates
  - Limited applications due to high modulus and brittleness
  - Marketed currently in combination with polymethylmethacrylate as bioactive bone cement and as implant coating to enhance bonding with bone
- Synthetic polymers
  - Classifications: natural versus synthetic and degradable versus nondegradable
  - Available examples
    - Collagen fiber with hydroxyapatite polymer-ceramic used as bone graft substitute for spine fusions
    - Resin-based products for spine fusions
    - Polylactic acid (PLA) and polyglycolic acid (PGA) degradable plates and screws
    - Poly(lactic-co-glycolic acid) compounds used as graft extenders

Osteoinductive Methods

- Osteoinductive materials induce cellular development through growth factors, which leads to bone formation.
- TGF-β family (transforming growth factor)
  - Bone morphogenic proteins: especially BMP-2, BMP-4, BMP-7 (OP-1)
- Insulin-like growth factors
- Fibroblastic growth factors
- Platelet-derived growth factors
- Demineralized bone matrix (allograft cocktail of growth factors and osteogenic proteins after bone mineral removed), available in numerous preparations alone or with ceramics and polymers

Pulsed Electromagnetic Fields

- The use of electromagnetic fields to treat nonunion is based on the discovery of electrical currents in bone that were generated in response to normal functioning mechanical loads.
- Pulsed electromagnetic fields are induced by a square wave generator (Faraday's law).
- Optimal frequency for bone growth: 15 to 30 Hz (extremely low frequency [ELF])
- Commonly used clinically: high-frequency induction waveforms 1 to 10 kHz at low frequency (1 to 100 Hz) (pulsed electromagnetic fields [PEMF])

Ultrasound

- Ultrasound is a form of mechanical energy that has been found to have a strong influence on biological activity.
  - Low-intensity ultrasound does not cause heating or destruction to tissues and is noninvasive.
    - Accelerates fracture healing with short (20-minute) daily treatments at 30 mW/cm^2
    - Utility in treating delayed unions or nonunions

SUGGESTED READING

Broadus AE. Mineral balance and homeostasis. In: Favus MJ, ed. Primer on the Metabolic Bone Diseases and Disorders of Mineral Metabolism, 4th ed. Philadelphia: Lippincott Williams & Wilkins, 1999:74–80.

Buckwalter JA, Glimcher MJ, Cooper RR, et al. Bone biology I: Structure, blood supply, cells, matrix, and mineralization. *AAOS Instr Course Lect* 1996;45:371–386.

Buckwalter JA, Glimcher MJ, Cooper RR, et al. Bone biology II: Formation, form, modeling, remodeling, and regulation of cell function. *AAOS Instr Course Lect* 1996;45:387–399.

Einhorn TA. Enhancement of fracture-healing. *J Bone Joint Surg [Am]* 1995;77:940–956.

Fung YC, ed. *Biomechanics: Mechanical Properties of Living Tissues.* New York: Spinger-Verlag, 1981.

Lane JM, Vigorita VJ. Osteoporosis. *J Bone Joint Surg [Am]* 1983;65:274–278.

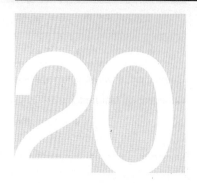

ARTICULAR CARTILAGE STRUCTURE, COMPOSITION, AND REPAIR

PETER J. ROUGHLEY
THOMAS V. SMALLMAN

Cartilage exists in the body as three types: hyaline cartilage, elastic cartilage, and fibrocartilage.

- Hyaline cartilage: characterized by type II collagen and aggregating proteoglycan
  - Skeletal: articular cartilage, costal cartilage, and growth plate
  - Extraskeletal: larynx, trachea, bronchi, and nose
- Elastic cartilage: characterized by preponderance of elastic fibers
  - Mainly in the ear and epiglottis
- Fibrocartilage: characterized by type I collagen and lower proteoglycan content than hyaline cartilage
  - Skeletal: meniscus of the knee, annulus fibrosus of the intervertebral discs

This chapter focuses on articular cartilage, whose single cell, the chondrocyte, is charged with all aspects of maintaining the structure. Growth plate cartilage, meniscus, and intervertebral disc are covered in separate chapters.

The unique avascular and alymphatic nature of articular cartilage makes it very durable but with minimal capacity for repair. Its aneural structure makes it liable to injury in an overuse or post-traumatic situation, as pain is not necessarily perceived.

An understanding of the cartilage response to cumulative wear, trauma, inflammation, and infection will allow the clinician to rationally treat cartilage disorders.

ARTICULAR CARTILAGE

A few joints in the body are fibrous (cranial sutures, tibiofibular syndesmosis) or fibrocartilaginous (symphysis pubis). However, most of the joints in the body are synovial and consist of hyaline articular cartilage covering the surface of bones where they meet in mobile joints. In the healthy young individual, articular cartilage has a white, lustrous, and smooth appearance. It is composed of living cells of only one cell type, the articular chondrocyte, supporting and maintaining an extracellular matrix.

TABLE 20-1 MATRIX AND CELLULAR FEATURES OF THREE ARTICULAR CARTILAGE REGIONS

	Articular Cartilage Region		
	Superficial/Tangential Zone	**Intermediate/Transitional Zone**	**Deep/Basal Zone**
Orientation of type II collagen fibrils	Parallel to surface	Oblique	Vertical
Chondrocyte features	Parallel to surface Flat shape High density, many cells	Random orientation Rounded shape Progressively lower density, fewer cells	Vertical columns (germinal layer)

Functions

- To provide a smooth surface compatible with friction-less motion
- To resist the compressive forces encountered across the joint under loading
  - This function is provided by the proteoglycan content.

Structure

- Morphologically, articular cartilage can be divided into three regions (Table 20-1), which can be distinguished by their differing orientation of type II collagen fibrils, orientation and cellular features of the chondrocytes, and histologic staining (Table 20-2).
  - Superficial collagen-rich tangential zone
  - Intermediate transitional zone
  - Deep/basal zone
- Morphologic correlation of articular cartilage on Hematoxylin and Eosin (H and E) stain (Fig. 20-1A)
  - Eosin the acidic stain in the two part H and E stain; tends to stain most proteins red since most proteins are weak bases (negatively charged)
  - Hematoxylin, a basic stain, characteristically stains the nucleic acids of the nuclei of cells, and appears blue
  - This histologic correlate of staining in articular cartilage with these two standard stains distinguishes three regions:
    - Superficial zone, containing the negatively charged protein, collagen, picks up the eosin and stains red

TABLE 20-2 HISTOLOGICAL PROPERTIES OF ARTICULAR CARTILAGE

	Histologic Stain	
	Fast green	**Safranin O**
Substance stained	Protein	Proteoglycans (polyanions)
Articular cartilage layer(s) stained	Tangential	Intermediate & deep

- Bone/cartilage junction with denser collagen anchoring elements, as well as the subchondral bone also stains red
- Intermediate and basal layers, rich in proteoglycans, pick up the basic hematoxlyin stain, and thus appear blue
- Special stains (see Table 20-2)
  - More apparent visualization of these layers is apparent with a "fast green/Safranin O stain"
  - Fast green stains the collagen green and thus green will predominate in the superficial layer and the bone/cartilage junction
  - Safranin O, a cationic dye, bonds to the polyanions of the proteoglycan and imparts a red color to the intermediate and deep layers.

Composition (Table 20-3)

- Mature articular cartilage contains about 5% of its volume as cells, the remainder being extracellular matrix.
- There is normally no mineral, and organic material accounts for about 30% of the matrix, with the remainder being water.
  - About 60% of the organic material is collagen, 25% is proteoglycan, and the remainder is a variety of matrix proteins.

Nerve and Vascular Supply

- Articular cartilage is characterized by having no nerves and no vascular system.
  - No nerves
    - Positive aspect: allows pain-free motion of the joints during normal use
    - Negative aspect: cartilage injury not perceived by the individual
  - No blood vessels
    - Nutrition and hydration for the tissue must arise from the synovial fluid by diffusion.
      - Clinical correlate: Cartilage exposed during surgery will rapidly dry, with resulting disruption of cell function, even leading to cell death, unless periodically bathed in fluid (every several minutes). The effect of drying on the matrix is not known.
    - No system for repair, as the usual microvascular source for cells in connective tissue repair is absent

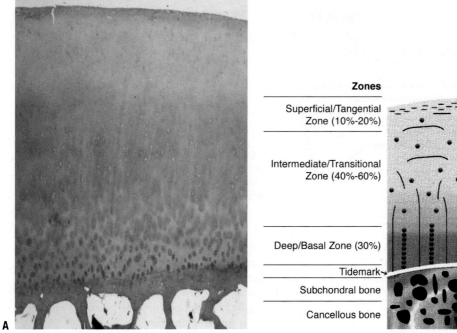
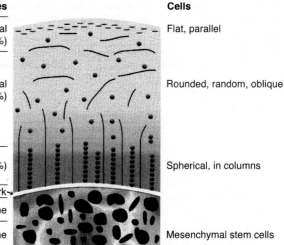

Figure 20-1   Cartilage morphology. (**A**) Superficial layer collagen stains red with eosin; intermediate layer proteoglycan stains bluish with hematoxylin. The basal layer with increasing collagen, binding the cartilage to bone and stains predominantly red with the eosin. The subchondral bone below, primarily collagen and mineral, stains densely red. (**B**) Diagram on the right outlines the corresponding zones and cellular morphology. (© 2003 American Academy of Orthopaedic Surgeons. Reprinted from the *Journal of the American Academy of Orthopaedic Surgeons*, Volume 11 (6), pp. 421–430.)

■ Clinical correlate: Incisions in cartilage (e.g., during arthroscopy) do not heal.
■ Chondrocytes undergo anaerobic metabolism and survive for several days in the body following death.
  ■ Clinical correlate: allows some cell viability in fresh tissue bulk allografting

TABLE 20-3 ADULT ARTICULAR CARTILAGE COMPOSITION

Component	Cartilage Content (%)
Cells	95
Matrix	5
Water	70
Mineral	—
Organic	30
Collagen	60
Proteogylcan	25
Protein	15

Collagens

Types and Functions

■ Collagens consist of three polypeptide chains that form a triple helix along at least part of their length.
■ They can be divided into fibrillar collagens (mainly types I, II, III, V, and XI) and nonfibrillar collagens (types IV, VI, VII, VIII, IX, and X).
■ The fibrillar collagens form the framework of connective tissues.
  ■ The fibrils consist of triple helical collagen molecules, arranged head to tail in linear arrays and side by side in a staggered manner (Fig. 20-2).
  ■ This staggered lateral arrangement gives the collagen fibril its characteristic cross-striated appearance when viewed in the electron microscope and contributes to its high tensile strength.
■ Nonfibrillar collagens serve both structural and nonstructural functions.
■ Different connective tissues contain different collagen types, reflecting their varied functions.
■ Fibrillar collagens in cartilage: types II and XI collagen
  ■ Types II and XI collagen occur in the same fibrils (see Fig. 20-2).
  ■ Type II collagen: 90% to 95% of total collagen, 10% of weight of cartilage
  ■ Type XI collagen: 5% to 10% of total collagen

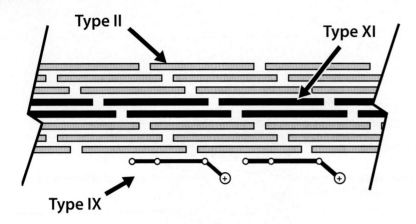

Type II

Type XI

Type IX

Figure 20-2   Cartilage collagens. Type II collagen provides the primary structural element (90%); type XI limits fibril diameter; type IX facilitates the interaction between the framework and the entrapped proteoglycan.

- ▥ While fibrillar itself, serves to limit fibril diameter of type II
- ▥ Nonfibrillar collagens in cartilage: type IX and X collagen
  - ▥ Type IX collagen
    - ▥ Resides on the surface of the fibrils
    - ▥ Facilitates interaction between the collagenous framework of the tissue and the interspersed proteoglycan
  - ▥ Type X collagen
    - ▥ Plays an integral role in the mineralization process in the growth plate
    - ▥ Site-specific immunostaining demonstrates localization that varies in noncalcified articular cartilage; animal work suggests that the presence of type X collagen may provide increased structural strength to normal articular cartilage.
    - ▥ In osteoarthritic and rheumatoid cartilage that is morphologically abnormal, there is expression of type X collagen; its role in normal articular cartilage is under investigation but has not yet been determined with certainty.
- ▥ Fibrocartilage contains type I collagen as its predominant fibrillar collagen, in common with most other connective tissues.

Collagen Turnover
- ▥ Physiologic conditions
  - ▥ Slow turnover: half-life of years
  - ▥ Net balance over time between formation and degradation
- ▥ Disease states
  - ▥ Shift to more rapid turnover disrupts the balance.
  - ▥ If the rate of degradation exceeds formation, then loss of collagen and proteoglycan ensues and degeneration follows.

Proteoglycans
- ▥ Proteoglycans are present in the extracellular matrix of all connective tissues, with the structure varying according to tissue.

- ▥ They consist of a central protein core to which sulfated glycosaminoglycans (chondroitin sulfate, dermatan sulfate, or keratan sulfate) are covalently attached.
- ▥ In articular cartilage, it is the proteoglycans that serve the major role in accomplishing the primary function of the tissue in resisting compressive loads.

Aggregating Proteoglycans (Fig. 20-3)
- ▥ Hyaline and elastic cartilages contain predominantly aggrecan, one of the aggregating proteoglycans, which, by definition, aggregate or interact with hyaluronic acid.
- ▥ Fibrocartilages do not contain as high an aggrecan content.

Structure
- ▥ Many aggrecan molecules link to a central molecule of hyaluronic acid by a link protein that is devoid of sulfated glycosaminoglycans.
- ▥ Aggrecan molecule
  - ▥ Long core protein with two types of glycosaminoglycan chains, chondroitin sulfate (100 per molecule) and keratan sulfate (60 per molecule), molecular weight 2,500,000 daltons, 90 percent carbohydrate
  - ▥ Aggrecan molecules account for 25% of the dry weight of cartilage.

Function
- ▥ Proteoglycan aggregates provide the tissue with its turgid nature that resists compression.

Nonaggregating Proteoglycans (see Fig. 20-3)
- ▥ All cartilages, in common with all soft tissues, also contain nonaggregating proteoglycans, which interact with collagen fibrils rather than hyaluronic acid, and function to stabilize the matrix.
- ▥ These are decorin, biglycan, fibromodulin, and lumican.
- ▥ They are much smaller than aggrecan and possess only a few dermatan sulfate (decorin and biglycan) or keratan sulfate (fibromodulin and lumican) chains.
- ▥ They mediate the interactions between adjacent collagen fibrils, or with other matrix components.

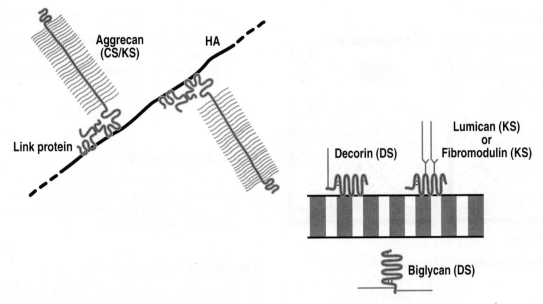

Figure 20-3 Cartilage proteoglycans. Aggrecan is the major aggregating proteoglycan (25% of dry weight); it is associated with compression and linked to hyaluronic acid (HA). The other proteoglycans are nonaggregating and associate with and stabilize collagen fibrils.

■ Cartilage also contains perlecan, a heparan sulfate proteoglycan normally associated with basement membrane, whose function is unknown.

The types of cartilage proteoglycans are summarized in Table 20-4.

BIOMECHANICS AND RESPONSE TO LOADING

The health of chondrocytes is closely related to joint loading and motion. Survival of the chondrocytes depends on adequate nutrition, and the passive diffusion of nutrients from the synovial fluid is aided by joint loading and motion. In general, dynamic (cyclic) loading is beneficial to matrix synthesis, whereas static loading is detrimental, causing a decrease in the synthesis of aggrecan and link proteins.

Cyclic Joint Loading

■ Promotes chondrocyte nutrition and function, stimulating the production and maintenance of the matrix
  ■ Cyclic loading clinical correlate: contributes to the beneficial effects of continuous passive motion (CPM)
  ■ Joint immobilization clinical correlate: Absence of this beneficial nutritional effect contributes to the cartilage atrophy observed upon prolonged joint underuse or immobilization.
■ Aggregating proteoglycans provide the articular cartilage with its resilience to compression, as compressive forces are counterbalanced by the focal increase in proteoglycan swelling potential (Fig. 20-4).
  ■ Serves to protect the chondrocytes from adverse forces
■ Compressibility is a function of the high hydrostatic pressure of cartilage.
  ■ Water content is not uniform throughout cartilage,

TABLE 20-4 AGGREGATING AND NONAGGREGATING PROTEOGLYCANS

Proteoglycan Type	Interaction	Function	Molecule(s)	Glycosaminoglycan Type
Aggregating	Hyaluronic acid	Resist compressive forces	Aggrecan	Chondroitin sulfate Keratan sulfate
Nonaggregating	Collagen fibrils	Stabilize collagen matrix	Decorin Biglycan Fibromodulin Lumican	Dermatan sulfate Dermatan sulfate Keratan sulfate Keratan sulfate
		Cell matrix interaction	Perlecan	Heparan sulfate

Synovial fluid

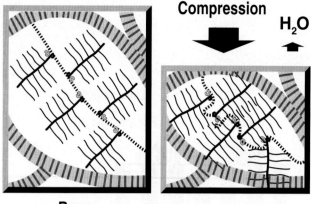

Requirements:
- High aggrecan content
- High GAG-SO$_4$ content
- Aggregate formation

Figure 20-4 Resistance to compression. On the left, articular cartilage is in equilibrium, with the swelling pressure of the proteoglycan balanced by the tensile force in the collagen fibril. With compression, water is squeezed out of the cartilage (taking waste metabolites with it); a new equilibrium is reached, with an increased swelling pressure of the proteoglycan balancing the applied compression. When the compression is removed, water is drawn in (along with nutrients) and the former steady state is achieved.

but rather is lower in the superficial layers and higher in the deeper layers.

■ Water squeezed out of cartilage by compression contributes to the thin boundary layer of liquid that reduces friction between the opposing articular surfaces.

■ Cartilage layers differ in their water flow and in their compressive strains (Fig. 20-5).

Static Joint Loading

■ Excessive loads or overuse cause chondrocytes to release proteolytic enzymes, which damage the proteoglycan and collagen, causing tissue degeneration and decreased ability to protect the cells.

Concept of Compressibility

■ Aggregating proteoglycans, highly sulfated, have a strong affinity for water and expand their molecular domain by drawing water and nutrients into the tissue.

■ As more water is drawn into the cartilage, the swelling potential of the proteoglycan decreases.

■ A balance is established wherein the outward swelling of the proteoglycan is resisted by stretching forces in the collagenous framework of the tissue.

■ Application of a load compresses the tissue, and water is displaced into the joint from the focally entrapped and large proteoglycan aggregates, creating a new equilibrium.

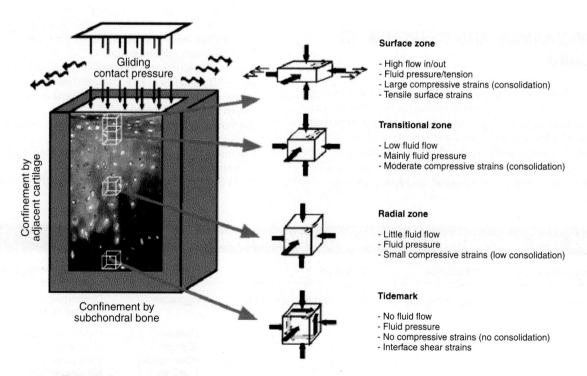

Figure 20-5 The mechanical environment of articular cartilage under intermittent joint loading and motion. (From Wong M, Carter DR. Articular cartilage functional histomorphology and mechanobiology: A research perspective. *Bone* 2003;33:1–13.)

- When the load is removed, water is drawn back into the cartilage, restoring the original equilibrium.
- Linked to the flux of water, nutrients move into, and waste products out of, the matrix.

MATRIX METABOLISM AND HOMEOSTASIS

Both the production of the extracellular matrix and its physiological regulation throughout life are controlled by the chondrocyte. Sequestered in the matrix, this cell receives its oxygen and nutrients by diffusion. The tissue pressure of oxygen is low, leading to the production of energy by glycolysis. Mechanical forces are sensed by the chondrocytes, which are linked to the matrix by integrins, cell surface-binding proteins.

Chondrocyte Function

- Conditioned by surface receptors, regulation of both anabolic and catabolic activities is carried out by these cells.
- The functions of the chondrocytes include growth and maintenance of the matrix, which is balanced by matrix degradation.
- Tissue formation (growth, synthesis): produce structural macromolecules (collagen and proteoglycan)
- Tissue turnover (degradation): produce secreted proteinases (including collagenases, gelatinases, stromelysins, and aggrecanases)

Chondrocyte Regulators: Hormones, Cytokines, Growth Factors

- Hormones: chemical messengers synthesized by specialized endocrine glands and transported to act on distant cells
- Cytokines: molecules commonly secreted by immune or other cells to act on damaged or infected tissue

- Growth factors: molecules synthesized and secreted by cells in a variety of tissues and generally act on nearby cells in a paracrine or autocrine fashion
  - Often secreted in an inactive form and may bind to extracellular matrix components, requiring proteolytic cleavage for activation and cell receptor binding
- Tissue formation (growth) regulators
  - Insulin-like growth factor-1; somatomedin-C
    - Increases collagen and proteoglycan synthesis
    - Synergistic with mechanical stimulation
  - Transforming growth factor beta (TGF-β)
    - Binds to specific cell surface receptors that activate intracellular pathways that regulate the expression of genes
    - Chondroprotective
    - Increases collagen and proteoglycan synthesis
    - Inhibits matrix degeneration and cell proliferation
  - BMP-2 and BMP-7 both increase proteoglycan synthesis and maintain chondrocyte phenotype.
- Tissue turnover (matrix degradation) regulators (Fig. 20-6)
  - Promoted by a variety of cytokines, such as interleukin-1 (IL-1) and tumor necrosis factor alpha (TNFα)
    - Both IL-1 and TNFα are implicated as mediators of inflammatory and degenerative arthritis.
  - Stimulate the secretion of specific collagenases that are part of a group of enzymes called matrix metalloproteinases (MMPs) from the chondrocytes
  - Inhibit synthesis of the structural macromolecules
- Homeostasis
  - Normally proteinase destruction is kept under control by the concomitant secretion of tissue inhibitor of metalloproteinases (TIMPs), which can inhibit the action of MMPs.
  - Clinical correlate: Drugs such as nonsteroidal anti-inflammatories (NSAIDs) and glucocorticoids used to treat arthritic joints retard cartilage degeneration by affecting the synthesis/degradation balance.

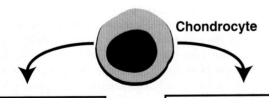

Chondrocyte

Degradation	**Synthesis**
Collagenases	Collagen
Gelatinases	Proteoglycan
Stromelysins	Proteins
Aggrecanases	
TIMPs	↑ growth factors, IGF-1
	TGF
↑ cytokines, IL-1	BMP2/7
TNFα	
	↓ cytokines, IL-1
↓ glucocorticoids	NSAIDs,
NSAIDs	glucocorticoids

Figure 20-6 Cartilage turnover. The chondrocyte is the only cell in cartilage. It supplies all of the molecules that make up this tissue: the collagen, the proteoglycan, and all of the other matrix proteins. It does so in response to a variety of growth factors, the most important being TGFβ, and insulin-like growth factor-1 (IGF-1, somatomedin-C). They stimulate the chondrocyte to make more matrix. The chondrocyte also supplies the enzymes needed for turnover. Turnover of cartilage during growth is needed for remodeling and maintenance. The enzymes include aggracanase and matrix metalloproteinases, including collagenase and stromelysin which may have a variety of activities, including collagenase, and stromelysin, which degrade the matrix. The chondrocyte also makes inhibitors of these enzymes called tissue inhibitor of metalloproteinases (TIMP). Normally a balance exists between synthesis and degradation. The TIMP system controls degradation.

However, some NSAIDs have an undesirable inhibitory effect on matrix synthesis by chondrocytes.

Chondrocytes and Drugs

- Drugs can interact with chondrocytes in such a way as to alter function.
  - Glucocorticoids
    - Controversial: Most suggest deleterious over chondroprotective effect
      - Inhibit chondrocyte proliferation and decrease both collagen and proteoglycan synthesis
      - Impair response to cytokines such as TGF-β
      - Little effect on cartilage degradation in osteoarthritis
      - Potent inhibitors of cyclooxygenase-2 (COX-2)
    - Preponderance of evidence suggests little long-lasting benefit and possible deleterious effects of steroid injections.
  - NSAIDs
    - NSAIDs reduce inflammation through reducing COX-2, but undesirable side effects are present due to the co-inhibition of the ubiquitous and constitutively produced COX-1.
    - COX enzymes catalyze the conversion of arachidonic acid and oxygen to prostaglandin H_2, the committed step in prostanoid biosynthesis; three isoforms exist:
      - COX-1: constitutive, exists in endothelium, stomach (promotes gastric mucosal protection), kidney (maintenance of renal blood flow and function), and platelets (promote aggregation)
      - COX-2: inducible isoform associated with the inflammatory response (increased prostaglandin E_2 in arthritis)
      - COX-3, an isoenzyme of COX-1, is a target for acetaminophen and other antipyretic/analgesic medications.
    - Inflammation in all forms of arthritis is associated with increased production of COX-2 in response to cytokine stimulation of synovial cells.
      - Prostaglandins produced by the action of COX-2 mediate the features of inflammation.
      - COX-2 is also a product of chondrocytes in the noninflammatory osteoarthritis joint, though its precise role is unclear.
    - Coxibs (specific inhibitors of COX-2) have demonstrated clinical efficacy in arthritis, but unfortunate and unforeseen side effects of these have reduced their availability.

ARTICULAR CARTILAGE, INFLAMMATION, AND AGING

Mechanism of Cartilage Destruction

- A global model of factors that might be operant in arthritis is outlined in Figure 20-7.

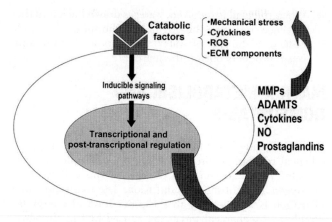

Figure 20-7 Pathways that modulate chondrocyte function in osteoarthritis (OA) are shown. Although the events that initiate cartilage destruction in OA are not defined, a number of potentially catabolic factors may interact with chondrocytes and induce signaling cascades that activate gene transcription and post-transcriptional modifications. These catabolic factors include pro-inflammatory cytokines, mechanical stress, reactive oxygen species (ROS), and extracellular matrix (ECM) components. These factors induce the synthesis of MMPs, aggrecanases (systemic nomenclature ADAMTS-4 and 5), cytokines, nitric oxide, and prostaglandins, which may feedback-regulate or amplify these responses, resulting in a vicious cycle leading to further destruction. (From Goldring MB, Berenbaum F. The regulation of chondrocyte function by proinflammatory mediators: prostaglandins and nitric oxide. *Clin Orthop Rel Res* 2004;(427S):S37–S46.)

Morphologic Changes/Radiographic Correlation

- Arthritic destruction of articular cartilage takes place mainly via the action of proteolytic enzymes.
- In the early stages of disease, loss of proteoglycan is reversible, whereas at later stages there is irreversible loss (Table 20-6).
- Intact cartilage consists of a balance between the containing forces of the collagen framework versus the expanding hydrostatic force of the contained proteoglycans (see Fig. 20-4).
- The earliest visible change in arthritis is loss of integrity of the collagen, resulting in tissue fibrillation and ultimate erosion to subchondral bone (see Table 20-6).
- Loss of proteoglycans from the matrix causes a loss of osmolality, with an increase in compressibility.
- The initial response to tissue loss is an anabolic, reparative reaction.
- Unfortunately, despite chondrocyte proliferation and increased collagen and proteoglycan synthesis, the exquisite and unique interrelationship that exists in cartilage is not so easily replicated.
- As the function of cartilage is protection from compressive load, the radiographic correlates to this process of cartilage loss involve first loss of joint space, then osteophyte formation, reflecting progressive remodeling to the increased load.
- Well-established pathways of cartilage destruction include the following (Fig. 20-8):

TABLE 20-5 MECHANISM OF CARTILAGE DESTRUCTION IN ARTHRITIS

Type	Origin	Disorder	Cause of Increased Proteolysis
Degenerative	Mechanical	Osteoarthritis	Normal matrix, abnormal load (misalignment, trauma, occupation) Abnormal matrix, normal load (chondrodysplasia, drug, synovitis)
Inflammatory	Microorganism	Septic	Microorganism within joint (infectious–bacterial, viral, fungal)
		Reactive	Bacterial infection at remote site (related antigen in joint)
	Autoimmune	Rheumatoid	Autoimmune recognition of cartilage degradation product? (type II collagen, aggrecan)
	Crystal	Gout	Sodium urate
		Pseudogout (chondrocalcinosis)	Calcium pyrophosphate

- Synovium and chondrocytes in osteoarthritis express TNF-α, which may be responsible for the inflammatory events, and IL-1, which promotes the cartilage degradation.
  - TNF-α
    - Predominantly secreted by macrophages
      - Expressed in osteoarthritic cartilage
      - Not expressed in normal articular cartilage
    - Shares many functions with IL-1, including suppression of proteoglycan synthesis, stimulation of collagen degradation, and induction of MMP expression, but appears to be less active than IL-1
    - Inhibits the synthesis of proteoglycans and type II collagen by promoting chondrocyte dedifferentiation and preventing cartilage repair
  - IL-1
    - Downregulates synthesis of collagen and proteoglycan
    - Upregulates synthesis of MMPs, the most important collagenases (MMP1 and MMP13)
      - Only enzymes able to degrade the collagen triple helix in cartilage
      - MMP13 cleaves epitopes in type II collagen in regions of matrix depletion in osteoarthritic cartilage and is 5 to 10 times more active than MMP1 or MMP8.
      - Upregulation is through an endogenous mediator, nitric oxide (see below).
    - Induces synthesis of aggrecanases (ADAMTS4 and ADAMTS5)
      - These degrade the core protein of the proteoglycan aggrecan, which then diffuses out of the cartilage.
- Prostaglandins and nitric oxide act as endogenous mediators of the actual damage.
  - Elevated in the articular cartilage, synovium, and synovial fluid of osteoarthritic and rheumatoid joints and serve as potential therapeutic targets for osteoarthritis
- Nitric oxide

TABLE 20-6 SEQUENTIAL MORPHOLOGIC AND RADIOGRAPHIC FINDINGS IN PROGRESSIVE ARTHRITIS

Stage of Arthritis	Morphologic Change	Radiographic Correlate
Early	Reversible loss of proteoglycans	No abnormalities
Intermediate	Permanent loss of proteoglycans Collagen breakdown Surface cracks and fibrillation	Joint space narrowing Osteophyte formation (progressive remodeling)
Advanced	Further loss of collagen framework Ultimately complete loss, leading to raw eburnated bone surface	Subchondral sclerosis (Wolff's law)

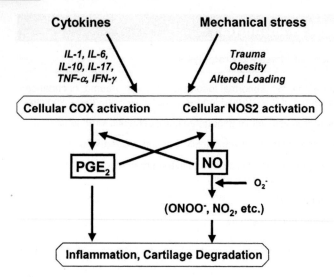

Figure 20-8 Pathways of interaction of mechanical stress and pro-inflammatory mediators. Increased concentrations of cytokines or alterations in the mechanical environment of the joint may activate COX2 and NOS2 in articular cartilage, increasing production of prostaglandins or NO. IL, interleukin; COX, cyclooxygenase enzyme; NO, nitric oxide; NOS, nitric oxide synthase; PGE_2, prostaglandin E_2; TFN-α, tumor necrosis factor-α; IFN-γ, interferon-γ. (From Guilak F, Fermor B, Keefe FJ, et al. The role of biomechanics and inflammation in cartilage injury and repair. *Clin Orthop Rel Res* 2004;(423):17–26.)

- Enzyme producing nitric oxide is nitric oxide synthase (NOS); exists in three forms
- NOS2 can produce high levels of nitric oxide and most commonly is associated with inflammation in arthritic disorders.
- Inhibition of nitric oxide production using NOS2-specific inhibitors can considerably reduce disease progression in animal models of osteoarthritis.
- Prostaglandin E_2
    - NSAIDs compete directly with arachidonic acid binding to the COX site and inhibit COX activity.
    - Aspirin covalently modifies and irreversibly inhibits COX.
    - Other NSAIDs such as ibuprofen and indomethacin act as reversible competitive inhibitors.

Cartilage Destruction in Clinical Situations (Table 20-5)

- Osteoarthritis (degenerative arthritis): Enzymes are released directly by the chondrocytes, due to abnormal forces acting on the cells.
- Inflammatory arthropathies: Same enzymes can also arise from the synovial cells; polymorphonuclear leukocytes possess a distinct collagenase (MMP8) and contain other proteinases (elastase and cathepsin G) able to degrade proteoglycan.
- Rheumatoid arthritis: Degradation products of cartilage matrix macromolecules are thought to initiate a T-cell–mediated autoimmune response, so exacerbating inflammation.

- Infectious arthritis: Bacterial collagenases may give rise to very rapid cartilage destruction because of their multiple sites of action along the collagen molecules.
- The mammalian collagenases cleave at only a single site in the fibrillar collagen molecule, and cleavage of the collagen fibril is a slow process. In contrast, most proteinases degrade aggrecans, and thus loss of proteoglycan aggrecan is a rapid process.

Fundamental Concept

- In general, it appears that if only proteoglycan loss occurs, the cartilage may regenerate a normal matrix over time, but once the collagen framework is damaged, the degenerative process is irreversible.

Susceptibility of Aggrecan and Stability of Collagen

Aggrecan

- Aggrecan is susceptible to damage by proteolytic enzymes.
- Figure 20-9 shows the structure of the proteoglycan with the aggrecan core protein, the keratan and chondroitin sulfate side chains, an interacting link protein that is an attachment to hyaluronic acid (HA).
- Proteinase cleaves aggrecan at sites unprotected by link protein.
    - The major proteinase is aggrecanase, and there are two known at this time.
        - Aggrecanase-1 (ADAMTS-4) and aggrecanase-2 (ADAMTS-5) are members of the disintegrin and metalloprotease with thrombospondin motifs (ADAMTS) protein family.
        - The link at the Glu373-ALA374 bond in the aggrecan core protein is cleaved, and the core protein plus the heavily negatively charged side chains are liberated into the tissue.
        - The free fragments, being negatively charged, are expressed rapidly from the negatively charged internal environment of the cartilage and into the synovial fluid.
- Hence, any damage to proteoglycans is rapidly detrimental to this tissue's physical properties. The only way to stop progression is relative rest (eliminate increased load) and treatment of the inflammation.

Collagen

- Collagen is difficult to damage; it resists proteolytic damage.
- Collagen can be cleaved by a series of collagenases, three of which are made in humans.
    - MMP1: made by most connective tissues for internal remodeling
    - MMP8: made by leukocytes, used in remodeling tissues following damage
    - MMP13: made by chondrocytes, used in cartilage; they cleave at only one site in the collagen molecule, in a very slow process; because the enzyme works at only one site, and because of the extensive cross-linking, the damage remains very localized, especially when the damage is being initiated at the chondrocyte level.

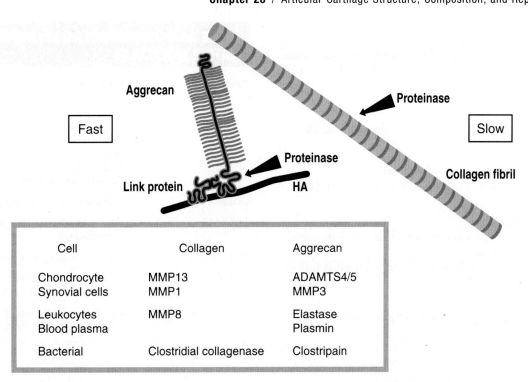

Cell	Collagen	Aggrecan
Chondrocyte	MMP13	ADAMTS4/5
Synovial cells	MMP1	MMP3
Leukocytes	MMP8	Elastase
Blood plasma		Plasmin
Bacterial	Clostridial collagenase	Clostripain

Figure 20-9 Arthritis: susceptibility of aggrecan and stability of collagen toward degradation. Aggrecan shows little resistance to proteolytic degradation, being rapidly cleaved by many proteinases adjacent to the hyaluronic acid (HA) binding domain of its core protein. In contrast, collagen, in the form of mature cross-linked collagen fibrils, is cleaved by only a few proteinases, and with the exception of the bacterial collagenases this is a slow event.

Relative Importance of Aggrecan and Collagen Damage in Clinical Situations

- Degenerative arthritis: Only the chondrocyte-initiated enzymes MMP13 and aggrecanase cause damage.
- Inflammation: Inflammatory cells invade the synovium, and both MMP1 and MMP13 become active. With acute inflammation, as in rheumatoid arthritis and infection, the damage is more rapid still because the leukocytes release MMP8 and elastase.
- Bleeding: Both in trauma and in hemophilia, blood plasma is released into the joint. Plasmin also acts on aggrecan to degrade it further.
- Bacterial infection: Bacteria can release collagenases that are very damaging to joints. The bacteria use collagen as food, and they therefore wish to generate extensive degradation. The collagenases from bacteria cleave each collagen molecule not at one site or even 10 sites, but rather at about 100 sites. They can lyse this molecule in a matter of minutes. Thus the bacterial damage is rapid and profound, and hence the necessity for very rapid diagnosis and treatment of bacterial arthritis.
- The hierarchy of damage to joints is hours to days for bacteria, months for inflammatory conditions, and years for degeneration.

Markers of Cartilage Metabolism (Box 20-1)

- The release of cartilage matrix components into the synovial fluid has been used to monitor disease status in the arthritic joint.

- Care must be taken in interpreting the meaning of increase in marker levels, as some reflect increased degradation (collagen cross-links and neoepitopes), some reflect increased or altered synthesis (collagens C-propeptide and chondroitin sulfate-neoepitopes), and others may reflect both (keratan sulfate-neoepitopes).

Examples of Markers
- Type II collagen markers (C-propeptide, telopeptide-derived cross-links and collagenase-derived neoepitopes)
- Aggrecan markers (KS- and CS-derived neoepitopes)

CARTILAGE REPAIR

- It is well accepted that lesions confined to the avascular articular cartilage have a very limited capacity for repair.

BOX 20-1 MARKERS OF CARTILAGE METABOLISM

Cartilage formation markers	Cartilage degradation markers
Type II collagen C-propeptide	KS, neoepitope (aggrecan)
CS-neoepitope (aggrecan)	COMP
	Type II collagen telopeptide cross-links
	Type II collagen/ collagenase neoepitope

■ However, when lesions penetrate the subchondral bone, a wound healing response is observed, as cells derived from the bone marrow fill the lesion and differentiate into chondrocytes. This observation forms the basis of surgical repair techniques.

Surgical Cartilage Repair Techniques (Table 20-7)

Drilling or Abrasion Chondroplasty
■ Techniques used to penetrate the subchondral bone

Periosteal Grafts
■ Periosteum is a source of cells that can differentiate into chondrocytes.
■ Used to repair cartilage in a more controlled fashion than drilling/abrasion

Chondrocytes or Differentiated Bone Marrow Stem Cell Implantation
■ Commercially available system has been developed that allows harvest of chondrocytes, with culturing, and then reimplantation under a periosteal flap.
■ Alternatively, the cells can be embedded in an artificial matrix for implantation in a lesion.
  ■ Matrices: collagen, hyaluronic acid, fibrin and synthetic polymers
■ Various growth factors have been used in these cell repair systems to promote matrix synthesis and stabilize the chondrocyte phenotype.

Osteochondral Grafts
■ Large frozen allografts with cryopreservation
■ Fresh osteochondral allografts implanted within a window of chondrocyte viability (7 days)
■ Small cylindrical osteochondral autografts can be harvested fresh and implanted in the same or other joints.
■ Chondrocyte survival in part determines long-term outcome.

TABLE 20-8 CHONDROPLASIAS: DEFECTS IN MATRIX MOLECULES

Gene	Disorder
COL2A1	Achondrogenesis type II
	Hypochondrogenesis
	Spondyloepiphyseal dysplasia
	Kniest dysplasia
	Stickler dysplasia
	Familial osteoarthritis
COL9A2	Multiple epiphyseal dysplasia type II
COL11A2	Stickler dysplasia (no eye involvement)
COL10A1	Schmid metaphyseal dysplasia
COMP	Pseudoachondroplasia
	Multiple epiphyseal dysplasia type I
Perlecan	Dyssegmental dysplasia
	Schwartz-Jampel syndrome

(Also see Fig. 15-2)

■ Early degenerative change is a consequence in part of a lack of survival.
■ An autoimmune response may complicate the result in bulk allograft situations.
■ A major problem in all repair systems is achieving integration between the repair cartilage and the surrounding normal cartilage.

CHONDRODYSTROPHIES

Functionally abnormal cartilage may result when a gene for one of the matrix macromolecules or for one of the cellular components involved in chondrocyte metabolism is defec-

TABLE 20-7 CARTILAGE REPAIR[a]

Mechanism of Repair	Technique	Main Limitations
Blood clot formation	Abrasion or drilling subchondral bone Microfracture	Phenotype stability
Cell implantation	Chondrocytes/marrow stem cells Artificial matrix for support or covering membrane for retention	Cell availability/ phenotype stability
Tissue transplantation	Osteochondral grafts Periosteal grafts	Tissue availability/ chondral integration

[a]Limitations regardless of technique may include cell or tissue availability, phenotype instability, chondral integration.

TABLE 20-9 CHONDRODYSPLASIAS: DEFECTS IN CELLULAR MOLECULES

Gene	Disorder
FGFR3	Achondroplasia
	Hypochondroplasia
	Thanotophoric dysplasia types I and II
PTHrPR	Jansen metaphyseal dysplasia
SOX9	Camptomelic dysplasia
SHOX	Dyschondrosteosis
DTDST	Diastrophic dysplasia
	Atelosteogenesis type II
	Achondrogenesis type IB
GAL & GALNS	Morquio syndrome
EXT1/2	Hereditary multiple exostosis

(Also see Fig. 15-2)

in a chondrodysplasia, and impairment in the function of the articular cartilage results in a premature familial osteoarthritis. Defects in the matrix molecules include the genes for type II collagen (COL2A1), type IX collagen (COL9A2), type X collagen (COL10A1), cartilage oligomeric protein (COMP), and perlecan (Table 20-8). Defects in cellular components include the genes for a growth factor receptor (FGFR3), a hormone receptor (PTHrPR), a sulfate transporter (DTDST), transcription factors (SOX9 and SHOX), and enzymes involved in glycosaminoglycan metabolism (GAL, GLCN6S, and EXT; Table 20-9). In many cases defects in the same gene can give rise to different clinical phenotypes (COL2A1 and FGFR3), depending on the site and type of mutation. It is also possible that defects in different genes can give rise to the same clinical phenotype, if the different gene products interact with one another (COL9A2 and COMP in multiple epiphyseal dysplasia) or if they are involved in regulating the same biochemical event (GAL and GALNS in Morquio syndrome).

SUGGESTED READING

Benjamin M, Evans EJ. Fibrocartilage. *J Anat* 1990;171:1–15.
Brooks PM. Clinical management of rheumatoid arthritis. *Lancet* 1993;341:286–290.
Bruckner P, van der Rest M. Structure and function of cartilage collagens. *Microscop Res Technique* 1994;28:378–384.
Buckwalter JA. Aging and degeneration of human intervertebral disc. *Spine* 1995;20:1307–1314.
Buckwalter JA, Mankin HJ. Articular cartilage repair and transplantation. *Arthritis Rheum* 1988;41:1331–1342.
Buckwalter JA, Mankin HJ. Articular cartilage. Tissue design and chondrocyte matrix interactions. *J Bone Joint Surg [Am]* 1997;79:600–611.
Caplan AI. Cartilage. *Scientific American* 1984;251:84–94.
Carney SL, Muir H. The structure and function of cartilage proteoglycans. *Physiol Rev* 1988;68:858–910.
Ghosh P. Nonsteroidal anti-inflammatory drugs and chondroprotection. *Drugs* 1993;46:834–846.
Hamerman D. Aging and osteoarthritis: basic mechanisms. *J Am Geriatr Soc* 1993;41:760–770.
Heinegard D, Oldberg A. Structure and biology of cartilage and bone matrix non-collagenous macromolecules. *FASEB J* 1989;3:2042–2051.
Hopwood JJ, Morris CP. The mucopolysaccharidoses; diagnosis, molecular genetics and treatment. *Mol Biol Med* 1990;7:381–404.
Horton WA. Progress in human chondrodysplasias. Molecular genetics. *Ann NY Acad Sci* 1996;785:150–159.
Jones AC, Doherty M. The treatment of osteoarthritis. *Br J Clin Pharmacol* 1992;33:357–363.
Kim YJ, Sah RLY, Grodzinsky AJ, et al. Mechanical regulation of cartilage biosynthetic behavior: Physical stimuli. *Arch Biochem Biophys* 1994;311:1–12.
Kuettner KE. Biochemistry of articular cartilage in heath and disease. *Clin Biochem* 1992;25:155–163.
Lohmander LS. Articular cartilage and osteoarthrosis. The role of molecular markers to monitor breakdown and disease. *J Anat* 1994;184:477–492.
Oegema TR. Biochemistry of the intervertebral disc. *Clinics Sports Med* 1993;12:419–439.
Roughley PJ, Lee ER. Cartilage proteoglycans: structure and potential functions. *Microscop Res Technique* 1994;28:385–397.
Sewell KL, Trentham DE. Pathogenesis of rheumatoid arthritis. *Lancet* 1993;341:283–286.
Spranger J, Winterpacht A, Zabel B. The type II collagenopathies: a spectrum of chondrodysplasias. *Eur J Pediatr* 1994;153:56–65.
Thomas JT, Ayad S, Grant ME. Cartilage collagens: Strategies for the study of their organization and expression in the extracellular matrix. *Ann Rheum Dis* 1994;53:488–496.
Toivanen A. Infection and arthritis. *Ann Med* 1994;26:245–248.

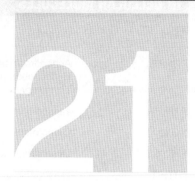

DIARTHRODIAL JOINTS

THOMAS V. SMALLMAN
KRIS SHEKITKA
DONALD FLEMMING

The objective of this chapter is to review briefly the development of joints and their normal structure and function and then to outline concisely the pathophysiology of arthritic disorders. Infectious arthritis is fully covered in Chapter 27, Infectious Disorders of Bone and Joints, and is not discussed here. The structure and function of hyaline cartilage and the cell biology of cartilage repair are covered in Chapter 20, Articular Cartilage Structure, Composition, and Repair. The reader might wish to review the key elements in this chapter prior to studying this section.

BACKGROUND

The articular system consists of:

- **Diarthrodial joints**: mobile joints consisting of hyaline cartilage covering juxtaposed bone ends surrounded by a capsule, the innermost layer of which is synovium
  - Factors to consider in joint motion
    - Joint geometry
    - Loading environment
    - Soft tissue and articular surface load sharing
  - Loading is accomplished through deformation of the whole joint complex.
- **Amphiarthroses**: less mobile structure consisting of a fibrocartilaginous plate between two bone ends covered by hyaline cartilage with an intervening "disc" material surrounded by a fibrous capsule
  - Examples include the symphysis pubis, the posterior superior two thirds of the sacroiliac joint (anterior inferior third is synovial), and the intervertebral disc (see Chapter 23).
  - Nature of intervening material determines the degree of motion achieved.
- **Syndesmoses**: nonmobile junction between bone ends, consisting of a simple fibrous connection
  - Examples include the distal tibiofibular joint and the skull sutures.

Disorders of joints are numerous. The essential steps of history, physical examination, problem definition, and investigation will usually lead the clinician to an ordered approach, a listing of options that leads to further inquiry, and usually an ultimate diagnosis. An understanding of normal growth and development of joints provides a basis on which to develop models for the pathophysiology of disease.

CLASSIFICATION

The classification of joint disorders is shown in Box 21-1.

DEVELOPMENT OF DIATHRODIAL JOINTS

(Limb bud development is reviewed in Chapter 14, Growth and Development of the Musculoskeletal System.)

In tribute to the late Donald E. Sweet, Director of Department of Orthopaedic Pathology, Armed Forces Institute of Pathology, Washington, DC.

I. Osteoarthritis
  A. Primary
  B. Secondary

II. Inflammatory Arthritis
  A. Rheumatoid arthritis
  B. Juvenile rheumatoid arthritis (Still's disease)
  C. Spondyloarthropathies
    1. Ankylosing spondylitis
    2. Reactive arthritis
    3. Psoriatic arthritis
    4. Arthritis associated with inflammatory bowel disease
    5. Undifferentiated

III. Infectious Arthritis
  A. Bacterial
  B. Granulomatous (tubercular, fungal, sarcoidosis)
  C. Lyme arthritis

IV. Metabolic
  A. Gout
  B. CPPD crystal deposition disease
  C. Ochronosis
  D. Hemophilia

V. Circulatory Disorders Affecting Joints
  A. Neuropathic arthropathy
  B. Avascular necrosis

VI. Anomalies
  A. Epiphysealis hemimelica

the central cartilage, mesenchymal cells continue to transform into all elements of the limb (skeletal muscle, ligaments, tendons, fat, vascular elements).

- Dense interzones, darker areas between the chondrified bone models, appear at 6 weeks and will become the joints (Fig. 21-1).
- Cavities within interzones appear at 10 weeks (Fig. 21-2).
- Mechanism of cavity formation: genetically determined enzymatic destruction with or without simple elaboration of synovial fluid; does not require activity of muscles, often occurs before adjacent muscles have formed or attached
- Persistence and maintenance of joints, once formed, require muscle action. Formation of the unique anatomy of each joint unfolds locally.
- All of the knee structures are present at 14 weeks. Menisci form as fibrocartilaginous semicircles with peripheral attachment; at no time in normal development are they complete discs separating the bone ends.
- All elements of the hip are formed at 4.5 months.

NORMAL STRUCTURE AND FUNCTION OF JOINTS

- Homeostasis in a diarthrodial joint involves important relationships between the three key components of the joint: articular cartilage, synovium, and subchondral bone.
  - Three important vectors of circulatory, mechanical, and metabolic influences are in constant interplay at any given time, affecting each of these components.

Articular Cartilage

- Articular cartilage is aneural and avascular, with diffusion from synovial fluid through the extracellular matrix being the route for its nutrition.

- Beginning during the sixth week, condensed cells in central mesenchyme within each limb bud become chondroblasts, making very primitive cartilage, so-called cartilage models of each bone.
- By end of the eighth week within each limb bud, beyond

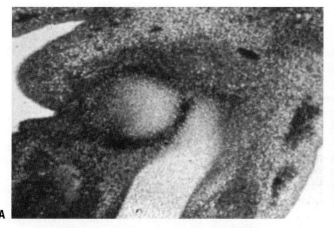
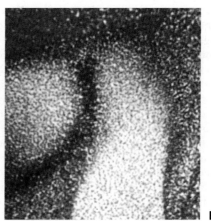

Figure 21-1 Limb bud. (**A**) Cross-section of limb bud shows early cartilage models, forming from mesenchymal cells that have modulated to form early cartilage. The dark area, the interzone between the cartilage models, is the joint anlage. (**B**) Higher-power view of the interzone shows that at this time (6 weeks), the interzone is a collection of primitive cells that have coalesced between the lighter-staining cartilage model bones.

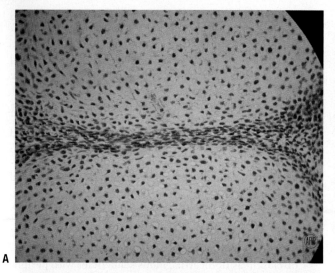

A

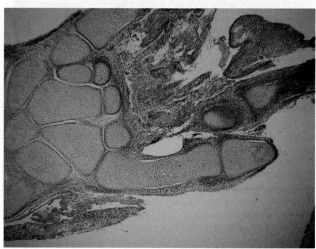

B

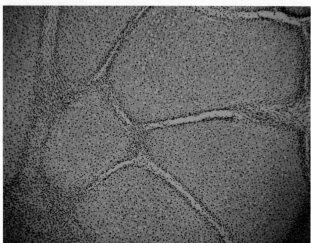

C

Figure 21-2   Synovial joint development. (**A**) Cells in the interzone flatten out and begin to secrete synovial fluid. The primitive cells, densely packed, are pushed apart by the fluid thus elaborated, and ultimately a joint space is created. On either side of the joint space the cells flatten out. (**B**) Section of the end of the limb but in an embryo (estimated 10 weeks). Portions of the thumb, index, and little finger as well as the carpal bone cartilage models are seen. Some joints have well-developed joint spaces, and some are at an earlier stage or the cut has missed the joint space. (**C**) At a higher power, some of the cartilage cells are beginning to hypertrophy. The interosseous ligaments between trapezium and capitate and between lunate and triquetrum are seen.

- Chondrocyte mediates all processes for articular cartilage: synthesis, maintenance, degradation, and repair.
- Repair is problematic (see Chapter 14) because the replacement material that results from the repair process lacks the normal architecture of the articular cartilage (see Fig. 20-1A in Chapter 20).
- Each joint is unique, reflecting its biomechanical tasks of motion, weight transmission, and stability. Inherent in the structure of each joint is conforming bony and articular surface anatomy, the synovial lining layer, ligaments and capsule with unique local geometry determined by the motion required, allowing recesses for accumulation and disposition of debris, and specialized fluid transport channels. The joint remodels throughout life, shedding material and cells from the surface of the articular cartilage, and replacing these cells with those arising from a growth zone located adjacent to the tidemark.
- Motion and activity within physiologic limits are essential. An appropriate exercise pattern throughout life promotes through Wolff's law the development and maintenance of optimal structure of bone, articular cartilage, ligaments, muscles, and tendons.

Synovium

- The role of the synovium is to maintain joint homeostasis and to provide the appropriate response in disease states. Synovium differs from true epithelium because it has no basement membrane, thus facilitating exchange of nutrients and other substances between the vascular system and the joint fluid.
- Three histologic types are described:
- Areolar synovium
  - Structure
    - Surface compact layer of collagen (types I and III) and synovial cells
    - Deeper layer is of fibrovascular matrix, vessels, nerves, migratory cells (mast cells and mononuclear cells), and ground substance, including dermatan sulfate and hyaluronic acid.
  - Three cell types exist:
    - Phagocytic cells (type A synoviocytes)
    - Maintenance cells (type B synoviocytes)
    - Intermediate forms (type C synoviocytes)
- Fibrous synovium
  - Present in transition zones adjacent to ligament surfaces

- Provides a conduit for neurovascular elements of the ligament
- Structure: surface compact zone denser and more flattened adjacent to the collagen lining; surface can be discontinuous
- Fatty or adipose synovium
  - Prototypical location is the fat pad of the knee; acts as mobile packing tissue, changing shape to match joint motion
    - Structure: Surface layer is collagen, surface lining cells, and neurovascular elements forming a continuous array with only a few very small gaps a few microns wide.
    - Deeper layer is fat and fibrous septa containing occasional synovial cells, vessels, and nerves.
    - Function of the fat pad of the knee may be much more complex than simple padding and protection, and may include roles in:
      - Paracrine function through the elaboration of cytokines
      - Mechanical function to condition motion between the patella, femur, and tibia
      - Neural function in proprioception, or in reactive neural inflammation through substance P fibers

Subchondral Bone

Each joint is a unique engine of force transmission. Dr. Sweet used an analogy in which one can think of the articular cartilage as representing the tire, the subchondral bone the rim, and the cancellous array the spokes. Cortical bone then acts as a deformable unit, accepting force and transmitting it to the metaphyseal cancellous array, which distributes the force uniformly to the articular cartilage (Fig. 21-3).

- Changes in the articular cartilage diminish its ability to absorb compressive loads, causing an alteration to the subchondral bone.
- Changes in the structure of subchondral bone can result in loss of structural support, exposing the cartilage chondrocytes to forces exceeding their tolerance.
  - In avascular necrosis (AVN), death of a portion of the subchondral plate leads to a reactive zone of granulation tissue in which osteoclastic activity leads to a loss of the bony supporting arch for cartilage, often leading to collapse and progressive arthritis.
  - In osteoarthritis, subchondral bone stiffens; it is not known whether this is primary or secondary to cartilage change.

Summary

- A diarthrodial joint can be considered a functioning unit, the integral elements of which are:
  - Articular cartilage
  - Synovium
  - Subchondral bone
  - Capsule/ligaments
  - Synovial fluid

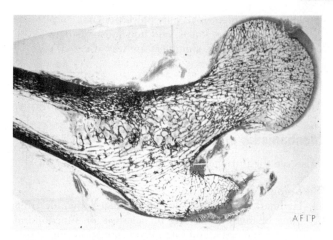

Figure 21-3   Proximal femur. Specimen from a patient with renal osteodystrophy, selected to show the bony structure: deformable cortex (which is osteopenic) linked to cancellous array to subchondral plate. Mechanical force from the cortex is linked to the cancellous trabeculae, which form a honeycomb-like pattern of interconnected bony plates, passing the force to the superiorly attached subchondral plate. Mechanical force is thus transmitted uniformly to the acetabulum. Not shown is a similar arrangement on the acetabular side where analogous cancellous trabecular arcs pass the force through the ilium to the sacroiliac joint.

- Any arthropathy will inevitably affect each of these elements.
- Beyond these inherent elements, to function appropriately, a joint requires motor support (e.g., skeletal muscle with intact innervation). Primary muscle (muscular dystrophy, inflammatory myopathies) and nerve disorders, both peripheral (nerve injury, peripheral neuropathies) and central (stroke), may lead to loss of motion and disordered joint function. In both instances, secondary atrophic changes occur in all of the elements of the associated joints; late degenerative disease may then follow. Disease in a joint leads to loss of function. Pain, instability, and loss of range of motion then lead to secondary changes in the supporting muscle groups, with disuse atrophy and weakness.

OSTEOARTHRITIS

Definition

- Osteoarthritis includes a heterogeneous group of conditions of multifactorial etiology, characterized by joint signs and symptoms, which are associated with defective integrity of articular cartilage, in addition to related changes in the underlying bone.
- Symptoms include aching, intermittent pain, stiffness, loss of motion, swelling (usually), and crepitus.

Epidemiology

- Prevalence increases progressively with age: 60% of men and 70% of women
- Leading cause of chronic disability at older age

- Joint involvement is usually polyarticular.
  - Hands, spine, knees, and hips most frequent
  - Wrists, elbows, shoulders are less affected.

Classification

Table 21-1 summarizes the classification of osteoarthritis.

Mechanisms of Joint Destruction

(Also see the introduction to this topic in Chapter 14.)

Pathologic Sequence
- Hallmark finding (late): loss of cartilage with underlying bony changes consisting of sclerosis of subchondral bone, bone cysts, and osteophyte formation (Fig. 21-4)
- The growth zone adjacent to the tidemark contributes to articular cartilage growth throughout life. Normal aging changes the contours of joints. Remodeling can add length (progressive), subtract from bone length (regressive), and add diameter (circumferential).
  - When the process is balanced, there is no disease.
  - When remodeling is unbalanced, the disease process of osteoarthritis occurs.
- Early
  - Often focal, osteoarthritis starts with superficial fibrillation and loss of small proteoglycans, decorin and biglycan (usually associated with fibrils at articular surface), and aggrecan (Fig. 21-5).
  - Increased type II collagen cleavage occurs by action of collagenase, aggrecan cleavage, and degradation of small proteoglycans.
- Intermediate

- Continued loss of proteoglycans, with increased fibrillation down to subchondral bone (see Fig. 21-5)
- Increase in number of degenerating chondrocytes, with cloning and regeneration of cells
- Late (see Fig. 21-4)
  - Mechanical abrasion of degenerative cartilage continues, with progressive loss of coverage so that the surface becomes eburnated. The loss of cartilage allows increased force to be transmitted to the subchondral plate. Increased bone formation (Wolff's law) then occurs, and over time the subchondral bone becomes sclerotic.
  - Subchondral cysts develop from two potential mechanisms:
    - Focal mesenchymal proliferation and accumulation of "stromal mucin" (myxoid change) in marrow fat
    - Surface cracks allow forced entry of joint fluid into the subchondral bone.
  - Proliferation of tufts of metaplastic cartilage along denuded bone create a new, mechanically inferior, cartilaginous joint surface (mechanism of "healing" seen after realignment osteotomy).
  - Cartilage fragments shed from surface may grow as metaplastic cartilage in the joint space concentrically; this may evoke secondary metaplastic cartilaginous change and mimic primary synovial osteochondromatosis.
  - Breakdown of cartilaginous fragments may induce an inflammatory response, including chondrogranulomas.
  - Hemorrhage of friable synovium may occur, producing hemosiderin staining of synovium over time.

TABLE 21-1 CLASSIFICATION OF OSTEOARTHRITIS

Type	Association	Presumed Mechanism
Primary	Genetic	Subtle abnormalities of articular cartilage
Secondary		
Mechanical	Post-traumatic; post–slipped capital femoral epiphysis	Damage to articular cartilage; joint incongruity
	Epiphyseal dysplasias	Abnormal articular cartilage; abnormal joint shape
	Blount's disease	Mechanism not known
	Overuse	Damage to articular cartilage
	Paget's disease	Joint incongruity; altered subchondral bone
	Joint instability (Ehlers-Danlos)	Damage to articular cartilage
Metabolic	Ochronosis; gout; CPPD crystal deposition disease	Abnormal metabolite (crystal) deposition in cartilage
	Hemochromatosis	Not known
	Acromegaly	Overgrowth of articular cartilage produces joint incongruity; cartilage may be abnormal.
Postinflammatory	Septic or inflammatory arthritis; hemophilia	Destruction of articular cartilage

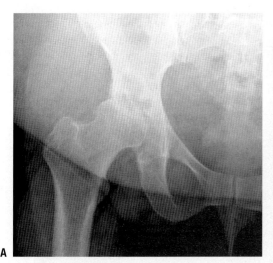 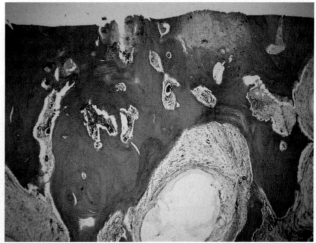

A   B

Figure 21-4 Osteoarthritic hip. (**A**) Radiograph showing advanced osteoarthritis with complete loss of surface cartilage, exposing dense subchondral bone. Numerous cysts are present filled with amorphous myxoid material. The bone adjacent to the cysts is sclerotic, representing altered mechanical force transmission around the area of the cyst normally filled with cancellous bone. (**B**) Photomicrograph showing advanced osteoarthritis with complete loss of surface cartilage, exposing dense subchondral bone. There is no definable articular cartilage present. Numerous cysts are present filled with amorphous myxoid material; the bone adjacent to the cysts is sclerotic, representing altered mechanical force transmission around the area of the cyst normally filled with cancellous bone.

Radiologic Findings (see Fig. 21-4)

- The classic findings are of joint space narrowing (reflecting loss of cartilage), subchondral sclerosis (increased bone formation secondary to increased force across the joint surface), osteophyte formation (progressive remodeling), and subchondral cyst formation (mechanism controversial, secondary to break in subchondral bone or arising as a result of metaplasia of subchondral marrow in the environment of increased mechanical force).

INFLAMMATORY ARTHRITIS

Mechanism

- Inflammatory arthritis is associated with specific recognition of antigenic triggers that are not fully known.
- Specific immune response occurs via two cellular mechanisms and requires initiation by antigen presenting cells, which present antigens to the lymphocytes.
  - *Humoral immunity* is mediated by B lymphocytes, which produce antibodies (Ab) responsible for recognition of foreign antigens, and their elimination with the aid of complement.
  - *Cellular immunity* is mediated by T lymphocytes, which recognize and eliminate intracellular antigens.
    - CD4 T cells (CD4 glycoprotein surface molecule) secrete cytokines.
    - CD8 T cells (CD8 glycoprotein surface molecule) kill antigen-bearing target cells.

- This process is governed by the MHC region of genes (HLA genes).

Cytokines

- A complex network of cytokines functions in initiating and perpetuating arthritis.
- These polypeptide signaling substances are produced by a host of cells, including synovial cells, chondrocytes, monocytes, macrophages, T lymphocytes, B lymphocytes, other connective tissue cells, and endothelial cells.

RHEUMATOID ARTHRITIS

Definition

- Rheumatoid arthritis is an immunologically mediated inflammatory disorder of synovial joints. It can have systemic manifestations, characterized by multiple joint involvement beginning with synovitis and later arthritis that can become chronic and disabling.

Epidemiology

- There is considerable variation of disease occurrence.
  - Highest prevalence (0.5% to 1%): Northern European, North American, some Native Americans
  - Intermediate prevalence (0.3% to 0.7%): Southern European
  - Low prevalence (0.1% to 0.5%): developing countries, rural Africa
- Multifactorial disease
  - Genetic susceptibility

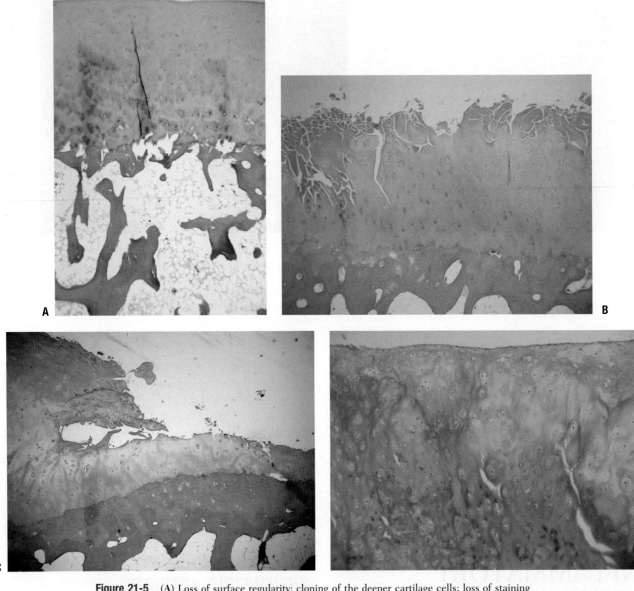

Figure 21-5   (**A**) Loss of surface regularity; cloning of the deeper cartilage cells; loss of staining pattern of proteoglycans; subchondral plate shows evidence of turnover with increased cement lines, and Howship's lacunae. (**B**) Further loss of surface regularity, and of proteoglycan staining pattern; the development of fissures; thickening of subchondral bone; cloning of chondrocytes in the basal layers. (**C**) There is fragmentation of the surface cartilage, with a small piece flaking off; the surface wear has left just a thin layer of articular cartilage remaining; the subchondral bone has become a solid plate of dense cortical bone. (**D**) The cartilage that flakes off can grow in the synovial fluid and become a "joint mouse"; calcification of the senescent cartilage in the loose body makes it radiographically visible, and it may mimic synovial osteochondromatosis, a metaplastic condition in which the synovial lining changes and islands of cartilaginous differentiation develop in the joint lining. This image shows the fibrocartilaginous surface of a joint mouse; the darker-staining deeper areas represent calcification of the cartilage.

- Environmental, lifestyle, and personal characteristics
    - Sex (female:male 2 to 3:1)
    - Age (onset fifth decade)
    - Positive factors associated with a reduced incidence
        - Hormonal (parity, pregnancy, oral contraceptives)
        - Dietary (fish, olive oil, cooked vegetables, omega-3 long chain polyunsaturated fatty acids)
    - Negative factors associated with an increased incidence
        - Smoking (increased incidence)
        - Infectious agents
        - Socioeconomic (low status worse)
        - Ethnic factors (higher prevalence in Northern Europe and North America)

Etiology

- Susceptible individual (genetic and immunological predisposition) plus trigger:
    - HLA-DR4 and DW4 are most prevalent phenotypes (80%).
    - Trigger is unknown; possibilities are environmental antigen (infection most likely) versus nonspecific local stimuli (trauma, infection, allergic reaction, immunologic materials).
    - For infectious model, Epstein-Barr virus or retroviruses are most likely initiators.

Pathophysiology

- Regardless of trigger, IgM is produced, directed against altered autologous IgG; leukocytes phagocytose the IgM/IgG complexes along with fibrin and complement; necrosis of these cells induces release of lysosomal enzymes, which cause an acute inflammatory reaction.
- Infectious trigger
    - Environmental antigen is attached to an antigen presenting cell macrophage and presented to T cell (CD4 phenotype is most populous in rheumatoid arthritis pannus).
    - CD4+ T cells produce numerous cytokines, the actions of which include:
        - Catabolic effects on cartilage
        - Activation of B cells, which differentiate into plasma cells producing IgG and IgM
- Noninfectious trigger
    - Nonspecific stimuli induce local changes that promote the differentiation of dendritic cells in the rheumatoid synovium; these cells present an autologous Ag to the T cell, which then initiate the disease process.
    - Progression continues as T cells clone, resulting in recruitment of other effector cells.

Clinical Features

- Diagnostic criteria are given in Box 21-2.
    - **Typical**: insidious malaise, fatigue, weakness, and

BOX 21-2 DIAGNOSTIC CRITERIA FOR RHEUMATOID ARTHRITIS

- Morning stiffness of at least 1 hour*
- Symmetrical joint swelling and involvement*
- Arthritis of hand joints (at least one area swollen in a wrist, metacarpophalangeal, or proximal interphalangeal joint)*
- Arthritis in at least three joint areas** with swelling or fluid*
- Subcutaneous nodules
- Radiographic changes typical of rheumatoid arthritis
- Positive rheumatoid factor

*Specified criteria: These four must be present for at least 6 weeks.
**Right or left proximal interphalangeal, metacarpophalangeal, wrist, elbow, knee, ankle, and metatarsophalangeal joints.

---

vague arthralgias for weeks, followed by joint pain, swelling, morning stiffness of several joints, usually wrists, proximal joints of fingers and toes, usually symmetric distribution; any other major joint can be involved.
- **Pauciarticular**: One third of patients have involvement of one or a few joints; then disease spreads to affect other joints, usually symmetrically.
- **Acute**: Some patients may have an acute onset with fever and multiple swollen painful joints.

Diagnosis

Physical Examination

Articular System
- Early: warmth, tenderness, swelling with boggy feel to synovium with cutaneous ruddy cyanotic hue; muscle weakness and atrophy adjacent to involved joints
- Late: Loss of motion, flexion contractures, ankylosis may occur with deformities of joints of hands and feet (swan-neck, boutonnière, cock-up toes, ulnar deviation of wrist and metacarpophalangeal bones).
- Spine: Cervical spine is often involved; lumbar spine is relatively spared.
    - **When considering surgery on a patient with RA, always rule out subluxation of the atlantoaxial joint; obtain a flexion/extension lateral to show instability of this joint; can produce compression of the spinal cord by the odontoid; look for symptoms and signs of cord compression: bladder dysfunction, sphincter laxity, circumanal hypesthesia, and long tract signs.**
- Popliteal (Baker's) cyst, often present, may rupture and mimic thrombophlebitis; both may coexist; investigation (Doppler/ultrasound, or venogram) is indicated.
- Rheumatoid nodules (necrobiotic granulomas) are present in 20% of patients—usually extensor surfaces of elbows, fingers, and other areas subject to pressure.

Systemic and Unique Local Features
- Pulmonary: diffuse interstitial fibrosis
- Cardiac: unusual, may involve vasculitis leading to in-

farction; granulomas may affect valves; pericarditis with tamponade may occur

- Reticuloendothelial system: Splenomegaly occurs in 10%; regional lymphadenopathy may also develop.
- Felty syndrome: rheumatoid arthritis + splenomegaly + neutropenia; appears in patients with longstanding disease; mechanism of neutropenia: antibodies to neutrophils, attachment of immune complexes to neutrophils and subsequent sequestration in spleen; marrow suppression
- Sjögren syndrome: Keratoconjunctivitis sicca (dry eyes + dry mouth + rheumatoid arthritis) occurs in ~15% of patients.

Synovial Fluid Aspiration
- Milky turbid appearance; 20,000 to 50,000 inflammatory cells/mm³ with 50% polys; in infection, there are >100,000 cells/mm³, of which >75% are polys.

Radiologic Findings
The radiological findings mirror the stage of the disease:

- Periarticular soft tissue swelling
- Bilateral symmetrical joint involvement
- Uniform loss of joint space
- Marginal erosions
- Juxta-articular osteoporosis
- Juxta-articular periostitis (not common, is more commonly associated with spondyloarthropathy)
- Large pseudocysts
- Joint deformity, including subluxation, dislocation, articular bony destruction, bony ankylosis, complete destruction of joint space

Figure 21-6A shows the radiology of a normal hand and wrist. This should be carefully examined and compared to Figure 21-6B, which shows the hand of a patient with rheumatoid arthritis, moderately advanced in the wrist and mildly involved in the digits.

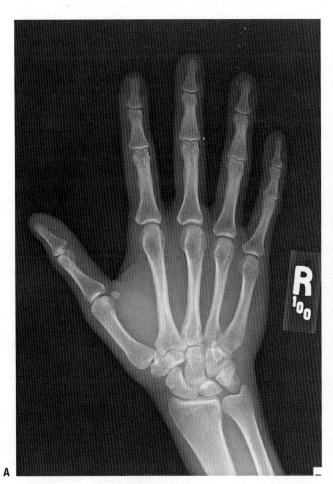
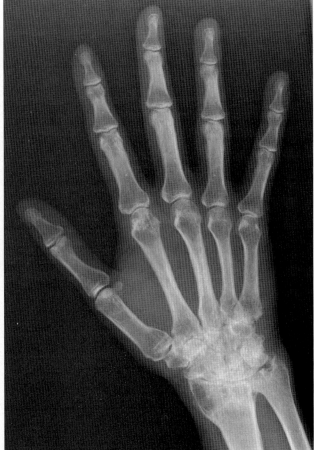

Figure 21-6 (A) Radiograph of a normal hand shows the numerous small joints of the hand with normal bone density, discrete joint spaces, and normal contour of adjacent soft tissues. (B) Radiograph of a hand with rheumatoid arthritis shows widespread juxta-articular osteopenia and early erosion (irregularity of the cortical surface) of both sides of the index metacarpal head at the level of the joint recess. The carpal joints show loss of cartilage space and a mottled sclerosis of the carpal bones with discrete circular zones of decreased density suggesting cyst formation. There are numerous focal areas of cortical lysis.

Pathologic Findings

- Chronic inflammatory synovitis attacks any synovial surface (joints, bursae, tenosynovial sheaths).
- Serum and synovial fluid contain immunoglobulins (mostly IgM) produced as antibodies to autologous IgG altered in some way in rheumatoid arthritis.
  - These immunoglobulins in serum are known as rheumatoid factor (RF) and are present in 70% of patients.

Synovium

- Nonsuppurative chronic inflammation of synovium with hypertrophy and hyperplasia of the synovial lining cells; the surface is papillary or villiform (Fig. 21-7)
- Scattered giant cells can be present among the synovial lining cells.
- Inflammation consists of infiltration of the synovial membrane by lymphocytes, plasma cells, and some mast cells; hyperplastic lymphoid follicles and a fibrinous exudate are present (see Fig. 21-7).
  - Plasma cells often contain cytoplasmic eosinophilic inclusions of immunoglobulin (Russell bodies).
  - In acute phase, polymorphonuclear leukocytes predominate.
  - Vasculitis may be prominent.
- Effects of synovial proliferation (Fig. 21-8)
  - Cartilage
    - Inflamed hypertrophied synovium (pannus) creeps over articular cartilage, depriving it of nutrition and enzymatically degrading the matrix; Figure 21-8 demonstrates these changes in articular cartilage even in the absence of an overlying pannus.
    - With complete loss of cartilage, the end result is fibrous or bony ankylosis.
  - Ligaments/capsule

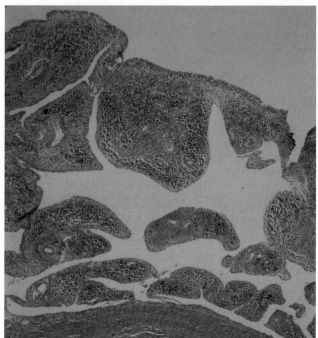

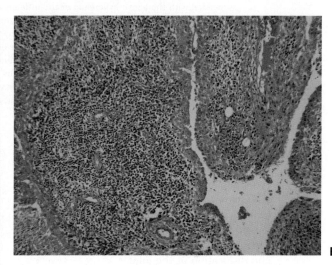

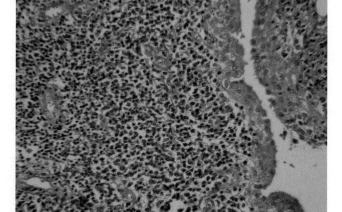

Figure 21-7 Rheumatoid arthritis. (**A**) Low-power view of nonspecific follicular synovitis with several rounded oval dark lymphoid aggregates beneath the synovial membrane. (**B**) Medium-power view showing the hyperplastic, nodular lymphoid aggregates typical of rheumatoid synovitis. Multiple lymphoid aggregates can produce a villonodular appearance to the synovium. Inflammation can vary but often is quite pronounced and accompanied by abundant fibrinous exudates (not evident in this field). These exudates can fill the inflamed joint, presenting as "rice bodies" at arthrotomy. The synovium is proliferative, appearing many cells thick. (**C**) High-power field showing cells involved in the lymphoid aggregate, a mixture of predominant lymphocytes, and a few plasma cells and histiocytes.

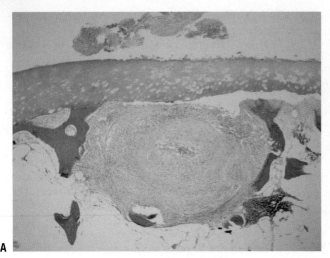 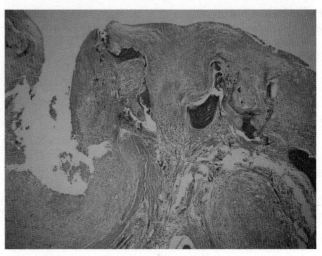

A   B

Figure 21-8   Rheumatoid arthritis in subchondral bone. **(A)** The chronic inflammatory process has reached the bone adjacent to the articular cartilage. Bone has been deleted (osteoclastic removal associated with the active hyperemia of the inflammatory process), and an inflammatory focus has replaced the marrow and bone. This has the appearance of a rheumatoid nodule with chronic inflammatory cells (type not apparent at this power) surrounding a zone of fibrinoid necrosis. There is a collection of fibrinous material in the joint space above. The articular cartilage is affected; it appears porous and shows increased cloning of cells and abnormal staining suggesting loss of proteoglycans. **(B)** View of severe rheumatoid arthritis with pannus destroying the articular surface and involving the medullary space. There is no recognizable articular surface. Shards of subchondral bone, with divot-like irregularities in the surfaces, Howship's lacunae, indicative of clast activity.

- Inflammatory tissue mass (pannus) is highly vascular, with an activated cellular mass producing cytokines as well as clastic cells, which themselves produce cytokines and enzymes producing tissue lysis.
- Destruction and weakening of the ligaments and capsule with resulting instability, subluxation, and dislocation of the joint
  - Subchondral bone
    - Subchondral bone is attacked by the pannus at the joint margins, producing radiographically apparent marginal erosions.
    - The active hyperemic flush pervades the entire juxta-articular region, inducing clastic removal of bone and explaining the juxta-articular osteopenia that accompanies inflammatory arthritides.
    - Vasculitis and inflammation can extend throughout the subchondral bone, inducing lysis of articular cartilage from below in addition to the effects of the pannus above (see Fig. 21-8).

Rheumatoid Nodule
- Can be the first indication of rheumatoid arthritis; locations: subcutaneous extensor surfaces, gastrointestinal tract, lungs, heart, and any synovial membrane
- Associated with vasculitis
- Irregularly shaped central necrobiotic zone of necrotic fibrinoid material, surrounded by a zone of pallisaded histiocytes and chronic inflammatory cells encircled by

dense fibrosis; vasculitis may be seen in surrounding tissue (Fig. 21-9)

JUVENILE INFLAMMATORY ARTHRITIS/ RHEUMATOID ARTHRITIS

Definition
- A chronic inflammatory arthritis of children similar to rheumatoid arthritis; often less severe, but with analogous radiologic and histologic findings

Diagnosis
Clinical Features
- Presentation varies:
  - 25% systemic presentation with self-limited course
    - Male > female
    - Median age of onset 5 years
    - High fever, nonpruritic erythematous macular or maculopapular rash in association with rash
    - Reticuloendothelial system involvement with lymphadenopathy, hepatosplenomegaly, pneumonitis, and pleuritis
    - Cardiac involvement with pericarditis and/or myocarditis (rarely)
    - 25% of patients have severe, destructive polyarthropathy.
    - Seronegative and antinuclear antibody (ANA) negative

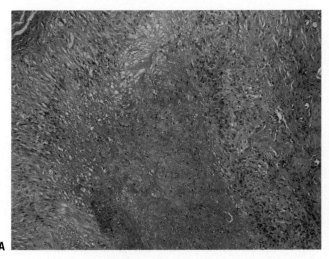
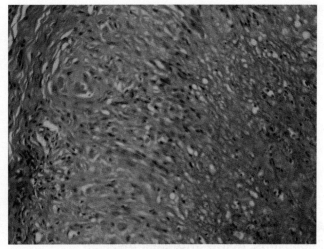

A   B

Figure 21-9   Rheumatoid nodule. (**A**) Close-up view of palisades of histiocytes of the rheumatoid nodule surrounding a central zone of amorphous fibrinous material. On the far left and right are spindle cells within the fibrous capsule. (**B**) Close-up of the transition: capsule on the left, palisading histiocytes in the middle, central zone of necrosis on the right. This picture of a rheumatoid nodule might be confused with a caseating granuloma of tuberculosis. Mycobacterial and other infectious granulomas generally have multinucleated giant cells and caseous necrosis (tends to appear more granular than the fibrinoid necrosis seen here).

- 30% pauciarticular disease
  - Female > male
  - Involvement of one or more joints, usually knees or ankles
  - Mild arthritis, excellent prognosis
  - Eye involvement is a problem, with 50% of patients having chronic iridocyclitis, which may progress to band keratopathy, cataracts, and loss of vision.
  - RF negative
  - ANA present in 50% to 60%
- 25% polyarthritic without systemic disease with good prognosis
  - Insidious onset, in small joints of hands and feet
  - Mainly affects young females (median onset 2 years)
  - RF negative
  - 25% are ANA positive.
  - Special techniques demonstrate IgG and IgA rheumatoid factors in more than half.
- 5% to 10% polyarticular with positive RF
  - Female > male
  - Median age at onset is 12.
  - Analogous to adult rheumatoid arthritis in clinical presentation and course.

JUVENILE INFLAMMATORY ARTHRITIS/ ANKYLOSING SPONDYLITIS

- May also present in childhood
- Represents 20% of children who present with juvenile-onset arthritis
- Male > female
- Median onset 10 years
- Present with early hip girdle symptoms
- Often iridocyclitis
- RF and ANA negative
- HLA-B27 positive in 75%, as compared to negative finding in other types of childhood arthritis

SPONDYLOARTHROPATHIES

- The spondyloarthropathies are a heterogeneous group of inflammatory diseases characterized by spinal and peripheral joint oligoarthritis, inflammation of the attachments of ligaments and tendons to bones (enthesitis), and, at times, mucocutaneous, ocular, and/or cardiac manifestations.
- They include:
  - Ankylosing spondylitis
  - Reactive arthritis, known previously as Reiter's syndrome
  - Psoriatic arthritis
  - Enteropathic arthritis (related to inflammatory bowel diseases, ulcerative colitis, or Crohn's disease)
  - Juvenile spondyloarthritis
  - Undifferentiated spondyloarthropathies (patients expressing elements but failing to fulfill accepted criteria for any of the above)
- Pathogenesis involves an inherent "early warning system" of the synovium that is acutely responsive to deposition of immunogenic fragments. This involves a humorally mediated process that initiates a cascade.
- Offending fragments could be immune complexes, mRNA/DNA from the initiating organism, or actual fragments of the microbe.

- The process of crossing vessel walls and synovial membrane can be assisted by adhesion molecules (integrins and selectins) on white blood cells carrying ingested pathogens or parts.
  - P-selectin shows affinity for attachment to synovium; may act as bridge allowing pathogenetic material into the cells, precipitating the synovial process.
- Presented with this immunogenic stimulus, antigen-specific CD4 T cells, synovial intimal lining macrophages, and B cells all participate in the production of key cytokines (tumor necrosis factor alpha [TNF-α], interleukins [ILs]), which initiate the inflammatory process.

Ankylosing Spondylitis (Rheumatoid Spondylitis, Marie-Strumpell Disease)

Definition
Ankylosing spondylitis is a chronic and usually progressive inflammatory disease involving the spine and adjacent soft tissues, sacroiliac joints almost always, hips and shoulders often, and other joints less frequently.

Epidemiology
- Male:female, 3 to 10:1
- Concordance rate in identical twins as high as 63% (compared to 23% in nonidentical twins)
- Histocompatibility testing shows HLA-B27 in >90% of patients versus 7% in the normal white population.
- Less frequent incidence of ankylosing spondylitis and HLA-B27 in blacks
- Prevalence of ankylosing spondylitis 1% in white population
- Ankylosing spondylitis is a disorder of the young, with onset in second or third decades.
- 20% of people who carry HLA-B27 will develop ankylosing spondylitis.

Diagnosis

Clinical Features
- Constitutional symptoms are mild in the absence of advanced disease.
  - Spine
    - Low back pain with stiffness, worse in morning; nocturnal back pain
    - Mimics sciatica in 10%
    - No evidence of nerve root irritation or compression initially
    - Progressive rigidity of the spine
    - Atlantoaxial subluxation and spinal cord compression less common than in rheumatoid arthritis
    - Cervical spine that has undergone multiple-level fusion is susceptible to fracture.
  - Peripheral joints
    - 25% of patients develop peripheral arthritis.
    - Hips can be severely involved with arthritis indistinguishable from osteoarthritis.

- Knees and heels may be involved.
- Anterior chest pain and pleuritic pain may occur (inflammation at insertion sites of costosternal and costovertebral muscles and at manubriosternal and sternoclavicular joints).
- Extra-articular manifestations
  - Ocular: Acute anterior uveitis (20% to 30%) may be initial indication of ankylosing spondylitis.
  - Cardiac: aortic valve incompetence (3%), may require replacement; cardiac conduction defects, may require pacemaker
  - Pulmonary: apical pulmonary fibrosis, chronic productive cough, and dyspnea
  - Renal: Amyloidosis may cause uremia.
  - Osseous: osteoporosis
  - Neurological: cauda equine syndrome (rare) late complication, possibly due to arachnoiditis or ischemia; slowly progressive; treatment problematic

Pathologic Findings
- Diarthroidal joints
  - Synovitis resembling rheumatoid arthritis begins in the apophyseal joints of the spine, costovertebral joints, and sacroiliac joints.
  - Same pathological findings in the hip, shoulder, and other peripheral joints
  - Bony erosions and cartilage destruction ensue, followed by ankylosis.
- Amphiarthrial joints
  - Intervertebral discs, manubriosternal joint, and symphysis pubis are invaded by granulation tissue.
  - The cartilage is destroyed, and local fibrosis and then ankylosis occur.

Radiologic Findings (Figs. 21-10 and 21-11)
- Vertebral bodies have squared margins (marginal erosion) or central cyst suggesting infection.
- Syndesmophytes at margins of vertebral bodies produce "bamboo spine" appearance (ossification of outer layers of annulus fibrosis); differential diagnosis with diffuse idiopathic skeletal hyperostosis: lack of ossification of anterior and posterior longitudinal ligaments in ankylosing spondylitis (see Fig. 21-11)
- Diffuse osteoporosis
- Fusion of sacroiliac joints
- Erosions and ossification of insertions of ligaments, tendons, and capsules into bone (spinous processes, greater trochanters, pelvis, and heels)
- Involvement of peripheral joints resembles osteoarthritis late.

Reactive Arthritis

Definition
- An arthritis that is preceded by an immunologic sensitization
- The term "Reiter's syndrome" applies only to the classic triad of arthritis, urethritis, and conjunctivitis.

Classification
For some organisms, the link between infection in locations other than the joints is clear. For others an associa-

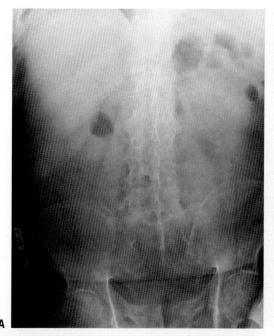

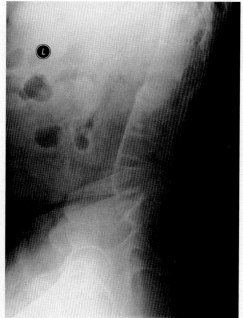

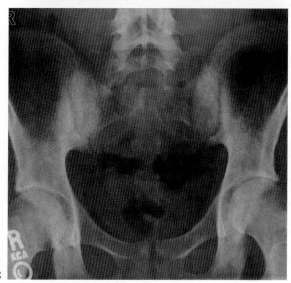

Figure 21-10 Ankylosing spondylitis. (**A**) Anterior-posterior view of lumbar spine shows ankylosis of the sacroiliac joints and the lumbar spine. There is joint space narrowing of the hip joints indicative of early secondary osteoarthritis. (**B**) Lateral view of the lumbar spine demonstrating ossification of the anterior longitudinal ligament, preservation of the disc spaces, and osteopenia of the vertebral bodies, the margins of which are "squared off." (**C**) A 27-year-old man with low back pain and ankylosing spondylitis. Anterior-posterior view of the pelvis shows erosions and sclerosis in a bilateral, symmetrical distribution typical of sacroiliitis of ankylosing spondylitis.

tion exists, but the role of the offending organism as a triggering agent of reactive arthritis is not well established; these organisms are marked with (?) in the classification.

- Urogenic with bacterial associations
  - *Chlamydia trachomatis*
  - *Mycoplasma genialium* (?)
  - *Ureaplasma urealyticum* (?)
  - *Neisseria gonorrhoeae* (?)
- Enterogenic with bacterial associations
  - *Salmonella* (various types)
  - *Shigella* (various types)
  - *Yersinia* (various types)
  - *Campylobacter* (various types)
  - *Clostridium difficile*
- Respiratory tract associated with bacterial associations

- Beta-hemolytic *Streptococcus* (?)
- *Chlamydia pneumoniae*
- Idiopathic: typical clinical presentation without a clear association with an established infection
  - The idiopathic group becomes smaller as more and more new associations are being reported.

Epidemiology

- Risk of reactive arthritis in an enteric infection caused by gram-negative microbes is 1% to 15%.
- HLA-B27 is detected with 5 to 10 times greater frequency in reactive arthritis patients than in the general population.
- Patients are usually young adults (mean age 30 to 40); disease is uncommon in children.

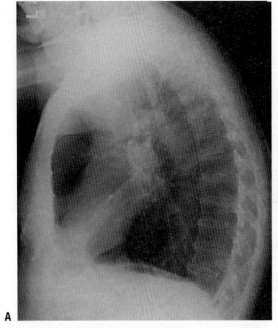

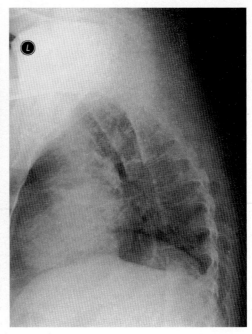

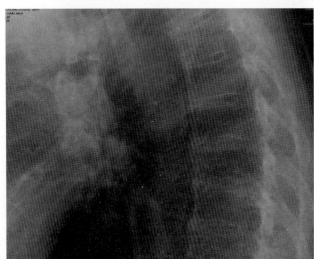

Figure 21-11   Diffuse idiopathic skeletal hyperostosis (DISH). (A) A 73-year-old man with typical manifestations of DISH in the thoracic spine. Lateral view of the thoracic spine shows anterior ossification extending over more than four contiguous vertebral bodies. The ossification is separated from the vertebral bodies by a lucency, indicating the density is in the anterior longitudinal ligament and soft tissues anterior to it. (B) Differential diagnosis: DISH versus ankylosing spondylitis. In this lateral view of ankylosing spondylitis, the anterior ossification merges with the vertebral body. The disc spaces are preserved. In DISH there is extensive calcification of the disc space, as is shown in the magnified view in (C).

Pathophysiology

■ Organisms or bacterial antigens disseminate to the joint, causing inflammation.

■ CD4 + T-cell response drives and supports the arthritic process.

■ Persistence of the microbial structures may be a function of:

   ■ Impaired elimination by a deficient cytokine reaction, such as poor T-helper response

   ■ Defective or aberrant function of HLA B-27

Diagnosis

Clinical Features

■ Onset of arthritis is 1 to 4 weeks after infection; triggering infection may be asymptomatic.

■ Asymmetric oligoarthritis, often large joints of lower ex-

tremities; 50% have arthritis in upper limbs; occasionally present in small joints of hands or feet

■ Associated features

   ■ Enthesitis/bursitis may be associated with arthritis or may be the initial presentation.

   ■ Eye findings are conjunctivitis (usually) or acute anterior uveitis (less frequently).

   ■ Skin rashes can present with several forms.

   ■ Nail changes may mimic those of psoriasis.

   ■ 30% have spondylitis with acute low back pain and buttock radiation.

■ Duration of the acute arthritis is a few months; in a small percentage, the symptoms become intermittent or chronic.

   ■ There are no specific radiologic or pathologic findings; the findings are analogous to mild rheumatoid arthritis.

Psoriatic Arthritis

Definition

- Psoriatic arthritis is a unique inflammatory arthritis associated with psoriasis; the pathology is analogous to that of rheumatoid arthritis.

Epidemiology

- Prevalence of psoriasis is 2% to 3%; prevalence of inflammatory arthritis among patients with psoriasis is ~30%.
- Genetic epidemiology suggests a unique status:
  - Psoriatic arthritis is associated with HLA class 1 alleles, rheumatoid arthritis with class 2 alleles.
- Patients with psoriatic arthritis are at increased risk of death; standardized mortality ratio of 1.62.

Diagnosis

Clinical Features

- The longer the duration of the psoriatic arthritis, the more it tends to become polyarticular.

- Arthritis may precede rash by many years.
- Five clinical patterns most relevant at time of disease onset
  - Distal predominant pattern
  - Oligoarticular asymmetrical
  - Polyarticular rheumatoid arthritis-like: 20% of patients over time develop a destructive arthritis; much more aggressive than previously thought.
  - Spondylitis
  - Arthritis mutilans
- The features of psoriatic arthritis and rheumatoid arthritis are compared in Table 21-2.
- Pathology of psoriatic arthritis is analogous to that of rheumatoid arthritis.

Enteropathic Arthritis (Associated with Ulcerative Colitis and Crohn's Disease)

- Enteropathic arthritis is a form of chronic, inflammatory arthritis associated with the occurrence of inflammatory bowel disease, usually ulcerative colitis or Crohn's disease.

TABLE 21-2 COMPARISON OF PSORIATIC ARTHRITIS AND RHEUMATIC ARTHRITIS

Feature	Psoriatic Arthritis	Rheumatoid Arthritis
Male:female ratio	Equal distribution	More common in women
Hand involvement	Distal joints; arthritis mutilans (resorption of phalanges, metacarpals, or metatarsals)	Metacarpophalangeal/proximal interphalangeal
Ray involvement	All joints of a single digit affected (on just one side, asymmetrical)	Same joints affected in both hands (symmetrical)
Erythema of affected joints	More	Less
Spinal involvement	Paravertebral ossification in lower thoracic, and lumbar regions, plus sacroiliac joints (40% have spondylitis)	Cervical spine most affected
Enthesitis	Yes	No
Tenderness	Mild	More severe
Rheumatoid nodules	No	Yes
Rheumatoid factor	13%	>80%
Radiologic features	Shortening of digits because of bone lysis, most severe form being telescoping of digits; bony fusion may occur, but usual feature is pencil-in-cup deformity; periosteal reactions; dactylitis (inflammation of entire digit) inflammation affecting both joints and tendons	Early: soft tissue swelling, juxta-articular osteopenia. Later: marginal erosions, joint space narrowing. Advanced: destruction of subchondral bone, diffuse osteoporosis, subluxation → dislocation.
Extra-articular features	Are those of the spondyloarthropathies: mucous membrane lesions, iritis, urethritis, diarrhea, aortic root dilatation, HLA-B27	Occur more often in men than women, late ("burned out"), in seropositive patients with more severe joint disease: include rheumatoid nodules, pleural and pulmonary inflammation leading to fibrosis, pericarditis, Sjögren syndrome (dry eyes, dry mouth, peripheral neuropathy, rheumatoid arthritis), Felty syndrome (rheumatoid arthritis, splenomegaly, granulocytopenia)

In general, severity of skin changes parallels the severity of the arthritis.

- The peak age of incidence is 15 to 35.
- About one in five people with Crohn's or ulcerative colitis will develop enteropathic arthritis; the arthritis can be peripheral or axial.

Peripheral
- 10% to 20% of patients with inflammatory bowel disease
- Male:female 1:1
- HLA-B27 association uncommon
- Coincides with inflammatory bowel disease activity
- Mainly affects lower limbs
- Asymmetric migration, relapsing oligoarthritis
- Lasts 2 to 6 weeks
- Radiographic changes rare

Axial
- 2% to 7% of patients with inflammatory bowel disease
- Male > female for spondylitis
- HLA-B27 association 50% to 70%
- Independent of inflammatory bowel disease activity; often precedes inflammatory bowel disease symptoms
- Gradual onset of low back pain
- Morning stiffness
- Pain worse with prolonged standing or sitting
- Pain improved by moderate activity
- Lasts <6 months

Undifferentiated Spondyloarthropathy

- An arthritis that lacks the specific features listed above for the other types of spondyloarthropathy is considered undifferentiated.

METABOLIC

PATHOPHYSIOLOGY OF CRYSTAL ARTHROPATHIES

- Monosodium urate and calcium pyrophosphate dihydrate (CPPD) crystals are responsible for:
  - Acute synovial inflammation
    - Interaction between crystals and synoviocytes (types A and B, infiltrating leukocytes)
    - Secretion of pro-inflammatory agents (IL-1β, TNF-α), and chemotactic factors (IL-8), leading to neutrophil invasion, activation, and further inflammatory response
  - Cartilage degradation
  - Bone lesions within the joint
- Cascades of activated proteins involve cytoplasmic membrane-related proteins (FAK complex, Src family tyrosine kinases), but also MAPK and NF-kB pathways, leading to nitric oxide, prostanoid, and cytokine production, and protease activation.

GOUT

Definition

- Inflammatory arthritis triggered by crystallization of uric acid within involved joints, characterized clinically by attacks of acute inflammation, and often associated with hyperuricemia

Epidemiology

- Prevalence <2% in men >30 years of age and in women >50 years of age; increased to 9% in men and 6% in women >80 years of age
- Incidence of primary gout (no diuretic exposure) has doubled over the past 20 years, probably due to the increasing incidence of obesity and other lifestyle factors.

Pathophysiology

Role of Urate Levels
- Uric acid exists as soluble urate at physiologic pH but precipitates at concentrations >8.0 ng/dL.
- There is a direct positive association between serum urate levels and a future risk of gout.

Urate Metabolism
- Urate balance depends on changes in diet, synthesis, and rate of secretion (Fig. 21-12).
- Dietary effects
  - Red meat, seafood, beer (++), liquor (+), and other sources: all increase serum level of uric acid
  - Vitamin C has a uricosuric effect.
- Increased synthesis can be primary or secondary.
  - Primary hyperuricemia (rare): due to an inherited error of metabolism resulting from an enzymatic defect of purine synthesis and/or in the renal excretion of uric acid
  - Secondary hyperuricemia: nongenetic disorders that increase the production of uric acid or that decrease the excretion of uric acid
    - Increased cell turnover in proliferative and inflammatory disorders (hematologic cancer and psoriasis)
- Excretion of urate is predominantly through the kidneys, less through gastrointestinal tract.

Diagnosis

Clinical Features

Acute Gout
- Usually monoarticular and, in the lower extremity, often the metatarsophalangeal joint of the great toe
- Characterized by severe pain, swelling, low-grade fever, and leukocytosis
- Precipitating events include trauma, recent surgical procedure, intercurrent illness.

Intercritical Gout
- Long asymptomatic periods occur, despite increased urate levels

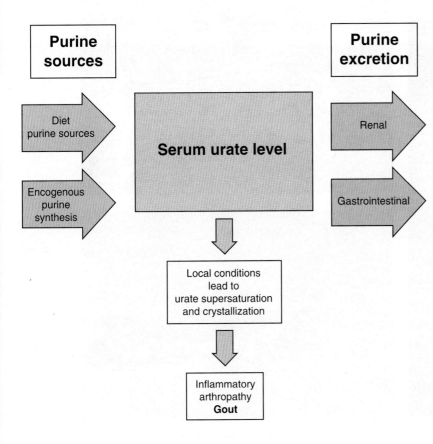

Figure 21-12 Gout is the result of supersaturation and crystallization of uric acid within the joints. The amount of urate in the body depends on the balance between dietary intake, synthesis, and excretion. Hyperuricemia results from the overproduction of urate (10%), underexcretion of urate (90%), or often a combination of the two.

Chronic Gout

■ Eventually widespread crystal deposition occurs throughout the body, particularly in the kidneys and adjacent to joints.

Radiologic Findings

■ Articular distribution of soft tissue swelling, marginal punched-out lesions with overhanging edges, with no regional osteopenia or reactive sclerosis (Fig. 21-13)

Pathologic Findings

■ To preserve crystals for identification, fixation in alcohol, hand processing, and using unstained sections are preferred over formalin fixation (urate crystals are water-soluble).
■ Synovial fluid (see Fig. 21-13)
   ■ Inflammatory exudate mimics infection.
   ■ Examination under polarized light reveals needle-like crystals with a strong negative birefringence.
   ■ Often crystals lie within polymorphonuclear leukocytes.
■ Synovium (see Fig. 21-13)
   ■ Inflammation, crystals lying within leukocytes
   ■ Tophi appear as granulomatous deposits of amorphous, proteinaceous material, bordered by fibrous tissue, histiocytes, and multinucleated giant cells.

CPPD CRYSTAL DEPOSITION DISEASE

Definition

■ Joint disorder induced by the deposition of calcium pyrophosphate dihydrate (CPPD) crystals in hyaline carti-

lage, fibrocartilage, and other soft tissue structures, characterized by acute, subacute, or chronic joint inflammation
■ Box 21-3 covers some terminology.

Epidemiology

■ Frequency is 1:1,000.
■ Rare before age 30; incidence increases with age, approaches 50% in patients >80
■ Female > male

Classification

■ Sporadic: middle-aged to elderly patient, with no sexual predominance
■ Hereditary: female predominance, occurs at an early age, more severe arthropathy
■ Secondary: hyperparathyroidism, hypothyroidism, gout, hemochromatosis, hypomagnesemia, hypophosphatasia

Diagnosis

Clinical Features

■ Six patterns have been described (Table 21-3).

Radiologic Findings

■ Calcification is seen in fibrocartilage, articular cartilage, capsule; appearance is punctuate or linear (Fig. 21-14).

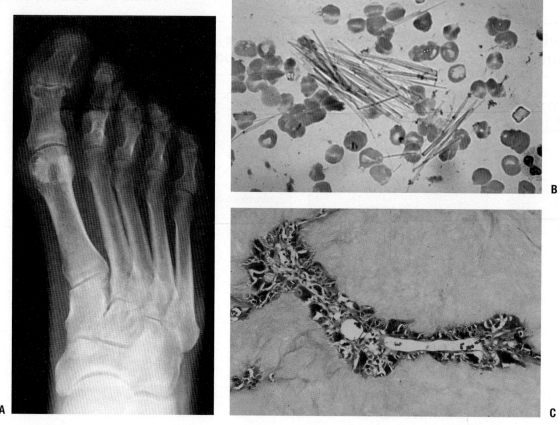

Figure 21-13 Gout. **(A)** A 58-year-old man with pain in the great toe and gout. Anterior-posterior view of the foot shows soft tissue swelling at the medial aspect of the first metatarsophalangeal and interphalangeal joints. Well-corticated erosions are seen at the medial aspect of these articulations as well. Note the relative preservation of joint space and mineralization. **(B)** Uric acid crystals. Synovial fluid sample contains needle-like crystals of uric acid. **(C)** Inflammatory reaction in gout. Surrounding and within a deposit of crystalline material is a thin layer of mononuclear and giant cells. A small vessel courses through this reaction.

BOX 21-3 CPPD CRYSTAL DEPOSITION DISEASE TERMS

Term	Definition
Chondrocalcinosis	General term describing pathologically or radiographically evident cartilage calcification; the crystals involved can be CPPD, dicalcium phosphate dihydrate, or calcium hydroxyapatite.
CPPDD	Calcium pyrophosphate dihydrate disease; exclusive term for the disorder associated with the presence only of CPPD crystals in or around joints
Dystrophic calcification	Calcification in injured tissues; deposition of calcium hydroxyapatite occurs in trauma and scleroderma; clinical examples include deposition in shoulder rotator cuff, other tendons, ligaments, bursae
Metastatic calcification	Increased levels of calcium or phosphates in the blood lead to widespread calcific deposition in kidneys, lungs, cornea, conjunctivae, vessels, dermis, and gastric mucosa; associated with: ■ Secondary hyperparathyroidism ■ Sarcoidosis ■ Metastatic disease ■ Myeloma ■ Hypermetabolic state + bed rest
Pseudogout	Gout-like clinical syndrome produced by CPPDD, characterized by intermittent acute attacks of arthritis
Pyrophosphate arthropathy	Particular form of structural joint damage that occurs in CPPDD, similar to osteoarthritis, but has some separate features, including an absence of cartilage calcification

TABLE 21-3 PATTERNS OF CPPD DEPOSITION DISEASE

Pattern	Prevalence	Description
Asymptomatic	10% to 20%	
Osteoarthitis	35% to 60%	Chronic, progressive, frequently bilateral and symmetrical, with distribution in knee, hip, metacarpophalangeal, elbow, ankle, wrist, and glenohumeral joints; flexion contractures of knee and elbow are common
Pseudogout	10% to 20%	May occur spontaneously or in association with trauma, concomitant medical illness (stroke, myocardial infarction, surgery, transfusion, intravenous fluid administration, institution of thyroxine replacement therapy, and joint lavage); mimics gout or infection with pain (less severe than gout), erythema, tenderness, and raised erythrocyte sedimentation rate; attacks are self-limited (duration days to weeks)
Rheumatoid arthritis	2% to 6%	Morning stiffness, fatigue, symmetric polyarthropathy, with synovial thickening, loss of range of motion, raised erythrocyte sedimentation rate; duration weeks to months
Charcot joint	<2%	Rapid, progressive destruction of large joint
Rare presentations		Ankylosing spondylitis, rheumatic fever, and trauma

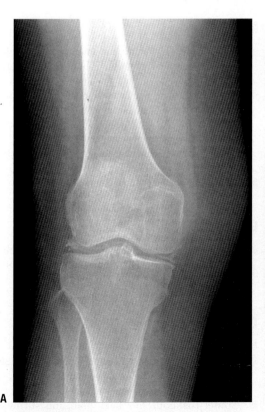
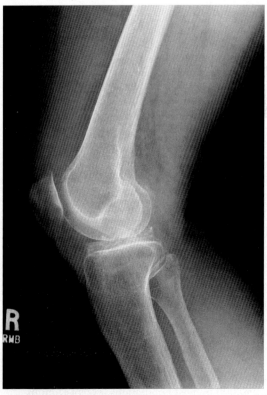

A   B

Figure 21-14 Knee with CPPD crystal deposition disease. Calcification of menisci, capsule, and articular cartilage accompanied by early osteoarthritic change (medial osteophyte formation).

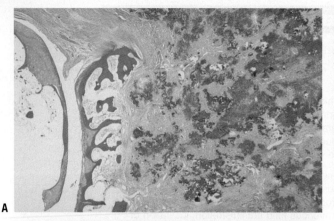

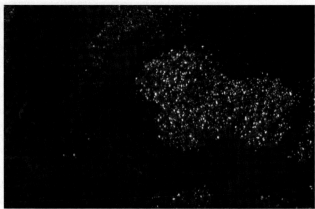

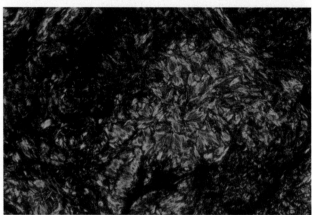

Figure 21-15 (**A**) Morphology of CPPD crystal deposition disease. Deposition of CPPD crystals in capsule adjacent to cortex, joint recess, and articular surface. (**B**) Photomicrograph of section using polarized light; refractive characteristics of rhomboidal CPPD crystals are shown. (**C**) For comparison, this section using polarized light shows the characteristics of uric acid crystals.

▪ May also be seen in symphysis pubis and intervertebral discs

Pathologic Findings
▪ Gross: chalky white deposits
▪ Micro (Fig. 21-15): In vascularized tissue, basophilic calcific deposits are surrounded by chronic inflammatory and giant cell reaction; in nonvascularized tissue, the reaction is absent.
▪ Crystal identification (see Fig. 21-15): rhomboidal-shaped crystals; weakly positive birefringence; crystals are best seen with polarized light on unstained sections.

OCHRONOSIS

Definition

▪ Ochronosis produces darkening of the connective tissues of the body and is caused by brown-black pigment composed of excess homogentisic acid (HGA) in patients with alkaptonuria.
▪ Musculoskeletal involvement leads to a severe arthropathy.
▪ Alkaptonuria: rare, autosomal-recessive disorder (prevalence <1:250,000 in most populations, except Dominican Republic and the Piestany region in Slovakia), characterized by the inability to metabolize HGA.

Metabolism

▪ Dietary phenylalanine and tryrosine are metabolized in liver and kidneys through HGA to acetoacetic acid and fumaric acid.
▪ In alkaptonuria, the enzyme homogentisic acid oxidase, a liver enzyme, is missing, allowing HGA to accumulate as alkapton, a black pigment; in urine, alkapton turns black on exposure to air; other connective tissues become progressively darkly stained (skin, sclerae, intervertebral discs, articular cartilage).
▪ Mechanism of arthropathy is not clear.

Genetics

▪ In somatic cell hybrids, HGA is located on chromosome 3, mapping to 3q21–q23 by fluorescent in situ hybridization.

Diagnosis

Clinical Features
▪ General: a progressive degenerative arthropathy, mainly affecting axial and weight-bearing joints, associated with extra-articular manifestations
▪ Spine: Insidious low back pain and stiffness begin in the 30s; occasionally an acute disc herniation provides the initial event leading to diagnosis.

- Peripheral joints: Knees, hips, and shoulders are most commonly involved; the usual presentation is of an aggressive osteoarthritis; occasionally, the process produces acute inflammation; small joints of the hands and feet are rarely involved.
- Tendinopathy: The tendons also become sites of alkapton deposition; tendinitis, rupture, with tendon calcification visible radiographically; Achilles tendon, rotator cuff are most commonly involved.
- Extra-articular manifestations: Pigmentation of sclerae and external ears allows early clinical diagnosis; alkapton pigment deposition in heart valves may lead to dysfunction, failure, and surgical replacement; stones may form in prostate and kidneys.

Radiologic Findings
- Spine: marked degenerative disc disease (disc space narrowing, endplate sclerosis, and osteophytosis), with excessive calcification of multiple intervertebral discs
- Peripheral joints: similar to osteoarthritis

Pathologic Findings
- Gross: brown-black discoloration of cartilage and disc
- Micro: disorganization similar to Charcot joint, with collections of brown-black shards of cartilage surrounded by fibrosis, histiocytic reaction, and chronic inflammation

HEMOPHILIA

Definition
- Hemophilic arthropathy produces a form of secondary osteoarthritis, the result of repeated hemorrhage into a joint.

Diagnosis

Clinical Features
- Acute hemorrhage: may be precipitated by minor trauma; typically involves knees, elbows, and ankles; presentation is of a hot, swollen, painful joint
- Chronic arthritis: a form of secondary osteoarthritis primarily affecting knees, elbows, ankles

Radiologic Findings
- Acute: joint effusion, soft tissue swelling
- Chronic: narrowed joint space, loss of cartilage, marginal erosions, multiple juxta-articular cysts, and progressive osteophyte formation; regional osteopenia (Fig. 21-16)

Pathologic Findings
- Chronic: Gross finding is dark-brown (mahogany) staining (from hemosiderin), with papillary proliferation of the synovial lining; hemosiderin staining within the synovium as well as the subsynovial tissue, which also shows chronic inflammation and fibrosis.

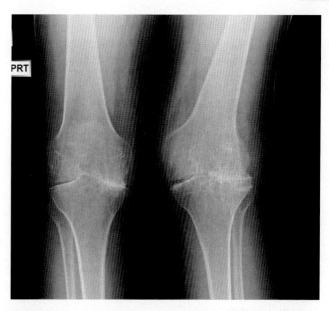

Figure 21-16   Hemophilia. A 34-year-old man with knee pain and hemophilia. Anterior-posterior view of the knees shows enlargement of the distal end of the femur and the proximal end of the tibia in response to hyperemia during development of the arthrosis. Severe joint space narrowing and secondary degenerative changes are seen. An erosion is present at the medial aspect of the left medial femoral condyle.

CIRCULATORY DISORDERS AFFECTING JOINTS

NEUROPATHIC ARTHROPATHY (CHARCOT JOINT)

Definition
- Neuropathic arthropathy is a chronic, progressive disease of bone, characterized ultimately by severe loss of joint architecture in a patient who has a neuropathy affecting the extremity.
- It can be rapidly progressive (within weeks), painful or painless, and can occur without weight bearing.

Epidemiology
- Distribution of joint involvement
  - *Diabetes: interphalangeal, metatarsophalangeal, and tarsal joints
  - *Tabes dorsalis: knees, hips, ankles, and lumbar spine
  - *Syringomyelia: shoulders, elbows, and cervical spine
- Other conditions associated with neuropathic arthropathy include *meningomyelocele, *congenital insensitivity to pain, *leprosy, and *peripheral nerve injuries.

Etiology

- Idiopathic: enigmatic association with indomethacin administration and intra-articular steroid injection
- Neuropathic: See the conditions listed above under Epidemiology (marked with *).

Pathophysiology

- The primary abnormality is a loss of vasomotor control in the region of a joint, secondary to the underlying neurologic disorder.
- The sequence then is:

1. A loss of coordination between arteriolar inflow and venous outflow occurs, with a marked increase on the arteriolar side.

2. Osteoclastic deletion of bone occurs in response to the high-flow state.

3. Juxta-articular osteopenia profoundly weakens the subchondral bone, leaving the articular cartilage without adequate bony support.

4. Fractures occur, liberating shards of bone and cartilage into the joint.

5. Aberrant articular cartilage incites a profound inflammatory response in soft tissue; a positive feedback cycle then ensues with further propagation of inflammation.

6. Inflammatory response also drives the hyperemic state, leading to further deletion of bone.

7. Repair is attempted with new bone formation about the joint and reinforcement of existing bone structures in the presence of ongoing weight bearing; this leads to visible periosteal reaction about the joint and sclerosis of existing juxta-articular bone.

Diagnosis

Differential Diagnosis
- Acute: cellulitis, acute gout, thrombophlebitis, osteomyelitis
- Chronic: osteomyelitis (may coexist with neuropathic arthropathy, especially in the presence of ulceration)
- Neuropathic neuropathy can mimic a neoplastic process clinically and radiographically.

Clinical Features
- Insidious presentation, usually in one joint, then progressing to others; an acute and painful onset suggests fracture
- Key clinical finding is that the *degree of discomfort is mild compared to the structural abnormality.*
- Erythema, local warmth, swelling, some tenderness, crepitus, instability, deformity

Radiologic Findings
- Plain films demonstrate the gross anatomy but are neither sensitive nor specific to separate neuropathic arthropathy from infection. Figure 21-17 shows neuropathic arthropathy of the foot in a diabetic.

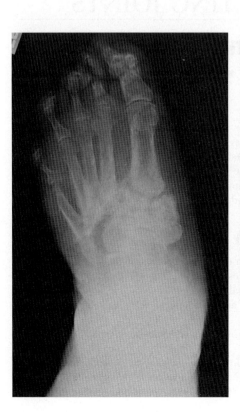
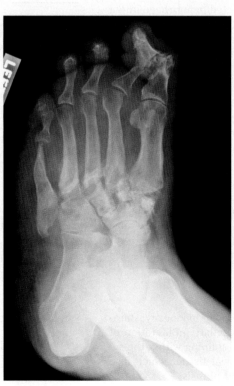

Figure 21-17 Neuropathic foot. Two radiographic views of the foot of a patient with polyneuropathy related to diabetes show extensive destruction of several joints. There is a loss of normal architecture of the midfoot with lateral subluxation of all of the metatarsals, subchondral sclerosis of the periarticular surfaces, as well as adjacent deposition of new bone. The great toe interphalangeal joint and the second toe proximal interphalangeal joints are subluxed; there has been destruction of bone adjacent to several joint surfaces. The fifth metatarsal shows "penciling" of the distal end, the end result of an inflammation-driven clastic removal of the outer layer of the cortex and the unbalanced deposition of endosteal bone to oppose this deletion.

- Regardless of the joint involved, the general features are:
    - Regional osteopenia, bone destruction, and periosteal reaction
        - Could be neuropathic arthropathy, osteomyelitis, or fracture without infection
    - Over time the appearance is one of:
        - Joint swelling
        - Subluxation or frank dislocation
        - Joint dissolution with debris and deformity
        - Regional osteopenia, local sclerosis

Pathologic Findings

- Mass-like, exuberant inflammatory process, usually mixed acute and chronic inflammation of synovium and subsynovial soft tissue with rich vascularity (granulation tissue-like)
- Numerous shards of bone and articular cartilage entrapped in soft tissue

AVASCULAR NECROSIS

- The importance of avascular necrosis is as a cause of secondary osteoarthritis.
- It can occur in multiple sites and in both children (e.g., Legg-Calvé-Perthes disease) and adults. (Also see Chapter 19.)

ANOMALIES

DYSPLASIA EPIPHYSEALIS HEMIMELICA (Trevor Disease)

Definition

- Dysplasia epiphysealis hemimelica is a rare congenital anomaly affecting the growth plates of the knee, talus, and tarsal navicular and first cuneiform joints.

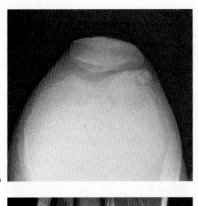
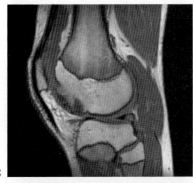
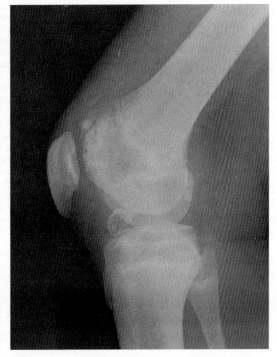
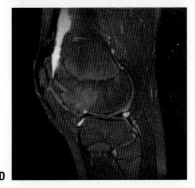

Figure 21-18　Dysplasia epiphysealis hemimelica (Trevor disease). A 14-year-old boy with atraumatic knee pain and locking and epiphyseal osteochondroma. Sunrise (**A**) and lateral (**B**) views of the knee show an osseous excrescence extending from the anterior aspect of the lateral femoral. Multiple osteochondral fragments project in the joint. Note the elongation of the inferior pole of the patella in response to chronically abnormal patellofemoral mechanics. Sagittal T1-weighted (**C**) and T2-weighted (**D**) images through the lateral femoral condyle show the lesion at the anterior aspect of the femoral condyle, with cortical and medullary continuity with underlying bone.

- It essentially consists of an epiphyseal osteochondroma that protrudes into the joint space.
- The medial side of the epiphysis is most commonly affected.

Epidemiology

- Incidence: 1:1,000,000
- No race predilection
- Male:female 3:1

Pathophysiology (Intra-articular Osteochondroma)

- Abnormality of the regulation of cartilage proliferation in the affected epiphysis, resulting in a cartilaginous exostosis.
- The morphology is that of benign cartilage over a base that resembles an osteochondroma.

Diagnosis

Differential Diagnosis
- Chondroblastoma, osteochondroma, enchondroma

Clinical Features
- Swelling and mechanical symptoms occur as the growing osteocartilaginous mass distorts the joint.
- Secondary changes include loss of motion, deformity, and atrophy of the supporting muscles.

Radiologic Findings (Fig. 21-18)
- The gross anatomy is of an exostosis, projecting and contiguous to the subchondral surface, covered by cartilage. The radiograph shows an abnormal projection of normal bone arising from the subchondral surface. Arising in childhood, the abnormal forces of this focal projection may cause secondary local changes in the adjacent articular structure.
- Magnetic resonance imaging will show the continuity of the base of the exostosis with the subchondral bone as well as abnormal signal in the cartilage cap in both the T1- and T2-weighted images.

SUGGESTED READING

Adams A, Lehman TJ. Update on the pathogenesis and treatment of systemic onset juvenile rheumatoid arthritis. *Curr Opin Rheumatol* 2005;17:612–616.

Bonnet CS, Walsh DA. Osteoarthritis, angiogenesis and inflammation. *Rheumatology (Oxford)* 2005;44:7–16.

Buckwalter JA, Brown TD. Joint injury, repair, and remodeling: Roles in post-traumatic osteoarthritis. *Clin Orthop Rel Res* 2004;7–16.

Buckwalter JA, Martin JA. Sports and osteoarthritis. *Curr Opin Rheumatol* 2004;16:634–639.

Choi HK, Mount DB, Reginato AM. Pathogenesis of gout. *Ann Intern Med* 2005;143:499–516.

Davis JC Jr. Understanding the role of tumor necrosis factor inhibition in ankylosing spondylitis. *Semin Arthritis Rheum* 2005;34:668–677.

Gladman DD, Antoni C, Mease P, et al. Psoriatic arthritis: Epidemiology, clinical features, course, and outcome. *Ann Rheum Dis* 2005;64:14–17.

Halverson PB, Derfus BA. Calcium crystal-induced inflammation. *Curr Opin Rheumatol* 2001;13:221–224.

Hammaker D, Sweeney S, Firestein GS. Signal transduction networks in rheumatoid arthritis. *Ann Rheum Dis* 2003;62:86–89.

Haugeberg G, Orstavik RE, Kvien TK. Effects of rheumatoid arthritis on bone. *Curr Opin Rheumatol* 2003;15:469–475.

Kim TH, Uhm WS, Inman RD. Pathogenesis of ankylosing spondylitis and reactive arthritis. *Curr Opin Rheumatol* 2005;17:400–405.

Kuo RS, Bellemore MC, Monsell FP, et al. Dysplasia epiphysealis hemimelica: Clinical features and management. *J Pediatr Orthop* 1998;18:543–548.

Liu-Bryan R, Liote F. Monosodium urate and calcium pyrophosphate dihydrate (CPPD) crystals, inflammation, and cellular signaling. *Joint Bone Spine* 2005;72:295–302.

Mannoni A, Selvi E, Lorenzini S, et al. Alkaptonuria, ochronosis, and ochronotic arthropathy. *Semin Arthritis Rheumatism* 2004;33:239–248.

Mohammed FF, Smookler DS, Khokha R. Metalloproteinases, inflammation, and rheumatoid arthritis. *Ann Rheum Dis* 2003;62:43–47.

Muller-Ladner U, Gay RE, Gay S. Activation of synoviocytes. *Curr Opin Rheumatol* 2000;12:186–194.

Reveille JD, Arnett FC. Spondyloarthritis: Update on pathogenesis and management. *Am J Med* 2005;118:592–603.

Steinbach LS, Resnick D. Calcium pyrophosphate dihydrate crystal deposition disease: Imaging perspectives. *Curr Probl Diagn Radiol* 2000;29:209–229.

Toivanen A, Toivanen P. Reactive arthritis. *Curr Opin Rheumatol* 2000;12:300–305.

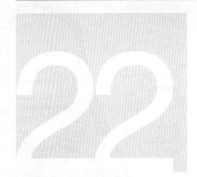

MENISCAL STRUCTURE, FUNCTION, REPAIR, AND REPLACEMENT

MARK C. DRAKOS
ANSWORTH A. ALLEN

The menisci are triangular wedges of fibrocartilage located on the medial and lateral aspects of the knee joint. They function to absorb shock and dissipate load between the distal femur and the proximal tibia. The knee may encounter forces two to four times body weight while walking and almost double that while running. Due to the high shear stresses that arise across the knee joint during activity, injury to the menisci is quite common. Epidemiologic studies indicate an annual incidence of meniscal tears of 60 to 70 per 100,000 people. In addition, these lesions are highly associated with both chronic and acute anterior cruciate ligament (ACL) tears as well as tibial plateau fractures. Initial treatment of these lesions is usually conservative. However, the natural history of meniscal tears depends on the specific location and characteristics of the tear within the meniscus. Due to the relatively avascular nature of the tissue, central injuries will often not heal. Repair and regeneration of normal cartilage is an area of increased interest in the orthopaedic community and a popular area for research. The focus of this chapter will be the anatomy, structure, and function of the menisci and how this pertains to potential treatments, including regeneration, repair, and replacement.

GROSS ANATOMY

The menisci of the knee joint were originally considered to be "functionless remnants of intra-articular leg muscles." We now know that these wedges of fibrocartilage play a critical role in normal knee kinematics. There are medial and lateral menisci, which are each divided into thirds: anterior horn, middle, and posterior horn. The anterior and posterior horns of each meniscus attach to intercondylar fossa (Figs. 22-1 and 22-2).

Medial Meniscus

- C-shaped
- ~3.5 cm in length
- Greater diameter than the lateral meniscus

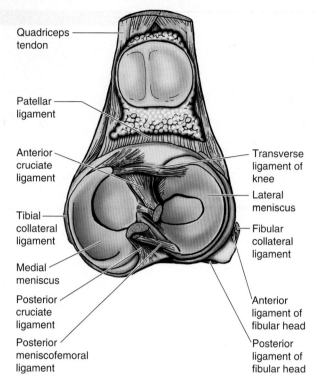

Figure 22-1 Superior view of the tibial plateau cruciate ligaments and menisci of the knee joint. (Courtesy of Dr. W. Kucharczyk, Chair of Medical Imaging, University of Toronto, and Clinical Director of Tri-Hospital Magnetic Resonance Centre, Toronto, Ontario, Canada.)

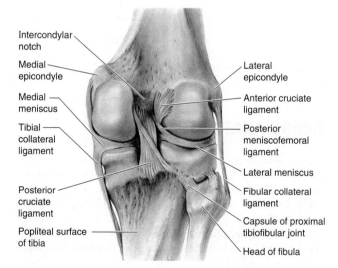

Figure 22-2 Posterior view of the knee demonstrating meniscofemoral ligaments. (Courtesy of Dr. W. Kucharczyk, Chair of Medical Imaging, University of Toronto, and Clinical Director of Tri-Hospital Magnetic Resonance Centre, Toronto, Ontario, Canada.)

- Posterior horn wider than anterior horn
- Coronary ligaments attach the meniscus to capsule.
- Deep bundle of the medial collateral ligament (MCL) is condensation of capsule that attaches to the meniscus at its midportion.
- Transverse meniscal ligament connects the anterior horns of the medial and lateral meniscus, but the attachment to anterior horn of the medial meniscus can be variable.
- Multiple attachments to medial meniscus are postulated to result in less mobility, to which the higher incidence of medial meniscal tears (three times as common as lateral meniscus) has been attributed.

Lateral Meniscus

- Semicircular
- Covers larger tibial surface area than medial meniscus
- Anterior and posterior horns are the same width.
- More mobile, weaker coronary ligament than medial meniscus
- No attachment to capsule in area of popliteal hiatus
- Meniscofemoral ligaments attach posterior horn of lateral meniscus to medial femoral condyle and posterior cruciate ligament (PCL).
  - Ligament of Humphrey is anterior to PCL.
  - Ligament of Wrisberg is posterior to PCL.
  - One or the other may be present, but not both, in 70% to 90%.

MICROSCOPIC ANATOMY AND HISTOLOGY

The meniscus is composed of a complex network of proteins, chondrocytes, water, and other matrix components, each of which plays a role in the biomechanics of the meniscus.

Meniscal Composition

- Predominant protein is collagen, which contributes 60% to 70% of the dry weight.
  - Specialized orientation to respond to large stresses (Fig. 22-3)
    - Peripheral fibers: arranged circumferentially following the contour of the meniscus
      - Woven in a mesh fashion superficially
      - Thicker and oriented more parallel at deeper layers
    - Radially oriented fibers: interposed fibers that act as "ties" to prevent longitudinal tears and provide structural stability. In addition, this arrangement helps the meniscus to function as a "wet sponge" (see below).
  - Primarily composed of type I collagen (90% of total collagen)
    - While mature cartilage has no progenitor cells, immature cartilage has a stem cell population, and it has been hypothesized that the stem cells

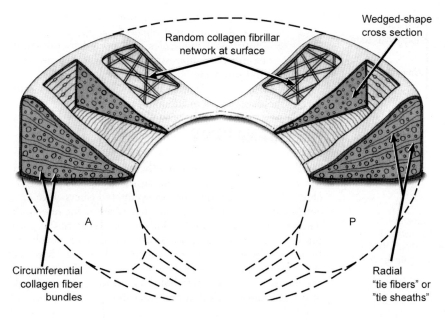

Figure 22-3   Collagen fiber ultrastructure and orientation within the meniscus.

differentiate into chondrocytes, which secrete type I collagen due to the tensile loads on the menisci.
- Less common collagen components: types II, III, V, VI
  - Larger proportion of type II collagen in the central, inner regions
- Remaining dry weight of the meniscus comes from other proteins, including proteoglycans and elastin.
  - Interaction of collagen and proteoglycans ("wet sponge" function): Aggregan, a common proteoglycan, combines with glycosaminoglycans to form a macromolecule that binds positively charged sodium ions. These ions then associate with the negative charge on the water molecules by hydrogen bonding. When a force that spreads the collagen fibrils apart is applied, these bonds are broken and water exudes from the tissue. When the force is relaxed, the water is drawn back into the cartilage by the electrostatic charge of the glycosaminoglycans. Thus, force is dissipated through the cyclic disruption and reformation of the hydrogen bonds with the glycosaminoglycans.
- Meniscal water content: 65% to 75%
- Cellular component: fibrochondrocytes
  - Terminology based on microscopic appearance as well as the fibrocartilaginous matrix that they synthesize
  - Secrete collagen, proteoglycans, and enzymes for cartilage metabolism
  - Differing morphologies based upon depth
    - Superficial zone: fusiform cells
    - Remainder: more rounded
  - Predominately anaerobic metabolism
    - Few mitochondria
    - Prevalent Golgi complexes and endoplasmic reticulum

VASCULAR ANATOMY

The vascularity of the menisci decreases precipitously after birth to assume its adult, relatively avascular composition by 10 years of age (Table 22-1). In the adult, only the peripheral third carries meaningful blood supply to either meniscus. The menisci derive their blood supply from the superior and inferior branches of the medial and lateral geniculate arteries as well as the middle geniculate artery. These vessels form a perimeniscal capillary plexus.

- A reflection of vascular synovial tissue gives a limited vascular supply to the peripheral 1 to 3 mm of the menisci.
  - In the adult form, Arnoczky and Warren demonstrated that the peripheral 10% to 25% of the lateral meniscus is vascularized.
  - The peripheral 10% to 30% of the medial meniscus is vascularized.
- Red-and-white classification system
  - Divides the meniscus into an inner, middle, and peripheral third (Figs. 22-4 and 22-5)
    - Inner third = white/white zone (poor healing potential for tears)
    - Middle third = red/white zone (intermediate healing potential)

TABLE 22-1 VASCULARITY OF THE MENISCI

Age	Vascularity
Birth	Entire meniscus
9 months old	Peripheral two thirds
10 years old to adult	Peripheral third

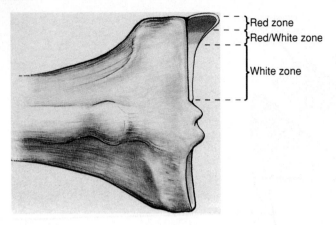

Figure 22-4 Distribution of healing zones within the meniscus. (From Miller MD, Warner JJP, Harner CD. Meniscal repair. In Fu FH, Harner CD, Vince KG. *Knee Surgery*. Baltimore: Williams & Wilkins, 1994.)

- Peripheral third = red/red zone (good healing potential)
  - Exception: Region of the lateral meniscus at the popliteal hiatus, which is devoid of capsular attachments, is avascular and effectively a watershed area, resulting in poor healing potential.
- Less vascular central two thirds depends upon synovial fluid and diffusion.
  - Joint fluid: ultrafiltrate of blood plasma combined with protein products
    - Protein products provide joint lubrication: hyaluronic acid, lubricin, collagenase, prostaglandins, and other enzymes.
    - Ultrafiltration removes red blood cells and clotting factors, prevents formation of intra-articular fibrin clot in response to injury.
      - Hemarthrosis associated with ACL reconstructions actually promotes healing of associated meniscal repairs.
  - Nutritional molecules transported by diffusion to intra-articular structures: proteins, glucose, and other metabolic molecules
- Joint forces help to distribute these nutrients into the deep layers of the meniscus.

NEUROANATOMY

Similar to the vascular supply, the neural elements within the menisci are distributed along the periphery. This includes both myelinated and unmyelinated fibers. Dye and colleagues mapped the internal structures of the knee and demonstrated that centrally located meniscal tissue gave minimal pain awareness. In contrast, the more peripheral tissues produced more pain awareness. Moreover, there are mechanoreceptors in the anterior and posterior horns of the menisci that may contribute to proprioceptive feedback at the extremes of flexion and extension.

FUNCTION AND BIOMECHANICS

To minimize contact stresses, the knee joint has a low coefficient of friction, on the order of 0.002. For comparison, the frictional coefficient of the knee is lower than that of ice on ice. Synovial fluid, fluid extrusion from the meniscal cartilage, elastic deformation of the articular cartilage, and fluid film formation all contribute to the normal kinematics of the knee. The menisci have several functions. They act as shock absorbers, minimize friction, share load, reduce contact stresses, limit extremes of motion, and have proprioceptive feedback mechanisms.

Shock Absorption/Load Distribution

- Menisci transfer 50% to 70% of the load with the knee in extension.

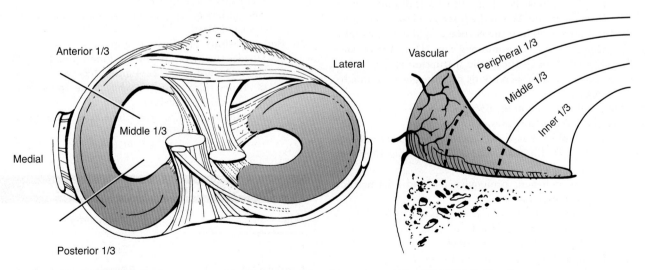

Figure 22-5 Superior view of healing zones within the meniscus. (After Siliski JM, Leffers D. Dislocations and soft tissue injuries about the knee. In Browner BD, Jupiter JB, Levine AM, et al, eds. *Skeletal Trauma*. Philadelphia: WB Saunders, 2003.)

- Menisci transfer 85% to 90% of the load with the knee in flexion.
- Shock absorption capacity is reduced by 20% after meniscectomy.

Decrease Contact Stresses

- After medial meniscectomy, there is a 50% to 70% decrease in femoral condyle contact area.
  - 100% increase in contact stresses
  - Relationship of shape of medial femoral condyle and medial tibial plateau (i.e., round on round) buffers the increased contact stress after meniscectomy.
- After lateral meniscectomy, there is a 40% to 50% decrease in femoral contact area.
  - 200% to 300% increase in contact stresses
  - Relationship of shape of lateral femoral condyle and lateral tibial plateau (i.e., flat on flat) results in a greater impact following meniscectomy than on the medial side.

Joint Stability

- Forces on medial meniscus are increased in ACL-deficient knee.
- Increase in anterior tibial translation by 58% with medial meniscectomy in ACL-deficient knee at 90 degrees of flexion

Excursion/Mechanoreceptors

- The excursion of the lateral and medial meniscus is determined by their attachments (anterior to posterior).
  - Medial meniscus: average excursion 5.1 mm
  - Lateral meniscus: average excursion 11.2 mm (fewer capsular attachments)
- Maximum excursion occurs at the extremes of flexion and extension, which provides proprioceptive information to the central nervous system through mechanoreceptors with type I and II nerve endings in anterior and posterior horns.

Joint Lubrication

- Increased conformity from menisci enhances viscous hydrodynamics for fluid-film lubrication and helps maintain low coefficient of friction.

Arthritis Prevention

- Implied by results after meniscectomy
- After meniscectomy: increased joint space narrowing, osteophyte formation, squaring of condyles, cyst formation

PATHOPHYSIOLOGY

There are several changes that occur with normal aging that lead to a decrease in the elasticity of the cartilage. The permeability of cartilage increases, which undermines its ability to absorb loads. The cartilage framework loses structure and total collagen content is decreased. Proteolytic enzymes such as metalloproteinase and cytokines such as IL-1 that have been implicated in the catabolism of cartilage are more prevalent.

Changes with Normal Aging

- Increased calcium pyrophosphate dehydrate crystals
- Decreased proteoglycan content (chondroitin and keratin sulfate; increased ratio of chondroitin 6 sulfate to chondroitin 4 sulfate)
- Decreased elasticity

Mechanical Tears

- Most common meniscal pathology (Table 22-2)
- Several classification systems (Figs. 22-6 and 22-7)
- Mechanisms of injury
  - Excessive shear force exceeding yield stress of cartilage
  - Normal forces acting on degenerative tissue
- Common tears and associated injuries
  - Most common: 81% oblique or vertical longitudinal
  - Prevalence of degenerative tears (especially posterior horns) increases with advancing age.

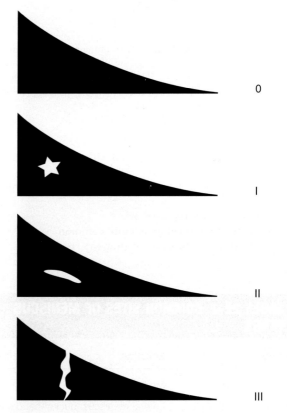

Figure 22-6 Magnetic resonance imaging classification of meniscal tears. (Thaete FL, Britton CA. Magnetic resonance imaging. In Fu FH, Harner CD, Vince KG, et al, eds. *Knee Surgery*. Philadelphia: Williams & Wilkins, 1994.)

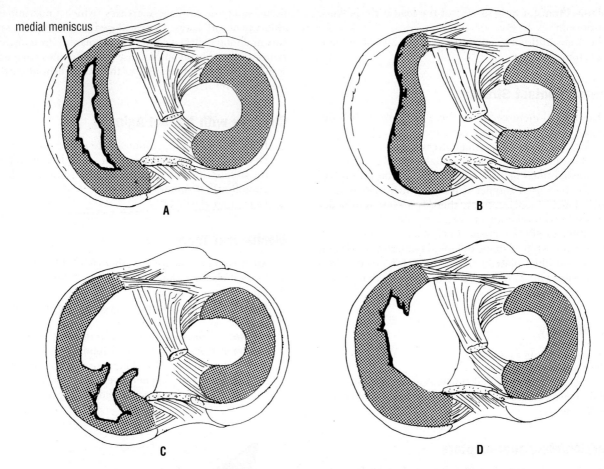

Figure 22-7   Tears of the medial meniscus of the knee joint. (**A**) Complete bucket-handle tear. (**B**) The meniscus is torn from its peripheral attachment. (**C**) Tear of the posterior portion of the meniscus. (**D**) Tear of the anterior portion of the meniscus. (From Snell RS. *Clinical Anatomy*, 7th ed. Philadelphia: Lippincott Williams & Wilkins, 2003.)

■   Acute ACL tears associated with bucket-handle lateral meniscus tears
■   Chronic ACL tears associated with medial meniscus tears
■ Parameniscal cysts
■   Lateral meniscal tears more common
■   Horizontal tears more common

TABLE 22-2 COMMON SITES OF MENISCUS TEARS

Injury	Location
Most common	Medial meniscus
Associated with ACL	Lateral meniscus: bucket-handle tear
Degenerative change	Tear of midbody and posterior horns
Meniscal cyst	Lateral meniscus, horizontal tear

TREATMENT

In most cases of meniscal tears, a trial of conservative management is an appropriate first-line treatment. The focus of therapy is to control symptoms and delay surgical intervention. Patient response to these modalities is often idiosyncratic and unpredictable. Given the relative lack of vascularity and neural supply, it is not surprising that not all meniscal tears cause symptoms. Some may heal spontaneously or remain asymptomatic.

Tears that May Not Require Operative Intervention

■   Short, stable vertical longitudinal tears (<1 cm)
■   Partial-thickness tears (<50%)
■   Small radial tears (<3 mm)

   The initial goals of therapy should be focused on minimizing pain and inflammation, increasing flexibility and strength, and optimizing function for activities of daily living. Nonoperative modalities include physical therapy, ac-

TABLE 22-3 SURGICAL INTERVENTION FOR MENISCAL LESIONS

Operative Treatment	Indications	Results
Total meniscectomy	Few, historical procedure	Poor outcomes, late osteoarthritic changes
Partial meniscectomy	Avascular region of meniscus, mechanical symptoms	Good immediate results, may be associated with late osteoarthritic changes
Open repair	Peripheral tears with other ligament injury, plateau fracture	Good results, may be more morbid than arthroscopic procedures for isolated tears
Arthroscopic repair	Peripheral tears, location in anterior-posterior plane will dictate technique	Different techniques including inside-out, outside-in, all inside, non-suture, and hybrid sutures. Many still do not heal with second-look arthroscopy, 20% revision rate, few good long-term data.
Meniscal transplantation	Previous total meniscectomy, early osteoarthritic changes, normal alignment	Good for pain relief in appropriately selected patients

tivity modification, heat/cold therapy, bracing, patient education, and topical, systemic, and intra-articular medications. However, many of these lesions persist and surgical intervention may be indicated, including meniscectomy, meniscal repair, and meniscal replacement (Table 22-3).

HEALING

In his original study, King demonstrated that for a meniscal tear to heal it must be located peripherally within the vascular zones of the meniscus. Furthermore, this blood supply must allow for all the inflammatory mediators essential to the healing response. This includes formation of a fibrin clot, resorption, and eventual fibrous scar tissue. Weiss reported on complete healing in 65% of stable vertical longitudinal tears at a follow-up arthroscopic examination. Moreover, radial tears that extend to the synovial fringe are healed with a fibrovascular scar tissue in 10 weeks (see Fig. 22-7). Similar to articular cartilage, this scar tissue does not retain all of the same biomechanical properties as the original meniscus. Some remodeling does occur, although the meniscus may never assume its original strength.

RESECTION

Despite medical intervention, symptoms such as clicking, joint line pain, and effusions often persist and require surgery to remove the offending agent.

Guidelines for Partial Meniscectomy

- All mobile fragments that can be pulled past the inner margin of the meniscus into the center of the joint
- Remaining meniscal rim should be smoothed to prevent further tearing and stress risers.
- A perfectly smooth rim is not necessary.
- A probe should be used repeatedly to gain information about the mobility and texture of the remaining rim.

- Meniscocapsular junction and peripheral meniscal rim should be protected.
- Both manual and motorized resection instruments should be used.
- In uncertain situations, more rather than less meniscal rim should be left.

This procedure will alleviate symptoms, but often at the cost of progression of degenerative disease. This dilemma has encouraged many physicians and scientists to search for interventions that can aid in healing, repair, regeneration, and in some cases replacement.

REPAIR

Meniscal repair is governed by the location and characteristics of a given meniscal tear. Tears within the red/red zone have the vascular supply to form a fibrin clot and subsequent scar. Lesions within the red/white zone have this capacity as well, albeit to a lesser extent. Lesions within the white/white zone do not have reparative capacity and will not heal even with excellent surgical technique. These lesions are a common indication for partial meniscectomy. Operative techniques for repair include open, arthroscopic, inside-out, outside-in, and all inside.

Criteria for Repair

- Complete vertical longitudinal tear >10 mm long
- Meniscal tear within the peripheral 10% to 30% of the meniscocapsular junction
- Meniscal tear that can be displaced by probing, thus demonstrating instability
- Meniscal tear without secondary degeneration or deformity
- Meniscal tear in an active patient
- Meniscal tear associated with concurrent ligament stabilization or in a ligamentously stable knee

Procedures to Augment Repair

- Accessory vascular channels from the periphery can be made to promote a healing response to central lesions.

- Meniscal trephination is a procedure through which horizontally oriented holes are made to provide a vascular channel while minimizing the detrimental biomechanical effects on the circumferentially oriented collagen fibers.
- Synovial abrasion can be used to provoke a vascular response.
- Exogenous fibrin clots have been shown to release chemotactic mediators that may stimulate dormant fibrochondrocytes to synthesize the matrix components necessary for meniscal repair.

REGENERATION

Similar to repair, results for regeneration after meniscectomy are closely tied to the vascular supply. Furthermore, the scar tissue that forms does not retain all the same biomechanical properties as the original meniscal tissue. Animal experiments have shown regeneration of "meniscal-like" tissue after total meniscectomy. This tissue remodels and by 7 months has the microscopic appearance of fibrocartilage. However, the radius of this tissue is only a fraction of the original meniscus. In addition, this was after total meniscectomy with excision into the peripheral vasculature. In specimens with subtotal meniscectomies or those with concomi-

tant synovectomies, meniscal regrowth was limited. The long-term function of the tissue that does regenerate is still a subject of controversy and has limited clinical applications at the current time. Many investigators have advocated collagen scaffolds on which to produce tissues. These products have yet to prove their efficacy in the orthopaedic community.

REPLACEMENT

Given the limited capacity of the injured meniscus to regenerate, many physicians have turned to meniscal transplantation as a potential solution. Several techniques have been described, but meniscal transplants with appropriately sized bone plugs have had good results (Fig. 22-8). Cryopreservation has been used to transplant allografts with viable fibrochondrocytes, which have a theoretically higher healing potential. However, studies comparing fresh, cryopreserved allografts and deep-frozen allografts showed similar incorporation features. Analysis 6 months postoperatively demonstrated a normal histologic pattern, normal tensile properties, increased water content, and decreased proteoglycan content. The long-term results are still a topic of debate. As with other transplant procedures, meniscal transplant

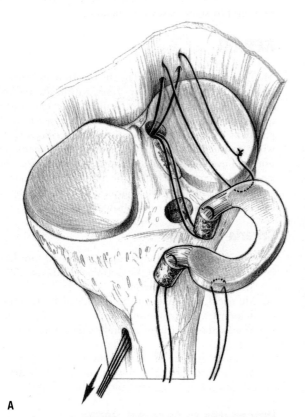

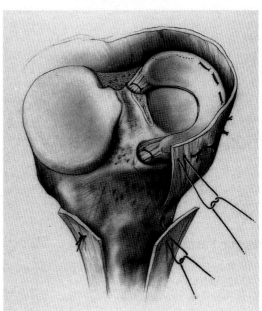

A   B

Figure 22-8   Diagram of a meniscal allograft transplant. (From Goble EM, Kane SM, Wilcox TR, et al. Meniscal allografts. In McGinty JB, Caspari RB, Jackson RW, et al, eds. *Operative Arthroscopy*. Philadelphia: Lippincott-Raven, 1996.)

does carry the risk of viral transmission: Nemzek and colleagues demonstrated the transmission of a virus in a feline model.

Criteria for Replacement

- Previous total or near-total meniscectomy
- Joint line pain
- Early osteoarthritic changes
- Normal anatomic alignment
- Ligamentously stable knee or amendable to ligament reconstruction

FUTURE DIRECTIONS

There are many exciting new therapies with the potential to change the way meniscal injuries are treated. Meniscal scaffolds continue to improve. Mesenchymal stem cells with regenerative capacity and their application to the meniscus are being studied. Gene therapy using recombinant retroviruses to deliver growth factors, cytokines, and other matrix components may also aid the regenerative process. Cultured fibrochondrocytes may also allow meniscal growth.

SUGGESTED READING

Boyd KT, Myers PT. Meniscus preservation; rationale, repair techniques and results. *Knee* 2003;10:1–11.

Day B, Mackenzie WG, Shim SS, et al. The vascular and nerve supply of the human meniscus. *Arthroscopy* 1985;1:58–62.

Greis PE, Bardana DD, Holmstrom MC, et al. Meniscal injury: I. Basic science and evaluation. *J Am Acad Orthop Surg* 2002;10:168–176.

Greis PE, Holmstrom MC, Bardana DD, et al. Meniscal injury: II. Management. *J Am Acad Orthop Surg* 2002;10:177–187.

Henning CE, Clark JR, Lynch MA, et al. Arthroscopic meniscus repair with a posterior incision. *AAOS Instr Course Lect* 1988;37:209–221.

McCarty EC, Marx RG, DeHaven KE. Meniscus repair: considerations in treatment and update of clinical results. *Clin Orthop Relat Res* 2002;122–134.

Rath E, Richmond JC. The menisci: basic science and advances in treatment. *Br J Sports Med* 2000;34:252–257.

Siliski JM, Leffers D. Dislocations and soft tissue injuries about the knee. In Browner BD, Jupiter JB, Levine AM, et al, eds. *Skeletal Trauma*. Philadelphia: WB Saunders, 2003.

Tria AJ, Klein KS. *An Illustrated Guide to the Knee.* New York: Churchill Livingstone, 1992.

Warren RF, Arnoczky SP, Wickiewicz TL. Anatomy of the knee. In Nicholas JA, Hershman EB. *The Lower Extremity and Spine in Sports Medicine.* St. Louis: Mosby, 1986:657–694.

Weiss CB, Lundberg M, Hamberg P, et al. Non-operative treatment of meniscal tears. *J Bone Joint Surg [Am]* 1989;71:811–822.

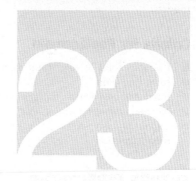

INTERVERTEBRAL DISC STRUCTURE, COMPOSITION, AND MECHANICAL FUNCTION

SAMUEL A. JOSEPH, JR.
PATRICK BOLAND

The spine can be considered a column of relatively rigid vertebrae connected by flexible intervertebral discs. Because of their flexibility, the intervertebral discs allow the spine to twist and bend throughout a wide range of postures. In addition to allowing flexibility, the intervertebral discs function in both absorbing energy and distributing loads applied to the spine. The unique structure and composition of the intervertebral disc allow for a wide array of mechanical functions to be performed. It is the disruption of this relationship that leads to intervertebral disc pathology.

ANATOMY, STRUCTURE, AND COMPOSITION

Anatomy

There are 23 discs in the human spine, which account for 20% to 30% of its length. Apart from the fused vertebrae of the sacrum and coccyx, the only vertebrae not connected by discs are the atlas and axis, which pivot at the specialized atlanto-axial joint, and the articulation between the atlas and the base of the skull, which articulate at the occipito-atlantal joint; this articulation also does not contain a disc (Fig. 23-1).

- Non-disc structures also connecting the vertebral bodies (Fig. 23-2)
    - Anterior and posterior longitudinal ligaments
    - Ligamenta flava
    - Interspinous ligaments
    - Supraspinous ligaments

Structure

- Shape
    - Roughly cylindrical
    - Most discs appear wedge-shaped because the anterior height is greater than posterior.
    - Cross-sectional area increases almost linearly from the cervical to lumbar segments.
    - Unlike cross-sectional area, disc height does not vary regularly along the length of the spine.

452

- Components
  - Nucleus pulposus: soft inner region
  - Anulus fibrosus: surrounding tough outer lamellae
    - Consists of 12 concentric coaxial lamellae that form a tube-like structure enclosing the nucleus
    - Arranged into a densely packed outer ring and an inner, larger fibrocartilaginous layer (Fig. 23-3)
- Vascularity: largest avascular organ in the body
  - Small blood vessels found on the surface of the outer anulus penetrate 1 to 2 mm at most.
  - Simple diffusion is the most important mechanism for small-molecule transport into the disc and appears to be the factor most responsible for limiting cell viability.
- Innervation: poorly innervated
  - Sensory nerves do not penetrate deeper than the outer third of the anulus.
  - Main afferent pathway involves the nerve to the vertebral body: sinuvertebral nerve (recurrent nerve of Luschka) (Fig. 23-4).

Composition

- Even though the discs may vary in size, they share the same basic structure and composition.
  - Two main structural components of the intervertebral disc
    - Collagen
      - Accounts for 70% of the dry weight of the anulus and <20% of the nucleus
      - Provides tensile strength
    - Proteoglycans
      - Account for a minimal percentage of the anulus but as much as 50% of the nucleus in the pediatric population
      - Provide stiffness, compressive strength, viscoelasticity
  - Collagen arrangement
    - Types I and II collagen fibrils
      - Distributed radially in opposing concentration gradients, with type II mostly in the nucleus pulposus and type I most concentrated in the exterior of the anulus
        - Anulus: I, II, III, V, VI, IX, X
        - Nucleus pulposus: II, VI, IX, X
    - Type I collagen provides strength to the tough lamellar sheets that are anchored into the bone of the adjacent vertebral bodies (Fig. 23-5).
  - Water: contained in the matrix of the disc and contributes approximately 65% to 80% of its total weight
  - Aggrecan is the main proteoglycan in the disc.
    - High density of negatively charged sulfate and carboxyl groups (cations) on the glycosaminoglycan chains that attract mainly Na+ (anions), which results in a cumulatively increased osmotic pressure of 1 to 3 atmospheres in the nucleus
    - Pressure gradient enables the disc to continually absorb water.
    - Hydration and swelling continue until it is restricted by the collagen network of the disc.

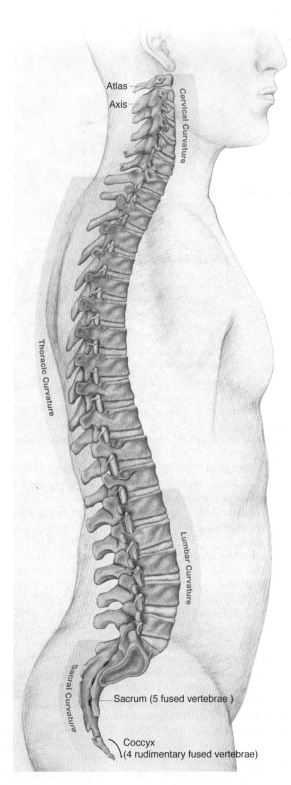

Figure 23-1   Lateral view of the human spine. (Asset provided by Anatomical Chart Co.)

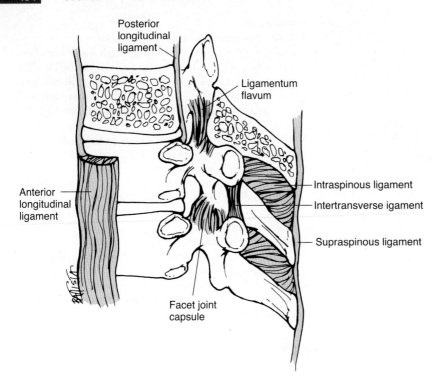

Figure 23-2 The ligaments supporting the thoracic spine consist of the capsular ligaments of the facet joints, the anterior and posterior longitudinal ligaments, the supraspinous and interspinous ligaments, the ligamentum flavum, and the intertransverse ligaments. (From Oatis CA. *Kinesiology: The Mechanics and Pathomechanics of Human Movement.* Baltimore: Lippincott Williams & Wilkins, 2003.)

■ Equilibrium between the aggrecan and collagen provides the load-bearing, compression-resisting tissue that holds the other units of the spine in correct position while allowing movement of the spinal column.

MECHANICAL FUNCTION

■ Withstands the significant forces of an upright posture
  ■ Forces up to 17,000 Newtons estimated in lumbar discs
  ■ Functions within a specialized unit called the *motion segment* (Fig. 23-6), where the basic motions of axial compression, torsional loading, and sagittal and

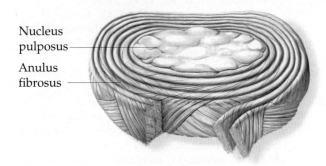

Nucleus pulposus

Anulus fibrosus

Figure 23-3 Structural features of an intervertebral disc. The nucleus pulposus is the central gelatinous cushioning part of the intervertebral disc enclosed in several layers of cartilaginous laminae. (Asset provided by Anatomical Chart Co.)

transverse bending or axial torsion occur (Fig. 23-7).
■ Biphasic viscoelastic behavior during loading (Table 23-1)
  ■ Mechanical loading causes fluid movement within the discs, which gives rise to time-dependent mechanical properties.
  ■ The less dense inner anulus and nucleus pulposus undergo larger volumetric changes in response to loads. This creates flow within the disc that dissipates the energy and causes viscoelastic creep.
  ■ The stiffer outer anulus converts this compressive load into hoop stresses while the inner layers act as a "shock absorber."
  ■ The high tensile modulus of the outer anulus helps to prevent any bulging of the disc from the loads applied.
  ■ Torques on the motion segment distort the shape of the anulus without altering the volume, while bending and compression cause disc bulging, volumetric changes, and endplate deformation.
■ Function of the cartilage endplate
  ■ The hydraulic permeability causes rapid fluid transport and less pressurization in response to loading.
  ■ This permeability provides a conduit for water to flow from and into the disc and thereby helps transfer loads in a uniform manner across the inner anulus and nucleus pulposus.

DISC AGING

Age-related deterioration of the intervertebral disc leads to two of the most common clinical disorders of the spine:

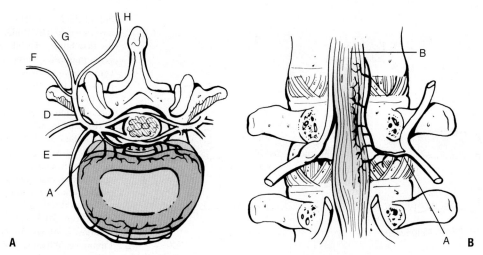

Figure 23-4 The innervation of the disc and facet joints. Sinuvertebral nerve and its branches innervate the dorsal portion of the disc (**A**) and posterior longitudinal ligament (**B**). The ventral ramus (**C**) branches to innervate the ventral disc and anterior longitudinal ligament (**E**). The dorsal ramus (**D**) branches into lateral (**F**), intermediate (**G**), and medial (**H**) branches. (From Wetzel FT. Microinnervation: Pain generators. In Bono CM, Garfin SR, eds. *Orthopaedic Surgery Essentials: Spine*. Philadelphia: Lippincott-Raven, 2004:272–277.)

degenerative disc disease and disc herniation. Changes in volume and shape are accompanied by gross morphologic and microstructural alterations (Table 23-2). The most extensive changes occur after the age of 20 in the nucleus pulposus, where the number of viable cells and the concentration of proteoglycans and water decline.

DEGENERATIVE DISC DISEASE

Disc degeneration is a multifactorial process that is complex and poorly understood. It is the result of an intricate rela-

tionship between cellular biology, mechanical factors, and genetics. Aging and degeneration of discs are separate processes: although all discs undergo aging, not all of them degenerate. The end stage of degeneration can be identified by imaging studies and gross examination, but accepted criteria for the diagnosis and the distinguishing factors between degeneration and aging have not been established. It is also unclear as to what degree the degenerative process contributes to pain. Currently disc degeneration is believed to be a source of chronic pain, and over 90% of surgical

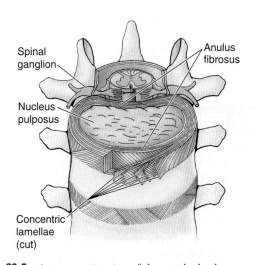

Figure 23-5 Anterosuperior view of the vertebral column, transversely sectioned through an intervertebral disc. The superficial layers of the anulus fibrosus have been cut and spread apart to show the direction of the fibers. (From Moore KL, Dalley AF. *Clinical Oriented Anatomy*, 5th ed. Baltimore: Lippincott Williams & Wilkins, 2006.)

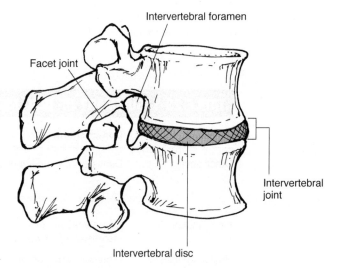

Figure 23-6 A motion segment consists of an intervertebral disc and the two adjacent vertebral bodies. (From Oatis CA. *Kinesiology: The Mechanics and Pathomechanics of Human Movement*. Baltimore: Lippincott Williams & Wilkins, 2004.)

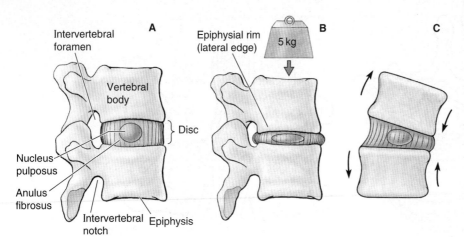

Figure 23-7 (A) The motion segment in cross-section. (B) Under axial compression, the disc bulges. Tensile stresses are generated in the outer anulus and compressive stresses in the nucleus pulposus. High fluid pressures are generated in the nucleus, causing extravasation of fluid. After the cessation of the axial loading, the osmotic pressure causes the extruded fluid to flow back into the disc, restoring its height. (C) Flexion or extension and lateral bending result in eccentric changes of the disc, which results in an alternating suction/extrusion action on the fluids into and out of the disc. (From Moore KL, Dalley AF. *Clinical Oriented Anatomy*, 5th ed. Baltimore: Lippincott Williams & Wilkins, 2006.)

spine procedures are performed because of consequences of the degenerative process.

- Degeneration appears to be the natural consequence of two scenarios:
    - Application of *normal loads* to a disc with *abnormal material properties*
    - Application of *abnormal loads* to disc with *normal material properties*

Biology of Degeneration

- Declining nutritional support is the most important event responsible for the changes in central disc cells and their matrices (Fig. 23-8).
    - Sequence of events resulting in loss of nutritional support
        - Increase in disc volume during growth results in relative decline in the vascular supply.
        - Decreased vascular supply results in impaired diffusion and convection that is necessary for the transport of nutrients and removal of waste.

- Loss of disc tissue results from the action of degradative enzymes within the disc and the inability of disc cells to maintain or restore their extracellular matrix.
    - Cause of this imbalance remains unknown.
    - Mediators of degradation
        - Proteolytic enzymes (cathepsin and lysozyme)
        - Inflammatory cytokine IL-1 decreases rate of proteoglycan production and increases rate of matrix breakdown.
- Extrinsic factors: mediate degeneration of the disc by nutritional and/or vascular means (Box 23-1)
- Mechanical environments
    - Overload hypothesis
        - Demanding mechanical environment produces local trauma of the disc that will be slow to heal due to slow turnover of the disc tissue.
        - Accumulation of injury and microtrauma progressively weakens the disc, making it more susceptible to further injury, thus starting a vicious cycle.
    - Hypomobility hypothesis

TABLE 23-1 SUMMARY OF DISC MECHANICAL FUNCTION

Structure	Composition	Function
Outer anulus	Dense concentric lamellae	Resist tensile loads Hydrostatic barrier that limits deformation Reduce strains across vertebral bodies
Inner anulus	Less dense lamellae Increased water content	"Shock absorbers": viscoelastic dissipation of force
Nucleus pulposus	High concentration of proteoglycans Increased water content	Resist axial compressive loads
Endplate	Hyaline cartilage	Transfer of axial loads to vertebral body

TABLE 23-2 AGE-RELATED CHANGES IN THE DISC

Age Group	Changes
Newborn	Distinct hyaline cartilage endplates Numerous perivascular and free nerve endings Small amounts of collagen in nucleus Small blood vessels present in outer lamellae Proteoglycan in nucleus similar to endplate
Childhood and adolescence	Disc volume and diameter increase. Blood vessels decrease in size and number. Increase in cartilaginous content of anulus Aggrecan becomes predominant proteoglycan.
Adult	Remaining peripheral vessels disappear. Inner anulus expands. Size of nucleus decreases. Myxomatous degeneration of anulus; loss of collagen fiber organization Fissures and cracks in lamellae Concentration of viable cells declines. Proteoglycan and water concentrations decrease. Collagen and noncollagenous protein concentrations increase. Decrease in structural integrity
Elderly	Inner anulus and nucleus become fibrocartilage. Few viable cells remain. Decrease in height

BOX 23-1 FACTORS INCREASING AGE-RELATED CHANGES

Nutritional Transport	Vascular Supply
Increased disc loading	Smoking
Immobilization	Vascular disease
Vibration	Diabetes
Spinal deformity	

- Hypomobility results in adaptive changes that may predispose to weakness and degeneration.
- Resultant weakness and degenerative changes can cause pain, which further reduces motion and initiates another vicious cycle.

- Genetics: plays a significant role in the variability of disc degeneration in the population samples studied to date (Box 23-2)
  - First reports of gene forms associated with intervertebral disc degeneration in humans were published in 1998.
    - Low magnetic resonance imaging (MRI) signal intensity of thoracic and lumbar discs (disc desiccation) associated with TaqItt-genotypes of the vitamin D-receptor gene
  - Several mechanisms have been suggested through which genetic factors could influence degenerative disc findings:
    - Size and shape of spinal structures
    - Intracellular processes that maintain disc function
  - Interactions of genetic and environmental factors are complex and continue to be an area of intense study.
- Diminished material and structural properties

As a consequence of degeneration-related alterations in structure and composition of disc tissues, changes occur in the material and structural properties of the components of the disc (Fig. 23-9). The degenerative changes in material properties are most profound in the nucleus and endplate.

- Nucleus pulposus
  - Shear modulus of the nucleus increases eight-fold (becomes stiffer).
  - This decrease in energy dissipation suggests that the nucleus pulposus undergoes a transition from fluid-like to solid-like behavior.
  - These alterations may be explained by the loss of water content and increase in tissue density.

Decreased diffusion of nutrients and waste removal

↓

Low oxygen tension

↓

Incomplete lactate concentration

↓

Decreased pH

↓

Compromised cell metabolism

↓

Cell death

Figure 23-8　Proposed pathway of cellular degeneration of the disc.

BOX 23-2 GENE FORMS ASSOCIATED WITH DISC DEGENERATION

Vitamin D receptor gene	Metalloproteinase-3
Collagen IX alleles	Aggrecan gene

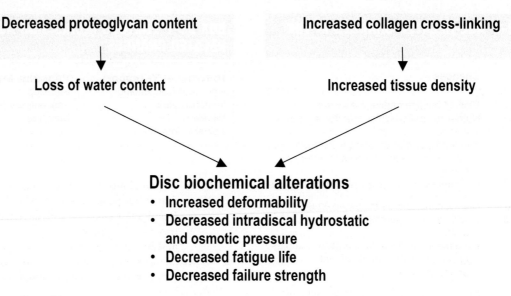

Figure 23-9   Biomechanical property changes of the degenerated disc.

This transition to more of a solid-like state suggests a more anisotropic (orientation-dependent) stress state with more non-uniform distribution of stresses.
- Anulus fibrosus
  - Significant increase in compressive modulus
  - Decrease in radial permeability
    - Decrease in permeability results from loss of water content and obstruction of pores with debris.
    - Diffusion of nutrients, which relies on this permeability, is hindered.
  - Moderate increase in shear modulus
- Endplate
  - Thinning, microfracture, or damage to the endplate increases its hydraulic permeability, which allows rapid fluid exudation with loading.
  - This leads to a more non-uniform distribution of load as well as higher shear stresses that result in damage to the disc.
  - These compositional and structural changes lead to non-uniform load transfers that result in high shear stresses and material failures.

Disc Degeneration and Back Pain

The relationship between disc degeneration and back pain is poorly understood. Many factors, including structural changes in the spine, soluble mediators that sensitize nerve endings, and nerve/vessel ingrowth into the outer anulus, have all been hypothesized to be possible causes of this chronic pain (Fig. 23-10).

- Changes in the mechanical properties of the disc lead to loss of spinal mobility and abnormal loading of the facet joints, spinal ligaments, and surrounding muscles.

- The altered alignment and relationship may contribute to spinal pain.
- The degenerated disc has been shown to produce cytokines and mediators that can sensitize surrounding nerve endings.
  - Tumor necrosis factor-alpha (TNF-α) has recently been suggested to play a role in discogenic pain.

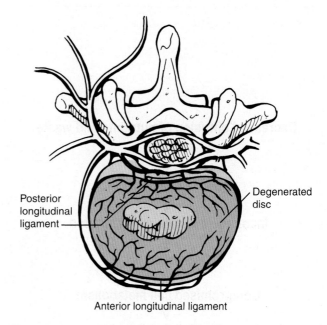

Figure 23-10   Pain fibers can penetrate more deeply into degenerated discs. These fibers may be accompanied by vascular ingrowth. (From Wetzel FT. Microinnervation: Pain generators. In Bono CM, Garfin SR, eds. *Orthopaedic Surgery Essentials: Spine*. Philadelphia: Lippincott-Raven, 2004:272–277.)

- TNF-α and other pro-inflammatory cytokines are a target of current research in pharmacologic intervention.

Medical Imaging

Obvious changes in disc morphology and matrix composition are observable with multiple imaging modalities. Although plain radiographs are nearly always the first step, computed tomography (CT) and MRI provide excellent detailed anatomic images of the spine. Prior to their development, more invasive techniques such as myelography, epidural venography, and epidurography were performed to evaluate intradiscal pathology.

- Early endplate changes preceding established degenerative disc diseases
  - Sclerosis, Schmorl's nodes, calcifications
  - Observed on both radiographs and MRI
- MRI is the advanced imaging modality of choice for intervertebral disc degeneration.
  - Characterizes many of the distinguishing features of the intervertebral disc
  - Does not distinguish between symptomatic and asymptomatic patients
  - Does not differentiate degeneration from age-related changes
  - Most sensitive MRI sign for disc degeneration: nucleus pulposus loses signal intensity on T2-weighted images
    - Loss of proteoglycans and dehydration occurring in degeneration
    - Seen as loss of signal intensity on T2-weighted images
- Plain x-ray and MRI changes of degeneration
  - Loss of disc height
  - Osteophyte formation

- Attributed to a compensation mechanism to distribute the increasing axial load and shear forces onto a larger bearing surface
- These osteophytes have been differentiated into two types: traction and claw.
  - Traction osteophytes result from abnormal shear and are a sign of instability.
  - Claw-type osteophytes represent traction at the site of osseous attachment (Sharpey fibers) of the anulus fibrosus.
- Radiographic correlates to morphological degree of degeneration
  - Plain film significant correlates: height loss, osteophytes, and intradiscal calcification (Table 23-3)
  - MRI correlative parameters: DEBIT (*d*isc *e*xtension *b*eyond the *i*nterspace), nucleus pulposus shape, anular tears, osteophytes, and endplate irregularity
- New and potentially useful imaging techniques for spine (continue to offer more opportunities to investigate and diagnose back pain and intervertebral disc degeneration)
  - Dynamic CT and MRI
  - Diffusion imaging
  - Magnetic resonance spectroscopy

DISC HERNIATION

- Definition: protrusion of tissue from the nucleus pulposus through a defect in the anulus fibrosus (Fig. 23-11)
- Early clinical course
  - Initially fragmentation rarely perceived due to poor innervation of disc
  - Back pain typically experienced as outer anulus becomes involved with extension of the fissure and fragmentation
  - With the herniation of the discal components, pressure on the anulus is transferred to the nerve root.

TABLE 23-3 THOMPSON GRADING SCHEME FOR GROSS MORPHOLOGY OF THE HUMAN LUMBAR INTERVERTEBRAL DISC

Grade	Nucleus	Anulus	Endplate	Vertebral Body
I	Bulging gel	Discrete fibrous lamellae	Hyaline, uniformly thick	Margins rounded
II	White fibrous tissue peripherally	Mucinous material between lamellae	Thickness irregular	Margins pointed
III	Consolidated fibrous tissue	Extensive mucinous infiltration; loss of anular–nuclear demarcation	Focal defects in cartilage	Early chondrophytes or osteophytes at margins
IV	Horizontal clefts parallel to endplate	Focal disruptions	Fibrocartilage extending from subchondral bone, irregularity and focal sclerosis in subchondral bone	Osteophytes <2 mm
V	Clefts extend through nucleus and anulus	—	Diffuse sclerosis	Osteophytes >2 mm

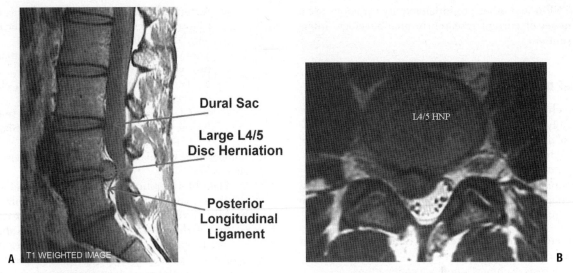

Figure 23-11   Lumbar microdiscectomy. MRI views of a large L4-5 disc herniation, sagittal (**A**) and axial (**B**). (From Koval KJ, Zuckerman, JD. *Atlas of Orthopaedic Surgery: A Multimedia Reference.* Philadelphia: Lippincott Williams & Wilkins, 2004.)

- Back pain is typically relieved at this point, yet the radiculopathy (sciatica) may increase in intensity.
- Later clinical course and outcome
  - In >90% of patients with symptomatic disc herniations, the pain subsides within 3 months.
  - In many people (28% to 35%), disc herniation occurs in the absence of symptoms. This relief of symptoms has theoretically been attributed to a spontaneous resorptive process that appears to be modulated by an inflammatory pathway.
- Histopathology and healing process
  - Herniated disc is surrounded by granulation tissues with an inflammatory cell infiltrate and newly formed vessels.
  - Neovascularization is related by MRI to the resorption of the herniated disc.
  - Infiltrating macrophages also play a crucial role in this resorption.
- Terminology from the North American Spine Society (NASS)
  - **Herniation**: localized displacement of disc material beyond the limits of the intervertebral disc space (Fig. 23-12). The disc material may be nucleus, car-

tilage, fragmented apophyseal bone, anular tissue, or any combination. The interspace is defined cranial and caudad by the vertebral endplates and peripherally by the outer edges of the vertebral ring apophyses (Fig. 23-13).

- **Anular tear**: localized radial, concentric, or horizontal disruption of the anulus without associated displacement of the disc material beyond the limits of the intervertebral disc space (see Fig. 23-12)
- **Extrusion**: In at least one plane, any one distance between the edges of the disc material beyond the disc space is greater than the distance between the edges of the base measured in the same plane; or when no continuity exists between the disc material beyond the disc space and that within the disc space (Fig. 23-14).
- **Protrusion**: The greatest plane, in any direction, between the edges of the disc material beyond the disc space is less than the distance between the edges and the base (see Fig. 23-14).
- Location of the herniation: Wiltse proposed a system of anatomic zones and levels to characterize the herniation (Figs. 23-15 and 23-16).

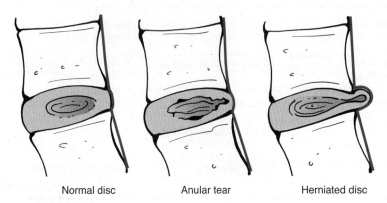

Normal disc   Anular tear   Herniated disc

Figure 23-12   Sagittal anatomic sections showing the differentiating features of anular tear and herniated disc. (After Milette PC, Fardon DF. Nomenclature and classification of lumbar disc pathology. *Spine* 2001;26: E93–E113.)

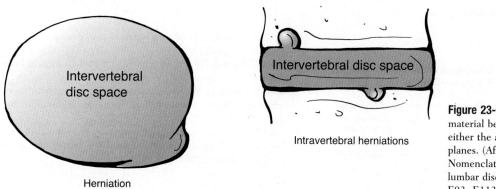

Intervertebral disc space

Intervertebral disc space

Herniation

Intravertebral herniations

Figure 23-13 Herniation of disc material beyond the interspace can be in either the axial or the caudad/cranial planes. (After Milette PC, Fardon DF. Nomenclature and classification of lumbar disc pathology. *Spine* 2001;26: E93–E113.)

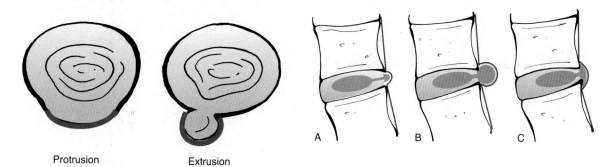

Protrusion

Extrusion

A   B   C

Figure 23-14 Differentiating characteristics of protrusion (**A**) and extrusion (**B,C**). (After Milette PC, Fardon DF. Nomenclature and classification of lumbar disc pathology. *Spine* 2001;26:E93–E113.)

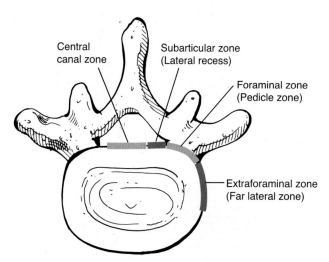

Central canal zone

Subarticular zone (Lateral recess)

Foraminal zone (Pedicle zone)

Extraforaminal zone (Far lateral zone)

Figure 23-15 The anatomic "zones" identified on axial images. (After Milette PC, Fardon DF. Nomenclature and classification of lumbar disc pathology. *Spine* 2001; 26:E93–E113.)

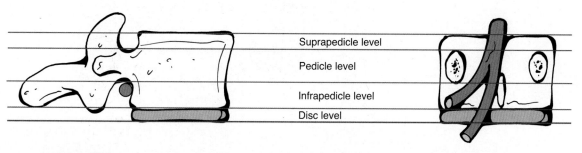

Suprapedicle level

Pedicle level

Infrapedicle level

Disc level

Figure 23-16 The anatomic "levels" identified on cranio–caudad images. (After Milette PC, Fardon DF. Nomenclature and classification of lumbar disc pathology. *Spine* 2001;26:E93–E113.)

SUGGESTED READING

Ashton-Millar JA, Schultz AB. Biomechanics of the human spine. In Mow VC, Hayes WC, eds. *Basic Orthopaedic Biomechanics*. Philadelphia: Lippincott-Raven, 1997:353–393.

Benneker LM, Heini PF, Anderson SE, et al. Correlation of radiographic and MRI parameters to morphological and biochemical assessment of intervertebral disc degeneration. *Eur Spine J* 2005;14:27–35.

Buckwalter JA, Einhorn TA, Simon SR, eds. *Orthopaedic Basic Science: Biology and Biomechanics of the Musculoskeletal System*. Rosemont, IL: AAOS, 1999.

Lotz JC. Animal models of intervertebral disc degeneration. *Spine* 2004;29:2742–2750.

Milette PC, Fardon DF. Nomenclature and classification of lumbar disc pathology. *Spine* 2001;26:E93–E113.

Stokes IAF, Iatridis JC. Mechanical conditions that accelerate intervertebral disc degeneration: overload versus immobilization. *Spine* 2004;29:2724–2732.

Wetzel FT. Microinnervation: pain generators. In Bono CM, Garfin SR, eds. *Orthopaedic Surgery Essentials: Spine*. Philadelphia: Lippincott-Raven, 2004:272–277.

TENDON AND LIGAMENT ANATOMY, BIOLOGY, AND BIOMECHANICS

BRIAN J. HARLEY
JOSEPH W. BERGMAN

Tendons and ligaments act as the bonds that tie the body together. Ligaments connect one bone to another at a joint, and tendons connect bone to muscle. While the specific natures of their tasks differ, tendons and ligaments share a great many features in their construction and function.

TENDON

TENDON ANATOMY, STRUCTURE, AND COMPOSITION

Gross Anatomy

Macrostructure
- Variable sizes and shapes: wide and flat to round and narrow
- The larger the muscle unit, and therefore the potential force, the larger diameter the corresponding tendon

- Unique features in regions of compression
  - Sheaths and bursa
    - Shield the tendon from abrasion and friction
  - Tendon assumes more of a cartilage-like appearance in these areas.
    - Synovial sheath
      - Encloses the path of the tendon
      - Provides a reservoir of fluid to hydrate and lubricate the tendon

Ultrastructure
- While variety is seen in tendon macrostructure, all tendons are organized with a similar ultrastructure (Fig. 24-1).
- Musculotendinous junction
  - Collagenous structure of the tendon blends with the muscle.
  - As the tendon fans out into the muscle, the collagen fibrils connect to the myocytes, allowing for the transmission of force from muscle to tendon.
- Epitenon

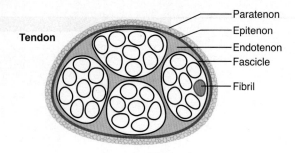

Tendon

- Paratenon
- Epitenon
- Endotenon
- Fascicle
- Fibril

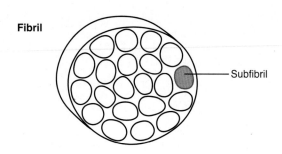

Fibril

- Subfibril

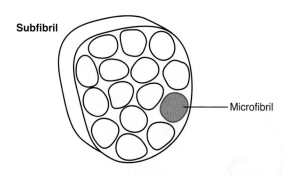

Subfibril

- Microfibril

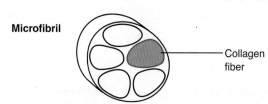

Microfibril

- Collagen fiber

Figure 24-1   Tendon ultrastructure.

- Layer of organized tissue that tightly encircles the entire surface of the tendon
- Endotenon
  - Layer of loose connective tissue between fascicles within a tendon
- Paratenon
  - Layer of loose areolar tissue that substitutes for a tendon sheath; serves a nutritional role
  - Present in tendons not enclosed within a fibrous sheath (e.g., Achilles tendon)
- Fibrils
  - Collagen molecules organized into microfibrils
  - Microfibrils assembled into subfibrils, fibrils, and fascicles
  - One or more fascicles compose a tendon.

Biochemistry

- Collagen
  - Primary component of tendon
  - Type I collagen predominates, typically representing up to 85% of the dry weight.
  - Other collagens in tendon: III, IV, V, VI
  - Collagen provides a strong molecule capable of transmitting tensile loads.
    - Constructed from tropocollagen, a triple-helical polypeptide molecule
    - Ends of tropocollagen overlap at regular intervals, giving the collagen fiber a banded appearance.
    - Primarily oriented in the direction of expected tensile force
    - Variety of fibers that travel in an oblique or perpendicular direction and tie the longitudinally oriented fascicles together
- Noncollagenous substances
  - Proteoglycans, proteins, and various supporting molecules, including elastin
  - Small variations in the concentrations of all these components are seen in tendons in differing locations and functions.
- Matrix
  - Proteoglycans and glycosaminoglycans
    - Ionic charge on the side chains of these molecules causes them to spread out and occupy as large a volume as possible.
    - Water molecules are strongly attracted by this structure and are strongly restrained within the tendon.
    - Presence of water bound to the proteoglycan molecules allows the tendon to resist compressive loads.
    - Compressive load passes through the water in much the way that the fluid inside a can of soda supports the thin walls surrounding it.
    - Resistance to fluid flow through the tendon also contributes greatly to its viscoelastic biomechanics.

Cellular Population

- As a consequence of the mechanical demands placed on the tendon, much of the structure of the tendon is composed of mechanical elements.
  - As a result, the tendon has a high structure to cellularity ratio.
- Tenocytes and tenoblasts
  - Spindle-shaped cells
  - Subjected to significant mechanical loads
  - Poorly supplied with blood and nutrients
  - Stimuli triggering cellular responses
    - Mechanical load
    - Electric potential
    - Various chemical and cytokine messengers
      - Transforming growth factor (TGF) and interleukin (IL) groups, as well as a variety of extracellular molecular fragments
  - Function: responsible for maintaining the collagen and proteoglycan matrix

- Normal tendon
  - Constant turnover of extracellular matrix in response to chemical and mechanical damage that occurs from normal day-to-day function
- Acute tendon injury
  - Inflammatory response (including lysis and removal of damaged molecules), followed by a regenerative, depositional phase (by tenocytes and tenoblasts)
  - Due to the paucicellular nature of tendon combined with areas of poor blood supply, it is possible for the cellular repair mechanism (tenocytes and tenoblasts) to become overwhelmed.
- Chronic tendon conditions
  - Inflammatory and lysis responses predominate.
  - Reparative response by tenocytes muted
  - Chronic tendinitis, tendinosis, and even tendon failure are manifestations of this state.

Blood Supply

- Vascular anatomy of tendons
  - Blood vessels exist within the epitenon and endotenon.
    - Fine areolar structures that surround tendon bundles and supply individual fibrils and fibers
  - Variable blood supply depending upon location within tendon
    - Variable amount of blood supply at origin and insertion
    - Myotendinous junction allows an increased microperforating blood supply to nourish a portion of the tendon extending away from the junction.
- Factors decreasing vascular incursion
  - Intense mechanical environment
  - Confined geometry of the tendon
  - Increased tensile and compressive forces within the extracellular matrix
- Secondary path for nutrition in poorly vascularized regions
  - Diffusion of nutrients and oxygen from the adjacent synovial layers

Innervation

- Neural elements within tendons
  - Two predominant mechanoreceptors, both of which sense pressure and tension within tendon
    - Rapidly adapting receptors: Pacinian corpuscles
    - Slow-adapting receptors: Ruffini endings
  - Free nerve endings less common
  - Sympathetic and parasympathetic innervation
- Importance of tendon innervation
  - Important for normal function
    - Proprioceptive receptors communicate with gamma-muscle-spindle system to modulate joint position.

- Recovery of mechanical function after an injury is not always accompanied by return of nervous function.
  - Unknown what effect this defect has on rehabilitation and musculotendinous action

TENDON BIOMECHANICS

Tendon acts as a relatively rigid connector between the motor unit of the muscle and the bone. Its first role is to transmit tensile forces created within the muscle to initiate and modulate motion. To accomplish this, tendon has one of the highest tensile strengths of any material in the body. Collagen has a high tensile strength (and high ultimate stress) along its longitudinal axis, and the parallel orientation of the collagen fibrils within tendon takes advantage of this strength. The clinical importance of these properties is evident when the biomechanical properties of the healing tissue in a tendon or ligament are compared to the intact state. The scar tissue is weaker, therefore reducing the material properties of a tendon. Increasing the total cross-sectional area of the tendon with this scar tissue may allow for the same structural properties, however.

Structural Properties of Tendons

- Describes the properties of the whole tissue complex, as in the entire tendon–bone insertion unit, in terms of force and displacement (Fig. 24-2)
  - **Strength**: overall force transmitted
  - **Stiffness**: ability of the structure to resist deformation when force (or load) is passed through it

Material Properties of Tendons

- Describes properties according to cross-sectional area, in terms of stress and strain (Fig. 24-3)

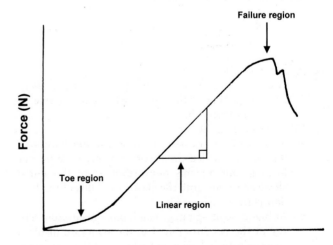

Figure 24-2 Typical force–displacement curve during low-load tensile testing of a tendon. A toe region exists representing the changes from crimp. The linear region represents the high stiffness obtained from full recruitment of collagen fibers. The failure region occurs with sequential loss of continuity of fibers.

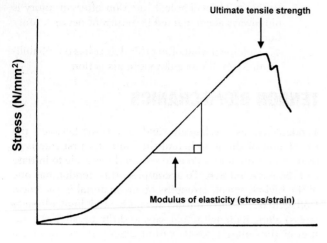

Figure 24-3 Typical stress–strain curve during low-load tensile testing of a tendon. The slope of the linear region represents the modulus of elasticity of the tendon. The ultimate tensile strength represents the stress at failure of continuity of the tendon.

- **Stress**: force divided by cross-sectional area
- **Strain**: amount of deformation of the structure divided by length over which the deformation takes place
- Useful for comparing tendons at various anatomic locations or comparing a healing tendon to an intact tendon, or when relating tendons to ligaments

Low-Load Tendon Mechanics

- The behavior of tendon at low loads reveals a degree of laxity that allows some movement through the tendon before load is passed to muscle.
- Crimp in tendons
  - At low loads, this "crimp" present in the collagen fibers straightens out before the collagen begins to conduct load (see Fig. 24-2).
- Steepening of force–deformation curve
  - Not all of the collagen is crimped equally, so there is a steepening of the force–deformation curve as more and more fibrils are recruited.
- Effect of loading rate
  - Most of the work performed on the mechanics of tendon has loaded the tissue at a very slow rate of loading, and in this quasi-static state the curve slowly steepens until the elastic modulus of the tendon is reached (see Fig. 24-3).
  - At higher loading rates, which more accurately represent the condition in vivo, the structure displays a viscoelastic behavior and acts as a stiffer structure.

Elastic Biomechanics

Structural and Material Properties

- An elastic substance is one in which a force and displacement and stress and strain are linearly related.

- Doubling a certain force will double the deformation.
- Doesn't matter if the force (load) is arrived at during loading or unloading

Elastic Properties

- Tendon demonstrates very important elastic behavior.
  - Any force generated by a muscle is transferred to the intended bone with virtually no energy wasted.
- Cycling between loaded and unloaded states does not waste energy.
  - Whatever energy is stored during loading of the material is released during its unloading.

Viscous Properties

- A purely viscous substance is one that will deform infinitely given a particular force.
- This is seen with fluids where rate of motion through the fluid is dependent on the force.

Viscoelastic Behavior

- A time-dependent property of material behavior whereby the tendon behaves partly as a viscous substance and partly as an elastic substance
- Interaction of the viscous and elastic properties during loading
  - The collagen fibers take up most of the force and the loaded fibers tend to squeeze together.
  - The water in the extracellular matrix resists this inward movement of the collagen fibers.
  - Typically the water would quickly be squeezed out of the tissue by the tension on the tendon.
    - The proteoglycans and glycosaminoglycans within the matrix act as a colloid attraction force to keep water within the tendon.
  - The rate at which a tendon is loaded is very important.
    - The more quickly a tensile load is placed on the tendon, the more effective is the resistance to outward flow of the water.
- Advantages of viscoelastic behavior in tendons
  - Load "sharing" between the elastic and viscous portions of the matrix
    - During very large loads, the viscous nature of the tendon absorbs and dissipates energy. This helps to protect the collagen from irreparable damage.
    - At lower, cyclic loads, the tendon behaves more as an energy-conserving, elastic material.
  - Energy conservation
    - One of the important functions of tendon is efficient transmission of energy. The most efficient way to transmit force is with a very stiff structure.
    - Within short time frames, the viscoelastic behavior of tendon causes it to act like a much stiffer and energy-conserving structure.
  - Loss of energy
    - Due to the properties of creep, force-relaxation, and mechanical hysteresis, upwards of 10% of total work is lost during normal cycles of loading and unloading.

TENDON INJURY, HEALING, AND REPAIR

Tendon dysfunction adversely affects overall orthopaedic health. Degenerative and/or traumatic injuries to tendons throughout the musculoskeletal system are a common cause of presentation to an orthopaedic surgeon.

Injury Mechanisms

Direct Trauma or Laceration
- Common example: laceration of the finger flexor tendon

Acute Application of Tensile Loads Exceeding the Strength of the Tendon
- Results in partial or complete ruptures of the tendon
- Distinct locations common
  - Avulsion of the tendon from its bone insertion
    - Healthy tendons can easily withstand tensile forces larger than the maximum force generated by the muscles or tolerated by the bones, so failures tend to occur at bony insertions.
    - Common example: distal biceps tendon avulsion
  - Midsubstance rupture
    - Generally pre-existing pathology at the site of a midsubstance rupture
    - Common example: Achilles tendon rupture
  - Disruption at the musculotendinous junction
    - Typically caused by a very forceful eccentric muscle contraction
    - Partial loss of continuity of the muscle fibers close to the junction (complete loss of continuity of tendon is uncommon)
    - Muscles that cross two joints appear to be more susceptible.
    - Spontaneous healing the norm; surgical repair unusual
    - Common example: hamstring tear (forceful hip flexion with the knee extended)

Fatigue/Overuse Conditions
- Repetitive loading of a tendon at loads well beneath its ultimate failure load can damage the tendon beyond its ability to repair the damage.
- Failure typically occurs at the site of tendon weakness.
  - Multifactorial etiology
  - Intrinsic and extrinsic causes
- Clinical examples of tendinous fatigue failure
  - Tendon coursing around a sharp turn
    - Damaged by constant friction by a harder material
    - Common example: posterior tibialis tendon rupture
  - Tendon compressed between two hard surfaces
    - Damage from abrasive wear
    - Common example: rotator cuff tendon tear
  - Chemical or enzymatic damage
    - Slow attenuation of tendon macrostructure
    - Generally associated with signs and symptoms of inflammation

- Common example: extensor tendon rupture in a patient with rheumatoid arthritis

Classification
Classification of intrinsic degenerative tendon disorders is covered in Table 24-1.

Clinical Presentation

Acute Injury
- Due to a single traumatic event
- No preceding symptoms
- May be subclinical pre-existing pathology in affected tendon, particularly if there is no externally applied direct impact to the tendon

Chronic Injury
- Etiology
  - Often thought of as "normal wear and tear" that exceeds the body's ability to repair it
  - Root cause of problem is twofold:
    - Pathologic changes within "at-risk" portions of the tendon
    - Limited metabolic potential of the host cells in these locations
- Factors that promote chronic injury
  - Increasing age
  - Conditions that impair normal vascularity (e.g., smoking)
- Clinical presentation
  - Insidious onset of clinical symptoms
  - Subacute worsening with extension of the tear
  - Swelling at the site of the affected tendon(s) is appreciated by a clinician only in superficial locations.
  - When chronic injury is caused by chemical/enzymatic damage from an inflammatory or autoimmune condition, patients generally complain of pain and crepitus before rupture.
    - If the inflammatory process is not abated, the tendon can be damaged to the point where rupture occurs with submaximal loading conditions.
    - In many patients with rheumatoid disease, the resultant tendon rupture is painless and manifests only as deformity and decreased function on physical examination.
- Histology of chronic tendon injury
  - Pre-existent tendon pathology typical
  - Abnormal tissue is usually seen in the portions of the tendon with the lowest strains, not the tissue under the highest tensile loads.
  - Suggests a "stress-shielding"–related atrophy
    - Internal and/or external shear forces can propagate into complete tears.

Tendon Healing

Tendon healing is a complex process with significant implications for clinical treatment. While the typical stages have been defined histologically, the exact molecular signaling

TABLE 24-1 CLASSIFICATION OF DEGENERATIVE TENDON DISORDERS

Diagnosis	Frequency	Pathological Findings

Tendinosis	Common
	Most frequent cause of tendon degeneration and failure
		Intratendinous degeneration
		  Collagen disorientation
		  Focal necrosis or calcification
		  Increased noncollagenous matrix
		  Proliferation of cellular elements
		  Mixture of neovascularization and poor blood supply

Tendinitis	Term frequently misused for tendinosis
	Commonly seen in inflammatory arthritides
		Symptomatic degeneration
		Hemorrhage and tearing
		Inflammatory and granulation tissue
		  Fibroblast proliferation
		  Marked inflammation in paratenon
		  Focal fibrin deposition with chronicity
		  Mucoid degeneration

Paratenonitis	Occurs where tendon rubs over bone/sheath Uncommon source of tendon rupture but can be very symptomatic	
Paratenonitis with tendinosis	Combination	Paratenonitis associated with intratendinous degeneration

and cellular control of the process remains poorly understood. Furthermore, the different anatomic locations can affect the success of the process.

Stages
Inflammation.
- Begins with hemorrhage at the time of tendon injury
- Lasts for about 5 days
- Inflammatory cytokines released and inflammatory cells recruited
- Resultant granulation tissue has no intrinsic strength.

Proliferation.
- Begins within 3 to 5 days of injury
- Continues until about 6 weeks after injury
- Copious deposition of immature collagen fibrils that do not resemble the anatomy of normal tendon
  - Greater levels of types II, V, and VI collagen than normal
- Fibroblasts migrate into wound.
  - Collagen is laid down in a haphazard fashion in first 2 weeks.
    - Fibers aligned perpendicular to the axis of tensile force
  - *Extrinsic healing* represents deposition from fibroblasts originating in the paratenon proliferating into the injury site.
  - *Intrinsic healing* represents deposition from fibroblasts within the epitenon and endotenon.

- Fibrous bridge connects the injured ends by 2 weeks.
  - Mechanical strength remains well below that of the native tendon.
- Gradual reorientation of the fibrils results in more normal-appearing microstructure over the last 4 weeks.
- Repetitive, low tensile loading of the tendon has been shown to improve the healing response during this stage.

The proliferative stage is of major importance. If the repair proceeds too slowly, the immature repair tissue will accumulate damage, leading to a chronic tendinitis state, gapping of the tendon ends, and possible failure. If this stage proceeds too vigorously, the tendon will scar to its sheath or other surrounding structures. Excessive scarring to the tendon will limit or deny its normal excursion. Scarring is a particular problem in areas where the healing tendon is in close association with a tendon sheath or retinacular restraint.

Remodeling.
- Begins at 6 weeks after injury and continues to beyond 1 year
- Encompasses two phases: consolidation and maturation phases
  - Previously disorganized collagen slowly becomes more organized.
  - Increased intermolecular bonding increases strength.
  - Little histological difference in vascularity and cellu-

lar organization compared to normal tendon 6 months after injury
- While this remodeling never results in the material properties of the original tendon, a structural strength approaching that of the original tendon can be realized.

Interventions and Repairs

Surgical Repair
- Surgical repair of a ruptured tendon accomplishes two ends:
    - Restoration of the musculotendinous unit function
    - Reduction of the gap between the healing ends: With close apposition throughout the healing stages, a more effective and stronger repair ensues.
- Timing
    - Repair is best performed within 2 weeks of injury.
    - Retraction and secondary fibrosis of the muscle seen after 2 weeks can prevent coaptation of the lacerated ends.
- Techniques
    - Key features of best techniques
        - Multiple suture strands
        - Some component of each strand placed perpendicular to the fascicle orientation to minimize cut-out
    - Specific techniques differ between the various sites of tendon injury.
    - Experts disagree on the "best technique" at any given site.
- Goals of the repair
    - Gain sufficient mechanical strength to minimize gapping of tendon ends
    - Allow some early motion

Postsurgical Care/Physical Therapy
- Benefits of early loads and motion on tendon healing
    - Monomeric collagen production, fibril orientation, and cross-linking are all enhanced by applied loads in the healing tendon.
    - Small amounts of motion applied early have been shown to reduce the amount of paratendinous adhesions, which can be detrimental to tendon gliding in the wound bed.
- Repairs of tendons with sheaths (e.g., flexor tendons in finger)
    - Early passive motion protocols and light active loading in the immediate postoperative period are encouraged.
    - Closely supervised by a trained therapist
    - Patient education and compliance is of utmost importance.
    - Risk of detrimental paratendinous adhesions far outweighs the risk of rupture with contemporary techniques.
- Repairs of tendons without sheaths (e.g., Achilles tendon)
    - Period of immobilization is often instituted.
    - Paratendinous adhesions are not as problematic to eventual outcome.
    - In the setting of an Achilles tendon rupture with ragged tendon ends after repair, a larger quantity of extrinsic paratendinous collagen production may be imperative to help offset the limited intrinsic healing that will occur early on. Later institution of active and passive motion protocols will generally provide the mechanical stimulation needed to stimulate adequate adhesive scar resorption.
- Modalities
    - Ultrasound, electrical field stimulation, and suction cupping are common techniques used by therapists
        - Used for resolution of adhesive scar formation in the postoperative period
    - Only anecdotal evidence demonstrating any benefit over more traditional stretching and passive motion protocols
        - No high-quality studies

LIGAMENT

LIGAMENT ANATOMY, STRUCTURE, AND COMPOSITION

Ligaments are responsible for the passive transmission of force between bones and are vital to joint stability. They connect one location on a bone across a joint to another bone and are generally short, flexible structures composed of fibrous tissue. As the force applied to the ligament increases, more fibers are recruited to resist the applied load. Ligaments are very similar to tendons with regard to their structure, but their differing role leads to a variety of unique features.

Macrostructure
- Variety of sizes and shapes
    - Correspond closely with the size and shape of the joint that they stabilize
- Most are located on the external surfaces of the joints and tend to be wide and thin.
    - Example: collateral ligaments of knee
- Some are located in protected positions within the articulation and shaped more like a cable.
    - Example: cruciate ligaments of knee
- All ligaments are composed of bands, or bundles.
    - Bundles are not distinct on gross inspection.
    - During physiologic motion, different bundles are recruited to maintain joint stability.
    - Depending upon the position of the joint, some portions of the ligament are minimally loaded, while other bundles are under high tension.

Ultrastructure
- Epiligament
    - Layer of organized tissue that tightly envelops the surface of the ligament and through which a neurovascular network enters the ligament.
- Endoligament
    - Layer of loose connective tissue between the fascicles
- Fascicles

- Ligaments, like tendons, are composed of a similar arrangement of microfibrils, subfibrils, and fascicles.
- One or more fascicles make up a ligament.
- Ligament–bone junction
  - Represents the critical region of load transfer from the ligament to the bone
  - It is a transitional zone with a complex arrangement.
  - There are two types of insertions:
    - *Direct*: insertion of ligament into bone only
      - Four morphologically distinct zones of transition: ligament → fibrocartilage → mineralized fibrocartilage → bone
    - *Indirect*: ligament fans out with connections into both bone and periosteum
      - Most common insertion type
      - Broader insertion zone
      - Superficial fibers insert into periosteum.
      - Deep fibers connect to bone obliquely via Shapey's fibers.

Biochemistry

Collagen

- Collagen represents about 70% of the dry weight of ligament.
- This is less than tendon and one of the most significant differences between tendons and ligaments (Table 24-2).
- Type I collagen predominates, with smaller proportions of types III, IV, V, and VI.
  - Slight variability in overall collagen composition between various ligaments is seen.
- On a microscopic level, the collagen is constructed somewhat different than tendon.
  - Ligaments experience a less uniform loading pattern.
  - There is a more varied arrangement in fiber direction.
  - There is variety in density and orientation of fibrils even among different ligaments.

Noncollagenous Substances

- Water is the primary component of ligament (70%).
- Remainder of the dry weight is composed of proteoglycans, fibronectin, and elastin.

Cellular Population

- There is a high structure to cellularity ratio.
- As with tendon, the fibroblasts within the extracellular matrix maintain the collagen and proteoglycan matrix. They are subject to significant mechanical loads and operate in a field of relative microvascularity. .
- There is constant turnover of the extracellular matrix in response to chemical and mechanical damage that occurs from normal day-to-day function.
- The cellular reaction is similar to tendon.

Blood Supply

Vascular Anatomy of Ligaments

- Host cells are supplied via a network of blood vessels located in the endoligamentous and epiligamentous tissue.
- Ligaments also receive a significant amount of blood supply at their insertions at bone.
- A uniform microvascular network travels along the epiligament, penetrating the ligament substance in a regular longitudinal pattern.
- Ligaments are shorter and subject to minimal excursion compared to tendons, so a more consistent microvascular supply exists.
  - A more uniform process of matrix synthesis and repair results.
  - This represents a difference when compared with tendon (see Table 24-2).

Innervation

- Neural elements within ligament
  - Generous nervous innervation within ligaments
  - Most are mechanoreceptors designed for detecting changes in pressure or tension.
  - Autonomic and nociceptive supply has also been documented.
- Importance of ligament innervation
  - Proprioceptive receptors form part of an important ligament–muscular feedback loop that helps modulate joint function.
    - The recovery of proprioceptive function after injury to a ligament is unpredictable and may contribute to altered rehabilitation and long-term ligament function.
  - Regulation of blood flow in the normal and injured ligament
    - Mechanism for control of inflammation or repair in periarticular tissue

TABLE 24-2 DIFFERENCES OF TENDONS AND LIGAMENT PROPERTIES

Property	Tendon	Ligament
Collagen composition	85%	70%
Fibril orientation	Uniform longitudinal	Varied, less uniform
Blood supply	Areas of reduced vascularity	Consistent microvascular system

LIGAMENT BIOMECHANICS

Ligaments act as relatively rigid connectors of joints that serve to stabilize and guide the bones through a range of motion. The first role of the ligament is to transmit tensile forces without failure, allowing for absorption of shock and dissipation of energy. Ligaments are only part of the equilibrium of compressive and tensile elements that ensure normal joint function. Furthermore, all the ligaments in a specific joint work together, and at any given time only distinct bundles of a given ligament are truly loaded. Early biomechanical testing of ligaments tended to isolate individual ligaments in vitro and involved nonphysiologic loading patterns; as such, much early biomechanical work is not truly indicative of ligament function in vivo.

Crimp

- Ligament accomplishes these tasks by having the same sort of microscopic "crimp" seen in tendons, only to a greater degree.
  - At low loads, this crimp straightens out and allows the ligament to accommodate a degree of lengthening or shortening of the ligament without generating large loads.
  - This is seen as a "toe" region on a force-displacement graph.
- There is a gradual steepening of the force–deformation curve as more and more fibrils are recruited.
  - As the amount of load in the ligament begins to rise sharply, the ligament provides more stability to the joint.

Variability

- The mechanical properties of ligaments closely correspond with anatomical location and in vivo loading conditions.

Ultimate Strength and Failure

- As the loaded collagen fibrils in ligament reach their point of maximal load, there is ultimate failure.

- Ligaments have a lower collagen content and a less uniform fibril and cross-linking arrangement than tendons.
  - More nonlinear load–deformation curve
  - Lower mechanical properties (ultimate tensile strength and elastic modulus) than tendons

Elastic Biomechanics

- Ligaments demonstrate increased elastic behavior compared to tendons.

Viscoelastic Behavior

- Allows for laxity that allows gradual assumption of force as the joint moves through a normal range of motion
  - Rapidly stiffens should an undesirable joint position occur
- Provides load sharing and energy conservation to protect ligaments
- The rate at which the ligament is loaded is important.
  - The more quickly a tensile load is placed, the more effective is the resistance to outward flow of the water.

LIGAMENT INJURY, HEALING, REPAIR, AND RECONSTRUCTION

In contrast to tendon injuries, ligament injury tends to occur by a single mechanism. The application of a load to a joint that exceeds the ultimate strength of part or all of the ligament results in loss of competence of the ligament. While the mechanism of injury is similar, the degree of injury to the ligament varies and has resulted in the following classification.

Clinical Presentation

- Relative degree of injury is given in Table 24-3.

Location of Disruption
- Midsubstance rupture
  - Most common location overall

TABLE 24-3 GRADING OF LIGAMENT INJURIES

Grade	Description
I	Mild strain with loss of continuity of some fibers: Ligament tender to palpation. Pain with stress testing of ligament, but no laxity
II	Moderate strain with partial loss of continuity of entire ligament: Ligament very tender to palpation, hemorrhage into adjacent joint. Pain with stress testing; obvious increase in laxity
III	Complete tear of the ligament in its entirety: Swelling and pain in area of rupture, hemorrhage into joint and soft tissues. Less pain with stress testing; marked increase in laxity

- Ligament is the weak link in the bone–ligament–bone construct.
- Rupture can occur at any location within the ligament.
  - Often very close to bone insertion
- Common example: ulnar collateral ligament of the thumb metacarpophalangeal joint
- Bony avulsions
  - Second most common location
  - Most common in skeletally immature patients
    - Growth plate represents weak link.
    - Common example: avulsion of medial epicondyle of elbow
  - Diagnosed by radiographs
  - A variable degree of subclinical failure in the ligament also evident
  - Good prognosis from surgical repair
    - Bone attachments generally easily reattached
    - Common example: avulsion of medial malleolus of ankle
- Chronic attenuation of ligament
  - Vast majority of ligament injuries occur after application of excessive traumatic force.
  - Chronic attenuation of ligament integrity occurs in conjunction with inflammatory disease.
  - Leads to slow loss of joint alignment and stability
    - Becomes progressively debilitating
    - Common example: rheumatoid degeneration of the metacarpophalangeal joints of the fingers

Ligament Healing

Ligament healing is similar to healing in most tissues in the body and nearly identical to the process in tendons (see section on tendon healing for description of stages).

Healing Environment
Vascular Supply
- More consistent vascular supply within torn ligaments than tendons
- Speculation that certain ligaments may fail to heal because of decreased vascularity and/or an environment inhospitable to the vascular response
  - All torn ligaments can generate an adequate hemorrhagic response.
  - Clinical example: anterior cruciate ligament of the knee, intra-articular location bathed in synovial fluid
- How far the healing progresses along the second stage (proliferation) seems to be the bigger variable, most dependent on mechanical environment.

Mechanical Environment
- Determines the quality of ligament healing during the proliferative stage
- Secondary stabilizing ligaments must minimize loading on the healing ligament for the progression of the healing process.
  - Minimization of gapping at the torn ends
- Institution of early and controlled joint motion further stimulates an ideal environment for ligament healing.
- Clinical example: isolated injury to the knee medial collateral ligament. Adequate secondary stabilizers (cruciate ligaments and capsule); generally heals with an early motion protocol.

Poor Healing Environment

- Secondary constraints cannot compensate for the function of the injured ligament.
  - Excessive loading stretches repair tissue.
  - Excessive gapping prevents tissue reorganization and vascular networks.
- Results in an incompetent repair and compromised joint stability long term
- Surgical intervention is most indicated in these instances.
  - Clinical example: anterior cruciate ligament of the knee—no adequate secondary stabilizer for the function of the ligament
- Joints that have suffered injury to more than one ligament will predictably have poorer restoration of stability and clinical function without surgical stabilization.
  - Clinical example: combined medial collateral and anterior cruciate injury

Outcomes
- Even when healing occurs in an ideal environment, normal ligamentous anatomy is not created.
- Healed ligament demonstrates subtle but significant differences when compared to normal ligament (Box 24-1).

Interventions and Repairs

Nonsurgical Treatment and Bracing
- A brief period of immobilization is often instituted as a first-line treatment for a ligamentous injury when the joint is anticipated to be stable.
  - Clinical example: elbow dislocation
- While joint contracture is obviously detrimental to eventual outcome, a short period of immobilization followed

---

BOX 24-1 DIFFERENCES IN LIGAMENT STRUCTURE AFTER HEALING

Histologic Changes
Increased cell density
Increased cell metabolic rate
Disorganized collagen

Biochemical Composition
Smaller collagen fibrils
Less type I collagen
Excess of glycosaminoglycans
Larger proteoglycans
Fewer cross-links

Biomechanical Properties
Mild loss of structural properties
Increased cross-sectional size
Moderate loss of mechanical properties
Increased creep

by a therapy program reliably leads to good clinical outcomes in certain predictable clinical situations.

- A program of active motion protocols in conjunction with a brace that minimizes detrimental loading of the healing ligament will generally provide the mechanical stimulation needed to maximize healing properties and stimulate adhesive scar resorption.
  - Clinical example: medial collateral ligament of knee injury

Surgical Repair

- Surgical repair of a ruptured ligament accomplishes two tasks:
  - Restores the ligament structural properties
    - A portion of the joint-stabilizing function of the ligament is restored.
    - Reduces loading-induced deformation of the early granulation tissue
    - May also reduce loads on partially injured secondary stabilizing ligaments within the same joint, increasing the likelihood of improved healing in these structures as well
  - Promotes apposition of the torn ligament ends for healing
    - Stronger repair with close apposition when compared with wide gaps.
    - No advantage to surgical repair when the torn ligament ends lay closely apposed naturally
    - If the joint retains adequate stability after ligament tear, surgical intervention may be detrimental to clinical outcomes.
- Preferred technique for ligament repair differs between various sites.
- In general, this is best accomplished via multiple suture strands.
- Suture anchor fixation or sutures through bone tunnels are most effective for repair of ligament back to bony origins.
- Even experts disagree on the "best technique" at any given site.
- Goals
  - Gain sufficient mechanical strength to initiate early motion protocols
  - Minimize gapping

Ligament Reconstruction

- In some instances, it is technically impossible to generate adequate stability or create sufficient apposition of torn ligament ends.
- In the setting of a joint with chronic ligament deficiency, imbrication of the poorly organized local scar tissue is ill advised.
  - Clinical example: chronic anterior cruciate ligament tear of the knee
- In these situations, ligament reconstruction with auto-

graft or allograft substitutes has been extensively described.

- Key features of these techniques

  1. Substitution of grafts with structural properties meeting or exceeding native ligament

  2. Secure graft fixation though bone tunnels

  3. Anatomic reapproximation of ligament–bone insertions

  4. "Isometric" placement: With increasing knowledge of fiber bundles, truly isometric graft placement is not possible for all knee positions.

  5. Ligament preconditioning: stress relaxation applied to graft before insertion and final tensioning

Postsurgical Care and Physical Therapy

- When compared with joint immobilization, motion applied to healing ligaments improves the biomechanical properties of the ligament in the following manner:
  - Increased size of scar
  - Increased size of collagen fibrils (little improvement in collagen fiber realignment, however)
  - Improved parallel sliding between fibers
  - Reduced synovial adhesions and adjacent connective tissue proliferation

SUGGESTED READING

Amiel D, Frank C, Harwood F, et al. Tendons and ligaments: A morphological and biochemical comparison. *J Orthop Res* 1984;1: 257–265.

Buckwalter JA, Einhorn TA, Sheldon SR, eds. *Orthopaedic Basic Science: Biology and Biomechanics of the Musculoskeletal System.* Rosemont, IL: AAOS Press, 2000.

Dienst M, Burks RT, Greis PE. Anatomy and biomechanics of the anterior cruciate ligament. *Orthop Clin North Am* 2002;33: 605–620.

Frank CB. Ligament healing: Current knowledge and clinical applications. *J Am Acad Orthop* 1996;4:74–83.

Gelberman RH, Woo SL, Lothringer K, et al. Effects of early intermittent passive mobilization on healing canine flexor tendons. *J Hand Surg [Am]* 1982;7:170–175.

Kirkendall DT, Garrett WE Jr. Clinical perspectives regarding eccentric muscle injury. *Clin Orthop* 2002;403S:S81–89.

Kjaer M. Role of extracellular matrix in adaptation of tendon and skeletal muscle to mechanical loading. *Physiol Rev* 2003;84:649–698.

Lin, TW, Cardenas L, Soslowsky LJ. Biomechanics of tendon injury and repair. *J Biomechanics* 2004;37:865–877.

Maffulli N, Wong J, Almekinders LC. Types and epidemiology of tendinopathy. *Clin Sports Med* 2003;22:675–692.

Maganaris CN, Narici MV, Almekinders LC, et al. Biomechanics and pathophysiology of overuse tendon injuries: ideas on insertional tendinopathy. *Sports Med* 2004;34:1005–1017.

Malcarney HL, Murrell GA. The rotator cuff: biological adaptations to its environment. *Sports Med* 2003;33:993–1002.

PERIPHERAL NERVE PHYSIOLOGY, ANATOMY, AND PATHOLOGY

SHIKHA SETHI
BRIAN J. HARLEY
CHRISTIAN CUSTODIO
MICHAEL STUBBLEFIELD

A comprehensive understanding of peripheral nerve anatomy and physiology is essential for understanding peripheral nerve pathophysiology and mechanisms of peripheral nerve injury and regeneration. Understanding peripheral nerve injury and cellular repair is critical to clinical management of operative nerve injury, microsurgical nerve repair, and emerging applications that target intrinsic nerve cell functions to assist in nerve regeneration.

PERIPHERAL NERVE ANATOMY

Gross Anatomy

General Organization
- 31 mixed spinal nerves emerge from the spinal cord:
  - 8 cervical
  - 12 thoracic
  - 5 lumbar
  - 5 sacral
  - 1 coccygeal
- Nerves emerge from the foramen of the vertebral bodies after the union of ventral and dorsal roots.
  - Autonomic, sensory, and motor fibers travel together in peripheral nerves to their destinations.
  - Nerves branch into dorsal and ventral rami upon exiting the foramen.
  - Dorsal rami
    - Small-caliber branches
    - Provide segmental innervation to dorsal paraspinal area
  - Ventral rami
    - Large-caliber branches
    - Cervical, lumbar, and sacral roots join together to form nerve plexuses to innervate the extremities.
    - Thoracic spinal nerves (except T1) <u>do not</u> form plexuses but instead provide segmental innervation to large areas of the ventral trunk.

Nerve Plexus
- Coalescence of multiple spinal nerve ventral rami
  - Fairly consistent anatomic connections and exchanges within plexuses
  - Each root level still innervates specific dermatomal and myotomal segments.
- At the distal aspect of the plexus, peripheral nerves form with representations from multiple spinal levels.
- Four consistent locations
  - Cervical plexus
    - First four cervical roots
  - Brachial plexus
    - Lower four cervical and first thoracic ventral rami
  - Lumbar plexus
    - First three and a part of the fourth lumbar ventral rami
  - Sacral plexus
    - All sacral rami along with the fifth and a part of the fourth lumbar ventral rami

Peripheral Nerves
- Each nerve may contain any combination of three possible nerve types:
  - Motor efferent fibers
    - Cell bodies in the spinal cord
    - Transmit motor information to muscles about when and how to act

- Motor unit: individual motor neuron and the specific group of muscle fibers it innervates
- Sensory afferent fibers
  - Cell bodies in dorsal root ganglia
  - Convey modality or quality, intensity, duration, and location of a stimulus from the periphery
  - Arise from specialized pain, thermal, tactile, and stretch (proprioceptive) receptors in the periphery
  - Terminal axons and presynaptic terminals for sensory fibers may be at the spinal level of the corresponding dorsal root ganglion or deeper in the central nervous system.
- Sympathetic fibers
  - Originate in the intermediolateral cell column in the thoracic and upper lumbar spinal cord
  - Synapse at variable levels of the paravertebral sympathetic ganglion and then travel as fibers within mixed spinal nerves to end organs such as sweat glands, blood vessels, and erector pili
  - Fibers join the spinal nerve and can then branch into ventral and dorsal primary rami.

Microanatomy

Nerves (Fig. 25-1)
- The normal peripheral nerve is composed of blood vessels, nerve fibers, and three levels of connective tissue within which the fibers and vessels lie.

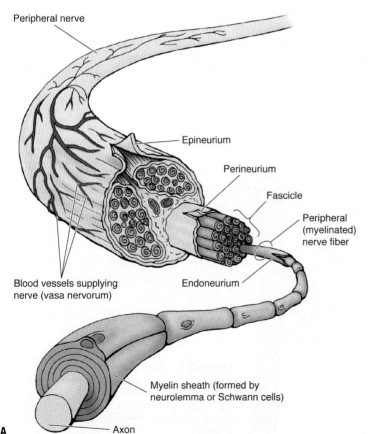

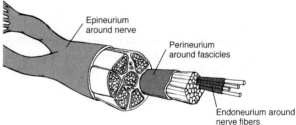

Figure 25-1 (A) Arrangement and ensheathment of peripheral, myelinated nerve fibers. All but the smallest peripheral nerves are arranged in bundles (fascicles), and the entire nerve is surrounded by the epineurium, a connective tissue sheath. Each small bundle of nerve fibers is also enclosed by a sheath, the perineurium. Individual nerve fibers have a delicate connective tissue covering, the endoneurium. The myelin sheath is formed by neurolemma (Schwann) cells. (B) Peripheral nerves are structured similarly to tendons, ligaments, and muscles, with long parallel fibers contained in bundles surrounded by connective tissue. (A from Moore KL, Dalley AF. *Clinically Oriented Anatomy*, 5th ed. Baltimore: Lippincott Williams & Wilkins, 2006. B from Hendrickson T. *Massage for Orthopedic Conditions*. Baltimore: Lippincott Williams & Wilkins, 2002.)

- Epineurium
  - Outermost connective tissue layer
  - Represents up to 50% of the cross-sectional area of the nerve trunk
  - Loose meshwork of collagen and elastin fibers and is generally thicker where a nerve crosses a joint
  - Well-developed vascular plexus runs within the epineurium.
  - Functions to protect the nerve fiber bundles, called fascicles, within the nerve
    - Tough <u>external epineurium</u> surrounds periphery of nerve.
    - Loose <u>internal epineurium</u> occupies space between fascicles.
- Perineurium
  - Thin, dense, multilayered connective tissue sheath that surrounds each fascicle
  - Tight basement membranes within the perineurium protect the endoneurial space by serving as a diffusion barrier.
  - Tensile strength of the perineurium helps maintain intrafascicular pressures.
  - Vascular structures traverse the perineurium obliquely to enter the endoneurial space.
- Endoneurium
  - Delicate collagenous matrix with fibroblasts, mast cells, and a capillary network
  - Surrounds individual myelinated nerve fibers or groups of unmyelinated nerve fibers within a fascicle

Fascicles

- All neurons within a peripheral nerve are bundled together into structures termed fascicles.
  - Fascicles are located within the internal epineurium.
  - Bounded by the perineurium

- Fascicles are often grouped together into a larger unit.
  - Inner interfascicular epineurium bounds grouped fascicles.
  - Grouped fascicles can be easily divided along internal epineurial planes.
- Major peripheral nerves will contain many grouped fascicles.
  - There is constant redistribution of fascicular organization along a peripheral nerve.
    - Interfascicular plexuses allow for interconnections.
  - Fascicles are more numerous and smaller where a nerve crosses a joint.
    - Smaller fascicles and more internal epineurium between them allows for increased protection of nerve fibers from external trauma and deformation.
- As the nerve gives off branches along its course, the fascicles divide (see Fig. 25-1).
  - Small terminal nerves contain only one or two fascicles.
    - Example: digital nerve

CELLULAR ANATOMY AND PHYSIOLOGY

Neurons (Fig. 25-2)

- Individual nerve fibers within the endoneurium of a peripheral nerve are termed neurons.
  - Neurons are extensions of a single nerve cell body.
- Neurons are broken down into four distinct regions:
  - Cell body
    - Contains the nucleus of the nerve cell
    - Metabolic center of the nerve cell
    - Dorsal root ganglion contains the cell body for sensory nerve fibers.
    - Motor nerve cell bodies are found in the anterior horn cells of the spinal cord.

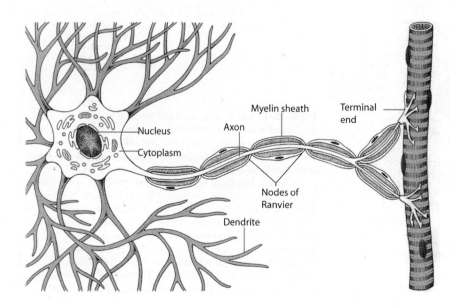

Figure 25-2 Neuron showing cell body, axon, dendrites, Schwann cells, myelin sheath, and nodes of Ranvier. (From Werner R, Benjamin BE. *A Massage Therapist's Guide to Pathology*, 2nd ed. Baltimore: Lippincott Williams & Wilkins.)

- Dendrites
  - Thin processes that branch off the cell body
  - Receive inhibitory or stimulatory synaptic input from other cells
    - Synapse with both central and peripheral nervous systems
    - This input allows modulation of peripheral nerve function.
- Axons
  - Each cell body gives rise to a single axon at its axon hillock.
  - Propagate electrical signals known as action potentials
    - Convey information over distances from cell bodies to nerve terminus
  - Axons may act at great distances from their cell bodies.
    - Example: Signal to extend great toe is generated in the motor cell bodies of the anterior horn cells of spinal nerve roots L5 and S1 and runs to the distal portion of the lower leg to innervate the extensor hallucis.
- Presynaptic nerve terminal
  - Located at the distal end of the axon
  - Action potential causes changes in ion exchange at terminus.
    - Release of neurotransmitter at the synaptic cleft or neuromuscular junction results.

Schwann Cells and Myelin Sheaths

- Specialized macroglial cells are called Schwann cells.
- Surround peripheral nerve axons and produce myelin
  - 70% lipid
  - 30% protein
  - High concentration of cholesterol and phospholipids
- Myelin provides electrical insulation for the electrical impulse.
  - Allows propagation of electrical impulses at faster speeds and at higher frequencies

Myelinated Axons

- Wrapped throughout their length by concentric, tight spirals of layers of the Schwann cell membrane
- Schwann cells line up end to end along the course of a single axon.
  - Entire length of the axon is surrounded.
  - Small spaces (up to 1.0 mm) between adjacent Schwann cells called nodes of Ranvier
  - Up to 500 Schwann cells may myelinate a single axon.

Unmyelinated Axons

- Surrounded as a group by processes of a single Schwann cell
- Conduction through these axons is comparatively slower.

Peripheral Nerves

- Contain both myelinated and unmyelinated fibers in an average ratio of 4:1 traveling within each fascicle

- Pathologic processes that disrupt the myelin sheath can slow conduction or cause focal conduction block.

Axoplasmic Transport

- Specialized transport processes within a nerve cell
  - All cellular proteins and neurotransmitters are produced in cell body.
  - Cell body may be at a significant distance from the terminal axon.
  - Multiple transport mechanisms
    - Fast and slow anterograde transport
      - Move cellular proteins from the cell body to the axon
    - Fast retrograde transport
      - Removes debris and breakdown products from the distal axon back to the cell body
  - Mechanisms proposed consist of carrier proteins binding to microtubules within the nerve cell.

ELECTROPHYSIOLOGY OF PERIPHERAL NERVES

Nerve cells communicate via electrical and chemical impulses. Ion exchanges between the microenvironment inside and around a nerve fiber create electrical potential differences in the nerve cell. When certain threshold levels are reached, events such as release of neurotransmitter vesicles, or initiation of an action potential, occur.

Resting Cell Membrane and Electrical State

- Neurons at rest have a negative potential within the cell between -50 and -80 mV.
  - Na^+ and Cl^- are concentrated on the outside of the neuron.
  - K^+ and organic anions are concentrated on the inside.
- Cell membrane is essentially impermeable to charged ions, except where specialized ion channels allow transit of charged ions.
- Net ion flux across the membrane at rest is zero.
  - Actively maintained by the Na^+/K^+ pump
- Excitatory and inhibitory neurons induce graded potentials in the nerve cell.
  - Act at cell body and dendrites
  - Membrane potential can become more or less negative as a result.
  - If sum of electrical activity received and processed reaches threshold, nerve depolarizes.

Depolarization

- Depolarizing "all-or-nothing" initiation of an action potential
  - Brief change in the properties of the neuron cell membrane occurs.
  - Na^+ channels open, causing net positive ions to

quickly accumulate within the nerve cell, and resting potential approaches neutral.
- Na^+/K^+ pump then begins to pump Na^+ out of the cell and restore resting negative potential to allow additional action potentials.
- Depolarization begins at the axon hillock.
  - Na^+ flows into this region of the axon first.
  - Adjacent areas of the axon become flooded with Na^+ and depolarize.
  - Depolarization propagates down the axon until the terminus is reached.

Saltatory Conduction

- Process of signal conduction in a myelinated axon
- Myelin insulates the nerve axon, allowing passive current flow to spread quickly through an area of myelination.

Nodes of Ranvier
- Unmyelinated spaces between adjacent Schwann cells on myelinated nerves
- Essential to fast impulse propagation
- Large density of voltage-gated Na^+ channels at nodes
- When depolarization reaches the node of Ranvier, these Na^+ channels open.
  - Na^+ flows into the axon.
  - Depolarizes the nodal region
  - Action potential quickly spreads through the next length of myelinated territory to the next node.

- Focal areas of demyelination can slow or stop saltatory conduction.
  - Example: Pressure on the peroneal nerve as it traverses around the fibular head can cause demyelination and a resultant mononeuropathy.

End-Organ Neurotransmission

- Depolarization in a nerve cell extends to the presynaptic terminal at the end of the axon.
- Depolarization in the presynaptic area allows nerve signal "communication" to the end organ.
  - Example: Calcium ion entry through voltage-gated calcium channels facilitates neurotransmitter release at the neuromuscular junction.

Classification of Nerve Fibers (Table 25-1)

- Nerve fibers characterized by Erlanger-Gasser or Lloyd-Hunt classification
  - Based on nerve fiber diameter and conduction velocity or function
  - Larger-diameter fibers typically have higher conduction velocities.

NERVE INJURY

Pathophysiology

- Efficient nerve transmission requires intact axons and myelin.

TABLE 25-1 NERVE FIBER TYPES

E-G Fiber Type	Lloyd Hunt	Myelin Status	Function	Diameter (mu)	Conduction velocity (m/s)
A-α	IA	M	Motor axons to muscles, muscle spindle proprioception	12–20	100
A-β	IB	M	Touch, pressure (sensory from tendons, Ruffini endings in skin)	5–12	30–70
	II	M	Mechanoreceptors (Meissner's and pacinian corpuscles)	5–15	30–80
A-γ		M	Motor to muscle spindle	3–6	15–30
A-δ	III	M	Pain and temperature	2–5	12–30
B		M	Preganglionic autonomic (white rami and cranial nerves III, VII, IX, X)	<3	3–15
C	IV	UM	Thermal pain, mechanoreceptor Postganglionic autonomic	0.3–1.3	0.5–2.3

E-G, Erlinger-Gasser; M, myelinated; UM, unmyelinated

- Injury to nerves can cause conduction slowing or failure of transmission.
- Nerve transmission may fail because of four possible mechanisms:
  - Axonal dysfunction
    - Example: nerve ischemia from tourniquet
    - Blocks oxidative metabolism needed to produce energy for nerve cell transport
    - Axonal transmission may recover soon after ischemia.
    - Axonal transport may take hours or up to a day longer to recover.
  - Axonal degradation (axonal neuropathy)
    - Can predominantly affect sensory or motor axons or both
    - Example: amyotrophic lateral sclerosis
    - Anterior horn cell degeneration producing preferentially motor dysfunction
  - Demyelination (demyelinating neuropathy)
    - Focal demyelination
      - Usually due to stretch or compression of nerve tissue
      - Usually at cutaneous sites where specific peripheral nerves run close to the skin surface and are vulnerable to injury
    - Generalized demyelination
      - Widespread slowing of conduction velocities
      - Example: Guillain-Barré syndrome
        - Acute inflammatory demyelinating polyneuropathy
        - Muscle weakness, pain, and in severe cases respiratory paralysis
  - Transport system disruption
    - Example: chemotherapeutic agents
    - Some agents interfere with microtubule assembly.
    - Axoplasmic transport affected
- Any combination of these disorders is possible.
  - Example: amyloidosis
  - Deposition of extracellular material between nerve fibers causes demyelination and loss of axonal continuity.

Anatomic Classifications of Nerve Injury

Radiculopathy
- Neuropathy of the nerve roots before they join to form spinal nerves
- Most radiculopathies are compressive.
  - Examples: herniated nucleus pulposus, spinal stenosis
- Noncompressive radiculopathies may be seen.
  - Examples: diabetes, sarcoidosis, amyloidosis, vasculitis, infections

Plexopathy
- Refers to nerve dysfunction at the nerve plexus
- Most result from blunt trauma.
  - Examples: brachial plexopathy
    - Sudden traction on arm from motorcycle accident

- Invasive breast cancer or lung cancer (Pancoast tumor)
- Radiation fibrosis from cancer treatment
- Idiopathic (Parsonage-Turner syndrome)

Peripheral Neuropathy
- Generic term used to describe a large and heterogeneous group of disorders affecting fibers distal to the plexus
- Large- and small-diameter motor and sensory fibers can be affected.
- Lesion can occur anywhere distal to the plexus.
  - To the neuromuscular junction for motor nerves
  - To the small intradermal fibers for sensory nerves
- Mixed motor and sensory axonal neuropathies are more common than pure motor or sensory neuropathies.
- Muscle weakness is usually more prominent distally, and sensory abnormalities are usually in a distal stocking-and-glove distribution.
  - Length-dependent dysfunction
  - Distal axon is affected more than the proximal axon.
  - Abnormality may be symmetric or asymmetric.
- Etiology of neuropathy includes multiple disorders that can be grouped broadly into the following categories:
  - Inherited
  - Traumatic
  - Compressive
  - Autoimmune
  - Toxic
  - Metabolic
  - Infectious
  - Idiopathic

Neuromuscular Junction Disorders
- A functioning neuromuscular junction is required for efficient and effective transfer of impulses from motor nerve to the muscle itself.
- Diseases affect synaptic transmission between motor nerve and muscle and can affect either the presynaptic or postsynaptic locations.
  - Presynaptic
    - Example: Botulinum toxin compromises release of acetylcholine from the nerve terminal of the motor axon.
  - Postsynaptic
    - Example: myasthenia gravis—antibodies to acetylcholine receptors on the postsynaptic muscle membrane

Complex Lesions: Multiple Anatomic Locations
- Neuropathies can coexist with radiculopathy and plexopathy.
  - Example: A patient with diabetes can have a combination of radiculopathy, plexopathy, and neuropathy (diabetic amyotrophy), median mononeuropathy at the wrist (carpal tunnel syndrome), mononeuropathy multiplex from vasculitis, distal symmetric polyneuropathy, or an isolated small-fiber neuropathy.

Electrodiagnostic Testing
- Frequently used in the assessment of peripheral nerve disorders

- Helps characterize and localize disorders
  - Differentiate mononeuropathies from mononeuropathy multiplex and distal symmetric polyneuropathies
  - Differentiate acute vs. chronic, axonal vs. demyelinating, and motor vs. sensory involvement
- Severity of a nerve lesion can often be determined.
  - Prognosis can sometimes be elucidated.
- Other disorders known to cause similar signs and symptoms can be excluded.

Traumatic Nerve Injury

- Direct trauma to the nerve may injure or sever the axons as well as the connective tissues surrounding the nerve fibers.
- Motor and sensory function of the nerve will be adversely affected.
  - Resultant dysfunction of muscles and loss of sensation
- Sympathetic fiber damage can induce dysfunction or hyperactivity of local sympathetic fibers.
  - Atrophy of skin and adnexal structures, changes in vascular and lymphatic flow
- Classification of traumatic nerve injury is based on the damage sustained by the nerve components and the ability for spontaneous recovery (Table 25-2).
  - Two schema widely used
  - *Seddon's classification* the first to characterize injury types
  - *Sunderland's classification* more precise

Grade I Injury (Neuropraxia)
- Mildest grade of traumatic nerve injury
- Dysfunction of conduction across a segment of a nerve
  - Conduction is evident in axon above and below site of injury.
- Axonal continuity preserved
  - Wallerian degeneration does not occur.
- Recovery is generally quick.
  - Pain and temperature return first, motor and fine touch last.
  - Recovery is complete within 3 to 4 months.
- Clinical example: median nerve stretched at the time of a distal radius fracture causing hand dysesthesias

Grade II Injury (Axonotmesis)
- Axon damage is seen but endoneurium is in continuity.
  - Wallerian degeneration occurs in distal axons.
  - Fibrillations and denervations evident in muscles
  - Neural connective tissue sheath, Schwann cells, and other supporting structures intact
- Recovery of motor and sensory is prolonged but generally complete.
  - Preservation of the connective tissue architecture guides axonal regeneration to reinnervate distal target organs.

Grade III Injury
- Axonal and endoneurial continuity is disrupted.
  - Perineurium is preserved.
  - Wallerian degeneration occurs in distal axons.
  - Fibrillations and denervations evident in muscles
- Recovery is prolonged and often incomplete.
  - When axons regenerate, they may enter an incorrect nerve sheath.
  - Intraneural scarring at site of injury obstructs axonal regrowth.

Grade IV Injury
- Axons and perineurial tissue are damaged but the epineurial nerve sheath is preserved.
- Neural scarring is common and adversely affects axonal regrowth and repair.
  - Axonal regeneration is still possible without surgical repair.

Grade V Injury (Neurotmesis)
- Endoneurium, perineurium, and epineurium are all disrupted or transected.
- Substantial perineural hemorrhage and scarring develop.
- Recovery through axonal regeneration cannot occur.
- Surgical repair is only effective way to allow for axonal regeneration.
- Clinical example: median nerve laceration at wrist with a knife

Grade VI Injury
- A sixth grade of injury has been proposed that more closely describes injury to nerve in vivo.

TABLE 25-2 SUNDERLAND AND SEDDON CLASSIFICATIONS OF TRAUMATIC NERVE INJURY

Sunderland	Seddon	Myelin	Axon	Endoneurium	Perineurium	Epineurium
I	Neuropraxia	+/−	−	−	−	−
II	Axonotmesis	+	+	−	−	−
III		+	+	+	−	−
IV		+	+	+	+	−
V	Neurotmesis	+	+	+	+	+

+ = damaged; − = intact without damage

- Complex injury that involves combinations of milder and more severe grades of nerve injury within a single nerve
- Recovery from grade VI injury is not uniform.
  - Varies across nerve segments and fascicles depending on the pattern of nerve injury
- Clinical example: radial nerve injury at level of humeral shaft fracture

Mechanisms of Traumatic Nerve Injury

- Eight mechanisms of traumatic injury to peripheral nerves are known. Each causes specific damage to the neuron, the Schwann cell, or the myelin sheath:
- Mechanical injury
  - Acute compression injury that can cause a focal demyelination
  - Typically results in a focal conduction block
  - Recovery occurs after remyelination of the axon.
    - Example: Prolonged use of a tourniquet may cause a mechanical injury.
  - If injury is severe enough or prolonged, axonal damage may also occur and recovery will be delayed.
    - Example: carpal tunnel syndrome
- Crush and percussion injury
  - Focal compression injury to the nerve induced by hematomas and/or compartment syndrome following a fracture
    - High pressure induced in the surrounding tissue compromises the vascular supply.
  - Neuronal ischemia leads to subsequent segmental demyelination, periaxonal and intramyelin edema, and axonal interruption of nerves.
    - Example: Delays in assessment and treatment of compartment syndrome can lead to nerve injury.
  - Double crush syndrome
    - A situation in which proximal compression injury renders the distal nerve more susceptible to compression injury
      - Likely a consequence of effects on axoplasmic transport
      - Example: carpal tunnel syndrome with a cervical radiculopathy
- Stretch injury
  - Nerve stretches approximately 10% to 20% before structural damage occurs.
  - Axonal injury results from acute lengthening greater than the nerve can tolerate.
  - Axons are disrupted over long segments of the nerve.
  - No disruption of epineurium is observed, so there is no clear role for surgical repair.
    - Example: Traction on peroneal nerve during knee dislocation causes a resultant foot drop.
- Laceration
  - Caused by blunt or penetrating trauma or combination thereof
  - Represents a progression of the stretch injury (type 3 above)
    - Stretch to the point where the nerve is grossly disrupted
    - Loss of continuity of both perineurium and epineurium
  - Nerves are not cleanly sectioned but are damaged in an irregular pattern over a large distance.
  - Nerve ends must be cut back to undamaged fascicles for successful repair.
    - Example: radial nerve laceration caused by open humerus fracture
- Transection
  - Associated with penetrating trauma, typically sharp edge
  - Nerves are partially or completely severed, with resultant epineurial disruption.
  - Direct surgical repair usually favorable with minimal resection of nerve ends
    - Examples: stab wound, glass lacerations, surgical incisions
- High-velocity trauma
  - Damage secondary to rapid tissue expansion in the track of a missile wound
  - Nerve injury a result of large amount of absorbed energy in surrounding tissue
  - Most frequently the nerve is not lacerated; rather, a mixed injury of axonotmesis and perineurial disruption.
    - Surgical repair is generally not required.
    - Example: gunshot wounds
- Cold injury
  - Several hours of exposure to temperatures between -2.5°C and 10°C will slow or stop axoplasmic transport.
    - Prolonged exposure may cause permanent damage to peripheral nerves.
  - Frostbite will likely lead to necrosis of peripheral nerves.
- Healing injury
  - Nerves can be damaged from the physiologic healing processes.
  - Adherence of nerves to scar tissue, fracture callus, or heterotopic bone may limit nerve gliding and a resultant decrease in function can be observed.

Pathophysiology of Nerve Injury

- After damage to a peripheral nerve, complex changes occur throughout the neuron.
- Cell body
  - Cell body and nucleolar swelling as well as nuclear eccentricity
  - The neuron shifts from nerve conduction mode to repair mode.
    - Increased production of cytoskeletal proteins and growth-associated proteins (GAPs)
    - Decreases in neurotransmitters and neurofilament proteins
- Site of injury
  - Immediate disruption of endoneurial and perineurial vessels, leading to hemorrhage, edema, and in-

creased vascular permeability with influx of inflammatory cells
- Changes in local tissue oxygenation and energy delivery negatively affect axonal transport and nerve conduction.
- The proximal segment of a transected nerve degenerates one or more internodal segments.
    - If the cell body survives, axonal sprouting begins.
- Wallerian degeneration
    - Structured process of breakdown in the distal segment that occurs with axonal disruption
    - *Axonal degeneration* initiated within hours of injury
        - Myelin breakdown and phagocytosis progress distally to the target organ.
    - Macrophages
        - Play important roles in phagocytosis of cellular and myelin debris and stimulation of Schwann cells
    - Schwann cells
        - Proliferate and create endoneurial tubes (bands of Bunger) for regeneration of axons
- Nerve conduction
    - Immediately after injury, stimulation proximal to the injured site will demonstrate a reduced compound muscle action potential (CMAP).
    - Distal CMAP amplitude will be normal immediately after injury.
    - Reduced amplitude on distal stimulation is observed by 7 days.
    - Spontaneous denervation potentials may be observed on electromyographic examination of affected muscles within 2 to 5 weeks.

NERVE REGENERATION AND REPAIR

Nerve recovery involves orderly degeneration followed by an orchestrated sequence of regeneration. The success of nerve regeneration is variable and highly dependent upon the age of the patient as well as the type of nerve injury. Little functional recovery will occur if the end organ has irreversibly atrophied by the time it is reinnervated, so the timing and location of nerve injury are also critical to outcomes.

Regeneration

- Axon regeneration occurs at rate of approximately 1 to 2 mm/day or 1 inch/month.
- Process begins with formation of multiple nerve "sprouts" at the proximal axon stump.
- Sprouts form a regenerating unit that contains multiple nonmyelinated axons surrounded by a single Schwann cell.
- Regenerating units must first elongate through the zone of injury.
    - Scar tissue density, increasing gap length, and axonal misdirection all negatively affect the process.
    - Several cytokines and nerve substances secreted by the distal end of the nerve and possibly by Schwann cells mediate the process.

- Axons that bridge the gap can then enter the distal endoneurial tubes.
    - The regenerating axon signals Schwann cells to begin myelination.

Reinnervation

- Functional recovery of nerve function is related to completeness of axonal regeneration and directed growth into the correct endoneurial tubes.
    - Lack of functional recovery is most likely a result of axon misdirection.
        - During neonatal development, selective reinnervation occurs as neurotropic factors guide axons to their target.
        - In adult models, this effect is greatly reduced and dependent upon nerve gap and axon orientation.
- Progress of the healing nerve can sometimes be monitored with an advancing Tinel's sign.
- Recovery of motor function is possible only when the distance from the site of trauma to the endplate in the muscle is short.
    - Irreversible motor endplate atrophy and permanent loss of functional muscle fibers occur 12 to 18 months after initial injury.
- Sensory function return after injury tends to follow a pattern of pain recovery first, followed by slow vibration sense, and then sensation to moving touch.
    - Smaller-diameter, unmyelinated fibers without specialized endplate receptors likely recover before the larger, myelinated fibers that carry sensation from specialized receptors.
    - Deep tendon reflexes may or may not recover, even after only partial nerve injury.

Operative Nerve Repair

- Nerve repair aims to reconstitute fascicular bundle organization after a transection or laceration.
    - Epineurial and group fascicular repair techniques have been described.
- Reconnecting the proximal and distal ends of severed nerve fibers is thought to speed recovery and improve reinnervation.
    - Repair reduces the gap and the distance axonal sprouts must navigate before connecting with distal endoneurial tubes.
    - Magnification in the form of a microscope is typically used to improve the accuracy of nerve repair.
    - Healthy proximal axons must be identified before coaptation begins.
- Nerve ends reconnected under excessive tension on the repair have been shown to have poorer functional outcomes.
    - Nerve graft material used to bridge gap distance
        - Nerve fibers
        - Silicone tubes

- ▪ Veins
- ▪ Bioengineered derived collagen tubes
- Even the most accurate surgical repair <u>does not</u> ensure that regenerating axons find their appropriate distal endoneurial tubes.
  - ▪ Repair of pure sensory nerves demonstrates reliable return of function.
    - ▪ Example: digital nerve of finger
  - ▪ Variable outcomes after repair of mixed nerves
    - ▪ Regenerating axons frequently reinnervate incorrect target organ.
    - ▪ Example: ulnar nerve in forearm
  - ▪ Poor outcomes observed from proximal nerve repair
    - ▪ Combination of axonal misdirection as well as end-organ atrophy during the lengthy regeneration process results in predictably poor distal functional return.
    - ▪ Example: brachial plexus
- Neurotropic factors are being studied as adjuncts to operative repair to assist regenerating axons to find their end-organ targets.

SUGGESTED READING

Chaudhry V, Glass JD, Griffin JW. Wallerian degeneration in peripheral nerve disease. *Neurol Clin* 1992;10(3):613–627.

Coleman M. Axon degeneration mechanisms: commonality amid diversity. *Nature Rev Neurosci* 2005;6(11):889–898.

Corfas G, Velardez MO, Ko CP, et al. Mechanisms and roles of axon-Schwann cell interactions. *J Neurosci* 2004;24(42):9250–9260.

Green DP, Hotchkiss RN, Pederson WC, eds. *Operative Hand Surgery*, 4th edition. Philadelphia: Churchill Livingstone, 1998.

Guzik BW, Goldstein LS. Microtubule-dependent transport in neurons: steps towards an understanding of regulation, function and dysfunction. *Curr Opin Cell Biol* 2004;16(4):443–450.

Johnson EO, Zoubos AB, Soucacos PN. Regeneration and repair of peripheral nerves. *Injury* 2005;36(Suppl 4):S24–29.

Lundborg G. Nerve regeneration and repair. A review. *Acta Orthop Scand* 1987;58:145–169.

Myers RR. Anatomy and microanatomy of peripheral nerve. *Neurosurg Clin North Am* 1991;2(1):1–20.

Sunderland S. The anatomy and physiology of nerve injury. *Muscle Nerve* 1990;13:771–784.

Sunderland S. The connective tissue of peripheral nerves. *Brain* 1965;88:841–854.

Whitwam JG. Classification of peripheral nerve fibres. An historical perspective. *Anaesthesia* 1976;31(4):494–503.

SKELETAL MUSCLE ANATOMY, PHYSIOLOGY, AND MECHANICS

BRYAN T. KELLY
WILLIAM J. ROBERTSON

MUSCLE STRUCTURE AND FUNCTION

Myofibrils and Connective Tissue

- **Myofibrils** represent the basic structural element of skeletal muscle (Fig. 26-1).
- Along with their innervating nerves, myofibrils are responsible for the contractile function of skeletal muscle.
- Myofibrils fuse together to form ribbon-like multinucleated cells called muscle fibers or myofibers.
    - Muscle fibers varying in length from a few millimeters to 50 cm.
    - Muscle is structurally organized by three connective tissue layers: the endomysium, perimysium, and epimysium (Table 26-1).
        - **Endomysium**: a delicate connective tissue layer (basement membrane) that surrounds each muscle fiber

- **Perimysium**: an enveloping connective tissue layer that bundles multiple muscle fibers to form larger fascicles
- **Epimysium**: a stronger, thick connective tissue sheath that combines and surrounds muscle fascicles to form the entire muscle belly
- This connective tissue framework allows individual muscle cells, nerves, and capillaries to work together during muscle contraction.

Intracellular Organelles and Architecture
- Below the layer of endomysium that covers each muscle fiber sits a plasma membrane called the sarcolemma (Fig. 26-2 and Table 26-2).
- The ends of each fiber are attached to the extracellular matrix (ECM) through the sarcolemma by way of protein molecules called integrins.

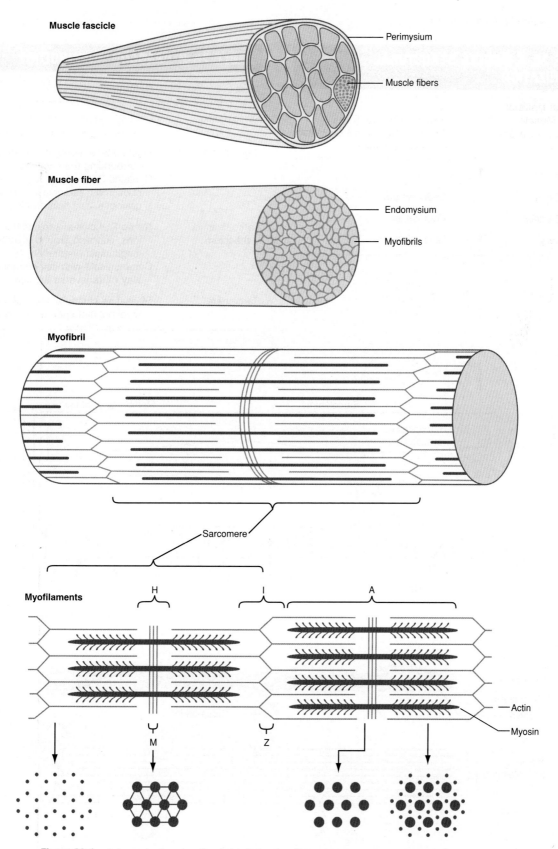

Figure 26-1 Schematic diagram of a skeletal muscle, showing a stepwise arrangement of its components. Myofibrils are composed of thin and thick myofilaments that provide the framework for muscle contraction. A muscle fiber (myofiber) is made up of numerous myofibrils covered in a delicate connective tissue layer (endomysium). Multiple muscle fibers are grouped into a muscle fascicle. The connective tissue surrounding each fascicle is called the perimysium. The fascicles, as a group, are surrounded by epimysium and form a skeletal muscle.

TABLE 26-1 MUSCLE STRUCTURAL ORGANIZATION

Structural Units of Skeletal Muscle Organized from Smallest to Largest	Separating Structures Between Structural Elements of Skeletal Muscle
Myofibrils	
Muscle fibers	Endomysium
Muscle fascicles	Perimysium
Muscle belly	Epimysium

TABLE 26-2 "SARCO" TERMINOLOGY

Term	Definition
Sarcolemma	Limiting plasma membrane surrounding individual muscle fibers (myofibers)
Sarcoplasm	Fluid material within the sarcolemma surrounding the myofibrils Contains Golgi apparatus, mitochondria, ribosomes, sarcoplasmic reticulum, glycogen, and lipid droplets
Sarcoplasmic reticulum	Network of closed sacs, rich in calcium ions, coursing around myofibrils in a longitudinal orientation Communicate with cell membrane by way of transverse tubules
Sarcomere	Repeating structural units of the myofibril that span between Z lines

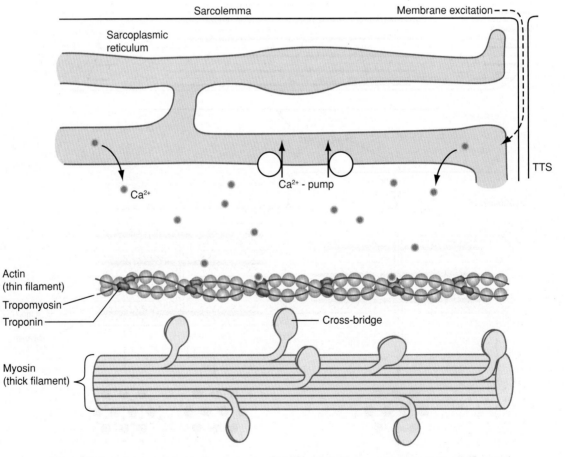

Figure 26-2 Schematic diagram showing some of the intracellular structures of an individual muscle fiber. Depolarization originating at the motor endplate travels down the sarcolemma membrane and continues via the transverse tubules (TTS) to the sarcoplasmic reticulum. A resultant depolarization of the calcium-rich sarcoplasmic reticulum releases calcium into the sarcoplasm, where at high concentrations it binds to troponin. A conformational change in troponin frees actin of tropomyosin and allows for actin-to-myosin cross-bridging.

■ Integrins are a family of adhesions receptors that provide muscle fibers with the strength to withstand tensile forces at the myotendinous junction (MTJ), while also playing vital roles such as cell-to-cell signaling, cell-to-ECM interactions, and signal transduction.

■ Within the sarcolemma there exists a fluid material, or sarcoplasm, that encompasses large numbers of longitudinally oriented myofibrils and numerous nuclei that compose each muscle fiber.

■ The sarcoplasm contains a Golgi apparatus, many mitochondria, ribosomes, sarcoplasmic reticulum, glycogen, and lipid droplets.

■ The sarcoplasmic reticulum is a network of closed sacs that course around the myofibrils in a primarily longitudinal direction.

  ■ These sacs are rich in calcium ions.

  ■ They communicate with the cell membrane by way of transverse tubules.

Myofibril Structural Composition (see Fig. 26-1)

■ Each myofibril exhibits periodic cross-striations.

■ These striations are alternating light and dark bands of isotropic and anisotropic materials, respectively, composed of repeating units called sarcomeres that spans from one Z line to the next Z line.

■ The light and dark bands of a sarcomere are created by overlapping thin and thick filaments, also termed **myofilaments.**

■ These thin and thick filaments are made up of specific proteins that, in the presence of calcium, are responsible for force production within the muscle.

Thin and Thick Filaments

Thin Filaments.

■ Thin filaments consist of three proteins (actin, tropomyosin, and troponin), which form the I band of a myofibril (see Fig. 26-2).

■ Major component of the thin filament is actin, consisting of two polymers:

  ■ G-actin, or globular actin

    ■ On binding with ATP, it polymerizes to the F form, or fibrous actin.

  ■ F-actin binds calcium tightly.

■ Actin has long, thin fibers attached to its surface that inhibit contraction by blocking actin and myosin cross-bridges. These fibers are called tropomyosin fibers and are attached to actin by troponin molecules.

■ Troponin is a three-subunit molecule (troponin-I, troponin-T, and troponin-C) that can bind actin, tropomyosin, and calcium, respectively. In the absence of adequate calcium levels, troponin binds tropomyosin to actin and inhibits contraction.

■ A high enough concentration of calcium within the sarcoplasm will allow calcium to bind to the troponin-C subunit. A conformational change then results in the other troponin subunits. These changes release the inhibitory effect of tropomyosin and allow actin and myosin interaction.

■ As the calcium concentration falls, the conformation of troponin reverts back to its inhibitory form, shifting tropomyosin to again stearicly inhibit cross-bridges.

Thick Filaments.

■ Formed by the muscle protein myosin

■ Thick filaments span the midportion of the sarcomere forming the A band of a myofibril.

■ I bands contain only thin filaments, whereas A bands contain both thick and thin filaments, except in the central H zone, where only thick filaments are present (see Fig. 26-1).

■ Myosin is the largest of the myofibril proteins, making up >50% of muscle mass.

■ Myosin molecule resembles a thin rod with two small, globular heads.

■ This globular end has significant ATPase activity in the presence of ionic calcium and serves as a cross-bridge, binding myosin with actin during muscle contraction.

Changes During Contraction.

■ When a muscle fiber contracts, each fiber and each sarcomere shortens.

■ Thick and thin filaments are arranged so that they can slide past each during contraction.

■ With maximal contraction a sarcomere shortens 20% to 50% of its normal resting length.

  ■ The I band becomes shorter and the H zone usually disappears.

  ■ The A band does not change in length during contraction or relaxation.

■ A sarcomere can extend to 120% of its length during passive stretching, and the I band becomes longer.

Neuromuscular Interaction

■ Each nerve cell axon branches many times, providing each muscle fiber with a point of contact called the motor endplate.

■ This single nerve axon and all of the muscle fibers it innervates constitute a motor unit.

Motor Unit

■ Both the size of the motor unit and the number of motor units within a given muscle are variable.

■ Muscles that require fine motor control and coordinated movements, such as the extraocular muscles, have small motor units.

■ Larger, more powerful muscles, such as the gastrocnemius muscle, have large motor units.

Stimulus for Muscle Contraction

■ The arrival of an electrical impulse at the terminal axon leads to an inflow of calcium ions.

■ Acetylcholine-containing vesicles fuse with the axon membrane and release acetylcholine into the synaptic cleft.

■ Acetylcholine binds to receptors on the muscle cell membrane, causing an inflow of current and depolarizing the motor endplate.

■ Sodium, potassium, and chloride ions move about

within transverse tubules to spread the impulse to the sarcoplasmic reticulum (see Fig. 26-2).

■ Depolarization of the sarcoplasmic reticulum causes a release of calcium ions into the sarcoplasm.

■ This in turn causes all filaments within a muscle fiber to contract together.

Muscle Contraction

■ Muscle contraction is initiated by the release of ionic calcium into the sarcoplasm.

■ In absence of calcium, troponin and tropomyosin interfere with the formation of active complexes between actin and myosin.

■ With the binding of free calcium, troponin undergoes a conformational change, releasing tropomyosin from actin and allowing the formation of cross-bridges between actin and myosin (see Fig. 26-2).

■ Intracellular calcium also activates the myosin–ATP complex, which motors the sliding action between actin and myosin.

■ Energy provided by ATP drives the pulling of the actin molecule past myosin, shortening the fibril.

■ As long as the calcium concentration in the cell is maintained at a high enough level, the myosin ATPase remains active, permitting the fibril to stay in its contracted form.

■ When the energizing impulse terminates, calcium is rapidly pumped out of the sarcoplasm.

■ As the calcium ion concentration drops, the calcium–troponin interaction is uncoupled.

■ Tropomyosin can again bind to actin, and the troponin–actin–tropomyosin B complex impedes cross-bridging between actin and myosin.

■ Calcium reuptake by the sarcoplasmic reticulum will not occur if there is insufficient ATP available, which may lead to muscle contraction without electrical stimulation, as is seen in rigor mortis.

FIBER TYPES AND ADAPTABILITY

■ In lower mammals and other animals, muscles are generally composed entirely of either type I or type II fibers.

■ Human muscle is made up of a mixture of type I and type II fibers.

■ Muscle fiber type depends not on any intrinsic feature of the fiber itself, but on the motor neuron supplying that fiber.

■ All muscle fibers supplied by one particular axon will be of either type I or type II.

■ There are significant differences in the fiber types.

Type I Fibers

■ Type I muscle fibers are rich in the enzymes necessary for oxidative metabolism and are darker in appearance.

■ Contain a higher concentration of mitochondria and more capillaries per fiber than type II muscle fibers

■ When stimulated, they have a slow contraction or "twitch" time.

■ These fibers have increased resistance to fatigue.

■ Type I fibers are well suited for activities related to physical effort requiring strength and endurance that depend on the metabolism of oxidative processes for energy.

Type II Fibers

■ Type II fibers obtain their energy through a much faster glycolytic process.

■ As glycogen stores are more rapidly depleted than oxygen supplies, type II fibers are less suited to continuous types of activity and are more suited to rapid alternating effort.

■ Those muscles most accustomed to slow, continuous work have a lower percentage of type II muscle fibers.

■ Type II fibers may be more prone to anatomic changes following altered energy demands than are type I.

■ Type II fibers tend to be smaller than type I in children and in adults who do not carry out strenuous physical exercise, although they increase in size with repeated physical demands on the muscle.

■ Type II fibers are subdivided into types IIa and IIb.
  ■ Type IIa fibers have an admixture of glycolytic and oxidative enzymes and show an intermediate twitch time.
  ■ Type IIb fibers (fast glycolytic fibers) have the largest motor unit size, have the fastest rate of contraction, and are most susceptible to fatigue.

Fiber Type Interconversion

■ It is generally accepted that the relative percentage of type I and type II fibers in humans is established genetically without a great deal of capacity for change.

■ Evidence does exist for a training-dependent interconversion of type IIa and IIb fibers.

■ Endurance training can result in an increased percentage of type IIa fibers at the expense of IIb fibers.

■ Likewise, strength training and burst exercises without an emphasis on endurance can lead to a percentage increase in type IIb fibers and corresponding decrease in type IIa fibers.

Muscle Injury

■ Type II muscle fibers are more susceptible to injury than type I fibers.

■ Other risk factors for injury include muscles that cross two joints and eccentric loading.

GROWTH AND DEVELOPMENT

Embryology of Skeletal Muscle

Myoblasts

■ Fusiform-shaped muscle progenitor cells that arise from the mesoderm cell population

■ Undergo mitosis in response to molecular signaling

■ When an adequate population of myoblasts exists, they fuse to form long multinucleated cells called myotubes.

Myotubes
- Precursor of eventual skeletal muscle fibers
- Continue to differentiate into large multinucleated cells called muscle fibers
- Skeletal muscle can be identified by the seventh week of gestation.

Longitudinal Growth of Skeletal Muscle
- Able to increase in length to accommodate for skeletal growth in the following ways:
  - In skeletally immature animals
    - Increasing muscle and tendon length: occurs at the musculotendinous junction rather than in the skeletal muscle midsubstance
    - Increasing the number of sarcomeres during longitudinal growth: individual sarcomere length remains relatively stable
  - In skeletally mature animals
    - The primary mechanism of muscle lengthening is elongation of the muscle belly.

Immobilization of Skeletal Muscle Under Stretch
- Initially muscle fibers lengthen and the sarcomeres stretch, resulting in an increased separation of the A bands and I bands compared to their normal state.
- Over several weeks, additional sarcomeres are added in series at the musculotendinous junction, allowing all sarcomeres to return to their normal length.
- This addition of sarcomeres results in muscles with increased protein and increased weight due to longitudinal growth rather than an increase in cross-sectional area.
- As little as 2 weeks of this type of immobilization shifts the length–tension curve to the right, resulting in less passive force generated in response to a given stretch.

ENERGETICS OF MUSCLE

Energy Sources for Skeletal Muscle

Adenosine Triphosphate (ATP)
- ATP is the immediate energy source for muscle contraction.
- Has two terminal high-energy bonds that, upon hydrolysis, provide a significant amount of chemical energy to drive biologic reactions
- The stepwise hydrolysis of these phosphate bonds produces: ATP → ADP + inorganic phosphate → AMP + inorganic phosphate

Creatine Phosphate (CP)
- Another source of high-energy phosphate bonds
- Cannot be used as direct energy source; used instead to produce ATP from ADP
- This reaction of ADP + CP → ATP + creatine is catalyzed by the muscle enzyme creatine kinase.

- The total energy available from ATP hydrolysis is approximately enough for a person to sprint for less than 50 yards.
- The total energy available from all the stored high-energy phosphate compounds is enough to sprint 200 yards.
- The ability to replenish ATP is the limiting factor in many aspects of athletic performance.
- Two metabolic pathways that maintain this ATP energy reservoir are the aerobic system and the anaerobic system.

Aerobic Metabolism
- The primary source for ATP when oxygen is available
- Uses glucose or fatty acids to produce ATP in large quantities
- Glucose is broken into two pyruvate molecules, which enter the Krebs cycle.
- Hydrogen molecules are removed from pyruvate and couple with oxygen to make water and release energy.
- This energy results in the generation of high-energy phosphates that are coupled to ADP to form ATP.
- The Krebs cycle results in 38 ATP from the oxidation of one glucose molecule.
- Glucose is stored in the muscle cell in the form of glycogen.

Anaerobic Metabolism
- The rapid hydrolysis of a glucose molecule into two molecules of lactic acid
- Releases enough energy to convert two ADP molecules into two ATP molecules
- The lactic acid produced causes acidosis and muscle fatigue.
- This is the system relied upon when a large amount of energy is needed for a relatively short period.

Fat
- Fat stores are abundant in the body and provide the largest potential source of energy.
- Usually stored as triglycerides, which consist of three separate fatty acids
- Variable-length fatty acid chains are cleaved by beta-oxidation into two carbon molecules called acetyl CoA.
  - Acetyl CoA enters the Krebs cycle.
- The amount of ADP converted to ATP is dependent on the size of the fatty acid chain.

Protein
- Under normal conditions, protein is not the primary source of fuel for muscle metabolism.
- Deamination of amino acids produces ketoacids, which enter the Krebs cycle.

Use of Energy Sources
- Anaerobic and aerobic systems function simultaneously and are not exclusive to any particular intensity level.
  - These systems are, however, different in how they can respond to a given activity level.

- Type I muscle fibers have a high concentration of aerobic enzymes.
- Type IIB muscle fibers have a high concentration of anaerobic enzymes.
- Type IIA muscle fibers have an intermediate level of both enzymes.
- Both carbohydrate and fat are used as energy sources for any activity level.
- Prolongation of aerobic exercise leads to a shift from the metabolism of stored glucose and glycogen to the oxidation of fatty acids.

MUSCLE MECHANICS

Length vs. Tension

- Passively stretched unstimulated muscle undergoes a period of lengthening before any tension develops.
- Tension in the passively stretched muscle then rises in a nonlinear manner and approaches significant levels with high strains.
- The length–tension relationship for active skeletal muscle is similar to that of cardiac muscle and can be explained by the myofibrillar ultrastructure.
- Actin and myosin overlap is required for force to be generated.
- In a lengthened position this overlap is reduced, as is the maximum force generated.
- As the sarcomere length decreases so does the cross-bridge overlap and the ability to generate force.
- However, with continued sarcomere shortening, the filaments will collide and again the ability to generate force is decreased.

Isometric Contraction

- With isometric (static) contraction, external muscle length does not change.
- Internally, however, within the fibril the distance between the Z lines does shorten.

Isotonic Contraction

- A constant internal force is produced and the muscle shortens.
- Also defined as a dynamic exercise with a constant load or resistance

Eccentric Contraction

- Contraction in which the external force applied is greater than the internal force of the muscle, which causes the muscle to lengthen while continuing to maintain tension
- Movement is controlled but not initiated.
- During an eccentric contraction, muscle can sustain greater tension than it can develop in isometric contraction at any given muscle length.
- Because greater tension is generated, muscles are more vulnerable to rupture during eccentric contraction.

Isokinetic Contraction

- Term means "constant force" and typically is used to describe dynamic exercise performed through the range of motion of a joint at constant velocity.
- Equipment used in isokinetic exercises accommodates the exerted force to maintain the specified velocity throughout the arc of motion.
- Because velocity does not change, the kinetic energy remains constant.
- Isokinetic contractions are not part of normal physiologic muscle function.

TRAINING EFFECTS ON MUSCLE

- Skeletal muscle is a highly adaptable tissue.
- Training can be aimed at increasing strength, endurance, and anaerobic or aerobic fitness.

Strength Training

- High-resistance, low-repetition (1 to 15) exercise leads to increased strength and increased muscle cross-sectional area.
- The majority of this size increase is likely due to muscle hypertrophy, but hyperplasia may also play a role.
- Results in increased contractile protein content
- Type II muscle fibers (higher in anaerobic metabolism) show a more pronounced hypertrophy than type I fibers.
- Neurologic component, resulting in improved motor unit recruitment and better synchronized muscle activation
- In poorly conditioned muscles, as few as 60% of the fibers fire simultaneously.
- Well-conditioned muscles may fire over 90% of the fibers simultaneously.
- Results in increased stores of energy-rich phosphagens

Endurance Training

- Aerobic training
- The challenge for the muscle is not to overcome high forces but rather to perform faster without fatigue.
- The goal is not to increase muscle size but instead to adapt to use energy more efficiently.
- Improvements in endurance result from better central and peripheral circulation and muscle metabolism.
- Cardiovascular gains
  - Larger stroke volume, resulting in a lower resting heart rate (fewer beats are need to deliver the same amount of blood)
  - Improved blood flow through arterioles to the muscles
  - Increased muscle capillaries, especially in type I muscles
  - These advances allow the muscle to use oxygen more efficiently.
- Muscle fiber changes
  - Mitochondria (important for oxidation) increase in size, number, and density.

- Oxidative enzymes increase in quantity.
- Adapt to use fatty acids more efficiently rather than glycogen

Aerobic (Sprint or Power) Training

- High-intensity exercise for a few seconds to 2 minutes
- Primarily driven by anaerobic metabolism
- Relies on available muscle stores of ATP and the ability to perform anaerobic glycolysis
- This training results in an increased level of stored phosphagens and an elevation in some enzymes involved in glycolysis.
- Almost exclusively seen in fast-twitch type II muscle fibers

MUSCLE INJURY AND REPAIR

Mechanisms of Skeletal Muscle Injury

- Can be caused by laceration, contusion, or strain
- The most common injuries occurring during sports, 90% of which are contusions or strains.
  - Contusions result from a heavy compressive force, such as a direct blow to the muscle, and typically occur in contact sports.
  - Strains result from an excessive tensile force on the muscle, resulting in complete or, more commonly, partial tears.
    - These tears usually occur near the myotendinous junction, where the terminal sarcomeres are stiffer.
    - Muscle strains are typically seen in muscles crossing two joints (gastrocnemius, rectus femoris, semitendinosus), where potentially higher length–tension values can occur.

Pathobiology of Muscle Injury

- Skeletal muscle heals via a repair process.
- Regardless of the underlying cause, the healing process is quite constant.
- Three phases of muscle injury have been identified:
  - Destruction phase
  - Repair phase
  - Remodeling phase

Destruction Phase

- Rupture and the ensuing necrosis of myofibers
  - Contused muscle tears at the point of impact, whereas muscle strains usually result in tears at the myotendinous junction.
  - The contusion injury is more superficial in a contracted muscle vs. deeper in an uncontracted muscle, where it is compressed against the underlying bone.
  - The characteristic length of myofibers predisposes them to widespread necrosis starting at the rupture site.

- The propagation of necrosis is halted within hours by myofiber structures called contraction bands that act like a system of fire doors, preventing further cell death.
- Hematoma formation between the ruptured muscle ends
  - Muscle fiber-associated blood vessels are torn, allowing inflammatory cells to gain access to the injury site.
- Inflammatory cell reaction
  - Macrophages and fibroblasts release chemotactic and growth factors.
  - In the acute phase, polymorphonuclear leukocytes (PMNs) are the most abundant cells at the injury site.
  - By the first day, PMNs are being replaced by macrophages that aid in the proteolysis and phagocytosis of the necrotic muscle tissue.

Repair and Remodeling Phase

- As the phagocytosis subsides, two simultaneous processes (regeneration and scar formation) begin.
  - Regeneration of disrupted myofibers
    - Although myofibers are considered postmitotic cells, undifferentiated reserve cells called satellite cells allow for restoration of the contractile unit following injury. During fetal development, a pool of these satellite cells is set aside underneath the basal lamina of each muscle fiber.
      - In responses to injury, these satellite cells proliferate and then differentiate into myoblasts.
      - Similar to their embryological development, myoblasts join together to form multinucleated myotubes.
      - Myotubes join with the injured ends of the myofibers, allowing them to regain their normal cross-striated appearance and structure over time
      - Both myofiber ends join to a connective tissue scar that has filled the injury gap by forming mini-myotendinous junctions with the scar periphery.
    - Mature skeletal muscle contains two major populations of satellite cells: committed and stem.
      - Committed satellite cells are ready to begin differentiation to myoblasts immediately upon muscle injury.
      - Stem satellite cells first undergo division before differentiation, providing another pool of satellite cells should subsequent injury occur to the same muscle.
  - Formation of the connective tissue scar
    - Immediately after injury the gap between the ruptured muscle fibers is filled with hematoma.
    - Early fibrin and fibronectin cross-linking forms granulation tissue within the gap that provides a foundation for arriving fibroblasts and most importantly the initial strength to withstand contractile forces.

■ Type III collagen is soon synthesized, and type I collagen synthesis is initiated a couple of days later.

■ This initially large connective tissue scar condenses efficiently into a small scar composed mainly of type I collagen.

■ Early on, this scar represents the weakest point of the injured skeletal muscle, but its tensile strength increases considerably with the production of type I collagen.

■ Approximately 10 days after injury, due to type I collagen cross-links, the scar is no longer the weakest link.

■ Rupture at this time most often occurs at the mini-myotendinous junction between the myofibers and scar.

■ The muscle still needs a relatively long time before its tensile strength is restored completely.

■ In reruptures or major trauma a dense scar tissue may result that acts as a barrier restricting myofiber regeneration.

■ With time, the connective tissue scar shrinks, bringing the myofiber ends closer to each other.

■ Whether these ends will ever fuse is still unknown.

■ Regenerating myofibers increase their tensile strength by reinforcing their adhesions to the extracellular matrix peripherally.

Classification

Table 26-3 covers the classification of muscle injuries.

Myositis Ossificans

■ A non-neoplastic formation of bone within skeletal muscle at a site of previous injury or hematoma

■ Relatively rare complication of muscle injury

■ Higher incidence in contact sports

■ Should be suspected if pain and swelling do not subside by 10 to 14 days after an injury

■ Radiographic detection of ectopic bone may be seen as early as 18 days after injury, but often the formation of ectopic bone lags behind symptoms for weeks.

TABLE 26-3 CLINICAL CLASSIFICATION OF MUSCLE INJURIES (STRAIN/CONTUSION)

Classification	Description
Mild (first degree)	Tear of only a few muscle fibers, minor swelling and discomfort, no or minimal strength loss
Moderate (second degree)	Greater damage with clear loss of function (decline in contractile ability)
Severe (third degree)	Full-thickness tear, virtual complete loss of muscle function

Delayed Muscle Soreness

■ Muscle pain typically occurring 48 to 72 hours after intense exercise (can begin several hours after exercise and peaks after 1 to 3 days)

■ Primarily associated with eccentric exercise and varies depending on intensity and duration

■ Strength loss and muscle swelling are common signs.

■ Structural changes typically occur.

■ Z-band streaming, A-band disruption, and myofibril misalignment

■ Most severe at 2 to 3 days after exercise and tend to occur primarily in type IIb fibers

■ Ultrastructural damage is thought to lead to edema formation within the muscle, which in turn results in soreness.

IMMOBILIZATION AND DISUSE

■ Muscle atrophy is among the initial changes seen with immobilization.

■ Atrophy results in a loss in muscle mass with associated reductions in muscle strength and endurance.

■ Decreased endurance, or higher fatigability, is associated with the diminished ability to utilize fat in aerobic pathways, decreased energy stores, and an increase in intramuscular lactic acid levels.

■ Muscle changes depend on the amount of time that the muscle is immobilized and the position of immobilization.

■ Muscles immobilized under no tension undergo more detrimental changes than those immobilized while stretched.

■ Muscles immobilized in a stretched position (i.e., hamstrings in a knee immobilizer) exhibit a decreased strength and cross-sectional area, but due to the addition of new contractile proteins and sarcomeres, the change in muscle mass is less pronounced.

■ Muscles immobilized in a shortened position can exhibit higher tensions for a given passive stretch, or stiffen.

Acutely Injured Skeletal Muscle

■ Advantages of early mobilization of an acutely injured muscle: shown to induce more rapid capillary ingrowth, results in better myofiber regeneration, produces more parallel myofiber orientation, and regains muscle strength more quickly

■ Disadvantages of early mobilization: associated with excessive scar formation at the injury site and increased rerupture rates

■ Advantage of immobilization for an acutely injured muscle: allows time for stronger, more efficient scar formation

■ Disadvantages of immobilization: can lead to muscle fiber atrophy, excessive deposition of connective tissue within muscle tissue, and a substantial delay in the recovery of muscle strength

Treatment Recommendations

- A short (3- to 5-day) period of relative immobilization, allowing the scar tissue and myofiber ends to gain the strength needed to withstand contractile forces and prevent reruptre
- After a few days, gradually, within the limits of pain, begin active mobilization that will enhance the penetration of muscle fibers through the connective tissue scar, limit the size of the permanent scar, facilitate the proper muscle fiber alignment, and restore the tensile strength of the muscle more rapidly.

HORMONAL EFFECTS ON SKELETAL MUSCLE

Insulin

- Insulin increases glucose and amino acid uptake by the muscle, increases glycogen synthesis and ribosomal protein synthesis, and decreases protein catabolism and the release of gluconeogenic amino acids.
  - Results in an anabolic effect, increasing both protein and carbohydrate stores within the muscle
- Insulin effects antagonized by glucocorticoids
  - Glucocorticoids accelerate protein degradation, decrease amino acid transport, and hinder protein synthesis.

Growth Hormone

- Produced in the pituitary gland
- By increasing muscle uptake of amino acids and protein synthesis, positively influences skeletal muscle synthesis
- Growth hormone leads to a metabolic shift that favors fatty acids metabolism, reducing amino acid and glucose breakdown within the skeletal muscle.
- Evidence exists for the direct interaction between growth hormone and skeletal muscle, as well as an indirect influence through somatomedins and insulin-like growth factors (IGF-I, IGF-II).
- Patients with excessively high growth hormone levels exhibit selective hypertrophy of type I muscle fibers and atrophy of type II fibers, often leading to weakness and fatigue.

Testosterone

- Anabolic; increases protein synthesis and decreases the rate of protein catabolism within the muscle fiber
- Testosterone and other androgens exert a growth-promoting influence on bone and skeletal muscle.
- Results in increased muscle size
- Androgens promote physeal closure of the long bones.

MUSCLE STRETCHING AND VISCOELASTICITY

- The viscoelastic properties of skeletal muscle help explain the improved range of motion and decreased stiffness seen after stretching and warm-up exercises.

Stress vs. Strain

- Muscle is viscoelastic (i.e., it exhibits a time-dependent stress-vs.-strain relationship).
- A certain muscle tension develops when stretched to a given length.
- With time this tension decreases.
- The phenomenon of diminished muscle stress with time is called stress relaxation.
- Muscle stretched quickly is stiffer than muscle stretched more slowly.
- Cold muscle is stiffer and therefore develops more tension than a warm muscle when stretched to a given length.

Creep

- Skeletal muscle also undergoes creep.
- Under a given load, muscle reaches an initial length and then slowly stretches with time.

ELECTROMYOGRAPHY (EMG)

- Means of detection and measurement of electrical currents passing across muscle cells
- An electrical representation of neuromuscular activation during muscle contraction
- Types of detecting electrodes
  - Skin electrodes
    - Applied to skin for use in detecting underlying muscle currents
    - Good for use in large muscle testing
  - Needle electrodes
    - Inserted directly into the muscle
    - Allow for the study of individual muscles and muscles not on the surface
- EMG provides an excellent representation of muscle activation but a less accurate picture of the force being exerted.
- EMG provides added insight into the muscles recruited during activities ranging from simple gait to complex movements.
- EMG can help in the diagnosis of neuromuscular pathology.
- In cases of neuropraxia
  - The nerve distal to the site of injury does not undergo necrosis.
  - Results in muscle silence and absent signal on EMG
- In cases of axonotmesis or neurotmesis
  - The axons distal to the injury undergo necrosis.
  - Leads to degeneration of the motor endplate over several weeks
  - This causes depolarization of the individual muscle fibers.
  - Needle electrodes can detect these smaller action potential or fibrillations, indicating muscle denervation.
  - With regrowth of axons across the site of injury, the muscle may become reinnervated.
  - Reinnervation leads to large atypical motor units that produce abnormally large muscle potentials.

■ EMG detection of these giant polyphasic action potentials provides the examiner with objective evidence of muscle reinnervation.

SUGGESTED READING

Appell HJ. Muscular atrophy following immobilisation. A review. Sports Med 1990;10(1):42–58.

Beiner JM, Jokl P. Muscle contusion injuries: current treatment options. J Am Acad Orthop Surg 2001;9(4):227–237.

Bloomfield SA. Changes in musculoskeletal structure and function with prolonged bed rest. Med Sci Sports Exerc 1997;29(2):197–206.

Caiozzo VJ, Utkan A, Chou R, et al. Effects of distraction on muscle length: mechanisms involved in sarcomerogenesis. Clin Orthop Relat Res 2002(403 Suppl):S133–145.

Deschenes MR. Effects of aging on muscle fibre type and size. Sports Med 2004;34(12):809–824.

Fitts RH, Widrick JJ. Muscle mechanics: adaptations with exercise-training. Exerc Sport Sci Rev 1996;24:427–473.

Garrett WE Jr. Muscle strain injuries. Am J Sports Med 1996;24(6 Suppl):S2–8.

Gollnick PD, Matoba H. The muscle fiber composition of skeletal muscle as a predictor of athletic success. An overview. Am J Sports Med 1984;12(3):212–217.

Green HJ, Jones S, Ball-Burnett ME, et al. Early muscular and metabolic adaptations to prolonged exercise training in humans. J Appl Physiol 1991;70(5):2032–2038.

Greiwe JS, Hickner RC, Hansen PA, et al. Effects of endurance exercise training on muscle glycogen accumulation in humans. J Appl Physiol 1999;87(1):222–226.

Hughes CT, Hasselman CT, Best TM, et al. Incomplete, intrasubstance strain injuries of the rectus femoris muscle. Am J Sports Med 1995;23(4):500–506.

Ingalls CP. Nature vs. nurture: can exercise really alter fiber type composition in human skeletal muscle? J Appl Physiol 2004;97(5):1591–1592.

Jarvinen TAH, Jarvinen TLN, Kaariainen M, et al. Muscle injuries: biology and treatment. Am J Sports Med 2005;33(5):745–764.

Kelso TB, Hodgson DR, Visscher AR, et al. Some properties of different skeletal muscle fiber types: comparison of reference bases. J Appl Physiol 1987;62(4):1436–1441.

Matoba H, Gollnick PD. Response of skeletal muscle to training. Sports Med 1984;1(3):240–251.

Nikolaou PK, Macdonald BL, Glisson RR, et al. Biomechanical and histological evaluation of muscle after controlled strain injury. Am J Sports Med 1987;15(1):9–14.

Noonan TJ, Garrett WE Jr. Muscle strain injury: diagnosis and treatment. J Am Acad Orthop Surg 1999;7(4):262–269.

Ryschon TW, Fowler MD, Wysong RE, et al. Efficiency of human skeletal muscle in vivo: comparison of isometric, concentric, and eccentric muscle action. J Appl Physiol 1997;83(3):867–874.

Seger JY, Thorstensson A. Effects of eccentric versus concentric training on thigh muscle strength and EMG. Int J Sports Med 2005;26(1):45–52.

Sheffield-Moore M, Urban RJ. An overview of the endocrinology of skeletal muscle. Trends Endocrinol Metab 2004;15(3):110–115.

Taylor DC, Dalton JD Jr, Seaber AV, et al. Experimental muscle strain injury. Early functional and structural deficits and the increased risk for reinjury. Am J Sports Med 1993;21(2):190–194.

Taylor DC, Dalton JD Jr, Seaber AV, et al. Viscoelastic properties of muscle-tendon units. The biomechanical effects of stretching. Am J Sports Med 1990;8(3):300–309.

Thompson LV. Skeletal muscle adaptations with age, inactivity, and therapeutic exercise. J Orthop Sports Phys Ther 2002;32(2):44–57.

Yarasheski KE, Campbell JA, Smith K, et al. Effect of growth hormone and resistance exercise on muscle growth in young men. Am J Physiol 1992;262(3 Pt 1):E261–267.

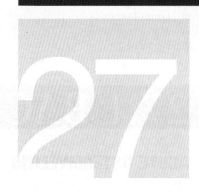

INFECTIOUS DISORDERS OF BONE AND JOINT

THOMAS V. SMALLMAN
KRIS SHEKITKA
DONALD FLEMMING
BRIAN J. HARLEY

The clinical presentation of infection is a function of time, location, and the nature of the organism and host. Acute bacterial disorders represent urgent clinical problems that, left untreated, may rapidly lead to joint destruction or bone infarction, sequestration, and development of chronic osteomyelitis. By contrast, the presentation of infection from some bacteria and all other types of organisms tends to be indolent. The clinical presentation, radiologic findings, and morphologic manifestations of osteomyelitis are influenced by the blood supply to bone and joint and by the structural architecture of bone, which is composed of living cells contained in a nonexpandable inorganic framework.

CLASSIFICATION

Infection in bone and joints can be classified by organism type, pathologic response, and presentation as follows:

- Bacterial
  - Acute

■ Subacute
■ Chronic
■ Granulomatous
■ Microangiopathic
■ Parasitic

This review will focus on specific disease mechanisms of the infectious diseases of bone and joint. In each instance, the type of organism and location, linked to the circulation and structure of bone and joint, will determine the presenting manifestations and prognosis.

27.1 BACTERIAL INFECTION

ACUTE OSTEOMYELITIS

■ Rapidly progressive pyogenic infection
■ Types
  ■ Hematogenous: usually in children with local trauma
  ■ Contiguous: from an open wound, surgical wound, or adjacent area of infection (ear infection, tooth abscess, furuncle)
■ Biologic response: a function of the inoculum (number and virulence of the organism) and the host response
■ Spectrum of disease outcomes
  ■ Control of the infection, with death of the organisms

■ Bacteria live in symbiosis with the host.
■ Bacteria overwhelm the host, causing initially local infection, then sepsis, and possibly death.
■ Common age ranges, clinical situations, organisms, and initial empiric treatment associated with musculoskeletal infection are listed in Table 27.1-1.
■ Bacteria develop an effective protective environment, an extracellular polysaccharide glycocalyx, within hours of adherence to bone, biomaterials, and tissue transplants.
  ■ Host defenses and antibiotics are excluded by this biofilm or slime.
  ■ Elements of the glycocalyx include a structure of

TABLE 27.1-1 TYPICAL ORGANISMS ASSOCIATED WITH AGE OR CLINICAL SITUATION

Age	Organism	Empiric TX
Neonate and infant	*Staphylococcus, Streptococcus,* and gram-negative bacteria	Nafcillin/oxicillin + third-generation cephalosporin *or* Vancomycin + third-generation cephalosporin
6 months to 3 years	*Staphylococcus, Streptococcus* (*Haemophilus influenzae* type B historically occurred in this age group but has all but been eliminated by immunization programs)	Nafcillin/oxicillin or vancomycin or clindamycin Add third-generation cephalosporin if Gram stain positive
3 years to adolescence	*Staphylococcus, Streptococcus*	Nafcillin/oxicillin or vancomycin or clindamycin Add third-generation cephalosporin if Gram stain positive
Prepubertal (9 to 12 years)	*Staphylococcus, Streptococcus, Pseudomonas aeruginosa* (if penetrating foot injury)	Nafcillin/oxicillin or vancomycin or clindamycin Aminoglycoside
Adolescence and adulthood	*Staphylococcus, Streptococcus, Neisseria gonorrhoeae* (monoarticular arthritis in sexually active patient)	Nafcillin/oxicillin or cefazolin or vancomycin Gram stain negative: ceftriaxone/cefotaxime/ceftizoxime Gram-positive cocci in clusters: nafcillin/oxacillin
Prosthetic implant	*Staphylococcus epidermidis* or coagulase-negative *Staphylococcus*	Treatment depends on the clinical situation.
Hospital-acquired	*Staphylococcus, Escherichia coli*	Nafcillin/oxacillin, ampicillin plus an aminoglycoside
Sickle cell anemia	*Staphylococcus, Salmonella*	Nafcillin/oxacillin, fluoroquinolones, or a third-generation cephalosporin
Hemodialysis patients, intravenous drug abusers	*Staphylococcus aureus, Staphylococcus epidermidis, Pseudomonas aeruginosa*	Nafcillin/oxacillin + ciprofloxacin

carbohydrate and protein, availability of Ca^{2+} and Mg^{2+}, and surface charge alterations to alter the host response.

HEMATOGENOUS OSTEOMYELITIS

Pathophysiology

- Acute hematogenous osteomyelitis usually presents in the metaphysis of a long bone in a growing child, often with a history of recent trauma.
- Postcapillary venous sinusoids of the metaphysis are a preferred environment for infection because of:
  - Venous pooling with low pO_2, turgid flow, and discontinuity of the endothelial lining of the sinusoidal vascular bed
  - Bacterial adherence to endothelial gaps
  - Recent trauma may alter local environmental factors.
  - Small vessel thrombosis further reduces host defenses.
- Sequence of events induced by the presence of bacteria in bone
  - Deposition of the organism at the postcapillary sinusoidal bed, invoking an acute inflammatory response
    - Increased local capillary permeability, polymorphonuclear (PMN) invasion, and edema
  - Opsonization, a precoating of the bacteria by opsonins, freely circulating serum molecules that are produced to attach to the surface of microbes, rendering them more attractive to phagocytes (examples of opsonins include IgG antibody and the C3b molecule of the complement system)
  - Ingestion of bacteria by polymorphs
  - If not contained by the initial immune response, the infection rapidly produces a compartment-like syndrome: raised intramedullary tissue pressure (from the edema) exceeds the arterial inflow pressure at the capillary level; this eliminates the arteriovenous pressure gradient that drives flow across the capillary, and flow ceases.
  - Ischemic necrosis then follows the spread of infection throughout the medullary space and through the cortex.
  - At the outer margin of the cortex, periosteum is lifted off by pus under pressure, severing the subperiosteal circulation.
  - Cortex is thus isolated from both endosteal and periosteal vascular sources, leading to cortical necrosis.

Diagnosis

Radiologic Features

- Radiography (Fig. 27.1-1) demonstrates the morphology, with the disease presentation limited to metaphysis and diaphysis, in the distribution of the circulatory beds of the nutrient artery and periosteum.
- Infected area creates an irregular zone of osteopenia in the metaphysis, with an external periosteal reaction.
- Mottled areas of cortical sclerosis in the predominately lytic area represent areas of cortical sequestration.

Clinical Findings

- Presentation is age dependent.
  - Neonates
    - Difficult diagnosis
    - Must be suspected in a neonate who is septic
    - Neonate may be afebrile.
    - Affected limb may be warm compared to opposite limb.
  - Children
    - Incidence higher in males
    - Child will look and feel ill.
    - Refusal to bear weight
    - Associated factors: recent trauma and infection elsewhere (middle ear infection, tooth abscess, cutaneous boil, or infected wound)
  - Adults
    - Advanced age and a variety of systemic factors predispose to the development of bone infection.
    - Acute vs. chronic infection clinical presentation
      - Typically, a patient with acute bacterial osteomyelitis may be acutely ill, with acute loss of function of an extremity.
      - The presence of chronic illness with an impaired immune system or partial treatment with oral antibiotics may mask the presence of infection in bone in adults, especially in the spine.
    - Spine infection often follows infection elsewhere (pneumonia, diverticulitis, cholecystitis, cystitis, pyelonephritis).
      - Pain is the predominant complaint: nonmechanical and localized
        - Lumbar spine 45%
        - Thoracic 35%
        - Cervical 20%
      - Half will have no fever or leukocytosis.
      - Spread of infection follows vascular supply with segmental arteries supplying disc and adjacent vertebrae.
      - *Staphylococcus aureus, Streptococcus,* and *Enterobacter* predominate.
- Talus and proximal radius are special cases. Hematogenous osteomyelitis can be a difficult diagnosis if bone is "hidden." Obtain early magnetic resonance imaging (MRI).
  - Proximal radius
    - Enveloped by supinator, acute infection will produce severe pain and forearm swelling and may present with a soft tissue compartment syndrome.
    - The presence of systemic signs and the absence of a traumatic cause for the raised tissue pressure should suggest the correct diagnosis.
    - MRI will confirm.
  - Talus
    - Infection will mimic cellulitis with pain and local erythema.

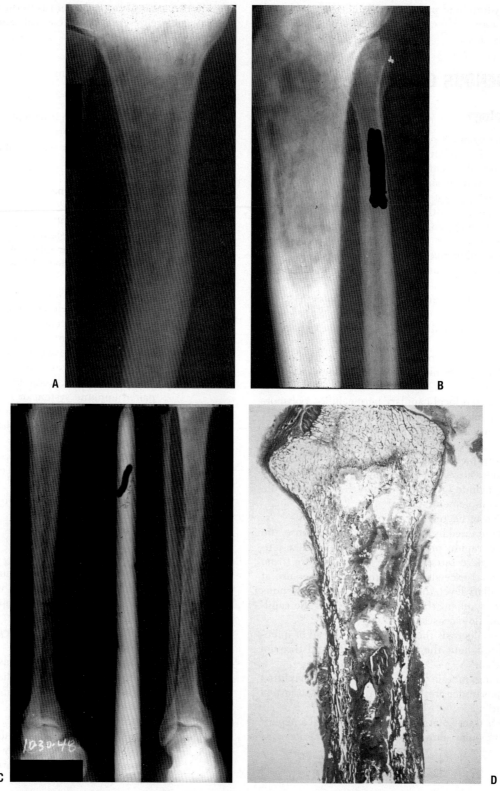

Figure 27.1-1 (**A,B**) Acute suppurative osteomyelitis. These radiographs show permeative changes and periosteal new bone formation that have taken more than 10 to 14 days to occur. Prior to this the earliest perceptible change would have been soft tissue swelling adjacent to the infected bone. (**C**) Over time, the areas of permeation become mottled as repair is attempted and the picture becomes that of early chronic osteomyelitis (here shown in a different case example). (**D**) Macrosection of proximal tibia shows the effect of acute osteomyelitis, with intramedullary accumulations of inflammatory exudates (purulent exudate). The cortex is permeated, and there is a large cortical sequestrum.

Chapter 27 / Infectious Disorders of Bone and Joint / Bacterial Infection   **499**

- Child will not bear weight; an ankle effusion may be sterile.
- The site of the infection can be confirmed early only by MRI.

Differential Diagnosis

- Osteomyelitis vs. Ewing sarcoma vs. eosinophilic granuloma (Langerhans cell histiocytosis)
- The linking of clinical, radiographic, and histopathologic findings is essential to establish the diagnosis.
  - Ewing sarcoma can perfectly mimic acute or subacute osteomyelitis with fever, malaise, leukocytosis, raised erythrocyte sedimentation rate (ESR), and a radiographic appearance of lysis with a periosteal reaction. Biopsy is needed to confirm the diagnosis.
  - Eosinophilic granuloma can mimic infection and tumor. The patient is usually not systemically ill. ESR may be elevated; the local findings can include pain and erythema; radiographic picture can be similar to acute osteomyelitis. Biopsy is necessary.

Diagnostic Principles

- Extent of disease
  - Physical findings
    - Bone tenderness on percussion helps localize infection.
    - Erythema, fluctuance, and, rarely, drainage in the acute setting
  - Laboratory parameters: complete blood count (CBC), ESR, C-reactive protein (CRP)
    - White blood cell (WBC) count with increased PMNs indicates infection but is present in only 50% of patients with infection.
    - ESR positive in 92% of pediatric patients with osteomyelitis
      - Time course: rises within 2 days of onset of infection, continues to rise for 3 to 5 days after onset of appropriate antibiotics, and returns to normal at 3 weeks
    - CRP elevated in 98% of pediatric patients with osteomyelitis; rises within 6 hours of onset of infection, peaks at 36 to 50 hours, and returns to normal 1 week after successful therapy
      - CRP is preferred for following both acute and chronic infection as it follows the time course of infection more closely.
    - Surgery delays normalization of both ESR and CRP.
  - Radiographs (see Fig. 27.1-1)
    - Initial radiographic sign of infection: soft tissue swelling; always consider tumor or fracture mimicking infection
    - Lucency occurs with active hyperemia, osteoclast action (Fig. 27.1-2).
    - Periosteal reaction begins at 2 weeks.
    - Sclerosis indicates either new bone formation on dead trabeculae or the presence of dead bone (sequestration), surrounded and made more apparent by contrast to living, osteopenic bone.
  - Technetium 99m (^{99m}Tc) bone scan assesses perfusion and osteoblastic activity; localizes pathology but is not specific.
  - Indium-11–labeled leukocyte scans differentiate infectious from noninfectious causes.
    - 83% to 85% sensitivity, 75% to 94% specificity
  - MRI can diagnose extent of disease and may show abscess formation.
    - Sensitivity close to 100%
    - Increased fluid content in marrow is a function of edema and hyperemia
      - Decreased marrow signal on T1-weighted images
      - Increased marrow signal on T2-weighted images
- Identify the organism.
  - Culture the aspirate and obtain cultures at the time of incision and drainage.
  - Treat empirically while awaiting culture results.
  - Positive Gram stain in one third of cases; highly specific, allows focused treatment.
  - Cultures are the gold standard for verifying infection and can be compromised by:
    - Prior antibiotic administration
    - Inadequate tissue sampling
    - Improper handling of specimens
  - Polymerase chain reaction (PCR) can amplify and detect bacterial DNA.
    - Allows early diagnosis compared to cultures
    - Results are not affected by concurrent use of antibiotics.
    - False-positive results can arise from contamination.

Treatment

- Treatment is based on identifying the extent of disease and identifying the organism, selecting and delivering appropriate antibiotic to the site, halting tissue destruction, and verifying response to treatment.

Nonsurgical Treatment

- Classical recommendations include empiric treatment after cultures; if no abscess and focal infection
  - Up to 6 weeks of parenteral antibiotic guided by ESR
  - Switch to oral antibiotic only if monitoring of serum bactericidal titers can be obtained.

Recent papers have suggested a more simplified approach for hematogenous acute osteomyelitis in a normal host:

- Shorter course of parenteral antibiotics (5 days)
- No monitoring of titers
- Shorter duration of therapy determined by normalization of the CRP and ESR (3 to 4 weeks)

Exceptions would include osteomyelitis in neonates, trauma, foreign bodies, the immunocompromised host, and gram-negative organisms.

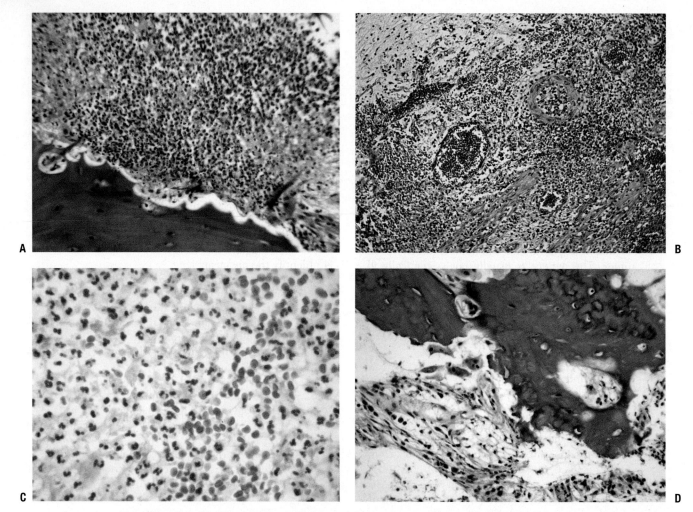

Figure 27.1-2 Acute inflammatory exudates. (A) Marrow is replaced by inflammatory cells (PMNs). Adjacent bone shows numerous Howship's lacunae, indicating brisk clast activity due to the effects of active hyperemia. (B) Higher magnification of acute osteomyelitis. No normal marrow is evident in this field; instead, the medullary space is filled with an acute inflammatory infiltrate. In the upper left corner is marrow that has been altered and shows an edematous reactive appearance to the stroma. (C) High magnification showing the cellular components of the inflammatory infiltrate: segmented neutrophils (PMNs) and extravasated red blood cells dominate the picture. (D) Acute osteomyelitis in bone showing marked effect of clasts on bone, numerous Howship's lacunae; the cellular infiltrate now shows a few lymphocytes and histiocytes.

Surgical Treatment

Indications

The classic indication of open drainage in virtually every case is changing. Given the simplified approach outlined above, the indications for surgery might include:

- Drainage of a large subperiosteal abscess
- Drainage of a metaphyseal cavity seen on the initial radiograph
- Failure of response to medical management after 36 to 48 hours
- Presence of sinus tract or sequestrum
- Osteomyelitis close to the intracapsular hip or shoulder

Surgical Technique
- Remove pus and debris.
- Fenestrate cortex.
- Remove nonviable bone (sequestrum).
- Preserve involucrum.

SUBACUTE OSTEOMYELITIS

Diagnosis

- Child presents with a painful limp with no or minimal constitutional symptoms.
- Fever mild or absent

- WBC often normal, ESR elevated in 50%
- Radiograph shows lytic lesion with or without a sclerotic border; in the classic Brodie's abscess the sclerotic border fades peripherally; the process can cross the physis, unlike acute osteomyelitis (Fig. 27.1-3).
- Differential diagnosis includes chondroblastoma (in epiphysis), osteoid osteoma.
  - Normal ESR in both conditions
  - Chondroblastoma rarely has sclerotic borders, may rarely have central mineralization.
  - Osteoid osteoma has more reactive bone unless close to joint; classic pain pattern worse at night and relieved dramatically by nonsteroidal anti-inflammatories (NSAIDs) in 70% of patients.

Treatment

- Treatment is surgical with débridement and curettage followed by appropriate antibiotics.

CHRONIC OSTEOMYELITIS

Pathophysiology

- Involves transition from acute inflammatory response, with granulation tissue, neutrophils, and microabscesses, to chronic inflammation, with lymphocytes, plasma cells, fibrosis, and bony reinforcement (Fig. 27.1-4)

Diagnosis

- Recurrent drainage from sinuses, fistulae, or ulcers
  - Usually there is a history of:
    - Acute osteomyelitis with inadequate treatment
    - Trauma with open wound or internal fixation
    - Local soft tissue spread in Cierny type C elderly patient (see below) (see Fig. 27.1-4)

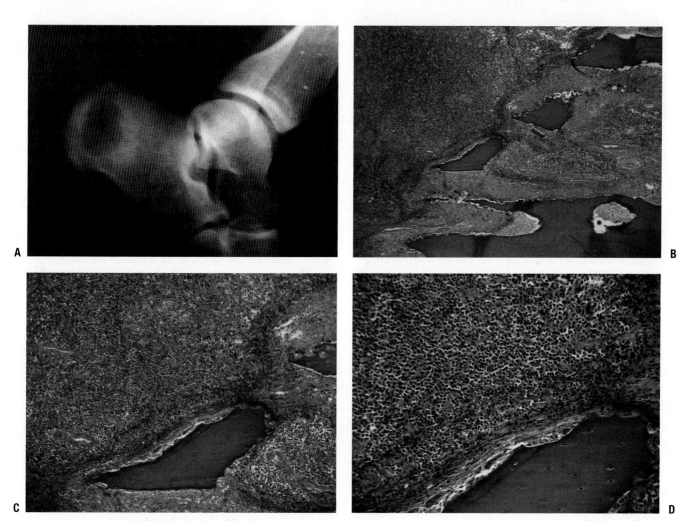

Figure 27.1-3   Brodie's abscess. (**A**) Radiograph showing lesion in calcaneus. A central zone of lysis is surrounded by a ring of dense reactive bone, with a fading external border. (**B–D**) Sequential images of a Brodie's abscess. (**B**) Low-power view reveals shards of bone that show marked evidence of clast activity; inflammatory infiltrate on the left, reactive zone on the right. (**C**) At medium power, numerous vessels are seen as well as the inflammatory exudate surrounding the trabecular bone. (**D**) High power reveals inflammatory exudate, vessels, fibrosis, and bone showing evidence of reaction. (*continued*)

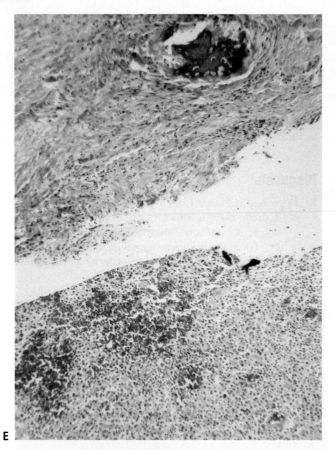

E

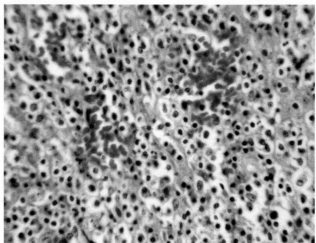

F

Figure 27.1-3 (continued) (E) Medium-power photomicrograph of a different case shows fibrotic wall of a Brodie's abscess in upper half of field. A single focus of reactive new bone formation is evident in this wall. Below, dense mixed inflammatory cells and blood vessels compose the central zone of the abscess. (F) High-magnification view of another case shows central zone of a Brodie's abscess with a mixed inflammatory infiltrate (lymphocytes, plasma cell, scattered PMNs) and red blood cells. Brown hemosiderin pigment can also be seen in a background of pink-staining fibrin.

■ Systemic symptoms are absent; may be present during flare of increased drainage.
  ■ Dead bone (microsequestra) is removed by osteoclasts or is cloaked with new lamellar bone, producing a radiographic picture of trabecular thickening; the random orientation of this bony response to the infection produces chaotic cement lines (so-called mosaic bone) also seen in Paget's disease (Fig. 27.1-5).
  ■ Cortical sequestration becomes enveloped by a periosteal response that matures (rapid woven bone deposition, followed by lamellar bone fill-in of the interstices), forming the involucrum.
  ■ Without treatment, infection heals by drainage to the exterior of the body; when treatment fails, pus seeks to drain through sinus tracts (cloaca). Over time (years), the tracts epithelialize (pseudo-epitheliomatous hyperplasia; Fig. 27.1-6); after many years, squamous cell carcinoma can occur along the tract.

Classification

Cierny and Mader have proposed a practical classification in which the extent of bone involvement is classified anatomically to allow appropriate intervention.

■ Clinical situations associated with each anatomic stage
  ■ Type I: medullary—after intramedullary rod

■ Type II: superficial—open wound perforation from outside
■ Type III: localized—after plate
■ Type IV: diffuse—progression from persistence of medullary, superficial, or localized infection
■ The physiologic status of the host determines the effectiveness of wound healing and thus the prognosis. The classification of the patient (host) includes:
■ A: normal host
■ B: compromised host
  ■ Local conditions limit perfusion, and systemic factors affect the immunologic, hematopoietic, and/or metabolic capabilities of the host. One attempts to optimize the patient prior to surgery by addressing all reversible factors locally and systemically.
    ■ Local adverse conditions
      ■ Chronic lymphedema
      ■ Venous stasis
      ■ Major vessel disease
      ■ Arteritis
      ■ Extensive scarring
      ■ Radiation fibrosis
    ■ Systemic factors
      ■ Malnutrition
      ■ Immunodeficiency
      ■ Chronic hypoxia
      ■ Malignancy
      ■ Diabetes mellitus

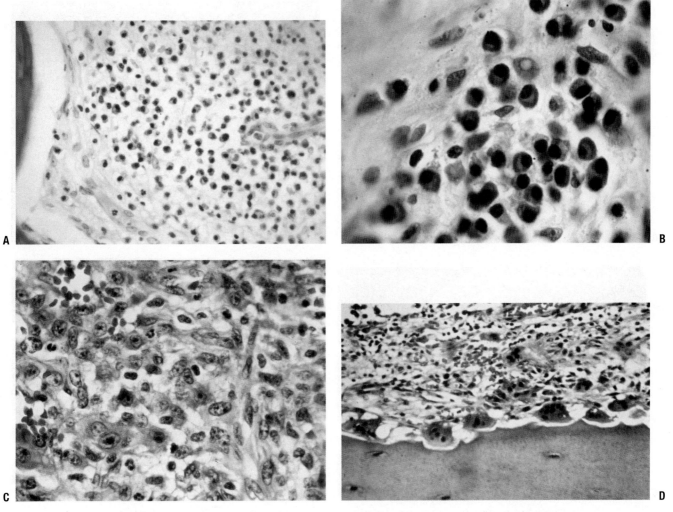

Figure 27.1-4 Chronic osteomyelitis. (**A**) The cellular players responding to the infection change over time. This photomicrograph shows a predominance of plasma cells (dark cytoplasm, perinuclear clear zone corresponding to the Golgi apparatus, and eccentric round nucleus) and lymphocytes (almost no cytoplasm, central nucleus). (**B**) Slide showing mostly plasma cells with a few scattered lymphocytes. (**C**) Plasma cells and histiocytes are present as part of the chronic inflammatory response regardless of cause. A histiocyte is a large cell with abundant cytoplasm (whose nucleus is vesicular; pale, dispersed chromatin pattern) and a large nucleolus. (**D**) A team of osteoclasts is seen lined up on and removing bone. The phenomenon of increased arterial blood flow brought to a region with associated osteoclastic activity is termed *active hyperemia* and was described by Dr. Lent Johnson.

- Advanced age
- Renal or liver failure
- Tobacco abuse
- C: multifactorial problem, not curable with acceptable morbidity; treatment deferred
  - Options are suppression with long-term antibiotics or amputation.
- Clinical stage is expressed by anatomic type and physiologic class, such as stage IVB (diffuse osteomyelitis in a compromised patient).

Diagnosis

- Determine extent of disease.
  - CBC, ESR, CRP: Obtain and follow throughout course.

- Radiographs
- ^{99m}Tc bone scan and indium-11–labeled leukocyte scans help determine the activity of the disease.
- Computed tomography (CT) scan useful for delineation of sequestrum and degree of union.
- MRI determines the extent of disease.
  - Fistula tracts
  - Extent of edema may exaggerate the zone of actual infection.

Treatment

- Determine extent of disease.
- Optimize host healing potential when possible.
- Obtain operative samples of deep specimens from multiple sites.

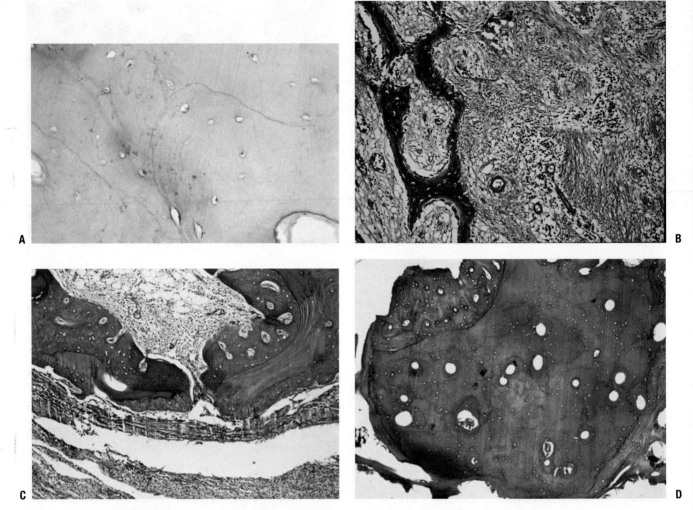

Figure 27.1-5 Chronic osteomyelitis. **(A)** High-power view of lamellar bone showing empty and enlarged lacunae, hallmarks of the enzymatic effect driven by the agonal osteocyte, termed *oncosis*. **(B)** A walling off of the infected area occurs, marked by fibrosis and periosteal woven bone formation. **(C)** Dead bone is either removed by clasts or cloaked by bone. Early on the appositional bone is woven, as shown here, or lamellar as the process slows down. Fibrous encapsulation is shown below. **(D)** Lamellar bone showing haphazard cement lines (mosaic bone) and woven bone apposition. This increased bone formation accounts for the mottled regions of sclerosis seen on radiographs.

- Eliminate the disease through intravenous antibiotics, surgical débridement.
- Reconstruct the area using flaps as necessary for soft tissue coverage, and delayed bone grafting (autograft, bone morphogenic proteins [BMP], allograft) and stabilization after infection is controlled.

Surgical Treatment

- Débridement: Approach as if resecting a locally aggressive benign tumor, erring on the side of resection back to normal tissue.
- Wound management
  - If compromised soft tissues are present, local or free muscle flaps will promote healing through:
    - Elimination of dead space
    - Soft tissue coverage
    - Improved vascularity

- Obtain multiple cultures: Culture results direct selection of antibiotic coverage, 3 to 6 weeks of intravenous treatment, plus or minus bone void fillers (polymethylmethacrylate [PMMA] with antibiotics or biodegradable material with antibiotics).
- Bone stabilization when necessary
  - External fixation: safest, allows distraction osteogenesis and bone transport; pin tract infection incidence is high
  - Repeat internal fixation: problematic given high rate of reactivation of the infection (20% to 50%)
  - Delayed reconstruction of bone voids
    - Autograft/BMP/allograft for cavitary defect
    - Structural autograft or bone transport for segmental defects
  - Augment healing with electrical stimulation or ultrasound.

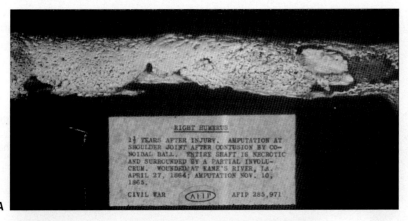

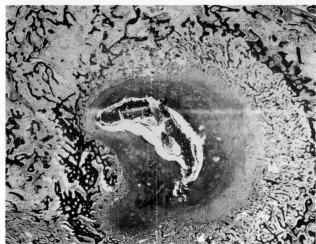

Figure 27.1-6 Chronic osteomyelitis. **(A)** Gross specimen of Civil War case from the Armed Forced Institute of Pathology museum. The sequestrated initial cortex (sequestrum) is cloaked by mature woven bone (involucrum); the openings in the involucrum are sites of purulent drainage to the exterior (cloacae). **(B)** Cross-section of a tibia with chronic osteomyelitis showing involucrum (layers of woven bone) surrounding an inflammatory exudate encompassing the necrotic intitial cortex (sequestrum).

■ Amputate when the situation is not reconstructable.

Complications
■ Long-term complications include sequestra, sinus tract formation, pathologic fracture, squamous cell carcinoma, and amyloidosis.

Squamous Cell Carcinoma
■ Occurs as a result of chronic irritation of draining sinus (1 to 55 years, mean 22 years)
■ Presents as a change in a longstanding setting of draining sinus: increasing pain, change in drainage or in appearance of a chronic ulcer; enlarging mass; pathological fracture
■ Incidence <2% of patients
■ Anatomic distribution: 85% in lower extremity
■ Radiograph may show new lucency in a longstanding area of mixed lysis and sclerosis.
■ Management is wide resection, often amputation.
■ Prognosis: 14% metastasis; 30% have regional node metastases

Amyloidosis
■ Deposits of a twisted β-pleated fibrillary protein occur in bone marrow and/or juxta-articular synovial tissue; rarely recognized clinically.

■ Common endpoint for multiple processes in addition to infection
■ Treatment and cure of the infection allows resolution of the amyloidosis.

SCLEROSING OSTEOMYELITIS OF GARRÉ

■ Localized control of an initial infection is followed by persistent repair with ongoing new bone formation; clinical presentation insidious with mild ache, local tenderness, no systemic symptoms or signs (Fig. 27.1-7).
■ Radiograph shows dense, progressive sclerosis.
■ Microscopy shows chronic inflammatory infiltrate, fibrovascular marrow, trabecular reinforcement.

CHRONIC RECURRENT MULTIFOCAL OSTEOMYELITIS

■ Age: children and adolescents
■ Clinical presentation: appears with multifocal minimal symptoms of localized pain, swelling, and low-grade fever; 70% of patients have pustulosis palmoplantaris

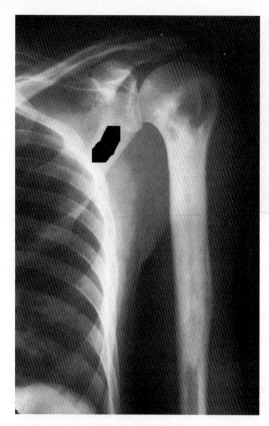

Figure 27.1-7 Sclerosing osteomyelitis of Garré. Repair predominates in this condition. The radiograph shows dense sclerosis throughout the humeral diaphysis.

- Distribution: Clavicle, distal femur, and distal tibia are most common sites.
- Laboratory evaluation: WBC and CRP are normal; ESR is elevated in all cases.
- Microbiology: Cultures for bacteria, mycobacteria, fungi are invariably negative.
- Radiographs: multiple metaphyseal lytic lesions with a thin rim of sclerosis
- Microscopy shows mixed acute and chronic inflammatory infiltrate with PMNs forming microabscesses; microsequestration with osteoclastic resorption is evident; adjacent marrow fibrovascular with chronic inflammatory infiltrate.
- Usually resolves spontaneously after years

SEPTIC ARTHRITIS

Etiology

Hematogenous Arthritis
- Most frequent cause of bacterial septic arthritis
  - Infants: hip most common; less commonly knee or ankle
  - Children and adults: knee most common
    - Debilitated older adult with inflammatory arthropathy is at risk.

Contiguous Arthritis
- Defined as extension of infection from adjacent acute osteomyelitis

Direct Arthritis
- Associated with surgery
- Traumatic introduction of bacteria (open wounds)
  - Hand infection in association with fist fights source of initially missed septic arthritis
  - Any open injury to the soft tissues directly overlying a joint necessitates débridement.

Pathophysiology

- Initiation
  - Inoculation of the organism activates the immune response.
  - Same sequence occurs as outlined in the discussion of the pathophysiology of osteomyelitis.
- Immune response
  - In joints, the profound immune response in the vascular synovium produces pain, swelling, erythema, and loss of motion.
- Cartilage destruction
  - In the swollen, avascular joint space, enzymes from bacteria, PMNs, and synovial cells cleave the glycosaminoglycan subunits of cartilage, which are then rapidly expelled from the cartilage.
  - Bacterial and host collagenases then break down the collagen with gross physical breakdown of the cartilage.
  - Loss of joint space on the radiograph correlates with this; regional osteopenia accompanies the reactive increased vascular flow to the periarticular region.

Diagnosis

Clinical Findings
- Classic presentation is "sick" patient with fever, pain, inability to use upper extremity (pseudoparalysis) or to bear weight on lower extremity.
  - Range of motion is markedly reduced and painful.
  - Resting position of maximal joint volume
    - Knee: flexion
    - Hip: flexion, external rotation, abduction
- To avoid irreversible joint destruction, timely diagnosis and treatment are mandatory.

Laboratory Findings
- WBC: elevated with shift to left
- ESR, CRP elevated in 90% of patients with septic arthritis

Radiologic Features
- Radiograph: effusion early progressing to joint space loss late; rare to have bony changes except regional osteopenia (Fig. 27.1-8)
- MRI: evaluates joint effusion, adjacent bone and soft tissue changes
- Ultrasound: can identify effusion

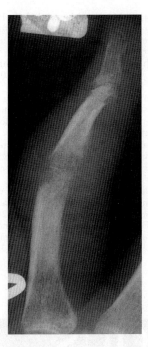

Figure 27.1-8   Septic arthritis. Loss of joint space occurs as a result of the dissolution of the articular cartilage. The infection extended under the subchondral plate. There is periosteal new bone formation and marked juxta-articular osteopenia.

- Scintigraphy can help with difficult diagnosis and identify multiple joint problems.
- Joint aspiration assisted when necessary by fluoroscopic or ultrasound guidance
  - Gram stain, cultures/sensitivity testing, WBC and differential, crystals
  - Thick fluid typically with WBC >50,000/ml (50%) and no crystals

Treatment

- Confirm diagnosis: joint fluid aspiration
- Initial surgical management: joint irrigation, open or arthroscopic
  - Drilling of adjacent metaphysis if osteomyelitis is present may be done.
- Intravenous antibiotics for 3 to 4 weeks (Table 27.1-2)
- Follow-up: clinical examination and ESR/CRP
  - Follow closely for prompt return of clinical findings to normal.
  - Persistent pain, swelling, and fever suggests return to operating room for second washout and débridement; do not hesitate to do this if minimal clinical response over 24 to 48 hours.
- Late diagnosis: If diagnosis is missed and joint destruction has occurred, initial surgical goal is to eliminate the infection; the long-term options are arthrodesis vs. arthroplasty, using precautions to lower the risk of recurrent infection.

TABLE 27.1-2 CLINICAL SPECTRUM OF SEPTIC ARTHRITIS

Age/Clinical Situation	Organisms	Empiric Management
Newborn to 3 months	Staphylococcus aureus, Streptococcus group B; less commonly Enterobacteriaceae, Neisseria gonorrhoeae	Nafcillin/oxacillin + third-generation cephalosporin; if organism is methicillin-resistant S. aureus, use vancomycin + antipseudomonal aminoglycoside (APAG)
Children (3 months to 14 years)	S. aureus, Streptococcus pyogenes, Streptococcus pneumoniae, Haemophilus influenzae, gram-negative bacilli, N. gonorrhoeae	Nafcillin/oxacillin + third-generation cephalosporin or vancomycin + third-generation cephalosporin
Acute monoarticular septic arthritis in sexually active adults; women > men	N. gonorrhoeae, S. aureus, streptococci, aerobic gram-negative bacilli	Gram-negative: ceftriaxone or cefotaxime or ceftizoxime Gram-positive cocci in clusters: nafcillin/oxacillin
Acute monoarticular septic arthritis in adults who are not sexually active	S. aureus, streptococci, aerobic gram-negative bacilli	Nafcillin/oxacillin + third-generation cephalosporin
Immunocompromised host	Gram-negative organisms, or unusual pathogens as mycobacteria or fungi	Depends on clinical situation
Intravenous drug users	S. aureus, Pseudomonas aeruginosa, Serratia marcescens	Nafcillin/oxacillin + antipseudomonal aminoglycoside (APAG)

SUGGESTED READING

Belli E, Matteini C, Andreano T. Sclerosing osteomyelitis of Garré periostitis ossificans. *J Craniofac Surg* 2002;13:765–768.

Berendt T, Byren I. Bone and joint infection. *Clin Med* 2004;4: 510–518.

Chambers JB, Forsythe DA, Bertrand S, et al. Retrospective review of osteoarticular infections in a pediatric sickle cell age group. *J Pediatr Orthop* 2000;20:682–685.

Chen CE, Ko JY, Wang JW, et al. Infection after intramedullary nailing of the femur. *J Trauma* 2003;55:338–344.

Cierny G III. Musculoskeletal sepsis chronic osteomyelitis: Results of treatment. *AAOS Instr Course Lect* 1990;39:495.

Cierny G III. A clinical staging system for adult osteomyelitis. *Contemp Orthop* 1985:10–17.

Darville T, Jacobs RF. Management of acute hematogenous osteomyelitis in children. *Pediatr Infect Dis J* 2004;23:255–257.

Duffy CM, Lam P, Ditchfield M, et al. Chronic recurrent multifocal osteomyelitis: review of orthopaedic complications at maturity. *J Pediatr Orthop* 2002;22(4):501–505.

Kocher MS, Mandiga R, Murphy JM, et al. A clinical practice guideline for treatment of septic arthritis in children: efficacy in improving process of care and effect on outcome of septic arthritis of the hip. *J Bone Joint Surg [Am]* 2003;85(6):994–999.

McGrory JE, Pritchard DJ, Unni KK, et al. Malignant lesions arising in chronic osteomyelitis. *Clin Orthop Rel Res* 1999;362:181–189.

Parsons B, Strauss E. Surgical management of chronic osteomyelitis. *Am J Surg* 2004;188(1A Suppl):57–66.

Patzakis MJ, Zalavrad C. Systemic disorders: Infection. In Vaccar AR, ed. *Orthopaedic Knowledge Update 8*. Rosemont, IL: American Academy of Orthopaedic Surgeons, 2005.

Rasool MN. Primary subacute haematogenous osteomyelitis in children. *J Bone Joint Surg [Br]* 2001;83(1):93–98.

Tetsworth K, Cierny G III. Osteomyelitis debridement techniques. Clin Orthop Rel Res 1999;360:87–96.

Vaccaro AR, Patzakis MJ, Zalavras C, eds. Systemic disorders, Chapter 20: Infection. In *Orthopaedic Knowledge Update 8*. Rosemont, IL: American Academy of Orthopaedic Surgeons, 2005:217–228.

Vinh TN, Sweet DE. Infectious diseases of bone and joint. In Connor DH, ed. *Pathology of Infectious Diseases* (2 volumes), 5th ed. Stamford, CT: Appleton & Lange, 1997, Vol. II, Ch. 182, pp. 1601–1631.

27.2 GRANULOMATOUS INFECTION

Granuloma is defined as a microscopic-sized aggregation of histiocytes and hypertrophied fibroblasts termed epithelioid cells, centrally located and rimmed by a chronic inflammatory infiltrate of lymphocytes and plasma cells (Fig. 27.2-1). The entire focus can be surrounded by a ring of fibrosis. Multinucleated giant cells, with a characteristic positioning of the nuclei at the periphery of the cell (foreign body or Langhans giant cells), are frequently present (Table 27.2-1). Over time the granuloma may be replaced by scarring and even calcification. In tuberculosis, the central area may undergo caseous (cheese-like) necrosis.

■ Conditions associated with granulomatous histology (see Fig. 27.2-1) include:
  ■ Infection by mycobacteria, fungi, or parasites
  ■ Foreign materials
  ■ Eosinophilic granuloma
  ■ Sarcoidosis

The response in bone is indolent, with slowly enlarging lytic defects in bone with smooth walls accommodating confluent, usually caseating granulomas.

■ Eosinophilic granuloma (Langerhans cell histiocytosis or Langerhans cell granulomatosis) only infrequently has clear-cut granulomatous histology (see Table 27.2-1). This disorder can progress with rapid local osteolysis (unique among granulomatous bone processes, which are usually indolent).

MYCOBACTERIAL OSTEOMYELITIS

■ Tuberculosis (TB) will be discussed in detail as the prototype disorder in this section.

Pathophysiology

General

■ Tubercle bacillus induces an acute inflammatory response on entry into host tissue that usually controls the infection, walling it off to form a primary complex; if infecting dose overwhelms the response, the infection persists and spreads; during the early stages, bacilli may move into the circulation and metastasize to central nervous system, bones, or liver.

■ PMNs, on ingesting the bacilli, may necrose and become engulfed by macrophages and mononuclear cells.

■ Macrophages adopt epithelioid morphology on accepting the lipids of the bacilli, or may aggregate to form Langhans giant cells, whose task is to digest and remove the bacilli; these cells may also be overcome by the bacillus, also necrosing and inducing further phagocytic activity. Necrosis of epithelioid and Langhans cells becomes confluent (caseating).

■ After 1 week, lymphocytes form a ring around the periphery of the lesion, forming a 1- to 2-mm nodule known as the tubercle.

■ During the second week caseation starts to occur, induced by the protein fraction of the tubercle bacilli.

■ Over time, the PMN response is replaced by chronic inflammatory round cell infiltration accompanied by a fibroblastic proliferation that is variable in degree around the tubercle (chronic inflammatory focus).

■ This immune response usually will control the infection, in essence walling it off, where it can lie dormant for a lifetime, potentially becoming active as old age and impaired immune response occur.

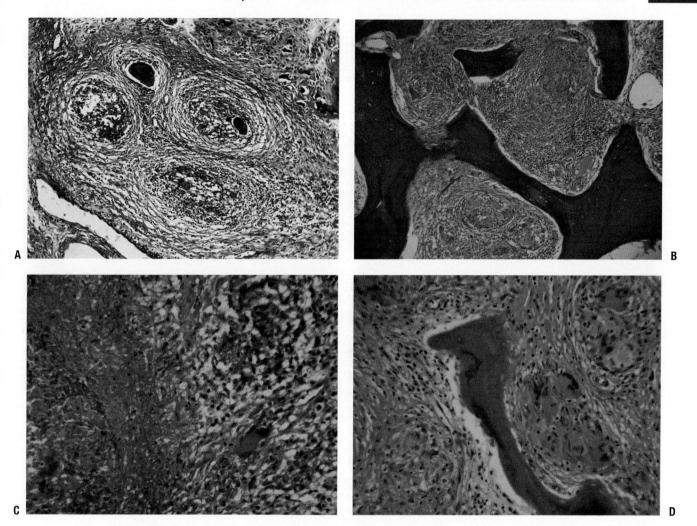

Figure 27.2-1 **Granuloma (TB).** **(A)** Granuloma formation is present. At this power, cellular detail is not visible, but there are four granulomas present, each within a ring of fibrosis. The center of the granuloma may manifest caseous necrosis; these granulomas are in the earliest stages of central necrosis. There are multinucleated giant cells of the Langhans or foreign body type frequently found in the granuloma. **(B,C)** **Caseating granuloma (TB).** **(B)** Here, granulomas are seen replacing normal marrow elements within bone. **(C)** Necrotic material is seen on the left, and the intermediate margin shows epithelioid cells centrally, with inflammatory cells (lymphocytes, plasma cells on the right, and a Langhans giant cell). Langhans cells have peripherally placed nuclei and are the cells to study carefully for the presence of acid-fast bacilli or fungi. **(D,E)** **Granulomatous osteomyelitis (foreign body).** Strictly speaking, a granuloma is a microscopic structure formed by two or more histiocytes or macrophages. They tend to have a nodular or circumscribed appearance and can be non-necrotizing or necrotizing. **(D)** In this photomicrograph, well-formed non-necrotizing (noncaseating) granulomas of histiocytes and multinucleated giant cells are evident, surrounded by fibrous connective tissue. Granulomas on hematoxylin and eosin stain are not specific, and their evaluation requires an evaluation of special stains and examination under polarized light (birefringent foreign particles are highlighted in this manner). (*continued*)

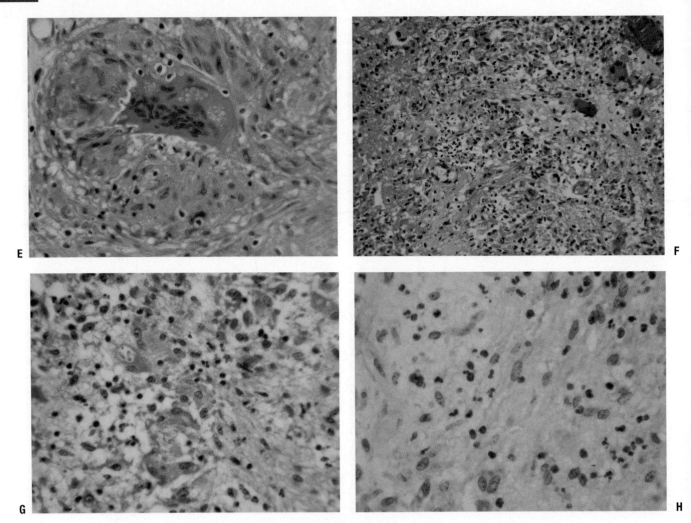

Figure 27.2-1 *(continued)*   (E) Higher-power view of **D** brings out the details of a single foreign body granuloma. Note the multinucleated giant cell and the surrounding plump mononuclear cells (histiocytes/macrophages). The vacuolated cytoplasm of the multinucleated giant cells underscores the brisk metabolic activity of these phagocytic cells. **(F–H) Granulomatous (fungal, mycotic) osteomyelitis secondary to Cryptococcus infection.** (F) This field shows a mixed inflammatory infiltrate with a few small discrete noncaseating granulomas composed of histiocytes and a few giant cells. Note the pale blue spherical structures within the cytoplasm of some of the histiocytes. Special stains (e.g., GMS and PAS stains) are useful for identification of the organism. (G) Higher-power view of **F** brings out the details of the histiocytes and multinucleated giant cells. A few gray-blue intracellular spherical bodies suspicious for fungi are noted. (H) Same view as in **G** with PAS stain (one fungal organism positive), which brings out a dark-pink spherical structure that is morphologically consistent with the yeast form of *Cryptococcus* species (this species has a capsule rich in mucin, which is readily stained by PAS).

■ Musculoskeletal lesions form by metastasis from 3 months to 3 years after the primary infection.

Spine
■ Children: Spine involvement begins in the vertebral body, usually anteriorly, then extends to adjacent disc and vertebral body.
■ Adults: Onset is beneath the periosteum under the anterior longitudinal ligament and may spread up and down the spine, bypassing some vertebrae to lodge at more than one level; disc space narrowing, vertebral body de-

struction, collapse with kyphosis, and eventual fusion may occur after 1 to 2 years.

Extraspinal
■ Unlike bacteria, TB does not produce proteolytic enzymes that aggressively destroy cartilage, affording more time to make the diagnosis before the joint is destroyed in tuberculous arthritis.
■ Bacillus lodges in synovium and proliferates, opposed by the immune process in sequence as outlined above.
  ■ The inflamed synovium enlarges to fill all recesses

TABLE 27.2-1 LANGHANS VERSUS LANGERHANS CELLS

	Langhans Cells	Langerhans Cells
Appearance	Giant cells with nuclei distributed around the periphery	Histiocytes with typical coffee-bean cleaved nuclei (NOT giant cells)
Associated conditions	Tuberculosis, foreign body granulomas	Langerhans cell histiocytosis or Langerhans cell granulomatosis or eosinophilic granuloma (older terminology)

of the joint, spreading over the cartilage from the periphery as a pannus, mechanically eliminating nutrition of the cartilage from the surface.
- Central joint space is preserved for months.
- Cold abscess
  - A marked exudative reaction consists of serum, PMNs, caseous material, bone debris, and tubercle bacilli.
  - This collection migrates under the influence of gravity and may present along the spine and pelvis, in the groins, or about involved joints.
  - It may present through the skin as a sinus or ulcer, which may then become secondarily infected, obscuring the diagnostic picture.
- Regional osteopenia
  - The inflammatory process induces an active hyperemia with osteoclastic deletion of bone, resulting in marked regional osteopenia.
- Kissing sequestrate
  - The inflammatory synovial mass invades weakened subchondral bone from the periphery.
  - Rarely, sequestration of the opposing joint surfaces can occur as a result of this bone destruction, leading to the radiographic picture of "kissing sequestrate."

Etiology

- Causative organisms include *Mycobacterium tuberculosis* (TB), *Mycobacterium leprae,* and environmental mycobacteria.
- Organisms grow on enriched medium slowly so that colonies appear at 2 to 4 weeks.
  - Acid-fast stain may reveal classic "red snappers."

Epidemiology

- One third of global population is infected with TB; most frequent cause of death and disability worldwide.
- U.S. statistics
  - 10 million are infected; 90% of new activated cases come from this pool.
  - In non-Hispanic whites, median age at diagnosis is 61; among minority groups it is 39.

- Americans >65 represent 6.5% of population but account for 26% of reported cases.
- 20% of new cases of TB have extrapulmonary disease.
- 33% of patients with TB and HIV have extrapulmonary disease.
- 1% to 3% of patients with TB develop musculoskeletal manifestations.

Diagnosis

Clinical Presentation
- Classic: Patient becomes insidiously ill and develops chronic local musculoskeletal pain, fever, and weight loss.
- Initial presentation may include:
  - Cold abscess: juxta-articular or paraspinal soft tissue mass without inflammation
  - Spinal involvement: may be truncal rigidity, muscle spasm, and neurological signs and deficit; spinal deformity (gibbus) is a late finding
  - TB arthritis: more common than TB osteomyelitis
  - Dactylitis: Small joints of the hands and feet are infrequently involved except in infancy, when digits may be involved with swelling.
  - Osseous disease: occurs by metastatic spread from an initial focus, usually the lungs, with involvement most often of spine (lower thoracic most frequent, with multiple vertebral bodies in 50% of cases), followed by pelvis in 12%, hip and femur 10%, knee and tibia 10%, hand, and any other joint
- Important clinical points
  - Diagnosis can be difficult in the elderly, whose presentation may initially be only nonspecific constitutional symptoms.
  - If you suspect musculoskeletal TB, check the lungs, kidneys, and gastrointestinal tract.

Radiologic Features
- No pathognomonic features
- Joints
  - Osteopenia and soft tissue swelling with minimal periosteal reaction early, then marginal deletion of subchondral bone on both sides of the joint with late loss of central joint space (Fig. 27.2-2)

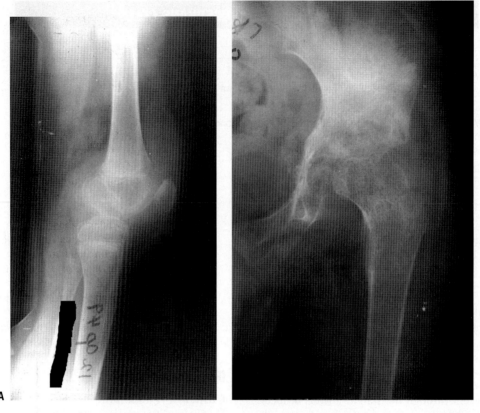

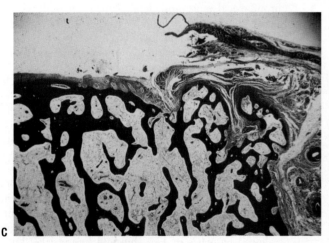

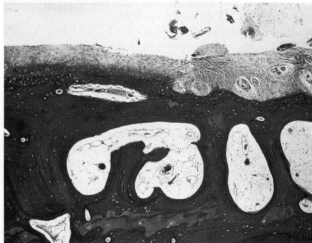

Figure 27.2-2 (**A**) TB of the knee. When TB first lodges in the synovium of a joint, it creates many tubercles (usually small, without caseation) and induces marked synovial proliferation. The suprapatellar pouch in this knee is filled with inflamed synovium with histology as in Figure 27.2-1. There is significant osteopenia. (**B–D**) TB of the hip. (**B**) Once the infection is established, the inflamed synovium invades the joint space from the margins, growing as a pannus as in rheumatoid arthritis, destroying the underlying cartilage by interfering with the diffusion of nutrients to the cartilage. The joint surface is usually preserved centrally until the process becomes much more advanced. Synovial pathology involves both sides of the joint. TB must be in the differential diagnosis for any periarticular disorder involving more than one bone around a joint area or marginal erosions. (**C**) Photomicrograph of the edge of a joint showing the pannus growing from the right onto the underlying articular cartilage. (**D**) This higher-power view shows complete destruction of the cartilage by the pannus.

- Subchondral cysts
- Enlargement of epiphysis
- Subchondral erosions may cross epiphysis in one third of children affected.
- Spine
  - Rarefaction of vertebral endplates
  - Increasing loss of disc height
  - Focal bony destruction with disc involved and late vertebral body collapse (Fig. 27.2-3)
  - Paravertebral soft tissue mass often present
  - Needle biopsy in HIV/TB patients must rule out other diseases such as Kaposi sarcoma.

MYCOTIC OSTEOMYELITIS

- Occurs mostly in immunocompromised patients or as opportunistic infections in individuals exposed to the specific contaminated environment (workers)
- Fungal infection mimics TB, so always culture for fungi if granulomatous pathology is found (see Fig. 27.2-1).
- Radiographic differential includes myeloma and metastasis (due to frequent multifocality).
- Relevant features of the fungal infections of the musculoskeletal system are outlined in Table 27.2-2.

SARCOIDOSIS

- A systemic granulomatous disorder of unknown cause; no known organism

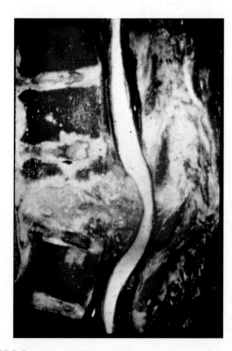

Figure 27.2-3   Gross specimen of TB of the spine. There is marked destruction of the bony architecture, with extension of the granulomatous process extending posterior to compress the cord. This degree of destruction can produce spinal deformity and paraplegia.

- Differential diagnosis in any clinical situation manifesting granulomatous histology

Diagnosis

Clinical Presentation

- Typical patient is an adult, more commonly African-American, age 20 to 40 years, with fever, fatigue, malaise, and weight loss.
- Affects lungs (90%), lymph nodes, skin, skeleton
  - Skeletal distribution: hand ("sausage fingers"), wrist, foot, skull, vertebral bodies, long bones, synovium
  - Typical musculoskeletal presentation: swollen, mildly painful fingers

Radiologic Features

- No large destructive lesions as seen more commonly with TB
- Mixed lysis and sclerosis is typical.
- Hands/feet: punched-out cortical lesions, with trabecular resorption (honeycomb lytic pattern) and linear endosteal sclerosis (acro-osteolysis; Fig. 27.2-4)

Laboratory Findings

- Elevated angiotensin-converting enzyme (ACE) derived from epithelioid cells
- Hypercalcemia arising from overproduction of 1-25-(OH)-D3, driven by activated pulmonary macrophages
- Cultures negative

Pathologic Findings

- Mimics TB but without caseation (see Fig. 27.2-4)
- Giant cells show nonspecific cytoplasmic inclusions.
  - Asteroid body: a central core of degenerating organelles encompassed by rays of collagen
  - Schaumann bodies: large, concentrically laminated concretions of a protein matrix impregnated with calcium and iron salts

Treatment

- Symptoms are usually self-limited. If severe, prolonged treatment with corticosteroids may be attempted.
- Immunosuppressive agents, such as methotrexate, azathioprine, and cyclophosphamide can be used.
- Rarely, some individuals with irreversible organ failure require organ transplantation.

RARE FORMS OF OSTEOMYELITIS

These conditions, whose relevant information is outlined in Table 27.2-3, include:

- Brucellosis
- Cat-scratch disease
- Microangiopathic osteomyelitis
  - Syphilis
  - Lyme disease
- Fibrosing osteomyelitis (fibrocystic)
  - Ecchinococcosis

TABLE 27.2-2 FUNGAL FORMS OF OSTEOMYELITIS

Organism	Entry	Skeletal Manifestations	Pathology	Diagnosis	Treatment
Blastomycoses dermatidis	Inhalation of conidia; they convert to yeast form in lungs and then disseminate systemically	Primary presentation in 10% with septic arthritis or osteomyelitis	Neutrophils ingest but cannot destroy organism; pus plus noncaseating granulomas termed pyogranulomas	Yeast forms: 8 to 15 mm, multinucleated (8 to 12), thick double-contoured cell walls; single broad-based budding	Amphotericin B; ketoconazole; surgery according to stage of disease
Histoplasmosis capsulatum; Midwestern and south-central U.S.	Inhalation of conidia from infected soil and bird droppings, same sequence as for *B. dermatidis*	African variant with skeletal infection 50% (*H. capsulatum diboisii*, large yeast, 10 to 15 mm); 50% incidence of skeletal lesion (skull, ribs, long bones, spine); eccentric, punched-out area of lysis	Suppurative areas mixed with epithelioid giant cell pyogranulomas; African histology contains large giant cells containing many yeast forms	Yeast forms 3- to 4-mm, spherical to oval, uninucleate, thin-walled, narrow-based budding	Primary: ketoconazole or itraconazole Secondary: amphotericin B for systemic, severe infection
Coccidioides immitis; arid regions of southwest U.S., Mexico, and Argentina	Same sequence as for *B. dermatidis* Infection—direct link to exposure 40%: symptomatic disease, usually lung 90% resolve 10% lung sequelae 1% have dissemination; of these one third have multisystem disease	Arthritis, tenosynovitis, osteomyelitis Lytic, unifocal in 60%, wide distribution; vertebral lesions often multiple, may spare the disc and extend to posterior elements and ribs. Joint lesions are unifocal in >90%; knee and ankle predominate.	In joints, primary response is neutrophils and macrophages, changing at 1 week to granulomatous inflammation to developing spherules; new endospores elicit a neutrophil response, initiating a new cycle.	In lungs conidia enlarge, become spherules 10 to 15 mm with thick double-contoured walls and many endospores, which then rupture.	Immobilization Synovectomy Oral ketoconazole, itraconazole, or amphotericin B systemic with or without intra-articular

(continued)

TABLE 27.2-2 (continued)

Organism	Entry	Skeletal Manifestations	Pathology	Diagnosis	Treatment
Cryptococcus neoformans; world-wide distribution	Soil fungus disseminated by excreta of pigeons produces asymptomatic lung infection in the immunocompetent host.	In immunodeficient may disseminate to central nervous system, skin, and bone. Bone lesions 5% to 10%: distribution—pelvis, femur, spine, tibia, and scapula, causing chronic pain and swelling in some; some are asymptomatic	Inflammatory response varies with usual lymphocytes and plasma cells, with or without large neutrophils and giant cells; granulomas absent usually.	Pleomorphic encapsulated yeast form, 2 to 20 mm, reproduces by budding.	In the absence of AIDS for disseminated disease, amphotericin B and flucytosine; surgery rarely used
Sporothrix schenckii; tropical America	Direct inoculation into the skin of hands or feet; rare inhalation	Typical in gardeners handling roses and sphagnum moss; local painless mobile nodule becomes red and soft and ulcerates; secondary lesions follow lymphatics; ulcers present for years; regional lymph nodes enlarge; local spread to bone/joint mimicking TB	Pyogranulomas	Dimorphic fungus: hyphal form in vitro at <37 degrees; in vivo, 2- to 6-mm oval to cigar-shaped yeast forms with unequal budding	Cutaneous treatment: saturated potassium iodide, 50 mg/day for 6 weeks. Surgery plus amphotericin B for bone and joint manifestations
Candidiasis	Systemic dissemination: neonates/immunocompromised patients. Cutaneous and mucous membrane portals	Hematogenous spread to bone and joint with a radiologic picture mimicking TB; clinical setting immunocompromised patients, neonates, rare case reports of candidal total joint infection	Mimics TB; combination of immune impairment and broad-spectrum antibiotics creates opportunity for pathogenicity.	>150 candida species exist, normally inhabit mucous membranes or damaged skin	Amphotericin B. Rarely surgery

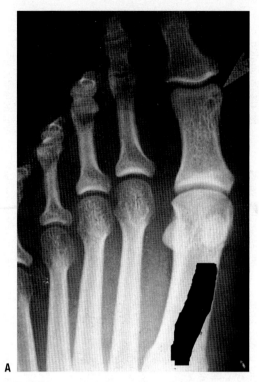

A

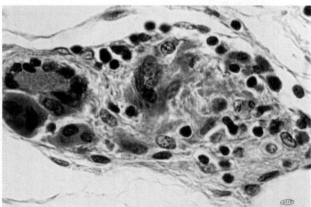

B

Figure 27.2-4   Boeck's sarcoid. (**A**) Radiograph shows a small lytic lesion with sclerotic borders in the proximal phalanx of the great toe. (**B**) A small tubercle in sarcoid, with each of the cellular elements of a granuloma demonstrated.

TABLE 27.2-3 RARE FORMS OF OSTEOMYELITIS

Organism	Entry	Clinical Manifestations	Pathology/Skeletal Involvement	Diagnosis	Treatment
Brucella (gram-negative coccobacilli)	Gastrointestinal: Goat's milk, *B. melitensis* Cow's milk, *B. abortus* Exposure to infected cattle, *B. abortus* Swine, *B. suis* Dogs, *B. canis*	**Acute (malignant) form:** overwhelming infection with fever, chills, collapse, reticuloendothelial system [RES] activation (lymphadenopathy, hepatosplenomegaly), delirium, coma, early death **Recurrent (undulant fever):** *B. melitensis* presents with flu-like symptoms with relapses. **Chronic (intermittent):** *B. abortus* (rare) presents with malaise, mild fever, weakness.	20% to 60% with septic arthritis, osteomyelitis, tenosynovitis, bursitis Sacroiliitis is most common location; TB-like spinal presentation in elderly. Radiographs mimic TB spinal and peripheral. Microscopy: *B. melitensis and suis*—necrotizing granulomas mimic TB. *B. abortus*—non-necrotizing granulomas mimic sarcoid.	Culture of blood, marrow, and infected tissue Serologic testing: serum agglutination or ELISA Difficult to stain and identify in infected tissue	Tetracycline with rifampin; *or* tetracycline with minocycline; *or* ciprofloxacin Surgery as indicated clinically
Cat-scratch disease (*Bartonella henselae*)	Skin puncture	Initial papule at inoculation site in 3 to 10 days, then regional lymphadenopathy (months to years), then systemic spread to RES and bone. Initial mild flu-like symptoms. Nodes may suppurate and drain through skin. Rare rash, conjunctivitis.	Bone involvement near skin lesions, mixed lysis/sclerosis. Microscopy: granulomas with rare giant cells, undergo necrosis with coalescence to form confluent microabscesses. Neutrophils common in early lesions.	Raised white blood cell count, erythrocyte sedimentation rate, eosinophilia (10% to 20%), positive skin test (90%), IFA Ab titer >1:64; positive culture; polymerase chain reaction (PCR) of DNA	No specific antibiotic therapy has proven useful. No treatment is indicated in normal host; self-limited condition. Symptomatic relief (no effect on duration of symptoms) with 5-day course of azithromycin. In immunocompromised host choices include trimethoprim–sulfamethoxazole; gentamicin; ciprofloxacin; rifampin.

(continued)

TABLE 27.2-3 (continued)

ORGANISM	Entry	Clinical Manifestations	Pathology/Skeletal Involvement	Diagnosis	Treatment
Syphilis (*Treponoma pallidum*, a spirochete)	**1. Direct:** Mucosal surface entry is followed by 3 stages: **a. Primary:** incubation 10 to 90 days, then chancre + regional lymph node enlargement (50%) **b. Secondary:** 6 to 24 weeks, systemic infection to every system ("*the great imitator*"), followed by *latency*, early phase (4 years) retaining infectiousness (25%) followed by late noninfectious latent syphilis **c. Tertiary:** years to decades, presents with gummas in any system **2. Indirect:** Congenital: intrauterine transmission from mother to child	**Direct syphilis** presents in the benign tertiary (gummatous) stage in the skeleton (50%) with bone pain (+/−) and local swelling without local signs of inflammation. **Indirect syphilis** may be: *Early* in first 2 years; infectious, resembles severe secondary syphilis in adult; *Late*, after 2 years; noninfectious; *Residual stigmata:* Hutchinson's teeth (centrally notched, widely spaced upper central incisors); "mulberry molars" (6-year molars with multiple cusps); abnormal facies (frontal bossing, saddle nose, poorly developed maxilla); saber shins (anterior tibial bowing). There are numerous other rare manifestations.	Skull, tibia (anterior aspect), clavicle are preferred sites of osteomyelitis. Inflammation is a periostitis with microangiitis, gummatous change, and granulomas, with possible spread to overlying skin and medullary space. Moth-eaten changes + sclerosis represent destruction induced by gummas (mimics chronic suppurative osteomyelitis). Septic arthritis of syphilis: painful, symmetric swelling of knee, elbow, ankle, shoulder, and wrist, with normal range of motion; spread is contiguous from osteomyelitis. **Early congenital syphilis:** symmetrical widespread osteochondritis and perichondritis affecting the most rapidly growing area (ends of cartilage model bones) progressing during first 6 months, then subsiding. Periostitis continues and becomes apparent between the ages of 5 and 20.	Serologic tests: rapid plasm reagin (RPR) test: reflects disease activity VDRL slide flocculation test: reflects the exact titer of serum regain antibody. Specific anti-treponemal antibody.: FTA-ABS is the standard test; *T. pallidum* hemagglutination tests (MHA-TP and TPHA) are convenient but less sensitive than the FTA-ABS test for detection of primary syphilis. Both the MHA-TP and FTA-ABS tests are very specific and have high positive predictive value when used for confirmation of positive reaginic tests.	Penicillin

(continued)

	Causative organism	3 clinical stages			Treatment
Lyme borreliosis; zoonosis transmitted by ticks, disease affecting skin, central nervous system, the heart, and joints	**Causative organism:** spirochete *Borrelia burgdorferi* - Northern hemisphere distribution - Reservoirs of spirochete are intermediate and small mammals, and birds. - Ticks transmit the organism to man; species is *Ixodes*, and geni include *dammini*, *pacificus*, and *scapularis* in North America	**3 clinical stages:** - Not all stages need appear, and they may overlap. **Stage I:** erythema migrans with centrifugal spread, 3 days to 16 weeks after tick bite, flu-like symptoms **Stage II:** weeks to months later, central nervous system, cardiac, skin, and joint symptoms appear. Other manifestations include lymphadenopathy, inflammatory eye disorders, hepatomegaly, testicular swelling, and hepatitis. **Stage III:** Chronic organ involvement affects joints (arthritis), skin, central nervous system, heart, muscles, and bone marrow.	In various organ systems the lesions are a chronic inflammatory infiltrate consisting of lymphocytes, plasma cells, and histiocytes. There is a microangiitis with perivascular cuffing by mononuclear cells resulting in an endarteritis obliterans, similar to syphilis. In joints the response is similar to rheumatoid arthritis histologically with a pannus invading the joint. The organism resides extracellularly but may attach to and invade some cells (fibroblasts and endothelial cells). *B. burgdorferi* activates inflammatory cytokines affecting joints (interleukin-1 and tumor necrosis factor alpha [TNF-α]). Possible immunogenetic predilection for Lyme disease in those with HLA-DR4 genotype.	Organism is difficult to culture. Identification is by silver stains and immunohistological techniques. Polymerase chain reaction testing is not yet validated. Culture and biopsy identification is thus difficult. Serologic testing: enzyme-linked immunosorbent assay (ELISA), indirect immunofluorescence assay (IFA), and Western blot. Stage I: less than half have detectable antibodies, mostly IgM. Stage II: 70% to 90% have antibodies, mostly IgG. Confirm with Western blot, and repeat if negative.	For systemic disease: doxycycline, cefuroxime axetil, or erythromycin. For arthritis, repeat 30-day courses of doxycycline, amoxicillin, plus probenecid.

TABLE 27.2-3 (continued)

ORGANISM	Entry	Clinical Manifestations	Pathology/Skeletal Involvement	Diagnosis	Treatment
Ecchinococcosis (hydatid cyst); parasitic infestation by a tapeworm	Ecchinococcosis species include *granulosis* (most common cause of unilocular hydatid cyst); *multilocularis* (causes multilocular cysts); *vogeli* (canine tapeworms); Disease of canines in which herbivores (sheep, deer, cattle) serve as intermediate host. Man inadvertently ingests tapeworm eggs from contaminated food or water.	Asymptomatic until cyst enlargement affects organ of involvement: liver, lungs, muscles, bones, kidneys, central nervous system, and spleen. There is a slow enlargement of the cyst with possible vague pressure effects; mass then can impinge, obstruct, or rupture. **In bone:** The cysts can be an incidental finding; mass effect: vague pain; pathologic fracture; vertebral body: nerve or cord compression.	Intraosseous lesion: large, multiloculated, distorted fluid-filled cyst, lined by gelatinous tissue, usually sterile. Early marrow response: Local marrow necrosis Mixed inflammatory infiltrate with eosinophils, and giant cells, hemosiderin deposits, and cholesterol crystals	ELISA or Western blot serology (>80% sensitive and specific for liver infection); radiology, ultrasound, computed tomography, and magnetic resonance imaging allow imaging of the cysts.	Surgical resection is the primary treatment. Medical management is indicated in patients with primary liver and lung cysts that are inoperable, or those who have multiple cysts. Benzimidazoles are used and the response rates are not encouraging (30% cure, 30% to 50% improvement with reduction in cyst size, and 20% to 40% no change).

SUGGESTED READING

Marchevsky AM, Damsker B, Green S, et al. The clinicopathological spectrum of non-tuberculous mycobacterial osteoarticular infections. *J Bone Joint Surg* [Am] 1985;67(6):925–929.

Rasool MN. Osseous manifestations of tuberculosis in children. *J Pediatr Orthop* 2001;21(6):749–755.

Sponseller PD, Malech HL, McCarthy EF, Jr, et al. Skeletal involvement in children who have chronic granulomatous disease. *J Bone Joint Surg* [Am] 1991;73(1):37–51.

Tuli SM. General principles of osteoarticular tuberculosis. *Clin Orthop Rel Res* 2002;398:11–19.

Zlitni M, Ezzaouia K, Lebib H, et al. Hydatid cyst of bone: diagnosis and treatment. *World J Surg* 2001;25(1):75–82.

27.3 INFECTION ASSOCIATED WITH NEUROPATHY

CHARCOT ARTHROPATHY

A wide spectrum of neurologic disorders are associated with the late development of neuropathic joint:

- Spinal cord level or higher
  - Syphilis (tabes dorsalis)
  - Syringomyelia
  - Meningomyelocele
  - Cerebral palsy
- Peripheral neuropathy
  - Diabetes
  - Leprosy
  - Alcohol abuse
  - Any other cause of peripheral neuropathy

Neuropathic joint (Charcot arthropathy) is defined as a progressive disease of bone and joints characterized by painless bone and joint destruction arising in limbs that have lost sensory and autonomic innervation.

Pathophysiology

The fundamental first step leading to joint and periarticular destruction is a profound regional osteopenia arising as a result of a loss of vasomotor control. A sustained regional hypervascular flush (active hyperemia) is associated with marked osteoclast activity. There is a loss of important structural subchondral bone with collapse under physiologic load of the affected joint. The loss of sensation to the region allows little perception of what is, in essence, a stress fracture situation. Normal weight bearing continues with mechanical displacement of shards of shredded and displaced articular cartilage, evoking a foreign body granulomatous response in the periarticular soft tissues. Once destruction has occurred, the biology of fracture healing occurs, modulated by the abnormal biomechanics of the region and ongoing abnormal vasoregulation. Over months to years the region may develop bony and soft tissue stability or may require surgery or external bracing to provide this.

Classification

A modified Eichenholtz classification is given in Table 27.3-1.

Diagnosis

Clinical Presentation

Acute
- The manifestations begin with synovitis and progressively involve instability, subluxation, dislocation, and complete destruction of the joint.
- The first manifestation of Charcot arthropathy can be swelling, erythema, warmth, and pain.
- Infection can be considered in the differential diagnosis for this presentation but is less likely the cause because the pain is not severe.
- Gout, inflammatory arthritis, and trauma are also considered in the differential.

Chronic
- The acute presentation may be missed or not perceived, and the patient may present with an established deformity.

Radiologic Findings
- Plain films (Fig. 21-17) can show an alarming degree of regional osteopenia and destruction of joint and periarticular structures. The destructive process can happen over a very short period (weeks).
- Once destruction has occurred, the radiographs will demonstrate the evolution over time of fracture healing in this region.

Diagnostic Work-up
- Recognition of the underlying neurological condition
- Cultures are negative in the acute presentation without skin breakdown.
- With an ulcer the issue becomes whether the ulcer is superficial or deep and involving bone, as per the Wagner ulcer classification (Table 27.3-2).

TABLE 27.3-1 MODIFIED EICHENHOLZ CLASSIFICATION OF CHARCOT ARTHROPATHY

Stage	Stage Name	Description
0	Clinical	Erythema, edema, increased temperature to foot
1	Fragmentation	Periarticular fractures, joint dislocation, instability, deformed foot
2	Coalescence	Reabsorption of bone debris, evolution of fracture healing process
3	Reparative	Stable foot, osseous healing complete

■ Biopsy will show shards of cartilage that characteristically evoke a marked foreign body granulomatous response in the adjacent periarticular soft tissues.

Treatment

■ Principles of management
■ Relief of pain

■ Treat any associated infection: rest, elevation, antibiotics (usually broad-spectrum), surgery as indicated by the clinical situation and investigations
■ Maintenance of stability
■ External supports (bracing must be judiciously applied and carefully monitored and adjusted to avoid skin problems)
■ Surgical procedures to return and maintain the

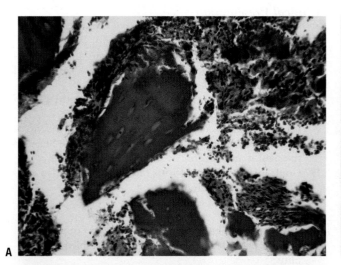
A

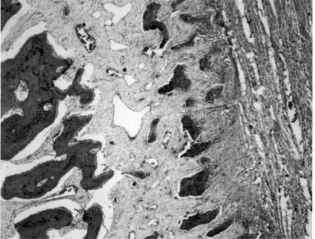
B

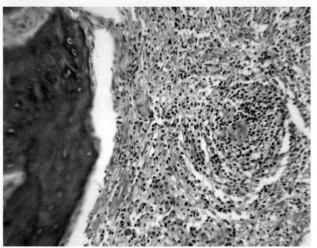
C

Figure 27.3-1 Congenital syphilis (severe periostitis). Three photos illustrate the severe inflammatory process produced by this infection. Marked chronic inflammation (lymphocytes and plasma cells with fewer histiocytes and a few multinucleated giant cells are seen in **A**, with an extensive periosteal new bone formation evident in **B**). The immature cortex has a cancellized look and is associated with marked chronic periostitis, gaping thin-walled blood vessels, vascular congestion, and thick-walled small blood vessels with endothelial hyperplasia (endarteritis obliterans can occur when the infection is severe). (**C**) Heavy perivascular plasma cell infiltration with vascular obliteration is a strong clue to rule out the possibility of syphilis (the Warthin Starry silver stain is helpful to look for the spirochetal organisms).

TABLE 27.3-2 WAGNER ULCER CLASSIFICATION FOR DIABETIC FEET

Grade	Description
1	Superficial diabetic ulcer
2	Ulcer extension to ligament, tendon, joint capsule, or deep fascia without abscess or osteomyelitis
3	Deep ulcer with abscess or osteomyelitis
4	Gangrene to portion of forefoot
5	Extensive gangrenous involvement of the foot

affected joint to physiologic alignment (osteotomy, arthrodesis)

DIABETIC FEET

This condition, a unique form of Charcot arthropathy, represents a significant burden on the health care system. Diabetes-related foot problems are the most common cause of hospitalization in patients with diabetes.

Etiology

The patient, systemically impaired, often presents with a benign indifference to a potentially catastrophic local problem. The sensory neuropathy plays a pivotal role: most ulcers and infection are the result of a break in the skin caused by unrecognized or unperceived pressure. With altered local mechanics (increased pressure over bony prominence) secondary to the process of neuropathic joint breakdown, a portal of entry is created and infection occurs. The following factors interact in the diabetic patient.

Angiopathy
- Combination of large vessel (atherosclerosis) and microvascular lesions is more severe and more prevalent and occurs at an earlier age than in the nondiabetic.
- Below the popliteal trifurcation the distal lesions of the arteries involve all three vessels in a ragged and widespread luminal narrowing that is more diffuse than the limited, discrete lesions of normal atherosclerosis.
  - Histologically lesions are in different layers: media in diabetics, intima in nondiabetics.
  - Explains the calcified, stovepipe appearance of vessels on plain film radiography

- There is no known anatomic lesion demonstrated to explain a "small vessel disease" in diabetics.

Neuropathy
- Typically distal and symmetric (glove-and-stocking)
- Reduced protective sensation, loss of proprioception, autonomic neuropathy, and motor neuropathy lead to altered skeletal structure, calluses, nail deformity, and skin breakdown.
  - Sensory neuropathy: the most important contributing factor to neuropathic fractures, skin breakdown, and ulceration; early identification of the sensory deficit is clinically important for all further management of the potential Charcot process
  - Autonomic neuropathy: Loss of regulation of skin temperature and sweating leads to dry, scaly, stiff skin that cracks easily, opening the portal for infection; loss of vessel autoregulation sets up the uncontrolled hyperemia that induces bone loss and subsequent fractures.
  - Motor neuropathy: leads to muscle imbalance, contractures, and subsequent prominences that become the sites of increased pressure and potential skin breakdown

Immunopathy
- Occurs at the cellular level, likely worsened by hyperglycemia
- Decreased chemotaxis, impaired intracellular killing
- Impaired lymphocyte transformation

Systemic Abnormalities
- Delayed wound healing secondary to malnutrition and to lack of control of hyperglycemia
- Indices that indicate whether the patient has adequate nutrition for wound healing:
  - Total lymphocyte count >1,500/mL
  - Total protein >6.2 g/dL
  - Albumin >3.5 g/dL

Dementia
- Often poor compliance

SUGGESTED READING

Brodsky JW. Evaluation of the diabetic foot. In Zuckerman JD, ed. AAOS Instructional Course Lectures 48. Rosemont, IL: American Academy of Orthopaedic Surgeons, 1999; Chapter 36, pp. 289–303.

Hill SL, Holtzman GI, Buse R. The effects of peripheral vascular disease with osteomyelitis in the diabetic foot. *Am J Surg* 1999;177(4): 282–286.

27.4 VIRAL DISORDERS

HUMAN IMMUNODEFICIENCY VIRUS INFECTION

The human immunodeficiency virus (HIV) pandemic has infected 56 million persons worldwide, including 20 million who have already died. An estimated 1.1 million persons in the United States have been infected with HIV. In the 3 years following the introduction of highly active antiretroviral therapy (HAART), mortality, AIDS, AIDS-defining diagnoses, and hospitalizations all decreased 60% to 80%. Despite the absence of a cure, the natural history of the disease has radically changed.

Surgical Complications and Outcomes

- Osteonecrosis and avascular necrosis
  - Associated with HIV-positive patients but may be related to the medical treatment
  - Femoral head most common site
- No prospective data are available on surgical morbidity and mortality.
  - Most clinical studies do not demonstrate an increased incidence of early postoperative complications in asymptomatic HIV-positive patients compared to the HIV-negative group.
  - Most orthopaedic studies do not show an increased incidence of early complications in symptomatic HIV-positive patients with CD4 counts >200 undergoing elective procedures.
  - Risk of infectious complications following emergent surgery is consistently higher in those with AIDS; incidence of late prosthetic implant infection may be somewhat higher, especially in hemophiliacs.
    - The experience reported in these studies may not be relevant to patients receiving current regimens of antiretroviral therapy.

VIRAL TRANSMISSION FROM MUSCULOSKELETAL ALLOGRAFTS

Hepatitis B virus, hepatitis C virus, and HIV can be transmitted through musculoskeletal allografts. A blood transfusion is more likely to transmit a viral disease than a bone allograft. Fresh-frozen, unprocessed bone appears to carry a higher risk of transmission.

SUGGESTED READING

Harrison WJ. HIV/AIDS in trauma and orthopaedic surgery. *J Bone Joint Surg* [Br] 2005;87(9):1178–1181.

Zalavras CG, Gupta N, Patzakis MJ, et al. Microbiology of osteomyelitis in patients infected with the human immunodeficiency virus. *Clin Orthop Rel Res* 2005;439:97–100.

NEOPLASIA

MATTHEW J. ALLEN

Neoplasia, literally *new growth*, is the result of disturbances in cell growth and/or survival. The clinical manifestation of this uncontrolled cell growth is the formation of a tumor. In some cases, for example in the lymph nodes or skin, the tumor may be palpable as a swelling or lump; in many cases, however, the tumor develops in an occult fashion and may be identified only after the patient presents with clinical symptoms. Definitive diagnosis of the lesion as a neoplasm depends on cytological or histological examination of a representative biopsy sample. At the same time, the pathologist will also determine whether the tumor is benign (unlikely to spread, or metastasize) or malignant (likely to metastasize). The term *cancer*, although generally used to describe all tumors, should be restricted to neoplastic lesions with malignant potential.

PREVALENCE

- Epidemiologic data for cancerous neoplasms, while only the tip of the iceberg in terms of overall neoplasms, are much more readily available.
  - Cancer is the second most common cause of death in the United States (heart disease remains the number-one cause of mortality).
  - According to the American Cancer Society, over 291,000 men and 273,000 women are expected to die as a result of cancer in 2006.
  - Breast and prostate cancers are the most common cancers, but lung cancer remains the most lethal.
  - Overall, the lifetime risk of developing cancer is 1 in 2 for men and women in the United States.

ETIOLOGY

It is generally accepted that some degree of chromosomal abnormality is required for cancer to develop. Most cancer cells display evidence of defects in either chromosome number or composition, and it is presumed that these genomic changes lie at the heart of the cancer phenotype. However, with relatively few exceptions, the mechanisms through which these alterations lead to cancer remain unclear. Cancer is a disease that develops by clonal expansion from a single abnormal cell. The underlying abnormality is typically genetic, but with successive cycles of cell division there is potential for additive damage through both genetic and nongenetic mechanisms. The end result of these changes is an expanding clone of cells that is unresponsive to normal growth controls.

LOSS OF NORMAL GROWTH CONTROL IN CANCER CELLS

Normal cellular growth is controlled by four major groups of regulatory proteins. Changes in the level of expression or in the genetic sequence of these regulatory proteins have the capacity to alter their function and, as a result, disturb normal cellular growth.

- Major groups of regulatory proteins are involved in normal cellular growth control.
  - Growth factors
    - Definition: circulating factors or local factors that act on cells with specific receptors

- Mechanisms of disturbance: Inappropriate expression (up- or down-regulation) can lead to uncontrolled cell growth.
  - Example: Disturbances in fibroblast growth factor (FGF) have been implicated in the development of sarcomas.
- Growth factor receptors
  - Definition: Typically expressed either on the cell surface or within the cytoplasm, these receptors bind and transduce external signals from growth factors into intracellular signals.
  - Mechanisms of disturbance: Disturbances in receptor activity may increase or decrease receptor numbers on the cell, or they may involve dysregulated receptors that are permanently "on," even in the absence of the growth factor signal.
    - Example: Overexpression of c-erb2/HER2 is implicated in breast cancer.
- Intracellular signaling proteins
  - Definition: These proteins transfer the signal from surface receptors to the nucleus, where the target is most often a nuclear transcription factor (see below).
  - Mechanisms of disturbance: Overactivity of these signaling proteins, for example as a result of constitutive overexpression of the gene, leads to uncontrolled nuclear signaling and activation of downstream genes, many of which regulate cellular growth and/or survival.
    - Example: Overexpression of the *ras* family of oncogenes is found in many tumors.
- Nuclear transcription factors
  - Definition: These control elements act directly on DNA, resulting in gene transcription.
  - Mechanisms of disturbance: In some cases chromosomal damage directly affects the expression of the transcription factor, while in others the effects are mediated via changes in the expression of tumor suppressor proteins.
    - Examples: A number of transcription factors have been implicated in human cancer, including E2F (involved in the cell cycle), p53, and MDM2 (see below).
- Downstream effects of mutations in any of these control elements
  - Depend on the nature of the affected gene and the extent of the change
    - Defects in one copy of a tumor suppressor gene may have no clinical consequence as long as the second copy is normal.
    - Defects in the androgen receptor may be silent in females but cause feminization in males.
    - In the most extreme cases, defects in just one copy of a gene may still lead to clinical disease.
      - Example: autosomal-dominant conditions such as achondroplasia (associated with a defective gene for the FGF3 receptor)

GENETIC ALTERATIONS IN CANCER

Mutations and Cancer

- Definition of mutation: changes in the normal sequence of DNA as a result of defects in DNA replication
- Causes of mutations
  - Endogenous defects in DNA replication and/or DNA repair
  - Exogenous factors such as radiation or chemical carcinogens
- Timing of mutations relative to cell division
  - Only at the time of DNA replication is damage converted into a change in the DNA sequence.
  - Nondividing cells are less susceptible to mutation than are cells that are highly proliferative (e.g., hematopoietic tissues, skin, intestinal tract).
- Targets for genetic mutation in cancer
  - Typically regulatory elements that affect cellular growth, differentiation, and survival (see above)
- Clinical importance of mutations
  - Associations between a particular cancer and a specific pattern of mutation exist.
  - Associations are rarely absolute.
    - Used in some cases to confirm histological diagnoses
      - Example: 11:22 translocation in Ewing sarcoma
  - It is common to find that an individual tumor contains multiple gene defects, and it is the combination of defects, rather than any single mutation, that determines the phenotype of the tumor in terms of growth, risk of metastasis, and response to therapy.
    - Examples: conventional osteosarcoma, chondrosarcoma

Cancer and the Cell Cycle

As described in Chapter 13, Cellular and Molecular Biology, the cell cycle is regulated by a complex series of control elements that ensure the integrity of the DNA, the accuracy of DNA replication, and the integrity of the cytoskeletal elements that facilitate the division of the two sets of DNA into the daughter cells. Disturbances in one or more of these control elements can lead to a spectrum of problems, including decreased proliferative capacity, abnormal cellular differentiation, resistance to apoptosis, or unchecked cellular proliferation. It is therefore not surprising that disturbances in the normal cell cycle lie at the heart of many human cancers.

Cyclins and Cyclin-Dependent Kinases (Cdks) (Fig. 28-1)

- Critical role in controlling the orderly progression of cells through the cell cycle
  - Mammalian species have at least 10 cyclins (cyclins A, B, C, etc.).
  - Cyclins cannot act alone.
    - Require activation by binding of a cyclin-dependent kinase (Cdk) to form Cdk–cyclin complex

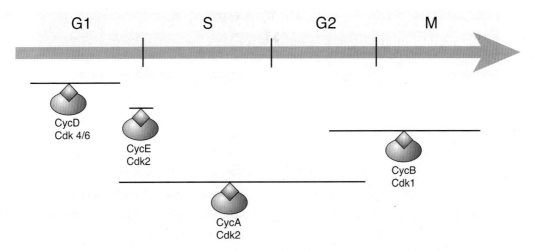

Figure 28-1   Regulation of the cell cycle by cyclins and cyclin-dependent kinases. The gray lines above each complex indicate the stages of the cell cycle during which they are most active.

- In mammalian species there are at least six Cdks (Cdk 1 through 6).
  - Subsequent phosphorylation of the Cdk within the Cdk–cyclin complex
  - Phosphorylating enzyme known as Cdk-activating kinase (CAK)
- Sequence in mammalian cells
  - Cell cycle initiated by binding of cyclin D to either Cdk4 or Cdk6
  - Final phase catalyzed by binding between cyclin B and Cdk1 to produce a complex known as mitosis-promoting factor (MPF)
- Control over cyclin–Cdk activity exerted through effects at multiple levels
  - Cyclin synthesis or breakdown
  - Cyclin–Cdk binding
  - CAK activity
  - Direct inhibition of Cdk activity by Cdk inhibitors

Proto-Oncogenes, Cellular Oncogenes, and Viral Oncogenes

- Oncogenes
  - DNA sequences that regulate the growth of tumor cells
  - Derived from proto-oncogenes
- Proto-oncogenes
  - DNA sequences in the healthy cell that encode transcription factors, intracellular signaling pathways, and receptors that control normal cellular growth, differentiation, and apoptosis
  - Importance of these genes as regulatory elements
    - Highlighted by the fact that they have been highly conserved throughout the course of evolution
    - Also strong homology between proto-oncogenes in different vertebrate species and even nonvertebrates (e.g., *Drosophila*, yeast species)

- Conversion of a proto-oncogene into an oncogene: This key step in cancer initiation involves activation through one of three mechanisms:
  - Point mutation: Changes in the nucleic acid sequence can render the gene product resistant to inhibitory elements.
  - Translocation: If the oncogene becomes associated with a new promoter, it may be expressed at abnormally high levels. Alternatively, combination of the oncogene with a gene sequence can lead to the formation of a fusion gene whose product can enhance cellular growth.
  - Amplification: production of multiple copies of the oncogene
- Specific important oncogenes (Table 28-1)
  - Many originally described in retroviruses known to be associated with neoplastic diseases in animals
    - Rous sarcoma virus
    - Avian erythroblastosis virus
  - Thought that these oncogenes were introduced into the viral genome when the viral DNA became integrated into the cellular DNA
    - Viral oncogene is capable of inducing cellular transformation directly because it has already been activated, either by mutations within its sequence or by the acquisition of multiple copies of the oncogene within the viral genome.

Tumor Suppressor Genes

Tumor suppressor genes encode proteins that regulate cell growth. Inhibition of tumor suppressor activity is associated with increased cell growth, genomic instability, and an increased susceptibility to cancer.

p53

- Normal role of p53 in healthy cells
  - Activated by DNA damage or hypoxia

TABLE 28-1 CELLULAR ONCOGENES AND THEIR ASSOCIATION WITH HUMAN CANCER

Oncogene	Function	Association with Human Cancer
erb-B1	Receptor for epidermal growth factor (EGF)	Bladder, lung, colon, breast carcinoma
erb-B2 (also known as *Her2/neu*)	Tyrosine kinase	Breast, ovarian, lung, pancreatic carcinoma
Sis	Growth factor (PDGF)	Non–small cell lung cancer
Src	Tyrosine kinase	Breast, pancreatic, colon carcinoma
ras family	G-protein	Colon, pancreas, lung, bladder carcinoma
bcl1	Cyclin D1	B-cell malignancies

- Protein product with multitude of diverse functions, perhaps best summarized as "guardian of the genome"
  - Functions as a transcription factor, regulating downstream genes involved in cell cycle arrest, DNA repair, and apoptosis
    - Major gene product induced by p53 is WAF1/CIP1/p21, inhibitor of Cdk-2
    - p21 activation blocks progression into the S phase.
- Dysfunction of p53 tumor suppressor gene
  - Mutations in p53 have been found in approximately 50% of all human cancers (Table 28-2).
  - Loss of p53 function induces genomic instability, impaired apoptosis, and diminished cell cycle restraint, all of which are critical elements favoring malignancy.
  - Loss of p53 activity confers resistance to apoptosis

and, as a result, decreases the sensitivity of tumor cells to radiation and chemotherapy.

Retinoblastoma (Rb)
- Normal role of Rb in healthy cells: inactivates cyclin–Cdk complexes that are required for transition through the G1/S checkpoint
- Dysfunction of Rb tumor suppressor gene: Initially described in the hereditary form of retinoblastoma, the Rb oncogene has subsequently been implicated in a variety of human cancers (see Table 28-2), including osteosarcoma.

MDM2
- Human homolog of the murine double minute 2 gene (MDM2), first identified as an amplified gene in a transformed mouse cell line
- Normal role of MDM2 in healthy cells

TABLE 28-2 TUMOR SUPPRESSOR GENES AND THEIR ASSOCIATION WITH HUMAN CANCER

Gene Product	Mechanism of Action	Association with Human Cancer
p53	Regulates cell cycle progression and apoptosis	Colon, lung, breast, esophagus, brain, liver; leukemia; osteosarcoma and rhabdomyosarcoma
Rb	Inactivates cyclin–Cdk complexes and stops cell cycle progression	Lung, bladder, breast carcinoma; osteosarcoma
MDM2	Downregulates p53 activity	Soft tissue sarcomas, metastatic osteosarcoma
BRCA1	Ubiquitin ligase activity	Early-onset breast and ovarian carcinoma

- Controls the activity of p53 via two distinct mechanisms
    - MDM2 binds to p53 and physically prevents it from activating target DNA sequences
    - MDM2 transfers a ubiquitin tag to p53, thereby marking it for degradation by the ubiquitin–proteasome system
- In response to DNA damage, p53 can activate MDM2 expression.
    - Since MDM2 inhibits p53 activity, negative feedback control loop is established.
- Dysfunction of MDM2: Overexpression of MDM2 leads to functional inactivation of p53.
    - Amplification of MDM2 has been reported in over one third of soft tissue sarcomas, as well as in a number of other cancers (see Table 28-2).
    - Even in the face of normal p53, constitutive overexpression of MDM2 appears to increase the risk of neoplastic transformation.

NONGENETIC ALTERATIONS IN CANCER

Although the vast majority of cancer research focuses on the role of chromosomal mutations, it is also possible to see changes in cell proliferation and differentiation in the absence of permanent changes in the DNA. Common examples would include tumor viruses and the hormonal environment to which tissues are exposed.

Tumor Viruses

- Both RNA viruses and DNA viruses have been implicated in cancer.
- Most of the information on RNA tumor viruses comes from naturally occurring diseases in animals (e.g., Rous sarcoma virus, avian erythroblastosis virus).
    - With the exception of human T-cell leukemia virus (HTLV-1), there does not appear to be a strong association between RNA viruses and cancer in humans.
- Of the DNA viruses that are linked to cancer, the most important associations appear to be between:
    - Epstein-Barr and Burkitt's lymphoma/nasopharyngeal carcinoma
    - Human papillomavirus and cervical cancer
    - Hepatitis B and hepatocellular carcinoma

Hormonal Factors

- Estrogen and cancer
    - Prolonged exposure to estrogens is a risk factor in the development of both breast and endometrial cancer.
        - Most of the evidence points toward estrogens as promoters rather than initiators of cancer.
            - By increasing the proliferative rate within target tissues, they increase the likelihood of developing genomic instability.
    - Approximately 70% of primary breast cancers express the estrogen receptor and are responsive to circulating estrogen.

- Androgens and prostate cancer
    - Androgens stimulate the growth of prostate cancer cells in vitro and in vivo.
- Hormonal-based therapies: Strategies that reduce endogenous hormone synthesis (e.g., by surgical or chemical ablation) or that interfere with receptor activation (e.g., selective estrogen receptor modifiers [SERMs]) are effective in the management of primary breast or prostate cancer.

CHEMICAL AND PHYSICAL AGENTS AS CAUSES OF CANCER

Many of the early studies on the etiology of cancer focused on environmental factors such as chemical and physical stimuli. Classic studies included those of Sir Percival Potts on skin cancer in chimney sweeps, the identification of bone cancer in women exposed to radium during the painting of watch faces, and the observation of a causal link between radiation exposure and leukemia. These studies led to the general concept of DNA as the target for damage in cancer, as well as to the concepts of promoters and initiators in the pathogenesis of cancer. The list of chemical/physical agents that are linked to cancer continues to grow. However, with the exception of the association between ionizing radiation and osteosarcoma, none appears to play a significant role in the development of musculoskeletal neoplasms.

IDENTIFYING AND CLASSIFYING CHROMOSOMAL ABNORMALITIES IN CANCER

Normal Human Genome and Cytogenetic Analysis

The normal human genome consists of 46 chromosomes: 22 pairs of autosomal chromosomes (one copy from each parent) and one pair of sex chromosomes (XY or XX). The identification of chromosomal abnormalities involves cytogenetic analysis. Traditionally this was performed by visual examination of the chromosomes in a so-called metaphase spread (the staining of chromosomes is most easily accomplished when cells are in the metaphase) and identification of gross abnormalities in either chromosome number (e.g., three copies of chromosome 21 in Down syndrome), size (e.g., abnormally short or long chromosomes are indicative of translocations), or staining pattern. However, these time-consuming techniques have now been revolutionized by the development of molecular techniques such as fluorescent in situ hybridization (FISH), in which fluorescent molecular probes are used to identify the location of specific sequences within the chromosomes.

Terminology Describing Normal and Abnormal Chromosomal Arrangements

- Chromosomes are identified by a number or, in the case of the sex chromosomes, a letter.

- Each chromosome is divided into arms:
  - Short arm = designated as *p*
  - Long arm = *q*
- Each arm is divided into regions.
- Each region is divided into bands.
  - Both regions and bands are numbered, with the numbers increasing with increasing distance from the middle of the chromosome (the centromere).
- Summary: CARB (Chromosome, Arm, Region, Band)
  - Accordingly, 13*q*13 refers to the third band on the first region on the long arm of chromosome 13.

Disturbances in the Normal Arrangement of Chromosomes

- Four mechanisms: translocation, point mutation, deletion, amplification
- Most common mechanism associated with malignancy is translocation, the result of two chromosomes breaking and sequences from one becoming incorporated into the other (Fig. 28-2).
  - Effects depend on the nature of the sequence that moves and on the location into which it moves.

- Clinically important examples of chromosomal translocations are summarized in Table 28-3.

Chromosomal Rearrangements in Sarcoma

As can be seen in Table 28-3, a number of translocations have been identified in sarcomas. The strong association between these rearrangements and the clinical tumor makes the identification of these translocations useful from a diagnostic perspective. The utility of this type of molecular diagnostic approach is such that it is becoming an integral part of the pathological confirmation and classification of sarcomas. Some of the specific sarcomas and their chromosomal rearrangements are reviewed below.

Ewing Sarcoma/Primitive Neuroectodermal Tumor (PNET)

- Products of t(11:22)
  - EWS/FLI1 fusion gene: over 90% of Ewing sarcoma/PNET lesions
  - EWS/ERG and EWS/ETV1 genes: ~5% of cases each
- Individual components

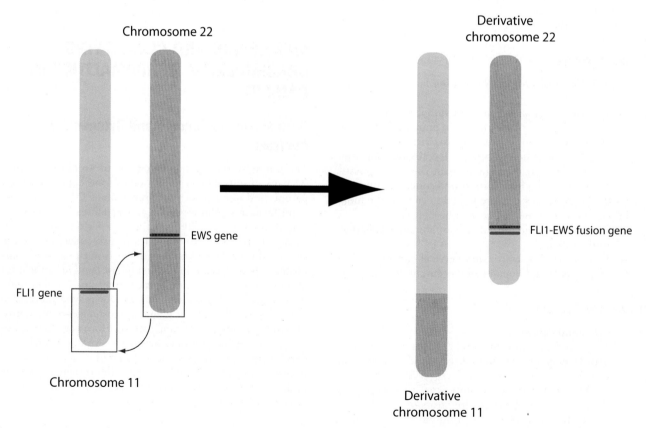

Figure 28-2   Terminology of chromosomal rearrangements. The chromosomes that are affected in the translocation are indicated in the first grouping, in parentheses, while the region/band information is contained in the second grouping, in square brackets. The entire sequence is preceded by the letter *t*, indicating a translocation. This particular rearrangement is seen in Ewing sarcoma.

TABLE 28-3 CHROMOSOMAL TRANSLOCATIONS ASSOCIATED WITH SPECIFIC HUMAN MUSCULOSKELETAL CANCERS AND CHRONIC MYELOID LEUKEMIA

Disease	Translocation(s)	Product(s)
Chronic myeloid leukemia	t(9:22) (q34:q11) (Philadelphia chromosome)	BCR-ABL
Ewing sarcoma/primitive neuroectodermal tumors (PNET)	t(11:22) (q24:q12)	EWS-FLI1 EWS-ERG EWS-ETV1
Synovial sarcoma	t(x:18) (p11:q11)	SYT-SSX
Desmoplastic/small round cell sarcoma	t(11:22) (q13:q12)	EWS-WT1
Myxoid/round cell liposarcoma	t(12:16) (q13:p11)	CHOP-TLS/FUS
	t(12:22) (q13:q12)	CHOP-EWS
Myxoid chondrosarcoma	t(9:22) (q31:q12)	EWS-TEC
Alveolar rhabdomyosarcoma	t(2:13) (q35–37:q14)	PAX3-FKHR

■ EWS gene: encodes a protein that binds RNA
■ FLI1, ERG, and ETV1: all members of the ETS family of transcription factors
■ Evidence of importance
  ■ EWS-FLI1 gene is capable of transforming cells in vitro.
  ■ Downregulation of EWS-FLI1 activity suppresses the growth of Ewing sarcoma cells in vitro.

Synovial Sarcoma

■ Products of t(x:18)
  ■ SYT gene on X chromosome translocates to involve one of two SSX genes on chromosome 18.
  ■ Present in nearly all synovial sarcomas
■ Individual components: SSX1 and SSX2 are DNA-binding proteins that regulate gene transcription.
■ Clinical relevance: The presence of SSX1 rather than SSX2 in the fusion gene appears to have prognostic importance.
  ■ 5-year survival for SYT-SSX2 is 48%, compared with 24% for patients with the SYT-SSX1 translocation.

Myxoid/Round Cell Liposarcoma

■ Products of t(12:16)
  ■ Fuses the CHOP gene on chromosome 12 with the TLS/FUS gene on chromosome 16
  ■ Present in over three quarters of myxoid/round cell liposarcoma lesions
■ Individual components
  ■ CHOP gene encodes a DNA transcription factor.
  ■ TLS encodes an activated transcription factor.
  ■ Targets for these transcription factors are not currently known.

FACTORS CONTROLLING THE GROWTH OF TUMORS

■ Vascularization
  ■ Vascularization is required for tumors >2 mm in diameter.
  ■ Antiangiogenic strategies (e.g., endostatin) show promise in retarding tumor growth.
■ pH
■ Oxygen tension
  ■ Local environment within/around many tumors can be hypoxic.
  ■ Hypoxia can decrease the effectiveness of standard cancer treatments such as chemotherapy or radiation therapy.
■ Endocrine, paracrine, and autocrine factors
  ■ Estrogen and androgen responsiveness of many breast and prostate cancers (see above)
  ■ Interleukin (IL)-6, released from bone marrow cells, is known to be a potent mitogen for multiple myeloma.
  ■ Transforming growth factor beta (TGF-β), insulin-like growth factor I (IGF-I), and IL-8 have all been implicated as factors that upregulate the growth of cancer cells within the skeleton.

TUMOR METASTASIS

Spread of the tumor away from its site of origin is known as metastasis. In most cancer patients, death results from the effects of the metastatic tumor rather than the primary tumor per se. What, then, is it that makes some tumors metastasize? The barriers to metastasis are immense; the tumor must first enter the systemic circulation (either vas-

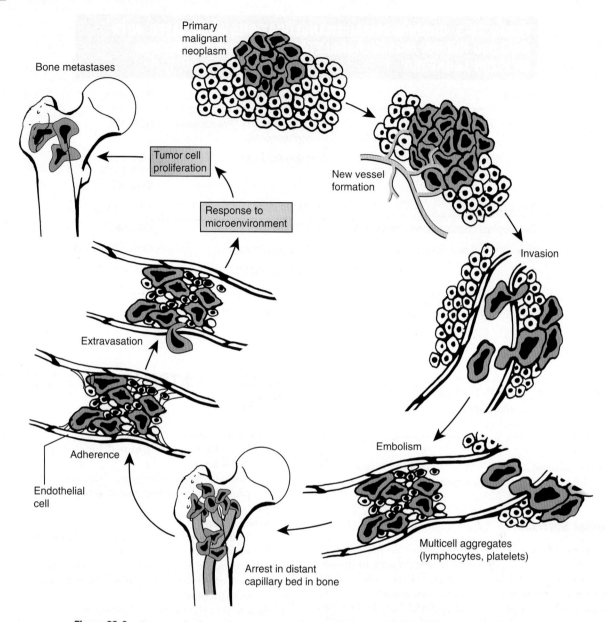

Primary
malignant
neoplasm

Bone metastases

Tumor cell
proliferation

New vessel
formation

Response to
microenvironment

Invasion

Extravasation

Adherence

Endothelial
cell

Embolism

Arrest in distant
capillary bed in bone

Multicell aggregates
(lymphocytes, platelets)

Figure 28-3   Steps involved in tumor metastasis. (Adapted by permission from Macmillan Publishers Ltd: Nature Reviews: Cancer. Mundy GR. Metastasis to bone: Causes, consequences and therapeutic opportunities. *Nat Rev Cancer* 2002;2:584–593.)

cular or lymphatic), then travel to target organs, exit the circulation, and then establish a new colony (Fig. 28-3).

Many solid tumors display predictable patterns of metastasis (e.g., bone, liver, and lung metastasis for many carcinomas), suggesting that the process of metastasis is far from random. A number of factors are now known to be important in controlling tumor cell metastasis (see Chapter 8: Metastatic Disease). Of particular interest within the context of musculoskeletal neoplasms are the matrix metalloproteinases (MMPs), which were discussed in Chapter 13. The clinical consequences of primary and secondary tumors on the skeleton were reviewed in Chapter 8, Metastatic Disease.

SUGGESTED READING

Antonescu CR. The role of genetic testing in soft tissue sarcoma. *Histopathology* 2006;48(1):13–21.

Kang Y, Siegel PM, Shu W, et al. A multigenic program mediating breast cancer metastasis to bone. *Cancer Cell* 2003;3(6):537–549.

Lazar A, Abruzzo LV, Pollock RE, et al. Molecular diagnosis of sarcomas: chromosomal translocations in sarcomas. *Arch Pathol Lab Med* 2006;130(8):1199–1207.

Mundy GR. Metastasis to bone: causes, consequences and therapeutic opportunities. *Nat Rev Cancer* 2002;2(8):584–593.

Schwartz GK, Shah MA. Targeting the cell cycle: a new approach to cancer therapy. *J Clin Oncol* 2005;23(36):9408–9421.

Steele RJ, Thompson AM, Hall PA, et al. The p53 tumour suppressor gene. *Br J Surg* 1998;85(11):1460–1467.

INDEX

Page numbers followed by *a* indicate an algorithm, those followed by *b* indicate a box, those in italics indicate a figure, and those followed by *t* indicate a table.

A

Abrasive wear, 371
Acceleration, 369
Achondroplasia, fibroblast growth
　　factors receptor gene mutation
　　in, 352
Acute osteomyelitis, 496–497, 496*t*
Adamantinoma
　　diagnosis of, 210–211
　　pathogenesis of, 209–210, *210*
　　treatment of, 211
Adenosine triphosphate (ATP), 489
Adhesive wear, 371
Adipocytic tumors, 298–299, *299*
　　See Lipoma, Liposarcoma
Adult fibrosarcoma, 299–300, *300*
Aerobic metabolism, 489
Allograft-prosthetic composite (APC),
　　for malignant bone lesions, 66,
　　67
Alveolar rhabdomyosarcoma, 302, *302*
Alveolar soft part sarcoma, 304, *304*
American Joint Committee on Cancer
　　(AJCC), soft tissue sarcomas
　　and, 36*t*
Anaerobic metabolism, 489
Aneurysmal bone cyst, 143–144, *145,*
　　146
Angiomatosis, 288, *290*
Angiosarcoma, 302–303, *303*
Ankylosing spondylitis, 430
Ankylosis spondylitis, 429. *See also*
　　Juvenile inflammatory arthritis
Ann Arbor staging system, 245*t*
Antibacterials, 387–388
　　clinical applications, 387–388
　　drug action mechanism
　　　classification, 387
Anticoagulants, 388, 388–389, *389*
　　aspirin, 388
　　factor Xa inhibitor (fondaparinux),
　　　389
　　heparin, 388–389
　　low-molecular-weight heparin, 389
　　warfarin, 388
Anti-inflammatory agents, 389
　　nonsteroidal anti-inflammatory
　　　drugs, 389, 389*t*
　　　COX-2 inhibitors, 389
　　　salicylates, 389
APC. *See* Allograft-prosthetic
　　composite
Apoptogenic signals, 312

Apoptosis, death of cells and, 311
　　detection of, 313–314
　　key steps in, 311–312, *312, 313*
　　molecular pathways of, 312–313
　　morphologic features in, 311, *311*
ARSE. *See* Arylsulfatase E gene
Arthritis
　　enteropathic, 433–434
　　inflammatory, 423
　　juvenile inflammatory
　　　definition of, 428
　　　diagnosis of, 428–429
　　prevention of, in menisci, 447
　　psoriatic, 433, 433*t*
　　reactive, 430–432
　　rheumatoid, 360, *361*
　　　clinical features of, 425, 425*b*
　　　definition of, 423
　　　diagnosis of, 425–428
　　　epidemiology of, 423–425
　　　etiology of, 425
　　　pathophysiology of, 425
　　septic, 506–508, *507*
Arthrogrypotic syndromes, 363
Articular cartilage
　　aggrecan susceptibility, 414, *415*
　　collagen stability, 414–415
　　collagens, 407–408, 407*t, 408*
　　composition of, 406, 407*t*
　　destruction of
　　　in clinical situations, 414
　　　mechanism, 412, 413*t*
　　functions of, 406
　　fundamental concept of, 414
　　metabolism markers, 415, 415*b*
　　morphologic changes in, 412–414,
　　　412*t, 414*
　　nerve supply to, 406–407
　　proteoglycans, 408–409, *409,* 409*t*
　　radiographic correlation, 412–414,
　　　412*t, 414*
　　repair of, 415–417, 416*t*
　　structure, 406, 406*t, 407*
　　vascular supply to, 406–407
Arylsulfatase E gene (ARSE), in
　　skeletal dysplasias
　　camptomelic dysplasia features, 358
　　chondrodysplasia punctata 1 X-linked
　　　recessive gene, 358
　　cysteine proteinase cathepsin K gene
　　　mutation, 358
　　SOX9 gene mutation, 358
Aspirin, 388

ATP. *See* Adenosine triphosphate
Autoimmune disorders
　　rheumatoid arthritis, 360, *361*
　　systemic lupus erythematosus, 360,
　　　360
Avascular necrosis, 441
Avulsive cortical irregularity, 149–151,
　　150, 151

B

Bcl-2 family members, 312–313
Becker muscular dystrophy, 363, 364*t*
Beckwith-Wiedemann syndrome
　　diagnosis of, 214–215
　　pathogenesis of, 214
　　　epidemiology of, 214
　　　etiology of, 214
　　　pathophysiology of, 214
　　treatment of, 215
Bending, 371
Bending stresses, 371
Beryllium oxide, osteosarcoma and, 4*b*
Biomaterials
　　ceramics
　　　characteristics of, 382
　　　definition of, 382, 386
　　　dense, 386
　　　functional types of, 382, 386
　　　in orthopaedics, 382, 383–385t
　　　porous, 385–386
　　　reabsorbable, 382, 386
　　metals/metallic alloys
　　　cobalt-based, 375–378
　　　implant manufacture, 373, 374*t*
　　　stainless steel, 378–379
　　　tantalum, 379
　　　titanium, 374–375
　　polymers
　　　bone cement, 381–382
　　　mechanical properties of, 381
　　　orthopaedic applications of, 381
　　　physical properties of, 380–381
　　　reabsorbable, 382
　　　synthesis, 379–380, 380*t*
　　　thermal properties of, 381
　　　UHMWPE issues, 381
Biomechanics
　　kinematics, 369
　　of ligaments, 471
　　material mechanical properties,
　　　369–371

calcitonin, 400
estrogen, 400
vitamin D, 400
mineralization, 397
osteonecrosis, 400–402
classification of, 400, 402t
diagnosis of, 400
intraosseous blood supply and, 400, 401b
pathogens of, 400
traumatic injury, 400
treatment of, 402
remodeling, 325, 328t, 398
bone growth, 398
skeletal maturity, 398
remodeling cellular mechanisms, 395–397
activation, 396, 396b
formation/mineralization, 396
regulation of, 397, 397b
resorption, 396
resting, 396
reversal/coupling, 396
Bony masses, painless, 6–7
diagnostic workup of, 6–7
differential diagnosis of, 6
history of, 6
physical examination of, 6
Brachytherapy, for soft tissue tumors, 90–91
Breast cancer, metastatic disease, medical management of, 109, 111
Bromodeoxyuridine (BrdU) labeling, 310, 311

C
Calcitonin, bone mineral homeostasis, 400
Cancellous bone, remodeling of, 342, 345, 346
Cancer, metastatic disease, medical management of
breast, 109, 111
lung, 111–112
prostate, 111
renal, 112
thyroid, 112
Carpal tunnel lesions, biopsy of, 47
Cartilage lesions
chondroblastoma, 135–138
chondromas, 126, 126
chondromyxoid fibroma, 138–139
enchondroma, 126–130
osteochondroma, 131–135
periosteal chondroma, 130–131
Cartilage oligomeric matrix protein (COMP) gene mutation, in skeletal dysplasias
multiple epiphyseal dysplasia, 356, 357
pseudoachondroplasia, 356
Caspase, 312
Cdks. See Cyclin-dependent kinases
Cell cycle
checkpoints in, 309–310, 310t

studying techniques of, 310–311, 311
bromodeoxyuridine labeling, 310, 311
Cell signaling
bone morphogenetic proteins, 315
cytokines, 314
cytoskeleton role, 317
fibroblast growth factor, 315
growth factors in, 314
insulin-like growth factors, 314
interleukin-1, 315
interleukin-6, 315
matrix interactions and, 316–317
platelet-derived growth factor, 314–315
prostaglandins, 315–316
transforming growth factor-beta, 315, 316
tumor necrosis factor-alpha, 315
via adhesion junctions, 316
Cells, death of
apoptosis, 311
detection of, 313–314
key steps in, 311–312, 312, 313
molecular pathways of, 312–313
morphologic features in, 311, 311
necrosis, 311
Cellular function
chondrocytes, 319–320
fibroblasts, 320
morphology, 317–320
musculoskeletal cell regulation differentiation, 318, 319, 319t, 320
common precursor pluripotential cell source, 318, 320
RANKL-OPG axis, 319, 319t, 320
ontogeny, 317–320
osteoblasts, 317, 317
osteoclasts, 318, 318–319
osteocytes, 317–318
Center of rotation, 369
Ceramics
characteristics of, 382
definition of, 382, 386
dense, 386
functional types of, 382, 386
in orthopaedics, 382, 383–385t
porous, 385–386
reabsorbable, 382, 386
Charcot arthropathy
classification of, 521, 522t
diagnosis of, 521–522, 522, 523
pathophysiology of, 521
treatment of, 522–523
Charcot joint. See Neuropathic arthropathy
Chemotherapy
for malignant bone lesions, 79–84
indications/contraindications for, 79–81
induction, 82
response, clinical assessment of, 82, 84, 85
response, pathologic assessment of, 82, 84

response, radiographic assessment of, 82, 84, 85
tailoring of, 84
types of, 81–82, 83b, 83t
for osteosarcoma, 185–186
for soft tissue sarcomas, 298
for soft tissue tumors, 91–92
doxorubicin, 91
ifosfamide, 92
indications/contraindications for, 91
Chondroblastoma
diagnosis of, 135–136, 136, 137
pathogenesis of, 135
treatment of, 138
Chondrocytes, 319–320
Chondrodysplasia punctata 1 X-linked recessive gene, 358
Chondrodystrophies, 416t, 417
Chondroitin sulfate, 392
Chondromas, 126, 126
Chondromyxoid fibroma, 13
diagnosis of, 138–139
pathogenesis of, 138
treatment of, 139
Chondro-osseous benign soft tissue tumors, soft tissue chondroma, 291, 291
Chondro-osseous tumors, 303
extraskeletal osteogenic sarcoma, 303, 303
Chondroprotective supplements, 391–392
chondroitin sulfate, 392
glucosamine, 392
hyaluronic acid, 392
Chondrosarcoma, 192t, 193
diagnosis of, 196–198, 197–199, 198b
pathogenesis of, 192–196, 193, 194, 195t, 196t
radiation therapy for, 86
treatment of, 198–201, 210t
CHOP. See Cyclophosphamide, hydroxydoxorubicin, Oncovin (vincristine), prednisone
Chordoma, radiation therapy for, 86
Chronic osteomyelitis
classification of, 502–503
diagnosis of, 501–502, 503, 504, 505
pathophysiology of, 501, 502
treatment of, 503–505
Chronic recurrent multifocal osteomyelitis, 505–506
Cisplatin, 83t
Clear cell sarcoma, 304–305
Cobalt-based alloys, 375–378
implant characteristics of, 376–378, 376b, 376t, 377t
metallurgy, 376
orthopaedic use of, 376
Collagen gene mutation, in skeletal dysplasias, 353–356
type II, 355, 357t
type I/osteogenesis imperfecta, 353–355, 354, 355, 356t

S

Salicylates, 389
Sarcoidosis, 513, *516*
Scapular lesions, biopsy of, 47
Schwann cells, 477
Schwannoma, 284, *285*
Sclerosing osteomyelitis of Garré, 505, *506*
Septic arthritis, 506–508, *507*
Seronegative spondyloarthropathies, 360–361, *361*
Shear, 371
Simple bone cyst, 141–143, *143*
Skeletal development, 321, 322t
Skeletal dysplasias
  arylsulfatase E gene, 358
    camptomelic dysplasia features, 358
      chondrodysplasia punctata 1 X-linked recessive gene, 358
      cysteine proteinase cathepsin K gene mutation, 358
      SOX9 gene mutation, 358
    cartilage oligomeric matrix protein gene mutation, 356
      multiple epiphyseal dysplasia, 356, 357
      pseudoachondroplasia, 356
  classification of, 352, 353
  collagen gene mutation, 353–356
    type II, 355, 357t
    type I/osteogenesis imperfecta, 353–355, *354, 355,* 356t
    type IX, 355
    type X, 355
    type XI, 355–356
  definition of, 350
  diastrophic dysplasia sulfate transporter gene mutation, 357–358
  epidemiology of, 350
  fibroblast growth factors receptor gene mutation, 352–353
    achondroplasia, 352
    hypochondroplasia, 352
    thanatophoric dysplasia, 353
  parathyroid hormone receptor 1 gene mutation, 356–357
Skeletal muscle benign tumors, rhabdomyoma, 286–287, *287*
Skeletal muscle tumors, 301–302
  alveolar rhabdomyosarcoma, 302, *302*
  embryonal rhabdomyosarcoma, 301–302
Skeletal muscles
  adaptability of, 488
  aerobic training, 491
  connective tissue, 484–487, *485, 486,* 486t
  delayed muscle soreness, 492
  development of, 488–489
  disuse of, 492–493
  eccentric contractions, 490
  electromyography, 493–495
  endurance training and, 490–491

energetics of, 489–490
fiber types, 488
function of, 484–488
growth of, 488–489
hormonal effects on, 493
  growth hormone, 493
  insulin, 493
  testosterone, 493
immobilization of, 492–493
injury to, 491–492
  classification of, 492, 492t
isokinetic contractions, 490
isometric contraction, 490
isotonic contraction, 490
mechanics of, 490
myofibrils, 484–487, *485, 486,* 486t
myositis ossificans, 492
neuromuscular interaction, 487–488
repair of, 491–492
strength training and, 490
stretching of, 493
structure of, 484–488
tension length, 490
training effects on, 490–491
viscoelasticity of, 493
Skinny needle. *See* Fine needle aspiration/biopsy
Smooth muscle benign soft tissue tumors, 286
  leiomyoma of deep soft tissue, 286, *286*
Smooth muscle tumors, 301
  leiomyosarcoma, 301, *301*
Soft tissue chondroma, 291, *291*
Soft tissue sarcomas
  adipocyte tumors, 298–299, *299*
    well-differentiated liposarcoma, 298–299, *299*
  chondro-osseous tumors, 303
    extraskeletal osteogenic sarcoma, 303, *303*
  diagnosis of, 296–297
    clinical findings in, 296
    diagnostic tools for, 297, 297t, 298t
    radiologic findings in, 297
  fibroblastic myofibroblastic tumors, 299–300
    adult fibrosarcoma, 299–300, *300*
    hemangiopericytoma, 299, *300*
    myxofibrosarcoma, 300, *300*
  fibrohistiocytic tumors, 300–301
    undifferentiated high-grade pleomorphic sarcoma, 300–301, *301*
  pathogenesis of, 294–296
    classification, 296
    epidemiology, 296
    etiology, 294, 296
    staging, 296, 296t
  peripheral nerve tumors, 303–304
    malignant peripheral nerve sheath tumor, 303–304, *304*
  skeletal muscle tumors, 301–302
    alveolar rhabdomyosarcoma, 302, *302*

embryonal rhabdomyosarcoma, 301–302
  smooth muscle tumors, 301
    leiomyosarcoma, 301, *301*
  treatment of, 297–298
    chemotherapy, 298
    radiation, 297–298
    results/outcome of, 298
    surgery, 297
  of uncertain differentiation, 304–305
    alveolar soft part sarcoma, 304, *304*
    clear cell sarcoma, 304–305
    epithelioid sarcoma, 304, *304*
    extraskeletal myxoid chondrosarcoma, 305, *305*
    synovial sarcoma, 305, *305*
  vascular tumors, 302–303
    angiosarcoma, 302–303, *303*
    epithelioid hemangioendothelioma, 302, *302*
  WHO classification of, 294, 295t
Soft tissue tumors
  benign
    cytogenetic alterations in, 29t
    molecular alterations in, 29t
  chemotherapy for, 91–92
    doxorubicin, 91
    ifosfamide, 92
    indications/contraindications for, 91
  diagnosis of, 29–32, 30t
    clinical features history, 30–31
    computed tomography, 31–32, 32
    magnetic resonance imaging, 32, 32t, 33–35
    physical examination and history, 30–32, 31–35, 32t
    plain radiographs, 31, *31*
    radiographic features, 31–32, 32–35
  inherited syndromes associated with, 30t
  malignant
    cytogenetic alterations in, 29t
    molecular alterations in, 29t
  pathogenesis of, 28–29
    classification of, 28–29
    developmental etiologic factors in, 29b
    epidemiology of, 28
    etiology of, 28, 29b
    pathophysiology of, 28, 29t, 30t
  radiation therapy for, 89–91, *90*
    brachytherapy, 90–91
    complications of, 91, 91f
    external beam, 90
    intraoperative, 91
  staging of, 32–36
    benign, 33
    intermediate, 33
    malignant, 33–36, 36t
  surgical management of, 87–89
    benign, 87, 87b
    malignant, 87
    margins, 87–89, 88
    principles of, 87, 88

treatment of, 208–209
Vascular tumors of soft tissue,
  302–303
  angiosarcoma, 302–303, *303*
  epithelioid hemangioendothelioma,
    302, *302*
Velocity, 369
Vincristine, 83*t*
Viruses, osteosarcoma and, 4*b*
Viscoelastic material properties, 370,
  370

Viscoelasticity, 370
Vitamin D, bone mineral homeostasis,
  400
v-Src gene. *See* Rous sarcoma virus

W
Warfarin, 388
Wear of materials, *370*, 370
Werner syndrome
  diagnosis of, 227–228

epidemiology of, 227
etiology of, 227
pathophysiology of, 227, 228
treatment of, 228

Y
Yield point, 369

Z
Zinc beryllium silicate, osteosarcoma
  and, 4*b*